Lippincott's Illustrated Q&A Review of

Anatomy and Embryology

H. Wayne Lambert, PhD

Associate Professor
Department of Neurobiology and Anatomy
West Virginia University School of Medicine
Robert C. Byrd Health Sciences Center
Morgantown, West Virginia

Lawrence E. Wineski, PhD

Professor
Department of Pathology and Anatomy
Morehouse School of Medicine
Atlanta, Georgia

With special contributions from:

Jeffery P. Hogg, MD

Professor
Departments of Radiology, Neurosurgery, and Neurology
West Virginia University School of Medicine
Morgantown, West Virginia

Pat Abramson

Research Media Specialist
Morehouse School of Medicine
Atlanta, Georgia

Bruce Palmer

Visual Technologist
Department of Neurobiology and Anatomy
West Virginia University School of Medicine
Morgantown, West Virginia

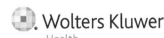. Wolters Kluwer | Lippincott Williams & Wilkins
Health

Philadelphia • Baltimore • New York • London
Buenos Aires • Hong Kong • Sydney • Tokyo

Acquisitions Editor: Crystal Taylor
Product Managers: Kelley A. Squazzo & Catherine A. Noonan
Designer: Doug Smock
Compositor: SPi Technologies

First Edition

351 West Camden Street   Two Commerce Square, 2001 Market street
Baltimore, MD 21201   Philadelphia, PA 19103 USA

Printed in the United States of America

Library of Congress Cataloging-in-Publication Data
Lambert, Harold Wayne, 1972–
   Lippincott's illustrated Q&A review of anatomy and embryology / H. Wayne Lambert, Lawrence E. Wineski ; with special contributions from Jeffery P. Hogg, Pat Abramson, Bruce Palmer. — 1st ed.
      p. ; cm.
   Includes index.
   ISBN 978-1-60547-315-4
   1. Human anatomy—Examinations, questions, etc. I. Wineski, Lawrence E. II. Title.
   [DNLM: 1. Anatomy—Examination Questions. 2. Embryology—Examination Questions. QS 18.2 L222L 2011]
   QM31.L36 2011
   611.0076—dc22

                                                                                2010008648

DISCLAIMER

Care has been taken to confirm the accuracy of the information present and to describe generally accepted practices. However, the authors, editors, and publisher are not responsible for errors or omissions or for any consequences from application of the information in this book and make no warranty, expressed or implied, with respect to the currency, completeness, or accuracy of the contents of the publication. Application of this information in a particular situation remains the professional responsibility of the practitioner; the clinical treatments described and recommended may not be considered absolute and universal recommendations.

   The authors, editors, and publisher have exerted every effort to ensure that drug selection and dosage set forth in this text are in accordance with the current recommendations and practice at the time of publication. However, in view of ongoing research, changes in government regulations, and the constant flow of information relating to drug therapy and drug reactions, the reader is urged to check the package insert for each drug for any change in indications and dosage and for added warnings and precautions. This is particularly important when the recommended agent is a new or infrequently employed drug.

   Some drugs and medical devices presented in this publication have Food and Drug Administration (FDA) clearance for limited use in restricted research settings. It is the responsibility of the health care provider to ascertain the FDA status of each drug or device planned for use in their clinical practice.

To purchase additional copies of this book, call our customer service department at (800) 638–3030 or fax orders to (301) 223–2320. International customers should call (301) 223–2300.

Visit Lippincott Williams & Wilkins on the Internet: http://www.lww.com. Lippincott Williams & Wilkins customer service representatives are available from 8:30 am to 6:00 pm, EST.

                                                                        15 14 13 12

Dedication

This book is dedicated to our students who make our jobs enjoyable
each and every year, our mentors who trained us and still serve as our role models,
and our families for their constant support and patience.

Preface

Lippincott's Illustrated Q&A Review of Anatomy and Embryology presents essential concepts of gross anatomy and embryology in a question-and-explanation format. This textbook will enable students to identify and clarify specific, high-yield information frequently tested in anatomy and embryology courses and board examinations. Therefore, this book is beneficial to professional students in the fields of allopathic, osteopathic, dental, and podiatric medicine. It is designed to prepare these students for course examinations and the Gross Anatomy and Embryology Subject Examination given by the National Board of Medical Examiners as well as prepare students for professional board examinations, such as the Step/Part 1 of the United States Medical Licensing Examination, the Comprehensive Osteopathic Medical Licensing Examination, the National Board Dental Examination, and the National Board of Podiatric Medical Examination.

All of the 424 clinical vignette-style questions located within the *Lippincott's Illustrated Q&A Review of Anatomy and Embryology* textbook are written such that one best answer is required. Detailed explanations of both the correct and incorrect answers are included to highlight frequently tested material, key concepts, and mnemonics to facilitate retention of information. Working through this textbook will help students develop their knowledge base, problem-solving skills, and integration of important clinical concepts. Because professional courses and board examinations often require interpretation of illustrations, over 200 high-quality photographs and line drawings are included within many of the questions. These illustrations portray clinical signs and symptoms, summarize information, and expose students to current radiologic imaging techniques, such as magnetic resonance imaging, computed tomography, and basic X-ray (or plain) films. For students taking medical, dental, podiatric, and allied health courses, the use of this review book and the online testing site will facilitate classroom learning and self-assessment in the fields of anatomy and embryology.

H. Wayne Lambert
Lawrence E. Wineski

Acknowledgments

We thank our many colleagues who have contributed to the development and completion of this textbook, whether they are aware of their contributions or not. We greatly appreciate the time, thought, ideas, critical review, support, mentoring, and encouragement from the following individuals.

Dr. Anne M. R. Agur, Professor in Division of Anatomy, Department of Surgery, Faculty of Medicine, University of Toronto, Toronto, Ontario, Canada

Dr. Heather J. Billings, Assistant Professor, Department of Neurobiology and Anatomy, West Virginia University School of Medicine, Morgantown, West Virginia

Dr. Ferrell R. Campbell, Professor, Department of Anatomical Sciences and Neurobiology, University of Louisville School of Medicine, Louisville, Kentucky

Dr. Arthur F. Dalley II, Professor of Cell and Developmental Biology, Vanderbilt University School of Medicine, Nashville, Tennessee

Dr. James F. Densler, Adjunct Clinical Associate Professor, Department of Surgery, Morehouse School of Medicine, Atlanta, Georgia

Dr. Richard D. Dey, Professor and Chair, Department of Neurobiology and Anatomy, West Virginia University School of Medicine, Morgantown, West Virginia

Mr. Sean Dodson, Third year medical student, West Virginia University School of Medicine, Morgantown, West Virginia

Dr. Martha L. Elks, Professor and Associate Dean for Medical Education, Morehouse School of Medicine, Atlanta, Georgia

Dr. Noelle Granger, Professor Emeritus, Department of Cell and Developmental Biology, University of North Carolina School of Medicine, Chapel Hill, North Carolina

Dr. Herbert C. Jones, Adjunct Clinical Professor, Department of Surgery, Morehouse School of Medicine, Atlanta, Georgia

Dr. Brian R. MacPherson, Professor, Department of Anatomy and Neurobiology, University of Kentucky College of Medicine, Lexington, Kentucky

Dr. James A. McCoy, Professor of Clinical Surgery and Director of Surgical Education, Morehouse School of Medicine, Atlanta, Georgia

Dr. Keith L Moore, Professor Emeritus in Division of Anatomy, Department of Surgery, Faculty of Medicine, University of Toronto, Toronto, Ontario, Canada

Dr. Peter R. MacLeish, Professor and Chair, Department of Neurobiology, Morehouse School of Medicine, Atlanta, Georgia

Dr. Douglas F. Paulsen, Professor, Department of Pathology and Anatomy, Morehouse School of Medicine, Atlanta, Georgia

Dr. Wojciech Pawlina, Professor and Chair, Department of Anatomy, Mayo Medical School, Rochester, Minnesota

Ms. Doris Pitts, Administrative Assistant, Department of Pathology and Anatomy, Morehouse School of Medicine, Atlanta, Georgia

Dr. Frank D. Reilly, Professor, Department of Neurobiology and Anatomy, West Virginia University School of Medicine, Morgantown, West Virginia

Dr. Thomas W. Sadler, Consultant, Birth Defects Prevention, Twin Bridges, Madison County, Montana

Dr. Virginia T. Lyons, Associate Professor, Department of Anatomy, Dartmouth Medical School, Hanover, New Hampshire

Dr. Peter J. Ward, Assistant Professor, Department of Anatomy, West Virginia School of Osteopathic Medicine, Lewisburg, West Virginia

We also extend our appreciation to the staff at Lippincott Williams & Wilkins for their guidance during the development of this textbook: Crystal Taylor, Acquisitions Editor; and Kelley Squazzo and Catherine Noonan, Product Managers.

H. Wayne Lambert
Lawrence E. Wineski

Contents

Chapter 1

General Principles

QUESTIONS

Select the single best answer.

I. Anatomical Directions and Movements

1 Which of the following is true of the anatomical position?
(A) The humerus is proximal to the scapula.
(B) The radius is medial to the ulna.
(C) The vertebral arch is ventral to the vertebral body.
(D) The femur is superior to the fibula.
(E) The phalanges of the foot are cranial to the metatarsals.

2 If the body were sectioned along a ___ plane, it would be divided into ___ portions.
(A) sagittal...anterior and posterior
(B) sagittal...superior and inferior
(C) coronal...superior and inferior
(D) coronal...right and left
(E) horizontal...superior and inferior

3 Which of the following is true of a median plane of the hand?
(A) It becomes a horizontal plane when the hand is medially rotated 90 degrees.
(B) It becomes a coronal plane when the brachium (upper arm) is laterally rotated 90 degrees and abducted 90 degrees.
(C) It is the same as a frontal plane.
(D) It remains a median plane regardless of limb or body position.
(E) It is oriented mediolaterally.

4 A radiologist wishes to image the body in a plane parallel to both scapulae. Which of the following choices best describes the desired sectioning?
(A) Horizontal section
(B) Transverse section
(C) Frontal section
(D) Sagittal section
(E) Oblique section

5 A young boy uses his right hand to screw-in a new light bulb. Which of the following terms best describes the screw-home movement of his forearm?

(A) Flexion
(B) Abduction
(C) Pronation
(D) Adduction
(E) Supination

II. Bones and Joints

6 Bones are often classified according to their shape and/or developmental pattern. Which of the following choices is an example of a flat bone?
(A) Humerus
(B) Sternum
(C) Hamate
(D) Maxilla
(E) Patella

7 In endochondral ossification, bone replaces most of an initial cartilage model. Which of the following refers to the part of a bone ossified from the primary ossification center?
(A) Diaphysis
(B) Epiphysis
(C) Metaphysis
(D) Epiphyseal plate
(E) Condyle

8 A 16-year-old boy crashes his mountain bike and suffers a fractured tibia. Which of the following damaged structures would most likely produce the acute pain emanating from the fractured tibia?
(A) Nerves in compact bone
(B) Nerves in trabecular bone
(C) Surrounding muscle and tendon receptors
(D) Periosteal nerves
(E) Vascular nerves

9 Which of the following is an example of a cartilaginous joint?
(A) Humeroulnar joint
(B) Middle radioulnar joint
(C) Intervertebral disc joint
(D) Cranial sutural joint
(E) Tibiotalar joint

1

10 Synovial joints allow free movement between their bony elements. They are classified into multiple subtypes according to the shape of the articulating surfaces and/or the degree of movement allowed. Which of the following synovial joint types permits multiaxial movement?

(A) Pivot
(B) Ball and socket
(C) Condyloid
(D) Saddle
(E) Hinge

11 In examining a radiograph of the right shoulder of a 32-year-old male car accident victim, the radiologist identifies the head of the humerus located below the coracoid process of the scapula in a subcoracoid position. Which of the following terms best describes the condition of the humerus?

(A) Avulsed
(B) Comminuted
(C) Dislocated
(D) Reduced
(E) Subluxated

III. Integument, Fascia, and Muscle

12 A physician delivers an intramuscular injection into the lateral aspect of the shoulder. Which of the following sequences describes the correct order of tissue layers pierced by the needle, passing from superficial to deep?

(A) Epidermis, dermis, superficial fascia, epimysium, deep fascia
(B) Dermis, epidermis, superficial fascia, deep fascia, epimysium
(C) Dermis, epidermis, superficial fascia, epimysium, deep fascia
(D) Epidermis, dermis, superficial fascia, deep fascia, epimysium
(E) Epidermis, superficial fascia, dermis, deep fascia, epimysium

13 A 20-year-old college student on spring break suffers a first-degree sunburn on her back and upper limbs. Which of the following integumentary structures/functions is most likely affected?

(A) Hair follicles
(B) Subcutaneous fat
(C) Vitamin A production
(D) Parasympathetic nerve endings
(E) General sensory nerve endings

14 A teenage boy breaks a pane of glass with his fist and receives a laceration to the posterior aspect of his wrist. He notices the tendons that cross his wrist lift out of place (or bowstring) when he extends his wrist. Which of the following structures was most likely cut by the broken glass?

(A) Investing deep fascia
(B) Intermuscular septum
(C) Bursa
(D) Retinaculum
(E) Synovial tendon sheath

15 A 17-year-old boy engages in an intensive weight-lifting program to build muscle strength. The growth of his muscles is the result of which of the following processes?

(A) Atrophy
(B) Hypertrophy
(C) Hyperplasia
(D) Tonus
(E) Shunting

16 During an exercise program, a physical therapist instructs her patient to flex his elbow. Which of the following terms describes the muscles that perform that desired action?

(A) Agonists
(B) Antagonists
(C) Fixators
(D) Proprioceptors
(E) Synergists

IV. Nervous System

17 Which of the following structures are innervated by somatic motor neurons?

(A) Meissner corpuscles
(B) Arrector pili muscles of hair follicles
(C) Myocardium of the left ventricle
(D) Wall of the axillary artery
(E) Semispinalis muscle

18 A 55-year-old woman presents with ulceration and pain in the skin around and including her right nipple. Her physician correctly identifies the affected area as that of the T4 dermatome. The pain this woman is suffering could be related to which of the following spinal segmental levels?

(A) T3 only
(B) T4 only
(C) T3 and T4
(D) T4 and T5
(E) T3, T4, and T5

19 A man exhibits anhydrosis (lack of sweating) and erythema (flushing) on his chest due to loss of sympathetic innervation. A thorough neurological analysis reveals dysfunction of presynaptic (preganglionic) sympathetic nerve cell bodies. Which of the following sites is most likely damaged in this patient?

(A) Brainstem
(B) Lateral gray horn of the spinal cord
(C) Sympathetic chain ganglia
(D) Prevertebral ganglia
(E) Dorsal root ganglia

20 A research scientist at a pharmaceutical company discovers a new drug that selectively blocks the release of norepinephrine from nerve endings. At which of the following sites would this drug have the greatest effect on normal synaptic transmission?

(A) Somatic neuron motor end plates
(B) Postsynaptic parasympathetic nerve terminals
(C) Postsynaptic sympathetic nerve terminals
(D) Synapses between presynaptic and postsynaptic parasympathetic neurons
(E) Synapses between presynaptic and postsynaptic sympathetic neurons

21 During removal of a neurogenic tumor in the posterior mediastinum, the indicated structure in the given diagram was damaged. What type of nerve fibers were affected by this iatrogenic injury?

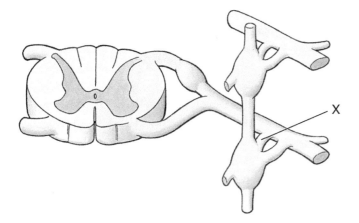

(A) Presynaptic sympathetic axons
(B) Presynaptic parasympathetic axons
(C) Postsynaptic sympathetic axons
(D) Postsynaptic parasympathetic axons
(E) Somatic motor axons

V. Cardiovascular and Lymphatic Systems

22 Which of the following is a characteristic feature of the venous system?
(A) The direction of blood flow in veins is away from the heart
(B) Veins in the limbs tend to be double or multiple vessels
(C) Veins are less abundant than arteries
(D) The walls of veins are thicker than those of their companion arteries
(E) Veins tend to spurt blood when cut

23 A 65-year-old woman develops blood clots in her lower limbs. If one of these were to break loose and flow through the venous system, it would embed in capillaries in which of the following locations?
(A) Brain
(B) Kidneys
(C) Lungs
(D) Liver
(E) Heart

24 A physician discovers that his 72-year-old patient is leaking blood from a vessel that normally carries oxygen-depleted blood. Which of the following vessels is most likely damaged?
(A) Pulmonary trunk
(B) Pulmonary veins
(C) Abdominal aorta
(D) Coronary arteries
(E) Common carotid arteries

25 Under normal conditions, lymphatic vessels periodically contain elevated amounts of fat droplets (chyle). The highest concentration of chyle is found in the lymphatics that drain which of the following organs?
(A) Small intestine
(B) Brain
(C) Heart
(D) Long bones
(E) Spleen

26 A surgeon mistakenly lacerates the thoracic duct during lung surgery. Which of the following would be the immediate consequence of this iatrogenic action?
(A) High blood pressure
(B) Low blood pressure
(C) Decreased immunity
(D) Chylothorax
(E) Lymphedema

VI. Medical Imaging

27 Assuming normal health and imaging conditions, which of the labeled structures in the given posteroanterior (PA) radiograph of the chest is the most radiopaque?

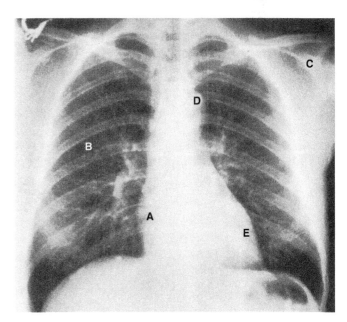

28 Which of the following medical imaging techniques utilizes a beam of X-rays to transilluminate the body?
(A) Computerized tomography (CT)
(B) Magnetic resonance imaging (MRI)
(C) Positron emission tomography (PET)
(D) Ultrasonography
(E) X-ray glasses

29 Which of the following statements is true regarding the resultant imagery in standard CT (computerized tomography) films?

(A) Air appears white
(B) Muscle appears black
(C) Bone appears white
(D) Fluids appear black
(E) Fat appears white

30 A radiologist orders a posteroanterior (PA) plain film of the chest. This image should provide the greatest resolution of which of the following structures?

(A) Transverse processes of vertebrae
(B) Heart
(C) Esophagus
(D) Primary bronchi
(E) Descending aorta

ANSWERS AND DISCUSSION

1 **The answer is D: The femur is superior to the fibula.** In the anatomical position, a person is standing erect, facing anterior (forward), with the upper limbs by the sides, the palms facing anterior, the lower limbs placed together with the soles on the ground, and the toes pointing anterior. In this position, the thigh is superior to (above) the lower leg. Thus, the femur is superior to both the tibia and fibula. **Choice A** (The humerus is proximal to the scapula) is incorrect. The humerus hangs from the lateral corner of the scapula; thus, it is lateral and inferior to the scapula. The humerus also may be described as distal to the scapula because it is further away from the attachment of the upper limb to the trunk. **Choice B** (The radius is medial to the ulna) is incorrect. The radius is the bone in the forearm located further away from the midline. Therefore, the radius is located lateral to the ulna. **Choice C** (The vertebral arch is ventral to the vertebral body) is incorrect. The vertebral arch, which is composed of the paired pedicles and laminae, is located dorsal (posterior; behind) to the body of the vertebra. **Choice E** (The phalanges of the foot are cranial to the metatarsals) is incorrect. The phalanges (toes) are positioned anterior to (or in front of) the metatarsals, which are located in the body of the foot. The phalanges also can be described as being distal to the metatarsals in that they are further away from the attachment/origin of the foot.

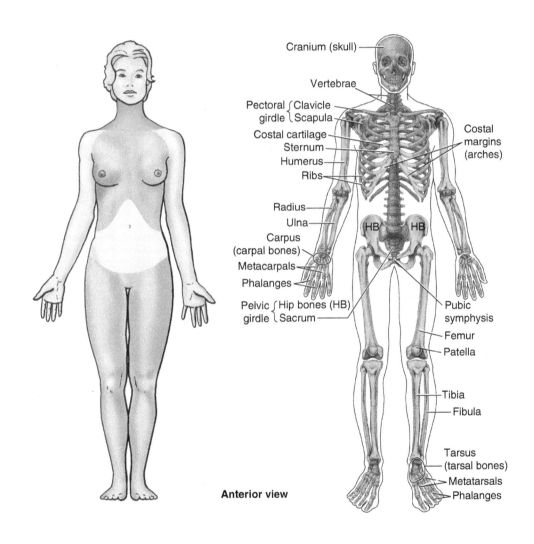

Anterior view

Cranium (skull)
Vertebrae
Pectoral girdle { Clavicle / Scapula
Costal cartilage
Sternum
Humerus
Ribs
Radius
Ulna
Carpus (carpal bones)
Metacarpals
Phalanges
Pelvic girdle { Hip bones (HB) / Sacrum
Costal margins (arches)
HB   HB
Pubic symphysis
Femur
Patella
Tibia
Fibula
Tarsus (tarsal bones)
Metatarsals
Phalanges

2 **The answer is E: horizontal...superior and inferior.** A horizontal plane lies perpendicular to both the median and coronal (frontal) planes. It divides the body into superior (upper) and inferior (lower) portions. **Choice A** (sagittal...anterior and posterior) is incorrect. A sagittal plane runs parallel to the median sagittal plane. It divides the body into right and left portions. **Choice B** (sagittal...superior and inferior) is incorrect. A sagittal plane runs parallel to the median sagittal plane. It divides the body into right and left portions. **Choice C** (coronal...superior and inferior) is incorrect. A coronal (or frontal) plane runs perpendicular to the median plane. It divides the body into anterior (front) and posterior (back) portions. **Choice D** (coronal...right and left) is incorrect. A coronal (or frontal) plane runs perpendicular to the median plane. It divides the body into anterior (front) and posterior (back) portions.

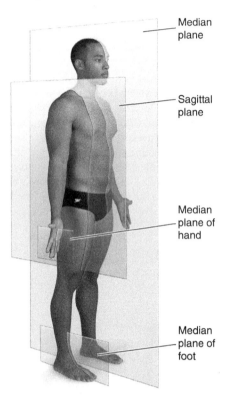

Median plane

Sagittal plane

Median plane of hand

Median plane of foot

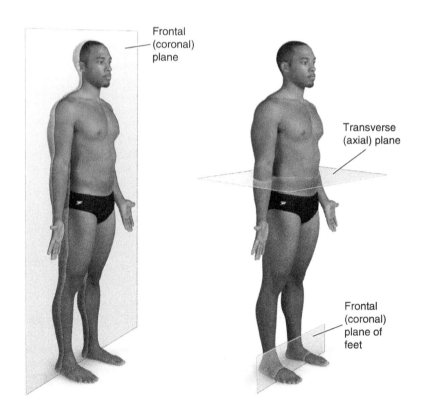

Frontal (coronal) plane

Transverse (axial) plane

Frontal (coronal) plane of feet

3   **The answer is D: It remains a median plane regardless of limb or body position.**   All anatomical descriptions are relative to the anatomical position. Thus, no matter how the body is moved or postured, the observer must transpose the body into the anatomical position in order to make accurate, uniform descriptions. **Choice A** (It becomes a horizontal plane when the hand is medially rotated 90 degrees) is incorrect. All anatomical descriptions are relative to the anatomical position and do not change

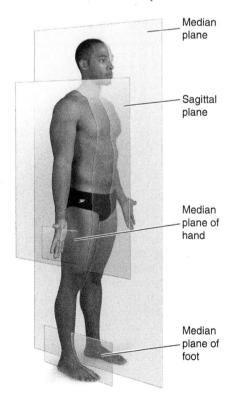

Median plane

Sagittal plane

Median plane of hand

Median plane of foot

with movement. **Choice B** (It becomes a coronal plane when the brachium [upper arm] is laterally rotated 90 degrees and abducted 90 degrees) is incorrect. All anatomical descriptions are relative to the anatomical position and do not change with movement. **Choice C** (It is the same as a frontal plane) is incorrect. A median plane is a vertical anteroposterior plane that runs through the central (median) plane of the body, dividing it into equal-sized right and left parts. In the hand, the median plane runs longitudinally through the third (middle) digit. A frontal plane is a mediolateral plane that divides the body into anterior (front) and posterior (back) parts. Thus, the median plane is perpendicular to the frontal plane. **Choice E** (It is oriented mediolaterally) is incorrect. A median plane is a vertical anteroposterior plane that runs through the central (median) plane of the body, dividing it into equal-sized right and left parts. In the hand, the median plane runs longitudinally through the third (middle) digit. A mediolateral (frontal; coronal) plane divides the body into anterior and posterior parts. Thus, a mediolateral plane is perpendicular to the median plane.

4   **The answer is C: Frontal section.**   The scapulae (shoulder blades) lie across the back. An imaging plane passing parallel to both these bones divides the body into anterior (front) and posterior (back) parts. A frontal (coronal) section divides the body into anterior (front) and posterior (back) portions. It runs perpendicular to the median and horizontal planes. **Choice A** (Horizontal section) is incorrect. A horizontal section passes at right angles to both the median and coronal planes, dividing the body into superior (upper) and inferior (lower) parts. **Choice B** (Transverse section) is incorrect. A transverse section (cross section) passes perpendicular to the long axis of a structure. While often the same as a horizontal section, it is not always equivalent. For example, a transverse section through the foot is equivalent to a coronal (frontal) section, dividing the foot into anterior and posterior parts. However, a horizontal section of the foot divides it into superior and inferior parts, as shown in the given illustration. **Choice D** (Sagittal section) is incorrect. A sagittal section runs parallel to the median plane of the body, dividing it into unequal right and left parts. **Choice E** (Oblique section) is incorrect. Oblique sections run at offset angles from the median, coronal, and horizontal planes. Horizontal sections of the abdomen produce mostly oblique (not transverse) sections of the small intestine because of the coiled nature of the bowel.

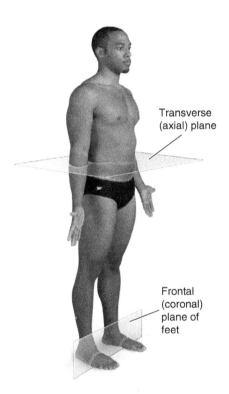

Transverse (axial) plane

Frontal (coronal) plane of feet

5 **The answer is E: Supination.** The screw-home movement is the clockwise motion that drives a screw into its receptacle, in this case the bulb into the socket. When using the right hand, the palm and forearm turn laterally and the palm moves from facing posterior to facing anterior, which is supination. **Choice A** (Flexion) is incorrect. Flexion is the action of decreasing the angle between parts while moving through the median or sagittal planes. **Choice B** (Abduction) is incorrect. Abduction refers to movements going away from the midline in the coronal plane. **Choice C** (Pronation) is incorrect. Pronation is the opposite of supination. When pronating the right hand, the palm and forearm turn medially so that the palm moves from facing anterior to facing posterior. In this case, right-handed pronation is a counter-clockwise movement that would unscrew the light bulb. However, when using the left hand, pronation produces the screw-home movement. **Choice D** (Adduction) is incorrect. Adduction refers to movements going toward the midline in the coronal plane.

6 **The answer is B: Sternum.** The sternum (breastbone) and the bones that form the cranial roof, or calvaria, are flat bones. These bones are typically located subcutaneously and are easily accessible. The sternum is a notable flat bone because it is relatively thick for this type of bone, and it is commonly used for collecting bone marrow. **Choice A** (Humerus) is incorrect. The humerus is a long bone. Long bones are usually elongated and tubular, with a distinct medullary (marrow) cavity. Long bones are characteristic of the limbs. **Choice C** (Hamate) is incorrect. The hamate is a short bone. Short bones do not have a medullary cavity. Short bones include the carpal bones of the wrist and the tarsal bones, located in the ankle. **Choice D** (Maxilla) is incorrect. The maxilla is an irregular bone, which makes up the "none-of-the-above" category. Irregular bones have shapes that are not readily classified as long, short, or flat. Examples of irregular bones include the facial bones (including the paired maxillae) and the vertebrae. **Choice E** (Patella) is incorrect. The patella (kneecap) is a sesamoid bone. This type of bone is formed within tendons. Sesamoid bones serve to protect tendons where they cross over joints and/or change the angle of tendons to improve their mechanical advantage at joints. The patella is the largest sesamoid bone. Other sesamoid bones are typically found at the bases of the thumb and the great toe.

7 **The answer is A: Diaphysis.** The diaphysis of a bone is the region that ossifies from the primary ossification center. This area typically corresponds to the main body of the bone model, which develops from the periosteal bud. In long bones, the diaphysis forms the shaft of the bone. **Choice B** (Epiphysis) is incorrect. The epiphysis is the region that ossifies from a secondary ossification center. There are usually at least two epiphyses in long bones, one at each end of the diaphysis. Additional epiphyses may occur in other areas, where they are often related to sites of attachment of muscles or ligaments. **Choice C** (Metaphysis) is incorrect. The metaphysis is the expanded end of the diaphysis adjacent to the epiphysis. In adult long bones, the metaphysis forms a transitional area between those two areas. **Choice D** (Epiphyseal plate) is incorrect. The epiphyseal plate is the cartilaginous growth zone between the diaphysis and the epiphysis in growing bones. When the epiphyseal plate ossifies, bone growth ceases and the diaphysis fuses with the epiphysis. In plain film X-rays showing immature bones, the epiphyseal plate appears as a distinct radiolucent zone. In mature bone, the ossified epiphyseal plate forms a dense seam that appears as a radiopaque epiphyseal line. **Choice E** (Condyle) is incorrect. A condyle is a rounded articular structure typically located at the epiphyseal end of a long bone (e.g., the head and capitulum of the humerus).

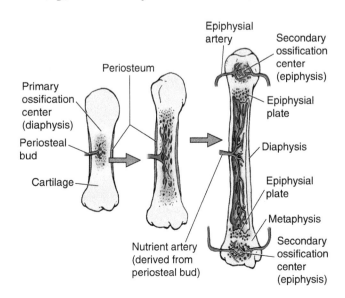

Epiphysial artery

Secondary ossification center (epiphysis)

Periosteum

Primary ossification center (diaphysis)

Periosteal bud

Cartilage

Epiphysial plate

Diaphysis

Epiphysial plate

Metaphysis

Nutrient artery (derived from periosteal bud)

Secondary ossification center (epiphysis)

8   **The answer is D: Periosteal nerves.**   The periosteum contains a dense population of pain fibers and is very sensitive to tearing, tension, or torsion. Thus, the severe pain associated with bone injury emanates mainly from trauma to the periosteum. **Choice A** (Nerves in compact bone) is incorrect. Bone tissue has relatively few sensory nerve endings, regardless of the type of bone. Thus, little (if any) pain would be derived from the fractured bone tissue. **Choice B** (Nerves in trabecular bone) is incorrect. Bone tissue has relatively few sensory nerve endings, regardless of the type of bone. Thus, little (if any) pain would be derived from the fractured bone tissue. **Choice C** (Surrounding muscle and tendon receptors) is incorrect. Pain from a bony fracture does not originate from surrounding muscle or tendon because the sensory receptors in those tissues are primarily proprioceptive (e.g., muscle spindles, Golgi tendon organs). However, if muscles and tendons are damaged as well, pain will emanate from these tissues as a secondary event. **Choice E** (Vascular nerves) is incorrect. Bones receive a rich vascular supply. However, the nerves that accompany the vessels are primarily vasomotor nerves that regulate blood flow and are controlled by the autonomic nervous system.

9   **The answer is C: Intervertebral disc joint.**   Three major classes of joints exist, based on the nature of the articulation: (1) Synovial, (2) Fibrous, and (3) Cartilaginous. In cartilaginous joints, the articulating bones are joined together by hyaline cartilage or fibrocartilage. The intervertebral discs are pads of largely fibrocartilage that bind together the bodies of adjacent vertebrae. Other examples include the pubic symphysis, the mental symphysis, and all epiphyseal plates. **Choice A** (Humeroulnar joint) is incorrect. The humeroulnar joint is a synovial joint, which is the most common joint type. In synovial joints, the articulating bones are linked by a joint capsule lined with a synovial membrane, which secretes lubricating synovial fluid into the potential joint cavity. Also, the articular bone surfaces are covered with articular cartilage. **Choice B** (Middle radioulnar joint) is incorrect. The middle radioulnar joint binds the shafts of the radius and ulna via an extensive fibrous membrane (the interosseous membrane). This joint is classified as a fibrous joint, in which the articulating elements are joined by fibrous tissue. In contrast, the proximal and distal radioulnar joints are synovial joints. **Choice D** (Cranial sutural joint) is incorrect. The cranial sutural joints bind together the flat bones of the cranium by very short fibers that form tightly bound suture-like connections. Thus, these joints are examples of fibrous joints. **Choice E** (Tibiotalar joint) is incorrect. The tibiotalar joint is a synovial joint, which is the most common joint type. In synovial joints, the articulating bones are linked by a joint capsule lined with a synovial membrane, which secretes lubricating synovial fluid into the potential joint cavity. Also, the articular bone surfaces are covered with articular cartilage.

10   **The answer is B: Ball and socket.**   Multiaxial movement occurs through several (more than two) axes or planes. In ball and socket joints, the rounded head of one bone moves in the concave socket of the other bone, such as the hip and shoulder (glenohumeral) joints. These highly mobile joints permit flexion-extension, abduction-adduction, medial and lateral rotation, and other more subtle motions. **Choice A** (Pivot) is incorrect. In pivot joints (e.g., the median atlanto-axial joint between the atlas [C1] and the dens of the axis [C2]; the proximal radioulnar joint between the head of the radius and the proximal end of the ulna), a rounded process of one bone fits into a relatively shallow socket of the other bone and is held in place by a strong ligament. Pivot joints allow only rotation about a single axis, and these movements are uniaxial or single planar. **Choice C** (Condyloid) is incorrect. In condyloid joints, the rounded (condylar) end of one bone moves in the shallow concave end of the other bone, such as the metacarpophalangeal joints. Movement is biaxial (through two planes); however, one movement typically is dominant. Some authors make a case that condyloid joints may be multiaxial, depending on the degree of movement argued for in the third plane. **Choice D** (Saddle) is incorrect. In saddle joints, the ends of the articulating bones are both concave and form a saddle-like junction. The movement here is biaxial (through two planes). The carpometacarpal joint located at the base of the thumb is a prime example. **Choice E** (Hinge) is incorrect. In hinge joints, the rounded end of one bone fits into the concave end of the other. The lateral sides of the joint are reinforced with strong collateral ligaments so that movement is essentially limited to a hinge-like, uniaxial plane. The humeroulnar (elbow) joint is a hinge joint.

11   **The answer is C: Dislocated.**   The head of the humerus normally articulates with the glenoid fossa of the scapula to form the glenohumeral (shoulder) joint. Therefore, the subcoracoid position is abnormal. A dislocation is a complete displacement of the bones at a joint. In this case, the head of the humerus is completely removed from its normal position. Repositioning of the humerus may require anesthesia and/or muscle relaxants

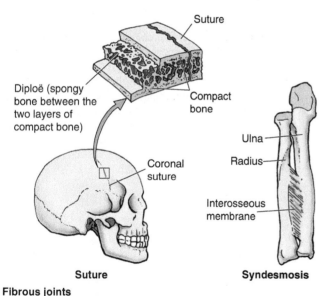

Suture

Diploë (spongy bone between the two layers of compact bone)

Compact bone

Coronal suture

Suture

Ulna

Radius

Interosseous membrane

Fibrous joints

Syndesmosis

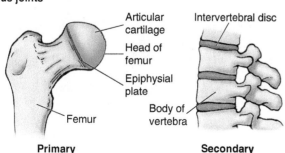

Articular cartilage

Head of femur

Epiphysial plate

Femur

Intervertebral disc

Body of vertebra

Primary

Secondary

Cartilaginous joints

administered to the patient. **Choice A** (Avulsed) is incorrect. An avulsion is a forced separation in which one part is torn away from its normal firm attachment to another. In immature bones, an epiphysis may be avulsed by the traction of attached muscles during high force production (e.g., the tibial tuberosity can be torn away from the tibia by the powerful action of the quadriceps muscles). Likewise, the roots of cervical spinal nerves can be torn from the spinal cord by the traction forces of certain neck injuries. **Choice B** (Comminuted) is incorrect. Comminution is the condition in which a structure, especially bone, is broken into several pieces. A comminuted fracture is one in which the damaged bone is broken into multiple fragments. **Choice D** (Reduced) is incorrect. Reduction refers to realigning abnormally separated parts. In this case, "reducing the humerus" indicates replacing the head back into its normal articular position with the glenoid fossa. Likewise, "reducing a fracture" means to reposition the broken ends of the fracture to set a bone. **Choice E** (Subluxated) is incorrect. A subluxation is an incomplete (partial) dislocation of the bones at a joint. Although the normal position of the bones is altered, there is still contact between the articular surfaces. Such conditions may reduce spontaneously.

12 **The answer is D: Epidermis, dermis, superficial fascia, deep fascia, epimysium.** The epidermis is the superficial cellular layer of the skin. The dermis is the deeper, dense connective tissue layer of the skin. The superficial fascia (subcutaneous tissue) is the fatty loose connective tissue layer that underlies the skin. The deep fascia is the relatively dense, fat-free connective tissue layer that lies deep to the skin and superficial fascia. The epimysium is a deep extension of the deep fascia that tightly invests the surface of individual muscles. **Choice A** (Epidermis, dermis, superficial fascia, epimysium, deep fascia) is incorrect. In this sequence, the epimysium incorrectly overlies the deep fascia. **Choice B** (Dermis, epidermis, superficial fascia, deep fascia, epimysium) is incorrect. Here, the dermis is incorrectly superficial to the epidermis. **Choice C** (Dermis, epidermis, superficial fascia, epimysium, deep fascia) is incorrect. Again, the dermis is incorrectly listed as the most superficial layer. Also, the epimysium incorrectly overlies the deep fascia. **Choice E** (Epidermis, superficial fascia, dermis, deep fascia, epimysium) is incorrect. In this sequence, the superficial fascia is incorrectly interposed between the epidermis and the dermis.

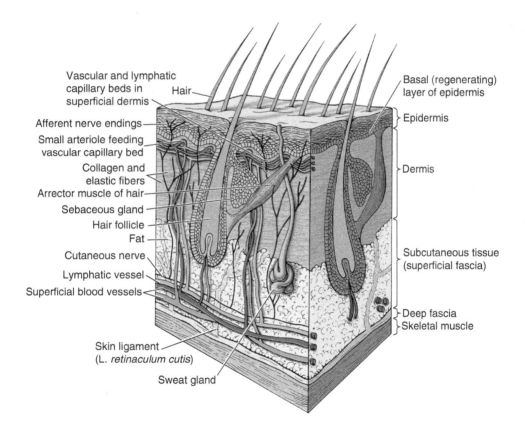

13 **The answer is E: General sensory nerve endings.** Burns are classified in increasing order of severity, according to the depth of damage to the skin. First-degree burns are superficial depth injuries (e.g., most sunburns) that damage only the epidermis. Second-degree burns are partial-thickness injuries that affect the epidermis and superficial part of the dermis. Third-degree burns are full-thickness injuries that damage the entire depth of the skin and may include deeper structures as well. General sensory (General Somatic Afferent; GSA) nerves are the general sensory nerves that register pain and other general

sensations in the body wall and limbs, including the skin. While most of these nerve endings are in the dermis, many do penetrate into the epidermis. Collectively, the general sensory fibers convey the pain derived from the sunburn. **Choice A** (Hair follicles) is incorrect. Hair follicles are embedded in deep extensions of the epidermis penetrating into the dermis and are not typically affected by first-degree burns, except possibly in their most superficial parts. **Choice B** (Subcutaneous fat) is incorrect. Subcutaneous tissue is located deep to the skin, largely in the superficial fascia. It could be damaged in third-degree burns, but not first- or second-degree burns. **Choice C** (Vitamin A production) is incorrect. The integument produces vitamin D, not vitamin A. **Choice D** (Parasympathetic nerve endings) is incorrect. Parasympathetic (visceral motor; General Visceral Efferent; GVE) nerves are distributed to the head, body cavities, and perineum. They are not found in the body wall and limbs.

14   **The answer is D: Retinaculum.**   A retinaculum is a thickened band of deep fascia that serves to hold tendons in place where they cross joints, as shown in the illustration. The presence of a retinaculum is important in muscle mechanics because it prevents tendons from lifting up out of place and bowstringing across the shortened joint angle created when the muscles crossing that joint contract. Because the tendons of the wrist lift out of place when the teenager extends his wrist, the retinaculum was damaged by the broken glass. **Choice A** (Investing deep fascia) is incorrect. The deep fascia is the relatively dense, organized connective tissue layer that lies deep to the skin and subcutaneous connective tissue (superficial fascia). Deep fascia is located in virtually all regions of the body, and deep extensions of this fascia may tightly enclose underlying structures (e.g., muscles, neurovascular bundles) to form investing deep fascia. Deep fascia may be specialized in certain places in order to serve specific functions (e.g., a retinaculum). **Choice B** (Intermuscular septum) is incorrect. An intermuscular septum is a deep, thickened extension of deep fascia that runs between muscles down to a central skeletal attachment. The organized arrangements of deep fascia, intermuscular septa, and skeleton, notably pronounced in the limbs, are termed osseo-fascial compartments. These compartments serve to group muscles with similar functions and generally similar innervation into larger working units. The compartment walls may add surface area for attachment of muscle fibers and aid in creating musculovenous pumps to return blood to the heart. **Choice C** (Bursa) is incorrect. A bursa is a closed, collapsed sac with a serous membrane lining that contains a thin film of synovial fluid. Bursae serve to decrease friction and facilitate movement between structures that rub against one another (e.g., between skin and bony projections; between tendons and bones). **Choice E** (Synovial tendon sheath) is incorrect. A synovial tendon sheath is a specialized, elongate bursa that encloses a tendon. These sheaths are common where tendons cross joints (e.g., wrist and ankle) and serve to decrease friction between the tendons and the bony surfaces.

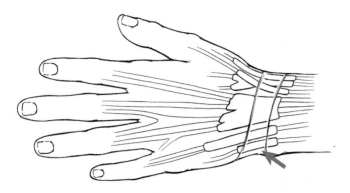

15   **The answer is B: Hypertrophy.**   Postnatal growth in size of skeletal muscles in response to exercise is the result of increased size (hypertrophy) of existing muscle fibers rather than the addition of new muscle fibers. Hypertrophy increases the number and size of myofibrils within individual muscle fibers. This growth increases the cross-sectional area of each fiber, thus each muscle, resulting in added muscle force production (strength). **Choice A** (Atrophy) is incorrect. Atrophy is the degenerative wasting of muscle tissue in which muscle fibers are gradually replaced by fat and connective tissue. Atrophy may be caused by denervation or disease. **Choice C** (Hyperplasia) is incorrect. Hyperplasia is the increase in number of muscle fibers (cells). This does not normally occur in postnatal growth of skeletal muscles. However, a limited form of hyperplasia may take place postnatally in response to muscle degeneration or trauma. In this case, new muscle cells may be derived from satellite cells located within the basement membrane of the muscle fibers. **Choice D** (Tonus) is incorrect. Tonus is the normal condition in which muscle fibers are almost always slightly contracted due to the intrinsic properties of the fibers and their motor nerves. Muscle tone does not produce movement, but it maintains muscle in a state of readiness and may assist in postural control. **Choice E** (Shunting) is incorrect. A shunt muscle is one that acts in parallel with its skeletal axis, thus maintaining joint integrity and resisting dislocation. In contrast, a spurt muscle is one that acts at an oblique angle to the skeletal axis, thus producing more rapid and mechanically efficient movement.

16   **The answer is A: Agonists.**   Muscles work in antagonistic pairings, that is, in opposition to one another. A muscle that performs a desired action is an agonist (prime mover). In this case, the muscles that act to flex the elbow are the agonists. **Choice B** (Antagonists) is incorrect. A muscle that acts in opposition to an agonist is an antagonist. During flexion of the elbow, muscles that extend the elbow are the antagonists. **Choice C** (Fixators) is incorrect. Fixators are muscles that act to stabilize a joint other than the joint the agonist is affecting. In this case, muscles that hold the shoulder (glenohumeral) joint steady while elbow flexion is occurring are the fixators. **Choice D** (Proprioceptors) is incorrect. Proprioception is sense of movement and position within the muscle. Muscle spindles are the proprioceptive organs in skeletal muscles that register positional information (e.g., stretch). **Choice E** (Synergists) is incorrect. Synergists are muscles that act to aid agonists. They may complement the action of an agonist or act as fixators at another joint. In this case, certain muscles that are weaker flexors than the agonists are considered synergists because they may assist in flexion to a lesser degree but are not the prime movers in producing flexion.

17   **The answer is E: Semispinalis muscle.**   The system of identifying functional components of nerves is used to organize neuron types according to their anatomical distribution, functional properties, and developmental patterns. Five defined functional components exist, including general sensory, visceral sensory, visceral motor, somatic motor, and special sensory. Somatic motor (General Somatic Efferent; GSE) neurons are motor neurons that supply skeletal muscles derived from embryonic myotomes, such as the semispinalis muscle in the back. **Choice A** (Meissner corpuscles) is incorrect. Meissner corpuscles are widely distributed (generalized) sensory receptors that carry general sensory (General Somatic Afferent; GSA) fibers from the body wall and limbs to the central nervous system. **Choice B** (Arrector pili muscles of hair follicles) is incorrect. The arrector pili muscles of hair follicles are smooth (involuntary) muscles, which are innervated by the autonomic nervous system. The neurons in the autonomic nervous system are designated as visceral motor (General Visceral Efferent; GVE) fibers. **Choice C** (Myocardium of the left ventricle) is incorrect. The myocardium of the entire heart is cardiac muscle innervated by the autonomic nervous system. Autonomic neurons are designated as visceral motor (GVE) neurons. **Choice D** (Wall of the axillary artery) is incorrect. The smooth (involuntary) muscle located in the walls of blood vessels, such as the axillary artery, is innervated by the visceral motor (GVE) neurons of the autonomic nervous system.

18 | **The answer is E: T3, T4, and T5.** A dermatome is the area of skin innervated by sensory fibers (i.e., by the dorsal root) from a single spinal segment. The classic anatomical dermatome map shown in the illustration indicates a barber-pole-like distribution of discrete bands of cutaneous territories. However, this standard map is somewhat deceiving in that there is actually considerable overlap between the dermatomes supplied by adjacent spinal cord segments. Thus, any one dermatome is actually supplied by three spinal segments: one major supplying segment plus two smaller supplying adjacent segments that overlap with the main segment. **Choice A** (T3 only) is incorrect. While this spinal segment contributes to the supply of the T4 dermatome (with T4 the major component), it does not account for the entire innervation. **Choice B** (T4 only) is incorrect. Damage to only the T4 dermatome would be hard to detect due to the overlap of innervation from the T3 and T5 spinal nerves. **Choice C** (T3 and T4) is incorrect. While this combination of damaged nerves more fully accounts for the supply of the T4 dermatome, it does not account for the entire supply due to the overlap of innervation from T5. **Choice D** (T4 and T5) is incorrect. While this combination of damaged nerves more fully accounts for the T4 dermatome, it does not account for the entire supply due to the overlap of innervation from T3.

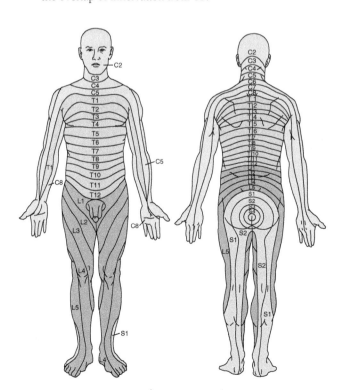

19 | **The answer is B: Lateral gray horn of the spinal cord.** Presynaptic sympathetic neurons originate in the pronounced lateral gray horn of the spinal cord, from spinal segments T1-L2 (or L3). Thus, the sympathetic division is described as having a thoracolumbar outflow. It is the sympathetic nerve fibers that are damaged in this patient, leading to the anhydrosis and erythema. **Choice A** (Brainstem) is incorrect. Nuclei-housing presynaptic parasympathetic neurons are associated with four cranial nerve outflow tracts in the brainstem: Oculomotor nerve (CN III); Facial nerve (CN VII); Glossopharyngeal nerve (CN IX); Vagus nerve (CN X). Because parasympathetic fibers emerge from both cranial and sacral levels of the central nervous system, this division is described as having a craniosacral outflow. **Choice C** (Sympathetic chain ganglia) is incorrect. The sympathetic chain ganglia, strung along the lateral sides of the vertebral column, contain the cell bodies of postsynaptic sympathetic neurons. These neurons project axons to the head and neck, body wall and limbs, and thoracic viscera. **Choice D** (Prevertebral ganglia) is incorrect. Prevertebral (preaortic) ganglia are located along the anterior aspect of the vertebral column and house mainly the cell bodies of postsynaptic sympathetic neurons. These cells project their axons to the abdominopelvic viscera and the external genitalia. **Choice E** (Dorsal root ganglia) is incorrect. Dorsal root (spinal) ganglia, located on each dorsal root of a spinal nerve, contain the cell bodies of general sensory (general somatic afferent; GSA) and visceral sensory (general visceral afferent; GVA) neurons. The axonal processes of these pseudounipolar cells originate as sensory receptors in the periphery and project to the dorsal grey horn in the spinal cord.

20 | **The answer is C: Postsynaptic sympathetic nerve terminals.** Postsynaptic sympathetic neurons typically release the neurotransmitter norepinephrine/noradrenaline from their endings, so the sympathetic division is described as a noradrenergic system. Blocking the release of norepinephrine would disrupt normal neurotransmission at these terminal sites. An important exception to this rule is that the postsynaptic sympathetic neurons supplying sweat glands typically release acetylcholine from their endings. **Choice A** (Somatic neuron motor end plates) is incorrect. The somatic motor neurons that supply skeletal muscle fibers utilize acetylcholine as their neurotransmitter at motor end plates. **Choice B** (Postsynaptic parasympathetic nerve terminals) is incorrect. Postsynaptic parasympathetic neurons typically release acetylcholine as the neurotransmitter at their endings, so the parasympathetic division is described as a cholinergic system. **Choice D** (Synapses between presynaptic and postsynaptic parasympathetic neurons) is incorrect. Both sympathetic and parasympathetic divisions utilize acetylcholine as the neurotransmitter between their presynaptic and postsynaptic cells. **Choice E** (Synapses between presynaptic and postsynaptic sympathetic neurons) is incorrect. Both sympathetic and parasympathetic divisions utilize acetylcholine as the neurotransmitter between their presynaptic and postsynaptic cells.

21 | **The answer is C: Postsynaptic sympathetic axons.** The indicated structure is a gray ramus communicans. Gray rami communicantes are located along the entire length of the sympathetic chain, connecting sympathetic chain ganglia with individual spinal nerves. They convey postsynaptic sympathetic fibers from the sympathetic chain to spinal nerves, for distribution to the body wall and limbs. **Choice A** (Presynaptic sympathetic axons) is incorrect. White rami communicantes convey presynaptic sympathetic axons from spinal nerves into the sympathetic chain ganglia. Postsynaptic sympathetic fibers were damaged by the surgeon within the gray ramus communicans. **Choice B** (Presynaptic parasympathetic axons) is incorrect. Nuclei housing presynaptic parasympathetic neurons are associated with four cranial nerve outflow tracts in the brainstem (Oculomotor nerve or CN III; Facial nerve or CN VII; Glossopharyngeal nerve or CN IX; Vagus nerve or CN X) and sacral levels S2-4. Because parasympathetic fibers emerge from both cranial and sacral levels of the central nervous system, this division of the autonomic nervous system is described as having a craniosacral outflow. Though presynaptic parasympathetic neurons reach the thorax via the vagus nerve (CN X), these fibers do not enter or leave the sympathetic chain, so cutting a gray ramus communicans would not damage these nerve fibers. **Choice D** (Postsynaptic parasympathetic axons) is incorrect. Parasympathetic fibers below the head travel through the vagus nerve or sacral spinal nerves, but these nerves carry presynaptic parasympathetic axons, which have no attachments to the sympathetic chain. The postsynaptic parasympathetic axons have their cell bodies in intrinsic ganglia, which lie within the organ that is being innervated. **Choice E** (Somatic motor axons) is incorrect. Somatic motor (General Somatic Efferent; GSE) neurons are motor neurons that supply skeletal muscles derived from embryonic myotomes. They reach skeletal muscles by traveling within the anterior (ventral) and posterior (dorsal) rami of spinal nerves. Remember, somatic motor axons do not enter or leave the sympathetic chain, so damaging a gray ramus communicans would not affect these nerve fibers.

22 **The answer is B: Veins in the limbs tend to be double or multiple vessels.** The veins in the limbs tend to occur as two or more smaller vessels tightly surrounding their accompanying artery. This feature is especially true of the deep vessels, where the veins are denoted as accompanying veins (venae comitantes). This arrangement works as a physiological countercurrent heat exchange mechanism, in which outflowing warmer arterial blood warms the inflowing cooler venous blood. **Choice A** (The direction of blood flow in veins is away from the heart) is incorrect. Regardless of any anatomical or physiological characteristics, veins always carry blood toward the heart. Conversely, arteries always carry blood away from the heart. This simple rule helps in interpreting issues with fetal-adult circulatory patterns and with many congenital anomalies. **Choice C** (Veins are less abundant than arteries) is incorrect. Veins are more abundant and more variable than arteries, thus often making them more challenging subjects. Furthermore, the venous system normally contains a significantly greater volume of systemic blood because of its greater surface area, typically greater wall diameters, and ability to expand. **Choice D** (The walls of veins are thicker than those of their companion arteries) is incorrect. Largely due to the lower blood pressure in the venous system, the walls of veins (especially the medium-sized veins) are thinner than their matching arteries. This characteristic is notable in the tunica media (the middle, mostly smooth muscle layer). **Choice E** (Veins tend to spurt blood when cut) is incorrect. Because of the lower blood pressure in the venous system and the less muscular walls, veins do not pulsate and do not spurt out blood when severed.

Thus, veins are not used for typical blood pressure and pulse readings. However, arteries are used for those purposes and do characteristically spurt blood when cut.

23 **The answer is C: Lungs.** Vascular drainage of the lower limbs is through the systemic veins and into the right side of the heart. The right heart sends blood to the lungs, where the first capillary beds are encountered. Thus, the clot (thrombus) would lodge in the capillary beds of the lungs, producing a thromboembolism. **Choice A** (Brain) is incorrect. Blood returning from the lower limbs must first pass through the pulmonary circuit of the heart (through the lungs) and then into the cranial systemic arterial circuit in order to reach the brain. **Choice B** (Kidneys) is incorrect. Blood returning from the lower limbs again must first pass through the pulmonary circuit of the heart (through the lungs) and into the descending aorta in order to reach the kidneys. **Choice D** (Liver) is incorrect. Venous blood entering the liver is derived from the drainage of the gut tube and spleen. This circuit constitutes the hepatic portal system. The systemic veins draining the lower limbs do not run through the hepatic portal system or liver. **Choice E** (Heart) is incorrect. Blood returning from the lower limbs must first pass through the pulmonary circuit of the heart (through the lungs), then through the left side of the heart, and into the ascending aorta in order to enter the coronary arteries and the heart wall.

24 **The answer is A: Pulmonary trunk.** The right side of the heart receives oxygen-depleted blood from the systemic and coronary veins. The pulmonary trunk is the large artery that drains the right ventricle and sends that blood to the lungs for aeration. Remember, the critical difference between arteries and veins is that arteries carry blood away from the heart, whereas veins carry blood toward the heart. In the systemic vessels, arterial blood is typically oxygen-rich and venous blood oxygen-poor. However, in the pulmonary circuit, that oxygenation relationship is reversed. **Choice B** (Pulmonary veins) is incorrect. The pulmonary veins carry oxygen-rich blood from the lungs to the left atrium. They represent the final step in the pulmonary circuit. **Choice C** (Abdominal aorta) is incorrect. The abdominal aorta conveys oxygen-rich blood to supply the abdomen, pelvis and perineum, and lower limbs. **Choice D** (Coronary arteries) is incorrect. The coronary arteries convey oxygen-rich blood to supply the myocardium of the heart. **Choice E** (Common carotid arteries) is incorrect. The common carotid arteries convey oxygen-rich blood to supply structures of the brain, head, and neck.

25 **The answer is A: Small intestine.** Lymphatic capillaries (lacteals) collect the lipids and lipid-soluble vitamins absorbed by the gut and send that chyle through larger lymphatic vessels to the thoracic duct. Thus, the greatest concentration of chyle is found in the intestinal lymphatics (e.g., those draining the small intestine) following meals. **Choice B** (Brain) is incorrect. The brain and spinal cord (i.e., the entire central nervous system) do not have a lymphatic drainage. The surplus tissue fluid from these organs drains into the cerebrospinal fluid rather than into lymphatic vessels. **Choice C** (Heart) is incorrect. The heart does not produce chyle. Its lymphatic drainage is via standard lymph capillaries to larger lymphatic vessels. **Choice D** (Long bones) is incorrect. Long bones have medullary cavities containing bone marrow and fat. However, these bones do not have a lymphatic drainage and do not produce chyle. **Choice E** (Spleen) is incorrect. The spleen does not produce chyle. Its lymphatic drainage is via standard lymph capillaries to larger lymphatic vessels.

26 **The answer is D: Chylothorax.** Because it is thin walled and often appears colorless, the thoracic duct may be difficult to recognize and is subject to accidental injury. If lacerated, lymph and chyle drain into the pleural cavity, creating a condition termed "chylothorax." If the thoracic duct requires ligation, lymph enters the venous system via alternative lymphatic vessels. **Choice A** (High blood pressure) is incorrect. Laceration of the thoracic duct does not in itself alter blood pressure relationships. **Choice B** (Low blood pressure) is incorrect. Laceration of the thoracic duct does not in itself alter blood pressure relationships. **Choice C** (Decreased immunity) is incorrect. Even though lymphocytes are produced by lymphatic organs and travel through lymph vessels, laceration of the thoracic duct does not result in compromised immunity. Again, the numerous alternative lymphatic drainage routes to the venous system offer effective lymph flow. **Choice E** (Lymphedema) is incorrect. Lymphedema (edema) is localized swelling caused by the buildup of tissue fluid when lymph does not drain. Cutting the thoracic duct allows lymph to drain out into body cavities but not to accumulate within tissues. If the thoracic duct were ligated or obstructed, edema would result from back pooling of tissue fluid.

27 **The answer is C: Coracoid process of the scapula.** The image is a conventional plain film radiograph of the thorax. This fundamental imaging technique utilizes a beam of X-rays to penetrate the body, producing an image of different degrees of light to dark on the X-ray film located past the body. The degrees of light to dark correspond to differing densities of tissue mass. Tissue that is relatively dense in mass (e.g., compact bone) absorbs more X-rays than less dense tissue (e.g., fat). As a result, fewer X-rays reach the silver salt emulsion in the X-ray film, and fewer grains of silver are developed when the film is processed. The areas where less silver is developed appear more white on the film and are referred to as "radiopaque". The areas where more silver is developed appear more black on the film and are referred to as "radiolucent". Therefore, dense tissue (e.g., compact bone, dental enamel) appears white and is radiopaque. The least dense substance (air) appears black and is radiolucent. Tissues of intermediate densities (e.g., fat, fluids, most organs, spongy bone) appear as varying shades of gray. In this radiograph, the coracoid process of the scapula (composed of both compact and spongy bone) is the densest of the labeled structures, is most radiopaque, and appears as a distinctly defined white image. **Choice A** (Right atrium) is incorrect. The right atrium produces an intermediate density, between the radiolucent lung and the radiopaque bone, so it appears on the X-ray as a shade of gray. **Choice B** (Right lung) is incorrect. Because the lung contains a large volume of air and is composed largely of spongy tissues, it typically appears black (radiolucent) on conventional plain films. **Choice D** (Arch of the aorta) is incorrect. The arch of the aorta produces an intermediate density, between the radiolucent lung and the radiopaque bone, so it appears on the X-ray as a shade of

gray. **Choice E** (Left ventricle) is incorrect. The left ventricle produces an intermediate density, between the radiolucent lung and the radiopaque bone, so it appears on the X-ray as a shade of gray.

28 **The answer is A: Computerized tomography (CT).** CT scans are produced by rotating a beam of X-rays in an arc or a circle around the body, measuring the energy absorptions of the beam in different tissues in a computer, and converting the differential energy absorptions into images. CT scans are very similar to plain film radiographs in that both use X-rays to image levels of radiodensity. However, CT images show radiographs that reconstruct horizontal sections of the body. **Choice B** (Magnetic resonance imaging [MRI]) is incorrect. MRIs are produced by pulsing radiowaves through the body in a scanner with a strong magnetic field. The signals, generated from the patient, are related to excitation of magnetically aligned free protons in different tissues. These are reconstructed into images, similar to CT scans. MRIs can reconstruct anatomy in any plane and are better than CT for tissue differentiation. **Choice C** (Positron emission tomography [PET]) is incorrect. PET is a form of nuclear medicine imaging. In this modality, the positrons emitted from very short half-life isotopes are scanned and computed into images, which can be viewed as whole organs or horizontal sections. PET scans are used to monitor the physiological functioning of organs. **Choice D** (Ultrasonography) is incorrect. Ultrasounds are produced by recording and reconstructing ultrasonic waves reflecting off tissues. A transducer in contact with the skin emits high frequency sound waves that pass through the body. These waves reflect off different tissues as differing echoes. The echoes are collected as electrical signals, which are converted into images. Ultrasonography is less expensive than CT or MRI, highly portable, produces real-time images, and can demonstrate motion and sound (Doppler Effect). **Choice E** (X-ray glasses) is incorrect. We hope no explanation is needed.

29 **The answer is C: Bone appears white.** Both plain film radiographs and CT scans utilize X-ray beams to penetrate the body and measure different levels of radiodensity. Thus, both techniques produce similar images. More radiodense tissue (e.g., compact bone) appears white, whereas less radiodense substances (e.g., air) appear black. Tissues of intermediate degrees of radiodensity appear as varying shades of gray. **Choice A** (Air appears white) is incorrect. Air is the least dense (most radiolucent) substance. Therefore, air appears black. **Choice B** (Muscle appears black) is incorrect. Muscle is composed of an intermediate density compared to the extremes of air, which appears black because it is the most radiolucent substance, and compact bone, which appears white because it is the most radiodense substance. Therefore, muscle would appear as a shade of gray in a standard CT scan. **Choice D** (Fluids appear black) is incorrect. Fluids are composed of an intermediate density compared to the extremes of air, which appears black because it is the most radiolucent substance, and compact bone, which appears white because it is the most radiodense substance. Therefore, fluids would appear as a shade of gray in a standard CT scan. **Choice E** (Fat appears white) is incorrect. Fat is composed of an intermediate density compared to the extremes of air, which appears black because it is the most radiolucent substance, and compact bone, which appears white because it is the most radiodense substance. Therefore, fat would appear as a shade of gray in a standard CT scan.

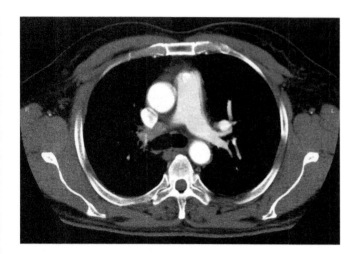

30   **The answer is B: Heart.**   The PA plain film is the standard radiographic view of the thorax, and probably the most commonly obtained medical image. In basic terminology, a PA radiograph is one in which the X-ray beam penetrates from the patient's posterior side to the anterior side, as shown in the given illustration. The X-ray projector is located posterior to the patient, and the X-ray film is positioned anterior. The part of the body under study should be as close as possible to the X-ray film in order to optimize the resolution of that part and minimize magnification artifacts. Thus, in the PA orientation, the heart is closest to the X-ray film and appears sharper than the other structures in question. **Choice A** (Transverse processes of the vertebrae) is incorrect. In the PA orientation, the vertebral column (being in the posterior aspect of the body) is further away from the X-ray film. Also, the vertebrae are in line with several other overlapping structures

(e.g., the heart, esophagus, and aorta) that add radiodensity and obscure the details of the individual structures. Imaging of the vertebrae would benefit best from a combination of AP (anteroposterior) and other angular projections that would allow better differentiation of these bones. **Choice C** (Esophagus) is incorrect. The esophagus lies further away from the X-ray film, so a PA plain film projection is not the optimal imaging technique for the esophagus. Remember, the esophagus occupies a position in the thorax that overlaps with other structures (heart, vertebral column) relative to a PA projection. **Choice D** (Primary bronchi) is incorrect. The primary bronchi lie further away from the X-ray film, so a PA plain film projection is not the optimal imaging technique for the primary bronchi. **Choice E** (Descending aorta) is incorrect. The descending aorta lies further away from the X-ray film, so a PA plain film projection is not the optimal imaging technique for the descending aorta. Remember, the part of the body under study should be as close as possible to the X-ray film in order to optimize the resolution of that part and minimize magnification artifacts.

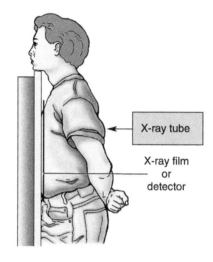

Chapter 2

Early Development

QUESTIONS

Select the single best answer.

1 A young couple hoping for a pregnancy buys an over-the-counter pregnancy kit. What substance will this test most likely detect?
(A) Early pregnancy factor (EPF)
(B) Human chorionic gonadotropin
(C) Progesterone
(D) Estrogen
(E) Luteinizing hormone (LH)

2 The given illustration depicts the passage of a human egg through the female reproductive tract from ovulation to implantation. These events occur during the 1st week of development. Fertilization normally occurs at which of the indicated steps?

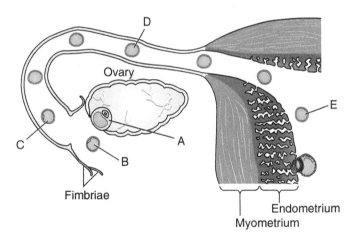

3 A 43-year-old pregnant woman at 16 weeks of gestation comes to her OB/GYN for a normal examination. During routine blood tests, her serum α-fetoprotein (AFP) concentration is markedly decreased for her gestational age. Which abnormality or condition will the physician need to rule out based upon these low AFP levels?

(A) Down syndrome
(B) Spina bifida
(C) Anencephaly
(D) Multifetal pregnancy
(E) Hepatocellular carcinoma

4 A 32-year-old pregnant woman at 30 weeks of gestation comes to her physician due to excess weight gain in a 2-week period. Ultrasonography reveals polyhydramnios. Which fetal abnormality is most likely responsible for the polyhydramnios?
(A) Bilateral kidney agenesis
(B) Urinary tract obstruction
(C) Uteroplacental insufficiency
(D) Hypoplastic lungs
(E) Esophageal atresia

5 Which structure is derived from the same embryonic primordia as the spinal (posterior root) ganglia?
(A) Adrenal medulla
(B) Kidney
(C) Liver
(D) Lungs
(E) Vertebrae

6 The given illustration shows a dorsal view of a human embryo. In the embryo, neurulation is well underway, and several distinct somites are present on each side of the neural tube. The development of the embryo depicted in this illustration is typical of which of the following embryonic periods?

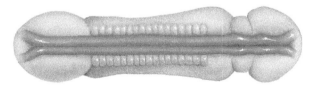

(A) Week 1
(B) Week 2
(C) Week 3
(D) Week 4
(E) Week 5

7 A male newborn suffers a complex of congenital defects involving malformation of the urinary and genital ducts. Examination of his family history reveals several members sharing a similar background of urinary and genital problems spanning three generations. These issues may be related to a genetic defect that is expressed in which of the following embryonic sites?

(A) Intermediate mesoderm
(B) Paraxial mesoderm
(C) Neural crest
(D) Surface ectoderm
(E) Yolk sac endoderm

8 In a 15-day embryo, the epiblast is capable of forming which of the following germ layers?

(A) Ectoderm only
(B) Ectoderm and mesoderm only
(C) Ectoderm and endoderm only
(D) Mesoderm and endoderm only
(E) Ectoderm, mesoderm, and endoderm

9 The given illustration represents a lateral view of an approximately 25-day-old human embryo. Disruption of further development of the structures indicated by the "X" could directly affect the formation of which of the following structures?

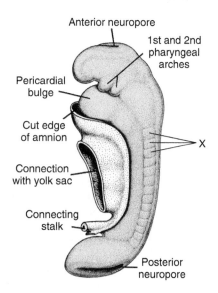

(A) Bones in the hand
(B) Skeletal muscles in the arm
(C) Body hair
(D) Lining of the intestines
(E) Melanocytes in the skin

10 A 28-year-old woman who does not know that she is pregnant undergoes a chemotherapy treatment at the end of her 1st week of pregnancy. Chemotherapy is associated with slowing the rate of mitosis in exposed cells, which is good in cancer treatment. However, this treatment may also have a negative influence on the implantation and growth of an embryo. In which of the following layers would a lowered rate of cell division be most likely to hinder implantation of the blastocyst?

(A) Amnioblast
(B) Epiblast
(C) Hypoblast
(D) Cytotrophoblast
(E) Syncytiotrophoblast

11 A 20-year-old woman is surprised to discover that she is pregnant. Following a review of her menstrual history and sexual activity, her physician determines that she is in the 4th week of pregnancy. Which of the following best describes the condition of the embryo at this time?

(A) Gastrulation is complete, resulting in two germ layers
(B) The embryo is entering a period of relative resistance to teratogenic substances
(C) Neurulation is nearly complete
(D) Somites have not yet formed
(E) The trophoblast is present, but the syncytiotrophoblast has not yet formed

12 A 4-month-old male infant presents with a "growing sore" located posterior to his left ear. This sore is diagnosed as a postauricular hemangioma, as seen in the given photo with the auricle pulled anterior. The cells forming the hemangioma are derived from which of the following cell layers?

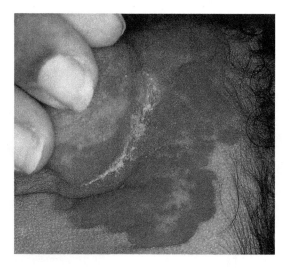

(A) Endoderm
(B) Neural crest
(C) Neuroectoderm
(D) Ectoderm
(E) Mesoderm

13 The notochord forms the initial axial skeletal element of the body and induces the formation of the neural plate. Which of the following structures is the sole postnatal remnant of the embryonic notochord?

(A) Spinal cord
(B) Nucleus pulposus
(C) Rib cage
(D) Anulus fibrosus
(E) Spinal meninges

14 A 22-year-old pregnant woman at 20 weeks of gestation comes to her OB/GYN for a scheduled prenatal examination. Routine blood tests indicate that her serum α-fetoprotein (AFP) concentration is markedly increased for her gestational age. Ultrasonography reveals a lower lumbar spina bifida in the fetus. During which weeks of gestation did this defect most likely occur?

(A) 1 to 2 weeks
(B) 4 to 6 weeks
(C) 9 to 11 weeks
(D) 12 to 15 weeks
(E) 16 to 19 weeks

15 A male infant presents with prune belly syndrome, as shown in the given photo. In this syndrome, the abdominal wall musculature is poorly developed, resulting in an abdominal wall so thin that the internal organs are visible and easily palpable. The muscles affected in this condition develop from which of the following embryonic sites?

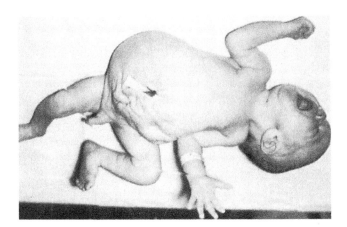

(A) Surface ectoderm
(B) Intermediate mesoderm
(C) Splanchnic mesoderm
(D) Epimere
(E) Hypomere

16 Which structure is derived from the same embryonic primordium as the kidney?

(A) Gonad
(B) Epidermis
(C) Pineal gland
(D) Liver
(E) Adrenal medulla

17 A developmental neurobiologist surgically removes the neural crest in the thoracic region of a chicken embryo immediately after closure of the neural tube. Which of the following cell types is most likely to be affected?

(A) Cardiac muscle cells
(B) Autonomic ganglia in the thoracic cavity
(C) Epithelial cells lining the lower respiratory tract
(D) Bone cells in the ribs
(E) Skeletal muscle cells in the thoracic wall

18 A married couple having difficulty with conception keeps a daily diary of the female's basal body temperature (BBT) throughout the month. On Friday, the woman noted a slight elevation in her BBT of approximately one-half to one degree Fahrenheit (one-quarter to one-half degree Celsius), which may indicate that she is ovulating. If her ovum, depicted on the right side in the given figure, is expelled into the peritoneal cavity from the ovary (ovulation), the secondary oocyte resides at what specific stage of meiosis?

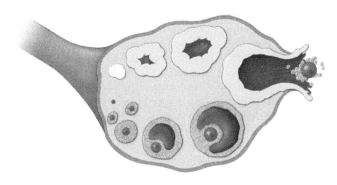

(A) Prophase of meiosis I
(B) Prophase of meiosis II
(C) Metaphase of meiosis I
(D) Metaphase of meiosis II
(E) Meiosis is completed at the time of ovulation

19 The amniotic cavity forms during the process of implantation of the blastocyst. The amniotic cavity forms within which of the following structures?

(A) Epiblast
(B) Hypoblast
(C) Cytotrophoblast
(D) Syncytiotrophoblast
(E) Maternal endometrium

20 A married woman who is having difficulty getting pregnant undergoes an endometrial function test (EFT), which determines that the endometrium of her uterus is not capable of implantation. Which of the following substances would likely increase the chances for implantation of the fertilized oocyte (or preimplantation embryo) into the uterine mucosa?

(A) Follicle-stimulating hormone
(B) Testosterone
(C) Progesterone
(D) Estrogen
(E) Luteinizing hormone

ANSWERS AND DISCUSSION

1   **The answer is B: Human chorionic gonadotropin.**   Early pregnancy detection kits most likely detect the level of human chorionic gonadotropin (hCG) in the female. hCG is a glycoprotein hormone produced by the syncytiotrophoblast to prevent the disintegration of the corpus luteum of the ovary. While hCG is a reliable marker of pregnancy, it cannot be detected until after implantation (6 to 12 days after fertilization), which results in false negatives if the test is performed during the very early stages of pregnancy. **Choice A** (Early pregnancy factor [EPF]) is incorrect. EPF is a protein believed to be the earliest possible marker of pregnancy. It is present in the maternal serum (blood plasma) shortly (24 to 48 hours) after fertilization. Though current methods for detecting EPF are highly accurate, this pregnancy test is costly. Therefore, modern over-the-counter pregnancy tests detect hCG, especially due to its presence in the urine of the pregnant woman. **Choice C** (Progesterone) is incorrect. Progesterone is a steroid hormone produced by the ovaries, brain, and placenta of pregnant females. In the menstrual cycle, progesterone production remains low until after ovulation. Then, the corpus luteum (the remnant of the collapsed ovarian follicle after ovulation) produces progesterone, which builds the lining of the uterus for implantation of the fertilized oocyte (preimplantation embryo). Though important for successful pregnancy, progesterone is not used to detect a pregnancy. **Choice D** (Estrogen) is incorrect. Estrogen is a steroid hormone produced by the developing follicles in the ovary, the corpus luteum, and the placenta. This hormone promotes the development of female secondary sex characteristics and is involved in the thickening of the endometrium. Though important for a normal menstrual cycle, estrogen is not used to detect a pregnancy. **Choice E** (Luteinizing hormone [LH]) is incorrect. LH is a glycoprotein that experiences an acute rise before ovulation in the menstrual cycle. Though important for the menstrual cycle, LH is not used to detect a pregnancy.

2   **The answer is C: Ampullary region of the uterine tube.** Fertilization normally occurs in the ampullary region of the uterine tube, which is the expanded distal end of the uterine tube, located in close proximity to the ovary. Only a minimal percentage (~1%) of sperm deposited in the vagina pass into the uterine cervix. After entering the uterus, sperm travel to the uterine tube and ultimately to its ampulla, which requires several hours. During this time, spermatozoa must undergo both the capacitation and the acrosome reaction to be able to fertilize the oocyte. The fertilized oocyte (zygote) moves through the uterine tube via peristaltic muscular contractions of the tube and ciliary action in the tubal mucosa. The zygote typically reaches the uterine cavity in approximately 3 to 4 days. **Choice A** (Preovulatory follicle) is incorrect. This labeled step represents the preovulatory follicle stage. At this point, the follicle is large and meiosis II has initiated. The surface of the ovary over the follicle bulges outward and breaks down in preparation for ovulation. Fertilization is not possible at this stage because the oocyte remains protected by the cell layers of the follicle and ovary. **Choice B** (Immediate postovulation) is incorrect. This labeled step represents the stage at which the oocyte has been released from the ovary (ovulation) and is starting to enter the uterine tube. Before ovulation, the

fimbriae at the distal (free) end of the uterine tube sweep the surface of the ovary, the uterine tube itself begins contracting rhythmically, and cilia on the tubal epithelium activate. These collective actions appear to draw the extruded oocyte into the uterine tube, where the cumulus oophorus cells fall away to better expose the oocyte for fertilization in the ampullary region. **Choice D** (2-cell stage) is incorrect. In this step, the zygote has achieved the two-cell stage of cleavage, about 30 hours postfertilization. The individual cells (blastomeres) continue to divide as the zygote proceeds down the tube. When it enters the uterine cavity (~3 to 4 days after fertilization), the zygote is typically at the 16-cell stage of division and is termed a morula (**L**: mulberry). The morula is composed of two parts: (1) the inner cell mass (embryoblast) which will become the embryo proper and (2) the outer cell mass (trophoblast) which contributes to formation of the placenta. **Choice E** (Early blastocyst stage) is incorrect. At about 4.5 days of development, the labeled zygote is at the early blastocyst stage, and it is located within the uterine cavity. At this stage, the zona pellucida has disappeared, which enables implantation to occur in the uterine mucosa.

3   **The answer is A: Down syndrome.**   In the serum AFP test, sometimes called the maternal serum AFP (MSAFP), a blood sample is drawn from the mother to check the levels of AFP. This blood test is most accurate when the initial sample is obtained between 16 and 18 weeks of gestation. AFP is a protein secreted by the fetal liver and fetal yolk sac and absorbed into the mother's blood. Decreased levels of MSAFP are associated with chromosomal defects, including Down syndrome (trisomy 21) and trisomy 18, which will need to be ruled out in this patient with additional tests, such as amniocentesis for chromosomal analysis. See the given figure of a karyotype of Down syndrome (trisomy 21), and note the encircled abnormality at chromosome 21. Pregnant women over the age of 35 have an increased incidence of having children with chromosomal abnormalities. Elevated levels of MSAFP are generally associated with neural tube defects. However, raised levels may also indicate other anomalies, including abdominal wall defects, esophageal and duodenal atresia, some renal and urinary tract anomalies, Turner syndrome, some low–birth-weight fetuses, placental complications, and a multifetal pregnancy. **Choice B** (Spina bifida) is incorrect. Spina bifida is a developmental defect involving incomplete closure of the embryonic neural tube, resulting in an incompletely formed spinal cord. In addition, the vertebrae overlying the open portion of the spinal cord do not fully form and remain unfused and open. This neural tube defect would lead to an elevated level of MSAFP, so it can be ruled out. **Choice C** (Anencephaly) is incorrect. Anencephaly is one of the most severe, typically fatal forms of a neural tube defect. Anencephaly is an incomplete closure of the cranial neural tube (i.e., the brain), accompanied by incomplete formation of the skull. This neural tube defect would lead to elevated MSAFP, so it can be ruled out. **Choice D** (Multifetal pregnancy) is incorrect. If the mother were carrying twins or triplets, the MSAFP would be elevated, which is not seen in this patient. **Choice E** (Hepatocellular carcinoma) is incorrect. Malignant hepatic cells produce the glycoprotein AFP. This patient has no history of liver problems, and the diagnosis of hepatocellular carcinoma is not valid because it would lead to elevated AFP levels.

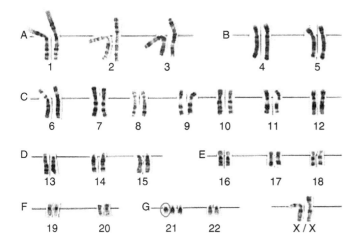

A — 1   2   3   B — 4   5

C — 6   7   8   9   10   11   12

D — 13   14   15   E — 16   17   18

F — 19   20   G — 21   22   X / X

are not derived from neural crest cells. **Choice E** (Vertebrae) is incorrect. The vertebrae are derived from paraxial mesoderm, specifically the sclerotome portions of the somites. They are not derived from neural crest cells.

4   **The answer is E: Esophageal atresia.**   Polyhydramnios is associated with the inability of the fetus to swallow because of esophageal atresia or anencephaly. Polyhydramnios can also be due to absorption defects such as duodenal atresia. The inability of the embryo to swallow amniotic fluid means that the fluid will not be absorbed into the fetal blood, removed by the placenta, and passed into the maternal blood. Therefore, the amount of fluid in the amniotic cavity is greater than normal causing polyhydramnios. **Choice A** (Bilateral kidney agenesis) is incorrect. Bilateral kidney agenesis would lead to reduced amniotic fluid volume (oligohydramnios) because the fetal kidneys, when present, increase the amniotic fluid volume through fetal urine production. **Choice B** (Urinary tract obstruction) is incorrect. Fetal urinary tract obstruction is defined as partial or complete obstruction of any portion of the urinary tract from the kidney to the urethra. This obstruction would not allow the fetal urine to enter the amniotic cavity, so this condition would lead to decreased amniotic fluid volume (oligohydramnios). **Choice C** (Uteroplacental insufficiency) is incorrect. Uteroplacental insufficiency is defined as insufficient blood flow to the placenta during pregnancy. This condition can negatively affect the fetus, leading to "fetal distress." However, uteroplacental insufficiency leads to oligohydramnios, which is not seen in this patient. **Choice D** (Hypoplastic lungs) is incorrect. Hypoplastic lungs are often caused by inadequate amounts of amniotic fluid (oligohydramnios). Swallowing of the amniotic fluid by the fetus promotes normal lung development, so hypoplastic lungs are associated with oligohydramnios, not polyhydramnios.

5   **The answer is A: Adrenal medulla.**   Both the spinal (posterior root) ganglia and the chromaffin cells of the adrenal medulla are derived from neural crest cells. Other structures derived from neural crest cells include C cells of the thyroid gland, odontoblasts, dermis in the face and neck, sympathetic chain ganglia, Schwann cells, glial cells, and melanocytes. **Choice B** (Kidney) is incorrect. The kidney is derived from intermediate mesoderm originating from a mesodermal ridge located along the posterior wall of the abdominal cavity. It is not derived from neural crest cells. **Choice C** (Liver) is incorrect. The liver appears in the middle of the 3rd week as an outgrowth of the endodermal epithelium at the distal end of the foregut. It is not derived from neural crest cells. **Choice D** (Lungs) is incorrect. The lungs develop from a single outgrowth of the endodermal epithelium from the ventral wall of the foregut. They

6   **The answer is D: Week 4.**   The illustration shows a dorsal view of a human embryo at approximately day 24 (during the 4th week) of development. Week 4 is characterized by most of neurulation, much of somite differentiation, the appearance of the pharyngeal (branchial) apparatus, and the appearance of the upper limb bud. Neurulation (the process of formation of the neural tube) begins late in week 3 with formation of the neural groove and neural folds. However, most of the process, including formation and completion of the neural tube, occurs during week 4. Likewise, segmentation of the paraxial mesoderm into somitomeres and somites begins late in week 3, with 4 to 7 somites formed at day 21. That number increases to 26 to 29 during week 4. Because somites appear at a very specific rate, their number can be used to determine the age of the embryo with great accuracy during weeks 3 to 5. This illustration shows nearly complete formation of the neural tube plus 17 defined somites, indicating the embryo is well into week 4. The pharyngeal arches and upper limb buds are not seen here, as they first appear later in the 4th week of embryonic development. **Choice A** (Week 1) is incorrect. Week 1 of embryonic development is characterized by the events of fertilization through implantation. Fertilization occurs in the ampullary part of the uterine tube. The zygote moves through the uterine tube, dividing into the morula (16-cell) stage by the time it enters the uterine cavity. Finally, it forms the blastocyst and begins implantation in the uterine mucosa by day 7. **Choice B** (Week 2) is incorrect. Week 2 of embryonic development features development of the bilaminar germ disc, which includes the completion of implantation of the embryo into the uterine mucosa and full development of the blastocyst. Remember to think of "twos" for week 2 of development. The blastocyst is composed of two main parts: the inner cell mass (embryoblast) and outer cell mass (trophoblast). The inner cell mass forms the embryo proper and differentiates into two parts that form a bilaminar disc: the epiblast and the hypoblast. The outer cell mass contributes to the formation of the placenta and differentiates into two parts: an inner cytotrophoblast and outer syncytiotrophoblast. **Choice C** (Week 3) is incorrect. Week 3 of embryonic development is characterized by the formation of the trilaminar germ disc. The featured event within this week of development is gastrulation, which results in formation of all three embryonic germ layers: ectoderm, mesoderm, and endoderm. Thus, we should remember "threes" for week 3. Weeks 3 to 8 are denoted as the embryonic period of development, which is the period of organogenesis during which the three germ layers form all tissues and organs. By the end of the 2nd month, the main organ systems are formed and the major external body features are established. Because organ primordia are very sensitive to teratogenic agents, weeks 3 to 8 of development are regarded as the sensitive period. If exposed to teratogens, gross structural organ defects can manifest during the period of organogenesis. **Choice E** (Week 5) is incorrect. Week 5 represents approximately the middle of the embryonic period of development, with organogenesis well underway. By the completion of week 5 of development, the embryo has developed significantly beyond the stages of neurulation and somite formation shown in the illustration. Also, the upper and lower limb buds have appeared and the pharyngeal apparatus is differentiating.

7   **The answer is A: Intermediate mesoderm.**   The urinary and genital systems both develop from the intermediate mesoderm. The intermediate mesoderm is a small zone that connects the paraxial and lateral plate mesodermal areas and also forms a longitudinal urogenital ridge. This urogenital ridge gives rise to the excretory parts of the urinary system, the gonad, and much of the genital duct work. Thus, defects in genetic signaling and/or teratogenic agents acting on the intermediate mesoderm may express themselves as various defects in the urogenital tracts. **Choice B** (Paraxial mesoderm) is incorrect. The paraxial mesoderm forms somites. These differentiate into sclerotome, dermatome, and myotome portions. The sclerotome gives rise to the vertebral column, the anulus fibrosus of the intervertebral discs, and the ribs. The dermatome forms the dermis and associated subcutaneous tissues of the skin. The myotomes give rise to the skeletal muscles in the body wall and limbs. **Choice C** (Neural crest) is incorrect. The neural crest forms a diverse assortment of structures spread widely across the body. This tissue separates off the neural folds and migrates into the neighboring mesoderm and beyond. Derivatives include autonomic ganglia, dorsal root ganglia, Schwann cells, arachnoid and pia meningeal layers, skeletal components of the pharyngeal arches and neurocranium, dentin of the teeth, parafollicular (C) cells in the thyroid gland, adrenal medullary (chromaffin) cells, melanocytes, and cells forming the aorticopulmonary septum in the heart. **Choice D** (Surface ectoderm) is incorrect. The ectoderm is the dorsal layer of the trilaminar germ disc. It forms the outer surface of the body and structures that form as invaginations from the surface. Derivatives include the epidermis (including the hair and nails), subcutaneous glands (including the mammary glands), dental enamel, the neural tube, and pituitary gland. Further, the linings of the stomodeum (primitive oral cavity) and proctodeum (primitive anal canal) are derived from surface ectoderm. **Choice E** (Yolk sac endoderm) is incorrect. The endoderm is the ventral layer of the trilaminar germ disc and forms the lining of the yolk sac. However, in humans, the yolk sac is vestigial, with a minor role in nutrition early in development. Of note, primordial germ cells (that originate in the epiblast) populate the proximal posterior wall of the yolk sac endoderm during week 3. These migrate into the genital ridges and induce the indifferent gonads to develop into either testes or ovaries. The great majority of the endoderm forms the epithelial lining of the gut tube and its derivatives (e.g., lower respiratory tract, urinary bladder and urethra, and middle ear cavity).

8   **The answer is E: Ectoderm, mesoderm, and endoderm.**   The epiblast is capable of forming all three germ layers (ectoderm, mesoderm, and endoderm) during gastrulation. Epiblast cells migrate to the primitive streak and invaginate into a space between the epiblast and the hypoblast. The given figure shows a cross section through the cranial region of the primitive streak at 15 days, illustrating the invagination of epiblast cells. The invaginating epiblast cells displace the hypoblast to create the definitive endoderm. Once the definitive endoderm is established, migrating epiblast cells also form the intraembryonic mesoderm. The remaining epiblast cells, which do not migrate through the primitive streak, remain in the epiblast to

form the ectoderm. Hence, the epiblast gives rise to all three germ layers in the embryo. **Choice A** (Ectoderm only) is incorrect. Cells of the epiblast that do not invaginate in the region of the primitive node and streak do remain behind to form the ectoderm. During gastrulation, however, the epiblast forms all three germ layers in the embryo: endoderm, mesoderm, and ectoderm. **Choice B** (Ectoderm and mesoderm only) is incorrect. The epiblast is capable of forming the ectoderm and mesoderm during gastrulation. However, some of these epiblast cells also displace the hypoblast to form the definitive endoderm. Hence, the epiblast gives rise to all three germ layers in the embryo. **Choice C** (Ectoderm and endoderm only) is incorrect. The epiblast is capable of forming the ectoderm and endoderm during gastrulation. However, migrating epiblast cells also form the intraembryonic mesoderm. Hence, the epiblast gives rise to all three germ layers in the embryo. **Choice D** (Mesoderm and endoderm only) is incorrect. The epiblast is capable of forming the mesoderm and endoderm during gastrulation. However, the remaining epiblast cells, which do not migrate through the primitive streak, remain in the epiblast to form the ectoderm. Hence, the epiblast gives rise to all three germ layers in the embryo.

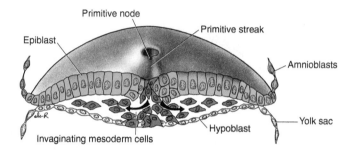

9   **The answer is B: Skeletal muscles in the arm.**   The structures indicated by the "X" are somites, which ultimately give rise to most of the skeletal muscles of the trunk and limbs, plus numerous other structures. Recall that the mesodermal germ layer segregates into three portions: paraxial, intermediate, and lateral plate. Somites form from the paraxial mesoderm and differentiate into myotome, dermatome, and sclerotome. Each myotome splits into a more dorsal epimere and a more ventral hypomere. The hypomere gives rise to the muscles in the anterolateral body wall and the limbs, whereas the epimere is related to the intrinsic muscles in the back. Thus, disruption of the development of the somites could cause malformations in the development of the muscles in the limbs. The dermatome forms the dermis and associated subcutaneous tissues of the skin. The sclerotome gives rise to the vertebral column, the anulus fibrosus portion of the intervertebral discs, and the ribs. **Choice A** (Bones in the hand) is incorrect. The bones and connective tissues in the limbs and the dermis in the body wall and limbs are derived from the parietal layer of lateral plate mesoderm. The lateral plate mesoderm splits into parietal (somatic) and visceral (splanchnic) layers related to the lateral body wall folds and incipient gut tube, respectively. The parietal mesoderm and overlying ectoderm form the ventrolateral body wall, including the limb buds. The visceral mesoderm contributes to the wall of the gut tube. **Choice C** (Body hair) is incorrect. The epidermis, including the hair and nails, is derived from the ectodermal germ layer. The ectoderm also gives rise to subcutaneous glands (such as sweat and sebaceous glands, including the mammary glands), lens of the eye, adenohypophysis, enamel of the teeth, olfactory placodes, and the neural tube. **Choice D** (Lining of the intestines) is incorrect. The epithelial lining of the gut tube is derived from the endodermal germ layer. However, the outer layers of the wall of the gut tube (including the smooth muscle) are formed mainly from the visceral layer of lateral plate mesoderm. Further, the linings of the stomodeum (primitive oral cavity) and proctodeum (primitive anal canal) are derived from surface ectoderm. **Choice E** (Melanocytes in the skin) is incorrect. Melanocytes in the skin and hair follicles are derived from the neural crest. This tissue originates at the crest of the neural folds (derived from the ectoderm), dissociates from the neural folds, and migrates into the neighboring mesoderm. Neural crest cells then migrate widely to form a diverse assortment of structures throughout the body.

10 **The answer is D: Cytotrophoblast.** The trophoblast forms the fetal part of the placenta, so it is concerned with implantation. The cytotrophoblast is the mitotically active inner part of the trophoblast, and it forms the primary chorionic villi that extend into the syncytiotrophoblast. The cytotrophoblast also provides the cells that migrate into the syncytiotrophoblast and allow it to expand. Thus, chemotherapy may directly affect mitotic activity in the cytotrophoblast, causing stunted growth of both it and the syncytiotrophoblast and possibly hindering implantation. **Choice A** (Amnioblast) is incorrect. Amnioblasts are the epiblast cells that line the amniotic cavity adjacent to the cytotrophoblast. They are mitotically active in the growth of the amniotic membrane; however, they are not involved in implantation. **Choice B** (Epiblast) is incorrect. The epiblast is the dorsal cell layer of the bilaminar germ disc. It contributes to the formation of the embryo proper. While certainly mitotically active, it is not involved in implantation. **Choice C** (Hypoblast) is incorrect. The hypoblast is the ventral cell layer of the bilaminar germ disc. It also contributes to the formation of the embryo proper. **Choice E** (Syncytiotrophoblast) is incorrect. The syncytiotrophoblast is the outer, multinucleated part of the trophoblast that is mitotically inactive. The syncytiotrophoblast erodes the maternal endometrium and contributes to the formation of the primitive uteroplacental circulation. However, its growth depends on incorporation of new cells from the active cytotrophoblast. Thus, chemotherapy in this case would not affect cell division within the syncytiotrophoblast.

11 **The answer is C: Neurulation is nearly complete.** Neurulation (the process of formation of the neural tube) begins late in week 3 with formation of the neural groove and neural folds. However, most of the process, including formation and completion of the neural tube, occurs during week 4. Additional major events during this week include much of somite differentiation, the appearance of the pharyngeal (branchial) apparatus, and the appearance of the upper limb bud. **Choice A** (Gastrulation is complete, resulting in two germ layers) is incorrect. Gastrulation is the process of formation of the trilaminar germ disc, that is, establishing the three germ layers: ectoderm, endoderm, and mesoderm. Gastrulation is the defining characteristic of week 3 of development. Remember "threes": three germ layers in week 3. **Choice B** (The embryo is entering a period of relative resistance to teratogenic substances) is incorrect. Weeks 3 to 8 constitute the embryonic period of development, which

is the period of organogenesis during which the three germ layers form all tissues and organs. By the end of week 8, the main organ systems are formed and the major external body features are established. This is also regarded as the sensitive period of development because the organ primordia are very sensitive to teratogenic agents. As a result, most gross structural organ defects are induced during this time. **Choice D** (Somites have not yet formed) is incorrect. Somite formation is normally well underway during the 4th week. Segmentation of the paraxial mesoderm into somitomeres and somites begins late in week 3, with 4 to 7 pairs of somites formed at the cranial end of the embryo at day 21. New somites are added in a craniocaudal sequence at a rate of about 3 pairs per day. There are typically 26 to 29 pairs by the end of week 4, increasing to 42 to 44 pairs at the end of week 5. Because somites appear at a very specific rate, their number can be used to determine the age of the embryo with great accuracy during weeks 3 to 5. **Choice E** (The trophoblast is present, but the syncytiotrophoblast has not yet formed) is incorrect. Differentiation of the trophoblast (the outer cell mass of the blastocyst) into cytotrophoblast and syncytiotrophoblast areas occurs early in week 2. These layers form the fetal component of the placenta and thus are critical to full implantation. At the same time, the embryoblast (the inner cell mass of the blastocyst) differentiates into the bilaminar germ disc, consisting of the epiblast and hypoblast.

12 **The answer is E: Mesoderm.** A hemangioma is a vascular tumor in which an abnormal proliferation of blood vessels leads to a mass resembling a neoplasm. Hemangiomas are mesodermal in origin, as they are formed by embryonic blood cells and the vascular endothelium formed by angioblasts, and may be present at birth. The mesoderm forms during gastrulation when invaginating epiblast cells form an additional germ layer between the endoderm and the ectoderm. The mesoderm has many notable derivatives, including muscle, connective tissue, bone, cartilage, blood cells, dermis of the skin, and organs, such as the kidney, spleen, and gonads. **Choice A** (Endoderm) is incorrect. Though the endoderm is not responsible for mesodermally derived hemangiomas, it does have many notable derivatives, including hepatocytes, acinar and islet cells of the pancreas, principal and oxyphil cells of the parathyroid gland, epithelial reticular cells of the thymus, and the epithelial lining of the gastrointestinal tract, trachea, bronchi, lungs, urinary bladder, and the female urethra (as well as most of the male urethra). **Choice B** (Neural crest) is incorrect. Though the neural crest is not responsible for mesodermally derived hemangiomas, it does have many notable derivatives, including the dentin of teeth, Schwann cells, ganglia, pia mater, arachnoid mater, chromaffin cells of the adrenal medulla, parafollicular (C) cells of the thyroid gland, melanocytes, and pharyngeal arch skeletal components. **Choice C** (Neuroectoderm) is incorrect. Though the neuroectoderm is not responsible for mesodermally derived hemangiomas, it does have many notable derivatives, including all the neurons within the central nervous system, neurohypophysis, pineal gland, astrocytes, oligodendrocytes, and the retina. **Choice D** (Ectoderm) is incorrect. Though the ectoderm is not responsible for mesodermally derived hemangiomas, it does have many notable derivatives, including the epidermis, hair, nails, sweat and sebaceous glands, lens of the eye, adenohypophysis, enamel of the teeth, and the olfactory placodes.

13 **The answer is B: Nucleus pulposus.** The notochord ("back string") is a solid fibrocellular cord that underlies the midline of the neural plate, induces the formation of the neural groove, and forms the template about which the axial skeleton develops. It is almost entirely replaced by sclerotomal cells that condense under the neural tube to form the bodies of the vertebrae. The only remnant of the notochord is the central core portion of each of the intervertebral discs, the nucleus pulposus. This hydrostatic structure is the component of the disc that herniates out of its normal position in cases of herniated ("slipped") discs. **Choice A** (Spinal cord) is incorrect. The spinal cord is the elongated caudal portion of the neural tube. The notochord lies ventral to the midline of the neural plate and induces formation of the neural groove, thus triggering formation of the neural tube. **Choice C** (Rib cage) is incorrect. The ribs develop from lateral processes of the primordial vertebrae. The paraxial mesoderm gives rise to somites, which give rise to sclerotomes. The sclerotomes condense around the neural tube and form the vertebral column. Each incipient vertebra gives rise to a pair of costal processes, which form ribs in the thoracic region. The costal processes also contribute to the formation of the transverse processes in the other vertebral regions. **Choice D** (Anulus fibrosus) is incorrect. The intervertebral discs are composed of two parts: the central nucleus pulposus and the peripheral anulus fibrosus. The anulus part of each disc is formed from the sclerotomal mesenchyme that also forms the vertebrae. It is the fibrocartilage structure that binds the vertebral bodies and stabilizes the position of the nucleus pulposus. **Choice E** (Spinal meninges) is incorrect. The entire neural tube is surrounded by three layers of membranes, the meninges. The outermost membrane, the dura mater, is derived from the mesoderm. The inner two membranes, the arachnoid and pia mater, are derived from the neural crest.

14 **The answer is B: 4 to 6 weeks.** Neurulation begins late in week 3. The posterior neuropore closes during week 4 (day 27). Failure of the posterior neuropore to close results in lower neural tube defects such as spina bifida. **Choice A** (1 to 2 weeks) is incorrect. The anterior neuropore closes at approximately day 25 of the 4th week, and the posterior neuropore also closes during week 4 (at ~day 27). Because neurulation has not yet begun during week 1 or 2, this period of development is not involved in the malformation leading to spina bifida. **Choice C** (9 to 11 weeks) is incorrect. Neurulation is complete as the posterior neuropore closes at ~day 27 of week 4 of development. So, weeks 9 to 11 of development are later than the time when a spina bifida occurs. **Choice D** (12 to 15 weeks) is incorrect. Neurulation is complete as the posterior neuropore closes at ~day 27 of week 4 of development. So, weeks 12 to 15 of development are later than the time when a spina bifida occurs. **Choice E** (16 to 19 weeks) is incorrect. Neurulation is complete as the posterior neuropore closes at ~day 27 of week 4 of development. So, weeks 16 to 19 of development are later than the time when a spina bifida occurs.

15 **The answer is E: Hypomere.** Skeletal muscles are derived from the paraxial mesoderm. Most of the paraxial mesoderm segregates into somites, which in turn give rise to myotome, dermatome, and sclerotome units. The myotome is the muscle-producing component. Each myotome splits into two segments: a more posterior epimere and a more anterior hypomere. The hypomere gives rise to the muscles in the anterolateral body wall (including the abdominal wall) and the limbs, whereas the epimere forms the intrinsic muscles of the back. The hypomere (and its derived muscles) is innervated by anterior (ventral) primary rami of spinal nerves. The epimere (and its derivatives) is supplied by posterior (dorsal) primary rami of spinal nerves. **Choice A** (Surface ectoderm) is incorrect. The ectoderm does not produce skeletal muscles. However, it does form a few small smooth muscles, for example, the dilator and sphincter muscles in the pupil of the eye. In general, the ectoderm forms the outer surface of the body and structures that form as invaginations from the surface, for example, the epidermis (including the hair and nails), subcutaneous glands (including the mammary glands), and the neural tube. **Choice B** (Intermediate mesoderm) is incorrect. Most of the urinary and genital systems develop from the intermediate mesoderm. This small zone connects the paraxial and lateral plate mesodermal areas. It gives rise to the excretory parts of the urinary system, the gonads, and much of the genital duct work. **Choice C** (Splanchnic mesoderm) is incorrect. The splanchnic mesoderm is the visceral layer of the lateral plate mesoderm. It becomes closely invested with the endoderm and gives rise to cardiac muscle that forms the myocardium and to the smooth muscle in the wall of the gut tube and its derivatives. **Choice D** (Epimere) is incorrect. The epimere is the posterior component of the myotome, which forms the deep (intrinsic) layer of back musculature. These muscles are supplied by posterior (dorsal) primary rami of spinal nerves. The abdominal wall musculature, affected in prune belly syndrome, develops from the hypomere, not the epimere.

16 **The answer is A: Gonad.** Both the kidneys and the gonads are derived from the intermediate mesoderm. This longitudinal dorsal ridge of mesoderm forms the urogenital ridge, which is involved with the formation of the future kidneys and gonads. **Choice B** (Epidermis) is incorrect. The epidermis is derived from the ectoderm, not the intermediate mesoderm. The ectoderm is also responsible for the formation of hair, nails, sweat and sebaceous glands, the lens of the eye, adenohypophysis, enamel of the teeth, and the olfactory placodes. **Choice C** (Pineal gland) is incorrect. The pineal gland is derived from the neuroectoderm, not the intermediate mesoderm. The neuroectoderm is also responsible for all the neurons within the central nervous system, neurohypophysis, astrocytes, oligodendrocytes, and the retina. **Choice D** (Liver) is incorrect. The liver is derived from the lateral plate mesoderm (specifically the splanchnic mesoderm), not the intermediate mesoderm. The lateral plate mesoderm is a thin plate of mesoderm in which large spaces (intraembryonic coelom) form. These spaces coalesce and divide the lateral plate mesoderm into the intraembryonic somatic mesoderm and the intraembryonic splanchnic (visceral) mesoderm. From the latter, the endocardium and myocardium of the heart, blood cells, endothelium of blood vessels, and the liver develop. **Choice E** (Adrenal medulla) is incorrect. The adrenal medulla is derived from the neural crest, not the intermediate mesoderm. The neural crest is also responsible for the formation of the dentin of the teeth, Schwann cells, ganglia, pia and arachnoid mater, parafollicular (C) cells of the thyroid gland, melanocytes, and pharyngeal arch skeletal components.

17 **The answer is B: Autonomic ganglia in the thoracic cavity.** All autonomic ganglia, plus the dorsal root ganglia, are derived from the neural crest. This tissue originates at the crest of the neural folds as they elevate and fuse to form the neural tube. The crest cells dissociate from the neural folds and migrate into the neighboring mesoderm. Subsequently, they migrate widely to form a diverse assortment of structures throughout the body. Other derivatives include (but are not limited to) Schwann cells, the arachnoid and pia meningeal layers, the skeletal components of the pharyngeal arches and neurocranium, dentin of the teeth, parafollicular (C) cells in the thyroid gland, adrenal medullary (chromaffin) cells, melanocytes, and cells forming the aorticopulmonary septum in the heart. **Choice A** (Cardiac muscle cells) is incorrect. Cardiac muscle is derived from the visceral layer of lateral plate mesoderm (splanchnic mesoderm) that surrounds the primitive paired endothelial heart tubes. During cardiogenesis, the heart tubes fuse into a single endocardial tube and the cardiac myoblasts form the thickened myocardium. **Choice C** (Epithelial cells lining the lower respiratory tract) is incorrect. The epithelium of the lower respiratory tract is formed from the endodermal germ layer. The lower respiratory tract consists of the larynx, trachea, and bronchi. During week 4, the respiratory diverticulum buds off the ventral wall of the primitive gut tube, which is lined with an endodermal epithelium. This diverticulum forms the lower respiratory tract that carries the lining derived from the gut tube. **Choice D** (Bone cells in the ribs) is incorrect. The ribs are derived from the paraxial mesoderm. The paraxial mesoderm forms somites, which in turn form sclerotome, dermatome, and myotome units. The sclerotomal mesenchyme condenses around the neural tube and forms the vertebral column and anulus fibrosus of the intervertebral discs. The individual vertebrae possess costal elements that expand to form ribs in the thoracic region. Thus, the ribs are also derived from sclerotome. **Choice E** (Skeletal muscle cells in the thoracic wall) is incorrect. The skeletal muscles in the thoracic wall (e.g., the intercostal muscles) are formed from the paraxial mesoderm via somites. The myotome portion of each somite splits into a more dorsal epimere and a more ventral hypomere. The hypomere gives rise to the muscles in the ventrolateral body wall (including the thoracic wall) and the limbs, whereas the epimere is related to the muscles in the back.

18 **The answer is D: Metaphase of meiosis II.** The secondary oocyte is arrested in metaphase of meiosis II about 3 hours before ovulation, and it will remain in this meiotic stage until fertilization occurs. **Choice A** (Prophase of meiosis I) is incorrect. Oogonia are formed in month 5 of a woman's fetal life. Of these 7 million oogonia, 5 million degenerate or become atretic before birth, leaving 2 million oogonia to differentiate into primary oocytes before birth. No oogonia are present at birth. The primary oocytes are dormant in prophase of meiosis I until puberty because they are surrounded by follicular cells, which secrete oocyte maturation inhibitor (OMI) that causes the arrest of meiosis I. **Choice B** (Prophase of meiosis II) is incorrect. After puberty, 5 to 15 primary oocytes will resume maturation (no longer dormant in prophase of meiosis I) with each ovarian cycle. Usually, only one primary oocyte will reach maturation with each cycle. This primary oocyte will complete meiosis I producing two daughter cells, a secondary oocyte (23 duplicated chromosomes

and almost all of the cytoplasm), and the first polar body (23 duplicated chromosomes and almost no cytoplasm). However, this secondary oocyte enters meiosis II and remains arrested in metaphase until (unless) fertilization occurs. **Choice C** (Metaphase of meiosis I) is incorrect. The ovulated secondary oocyte is arrested in metaphase of meiosis II until fertilization. This secondary oocyte has already completed meiosis I, so it cannot be in the metaphase stage of meiosis I. **Choice E** (Meiosis is completed at the time of ovulation) is incorrect. The ovulated secondary oocyte is arrested in metaphase of meiosis II until fertilization. Meiosis is only completed if fertilization occurs. If fertilization does not occur, the ovulated secondary oocyte will degenerate approximately 24 hours after ovulation.

19 **The answer is A: Epiblast.** The blastocyst typically begins implantation into the uterine wall by day 7. At this time, it consists of an inner cell mass (the embryoblast) and outer cell mass (the trophoblast). Characteristic of week 2, the embryoblast differentiates into the bilaminar germ disc. This consists of two cell layers, a dorsal epiblast and a ventral hypoblast. Splits develop between the epiblast cells and then coalesce and enlarge into a single amniotic cavity. Thus, the amniotic cavity is lined with epiblast cells and is located on the dorsal aspect of the embryo. Remember, the inner cell mass becomes the embryo proper, whereas the outer cell mass becomes the fetal part of the placenta. **Choice B** (Hypoblast) is incorrect. Hypoblast cells migrate outward to line the inner surface of the cytotrophoblast. Together, they demarcate the exocoelomic cavity (primitive yolk sac). With further development, the primitive yolk sac is reduced in size. Its remnant becomes the secondary yolk sac (definitive yolk sac), which will give rise to the gut tube. **Choice C** (Cytotrophoblast) is incorrect. The outer cell mass (trophoblast) differentiates into two portions: an inner cytotrophoblast and outer syncytiotrophoblast. The cytotrophoblast is mitotically active. It contributes to the wall of the primitive yolk sac, forms the primary chorionic villi that extend into the syncytiotrophoblast, and provides cells that migrate into the syncytiotrophoblast and allow it to expand. **Choice D** (Syncytiotrophoblast) is incorrect. This is the tissue zone that invades and erodes maternal tissues. It roots into the endometrium to form lacunae filled with maternal blood and glandular secretions. This lacunar network forms the primitive uteroplacental circulation. **Choice E** (Maternal endometrium) is incorrect. This provides the maternal site of implantation. Eroded endometrial blood vessels and glands leak into the lacunar network of the syncytiotrophoblast as part of the early uteroplacental circulation.

20 **The answer is C: Progesterone.** Progesterone is a steroid hormone produced by the ovaries, brain, and placenta of pregnant females. In the menstrual cycle, progesterone production remains low until after ovulation. The corpus luteum (the remnant of the collapsed ovarian follicle after ovulation) produces progesterone, which halts endometrial proliferation and builds the endometrial lining of the uterus in preparation for implantation of the fertilized oocyte (zygote). Therefore, progesterone supplementation would increase the chances for implantation of the fertilized oocyte into the uterine mucosa of this patient. **Choice A** (Follicle-stimulating hormone) is incorrect. Follicle-stimulating hormone (FSH), a glycoprotein secreted within the anterior pituitary, stimulates the maturation of ovarian follicles. Because increased serum levels of progesterone and estrogen suppress its release, FSH levels remain low during the buildup of the endometrial lining of the uterus, which is crucial for implantation. Also, the production of FSH peaks approximately 3 days after menstruation because serum levels of progesterone and estrogen are low. Therefore, FSH supplementation would decrease the chances for implantation of the fertilized oocyte into the uterine mucosa. **Choice B** (Testosterone) is incorrect. Testosterone is a steroid hormone secreted by the ovaries and the adrenal gland in females. Approximately 10 to 20 times less testosterone is produced in females compared to males, and it has been used to treat postmenopausal symptoms such as decreased libido. Because testosterone has more of a behavioral effect on females than a physiological one, testosterone supplementation would not increase the chances for implantation of the fertilized oocyte into the uterine mucosa. **Choice D** (Estrogen) is incorrect. Estrogen is a steroid hormone produced by the developing follicles in the ovary, the corpus luteum, and the placenta. This hormone promotes the development of female secondary sex characteristics and is involved in the thickening of the endometrium by triggering the endometrial cells to divide and proliferate. However, progesterone halts endometrial proliferation and promotes transformation of the endometrium into a receptive platform for implantation to occur. **Choice E** (Luteinizing hormone) is incorrect. In the menstrual cycle, a surge of luteinizing hormone (LH), a glycoprotein produced by the anterior pituitary, triggers ovulation. It also may play a role in converting the remnants of the collapsed ovarian follicle into the corpus luteum, which ultimately produces the progesterone responsible for building the endometrial lining of the uterus in preparation for implantation. However, the secretion of LH during implantation, which normally occurs 7 days after fertilization, remains at a basal level. Therefore, LH supplementation would not increase the chances for implantation of the fertilized oocyte into the uterine mucosa.

Chapter 3

Thorax

QUESTIONS

Select the single best answer.

1 A 54-year-old man presents with loss of sympathetic innervation to the left side of his head, characteristic of Horner syndrome. An MRI revealed a left-sided pulmonary sulcus tumor with a location approximated by the black dot to which the arrow is pointing in the given photo. What structure is most likely compromised by the tumor?

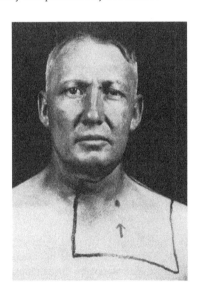

(A) Cervical anterior roots
(B) Thoracic posterior primary rami
(C) Thoracic posterior roots
(D) Thoracic anterior roots
(E) Thoracic gray rami communicantes

2 A 23-year-old man is stabbed in a bar fight. The blade of the knife enters his chest in the left 5th intercostal space, just lateral to the sternum, and pierces to a depth of approximately 4 cm. What structure is most likely damaged?
(A) Left lung
(B) Pulmonary trunk
(C) Left bronchus
(D) Stomach
(E) Pericardium

3 The given coronary artery angiogram is from a 68-year-old man with recurrent angina. It reveals 90% stenosis of the left anterior descending (LAD) artery, indicated by the white arrow. Based upon this finding, which portion of the heart is most likely susceptible to ischemic damage?

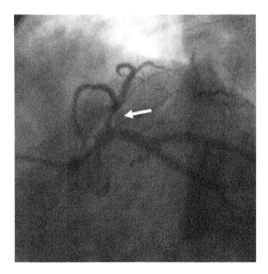

(A) Anterior two thirds of interventricular septum
(B) Posterior one third of interventricular septum
(C) Atrioventricular (AV) node
(D) Diaphragmatic surface of left ventricle
(E) Right atrium

4 A child is born at home without difficulty. Two weeks later, the mother takes the infant to her doctor, reporting that he "turns blue" when he cries. Physical examination reveals the infant is cyanotic and has a distinct systolic heart murmur. The physician suspects the baby has a tetralogy of Fallot (TOF). Which of the following conditions is a component of this syndrome?
(A) Transposition of the great vessels
(B) Hypertrophy of the left ventricle
(C) Interatrial septal defect
(D) Pulmonary infundibular stenosis
(E) Aortic valvular atresia

5 An 87-year-old woman with a history of metastatic adenocarcinoma of the breast presents with difficulty in breathing. A plain chest film reveals massive left pleural effusion, as noted in the photo. The physician chooses to drain the fluid with a thoracentesis. What is the proper location for placement of the cannula (hollow needle) to drain the pleural effusion?

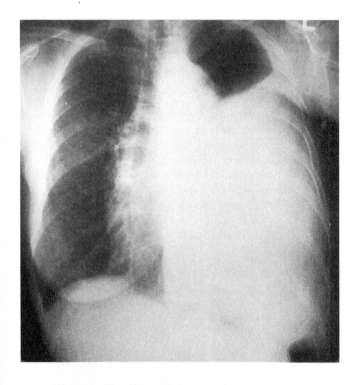

(A) Midaxillary line—6th intercostal space
(B) Midaxillary line—9th intercostal space
(C) Parasternal line—6th intercostal space
(D) Parasternal line—2nd intercostal space
(E) Midclavicular line—5th intercostal space

6 An early term embryo spontaneously aborts due to incomplete lateral body wall folding and failure of the primitive paired endocardial tubes to merge and form the primitive heart tube. The endocardial tubes are derived from which of the following embryonic sources?

(A) Paraxial mesoderm
(B) Intermediate mesoderm
(C) Splanchnic mesoderm
(D) Parietal mesoderm
(E) Extraembryonic mesoderm

7 A 22-year-old woman gives birth to an infant with an abnormally small coronary sinus that limits cardiac venous drainage. The coronary sinus is derived from which of the labeled structures in the given diagram of the primitive heart?

Cranial

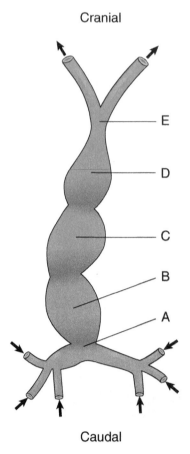

Caudal

8 Disruption of parasympathetic input to the thorax may be related to damage to which of the following structures?

(A) Cervical paravertebral ganglia
(B) Greater splanchnic nerves
(C) Gray rami communicantes
(D) Vagus nerves
(E) Intercostal nerves

9 A 40-year-old man goes to his family physician for an annual examination. Which of the following locations is ideal for placement of the stethoscope for auscultation of the tricuspid valve of the heart?

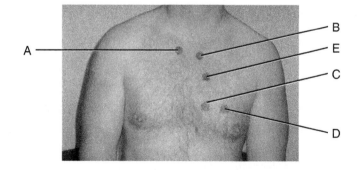

10 Which of the following congenital defects is the direct outcome of malformation of the spiral partitioning of the conus cordis and truncus arteriosus?

(A) Double aortic arch

(B) Transposition of the great vessels

(C) Patent foramen ovale

(D) Ventricular septal defect (VSD)

(E) Ectopia cordis

11 A 56-year-old construction worker comes to his family physician complaining of pain in the neck and shoulder, numbness and tingling in the right fingers, and a weak grip in his right hand. His symptoms are exacerbated by carrying heavy objects on his right shoulder. The given plain X-ray film indicates the presence of a right cervical (C7) rib in close approximation to the proximal part of the first rib. Given the signs and symptoms of this patient, what structure is most likely impinged by the cervical rib?

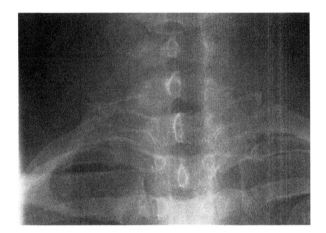

(A) Right common carotid artery

(B) Brachiocephalic trunk

(C) Right subclavian artery

(D) Vertebral artery

(E) Right brachiocephalic vein

12 A 7-year-old boy with Down syndrome underwent surgery to repair a congenital ventricular septal defect. During this procedure, iatrogenic injury to the coronary artery supplying the conduction system of the heart, including the sinuatrial (SA) and atrioventricular (AV) nodes, occurred, resulting in a heart block. What artery was most likely damaged by the surgeon?

(A) Anterior interventricular

(B) Left marginal

(C) Left coronary

(D) Right coronary

(E) Circumflex branch

13 During a newborn examination, a pediatrician is unable to detect a pulse in the groin or legs of an infant and notes the lower extremities are cold to the touch. The pulse and blood pressure of the upper limbs are significantly elevated from normal. A pediatric cardiologist performs an echocardiogram and other imaging. The given sagittal MRI verifies the presence of what specific anomaly, as indicated by the white arrowhead?

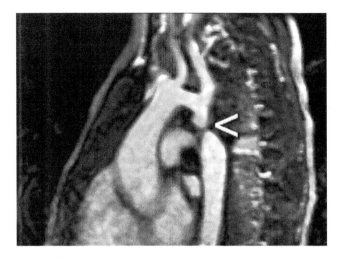

(A) Coarctation of the aorta

(B) Tetralogy of Fallot

(C) Ventricular septal defect (VSD)

(D) Atrial septal defect (ASD)

(E) Transposition of the great vessels

14 A pregnant woman is in a car accident and goes into premature labor. Her fetus is approximately 24 weeks in gestation. Her physicians administer her steroids and try to delay the birth of her baby. The survival rate of a premature baby rises significantly if the baby can reach 28 weeks gestation mainly due to the maturation of the lungs. What stage of lung maturation are the doctors hoping to reach, in which the blood-air barrier is beginning to be established?

(A) Embryonic period

(B) Pseudoglandular period

(C) Canalicular period

(D) Terminal sac period

(E) Alveolar period

15 A preterm neonate chokes and coughs throughout her first feeding with her mother with the breast milk regurgitating from the infant's mouth and nose. Noticing the difficulty feeding, a pediatrician tries to pass a catheter into the baby's stomach and meets resistance. A chest film is taken of the baby while in an incubator. The given radiograph reveals the location of the radiopaque catheter, shows no air within the stomach of the infant, and verifies normal lungs. What is the most likely diagnosis based upon the results of the X-ray?

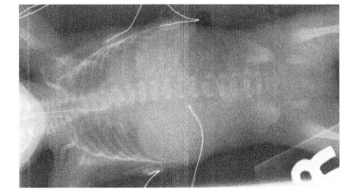

(A) Pyloric stenosis
(B) Tracheoesophageal fistula (TEF)
(C) Large bowel obstruction
(D) Respiratory distress syndrome (RDS)
(E) Esophageal atresia

16 A genetic coding defect in an early embryo results in absence of the lower part of the vertical portion of the cross of the endocardial cushions in the developing heart. Which of the following malformations is most likely present?
(A) Atrial septal defect
(B) Membranous ventricular septal defect (VSD)
(C) Transposition of the great vessels
(D) Tricuspid stenosis
(E) Muscular ventricular septal defect

17 Which of the labeled structures in the given CT scan of the thorax indicates the left main bronchus?

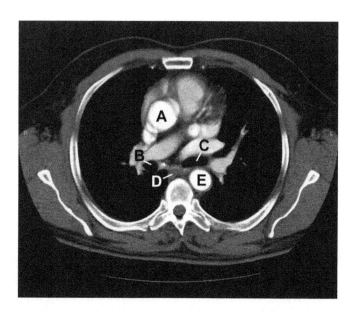

18 A 14-year-old girl is having difficulty swallowing. Her case history reveals she has mitral valve stenosis related to rheumatic fever. Which of the following structures is most likely compressing the esophagus?
(A) Right atrium
(B) Left atrium
(C) Arch of the aorta
(D) Pulmonary trunk
(E) Superior vena cava

19 A newborn baby is diagnosed with tricuspid atresia. The given echocardiographic apical four-chamber view shows the abnormal valve plus its typical associated defects: a widely patent foramen ovale (double arrows), ventricular septal defect (single arrow), hypoplastic right ventricle, and hypertrophied left ventricle. The patent foramen ovale most likely reflects a developmental failure of which of the following structures?

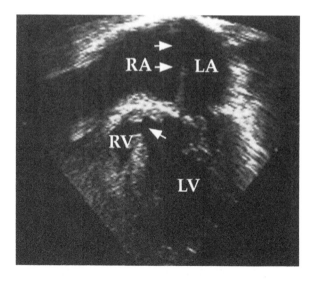

(A) Endocardial cushions
(B) Valve of the coronary sinus
(C) Ostium primum
(D) Septum secundum
(E) Septum spurium

20 A 46-year-old postal worker was exposed unknowingly to the powdered form of bacteria *Bacillus anthracis* (anthrax). He comes to the ER with flu-like symptoms, including fever, chills, fatigue, headache, chest pain, and shortness of breath. A chest X-ray shows an abnormally wide space between the lungs. Enlargement of which of the following structures is the most likely cause of the widened mediastinum in this patient?
(A) Aortic aneurysm rupture
(B) Lymph nodes
(C) Thymus
(D) Respiratory bronchioles
(E) Heart

21 A 12-year-old boy suffers an enlarging neurogenic tumor in the right posterior mediastinum, as shown in the given lateral view radiograph. This growth causes multiple lesions of the right thoracic sympathetic trunk below the T5 chain ganglion. Which of the following functions is most likely compromised?

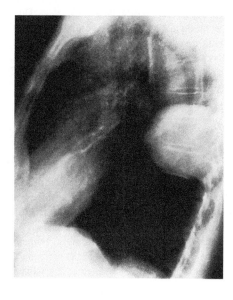

(A) Ability to produce cardiac deceleration

(B) Secretion of epinephrine

(C) Secretion of gastric juices

(D) Ability to produce bronchoconstriction

(E) Vasodilation of the coronary arteries

22 Diabetes mellitus is a disease characterized by elevated blood glucose levels (hyperglycemia). Persistent hyperglycemia is associated with degeneration of Schwann cells, followed by axonal damage. In the autonomic nervous system, the structures most susceptible to damage are the relatively smaller, nonmyelinated, postsynaptic axons. Which of the following structures are most likely to contain autonomic axons damaged secondary to diabetes mellitus?

(A) Greater splanchnic nerves

(B) Lumbar splanchnic nerves

(C) Pelvic splanchnic nerves

(D) Cardiac nerve branches of the cervical sympathetic ganglia

(E) Cardiac nerve branches of the vagus nerve

23 The structure indicated with the "X" on the given axial CT scan is which of the following structures?

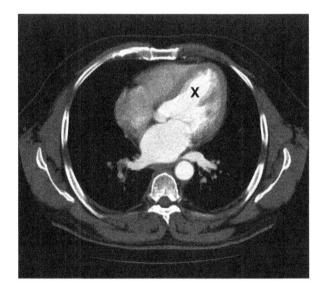

(A) Ventricular septum

(B) Right ventricle

(C) Right atrium

(D) Left ventricle

(E) Left atrium

24 During a surgery rotation, a 3rd year medical student is asked by a cardiovascular surgeon to explain what "left coronary dominance" means in relation to the left coronary artery. Which of the following explanations should be given by an astute student?

(A) It gives rise to the anterior interventricular (IV) artery

(B) It is derived from the left 6th aortic arch

(C) It supplies the right border of the heart

(D) It gives rise to the posterior interventricular artery

(E) It supplies the margin of the heart

25 One finding during autopsy of a newborn infant that died soon after birth is a significant ventricular septal defect at the upper end of the interventricular septum, as shown in the given photo. This malformation may have been related to maldevelopment of which of the following embryonic structures?

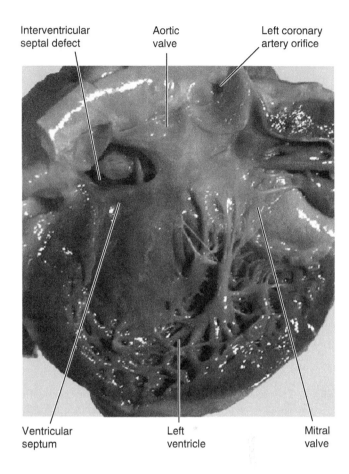

(A) Septum secundum

(B) Bulbus cordis

(C) Endocardial cushions

(D) Truncus arteriosus

(E) Sinus venosus

26 A young medical student finds herself at a moment of great relaxation during her pre-exam meditation. Which of the following events is characteristic of the inspiratory phase of normal, quiet respiration?

(A) Diaphragm flattens

(B) Intercostal muscles relax

(C) Ribs lower

(D) Abdominal wall muscles contract

(E) Horizontal dimension of the rib cage decreases

27 A male baby is born with Down syndrome (trisomy 21) and associated cardiac defects. The given apical four-chamber view echocardiogram shows a complete atrioventricular canal defect that includes a primum atrial septal defect and a posterior inlet ventricular septal defect. What embryonic structures normally fuse to close the foramen primum?

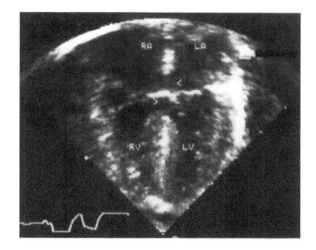

(A) Septum secundum and the septum primum
(B) Septum secundum and the fused endocardial cushions
(C) Septum primum and the fused endocardial cushions
(D) Septum primum and the septum spurium
(E) Left inferior and right superior truncus swellings

28 Which of the following components of the respiratory tract would be directly affected by a developmental failure of normal differentiation of the foregut endoderm?
(A) Nasal epithelium
(B) Intrinsic laryngeal muscles
(C) Bronchial cartilages
(D) Trachealis muscle
(E) Alveoli

29 A 25-year-old man is brought to the emergency room after suffering a deep stab wound directly through the right 5th intercostal space in the midclavicular line. Which of the following structures is most likely pierced?
(A) Superior lobe of the lung
(B) Lingula of the lung
(C) Inferior lobe of the lung
(D) Apex of the lung
(E) Middle lobe of the lung

30 Which of the labeled structures in the given PA radiograph of the chest indicates the right atrium?

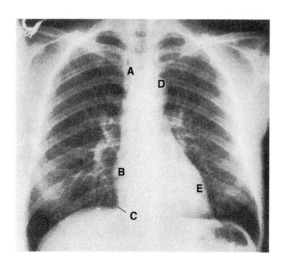

31 A radiologist is examining a series of contrast-enhanced CT scans of a patient's thorax in evaluating findings of a hypertrophied right heart. Which of the following structures is located in the pathologically enlarged right atrium?
(A) Opening of the coronary sinus
(B) Openings of the pulmonary veins
(C) Septomarginal trabecula
(D) Openings of the coronary arteries
(E) Trabeculae carneae

32 Atropine is a drug that acts to block stimulation of the receptors targeted by postsynaptic parasympathetic neurons. When it takes effect, atropine acts to do which of the following?
(A) Paralyze the diaphragm
(B) Stimulate bronchoconstriction
(C) Increase sweat gland secretions
(D) Paralyze the intercostal muscles
(E) Increase heart rate

33 A 24-year-old man who has been overweight and sedentary most of his life experiences shortness of breath and cyanosis on exertion when he attempts to start an exercise program for the first time. A thorough physical examination by his physician reveals an aortic valve defect and an aortic murmur. This murmur is best detected with the stethoscope placed over which of the indicated sites?

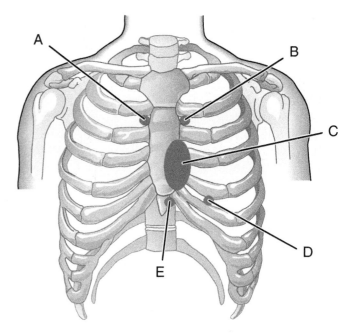

34 A newborn infant has difficulty breathing and swallowing. Radiographic examination reveals constrictions of both the trachea and esophagus in the same plane. Which of the following congenital malformations is the most likely cause of this condition?
(A) Double aortic arch
(B) Persistent right 2nd aortic arch
(C) Coarctation of the aorta
(D) Patent ductus arteriosus
(E) Persistent left 4th aortic arch

35 A 2-year-old boy comes to the ER due to accidental inhalation of a peanut. Which of the following sites is the most likely location for the aspirated peanut in the thorax?
(A) Larynx
(B) Carina of the trachea
(C) Left main bronchus
(D) Right main bronchus
(E) Right upper lobar bronchus

36 A 23-year-old man was brought to the ER barely conscious but in great discomfort after being wounded by an ice pick in the anterior chest. His doctor records the entry wound as the fifth intercostal space, immediately left of the sternum. She also notes the veins of the face and neck are engorged with blood. The given chest X-ray showed massive enlargement of the patient's cardiac silhouette. Which of the following structures is most likely damaged due to the entry site of the ice pick?

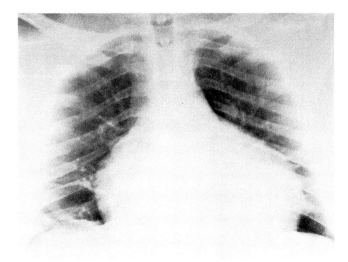

(A) Right atrium
(B) Left atrium
(C) Aortic arch
(D) Left ventricle
(E) Right ventricle

37 A 65-year-old man presents with a swollen neck, marked edema in both upper limbs, and engorged and prominent intercostal veins. Subsequent examination reveals a tumor in his right lung. The tumor is likely compressing structures in which of the following regions?

(A) Anterior mediastinum
(B) Posterior mediastinum
(C) Superior mediastinum
(D) Hilum of the lung
(E) Vena caval foramen of the diaphragm

38 An infant is born with an abnormally thin wall in the smooth part of the right atrium. This condition may be related to underdevelopment of which of the following embryonic structures?
(A) Pulmonary trunk
(B) Conus cordis
(C) Sinus venosus
(D) Truncus arteriosus
(E) Ascending aorta

39 A 58-year-old woman presents with acute abdominal pain, which radiates superior to the right shoulder region. The given CT reveals a large hepatic abscess. Which of the following nerves conveys the visceral sensory fibers involved with the pain specific to the right shoulder region?

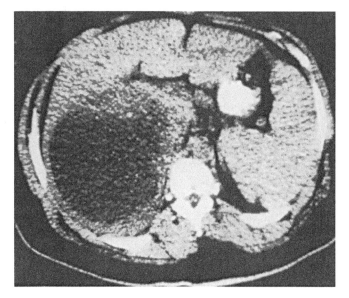

(A) Greater splanchnic nerve
(B) Lesser splanchnic nerve
(C) Least splanchnic nerve
(D) Phrenic nerve
(E) Vagus nerve

40 A 4-year-old boy presents with hypertension in the upper extremities and a diminished femoral pulse and pressure. Radiologic imaging reveals a postductal coarctation of the aorta. Which of the following is the most characteristic feature of this condition?
(A) Patent ductus arteriosus
(B) Closed ductus arteriosus
(C) Patent ductus venosus
(D) Patent foramen ovale
(E) Stenotic aortic valve

41 In preparing for his Board Certification in thoracic surgery, a surgeon reviews the geographic relations of critical structures in the chest. Which of the following is correct regarding the relationships of the vagus nerves in their passage through the thorax?
(A) Right vagus passes onto the anterior aspect of the esophagus to become the anterior vagus
(B) Left vagus passes through the anterior mediastinum
(C) Right vagus passes posterior to the root of the lung
(D) Left vagus passes across the posterior side of the aortic arch
(E) Right vagus passes through the middle mediastinum

42 A 59-year-old woman is brought to the ER in respiratory distress after her abdomen impacted the steering wheel in a motor vehicle accident. Auscultation of the left chest reveals the absence of audible breath sounds, but the presence of bowel sounds is noted. The given chest X-ray reveals radiopacity in her lower left hemithorax and a rightward mediastinal shift. Which of the following diagnoses would best explain the patient's presentation?

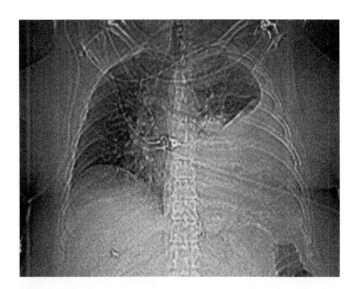

(A) Tension pneumothorax
(B) Hemopneumothorax
(C) Diaphragmatic hernia
(D) Emphysema
(E) Left lower lobe pneumonia

43 A 7-day-old newborn with a diagnosis of patent ductus arteriosus undergoes surgery to ligate the ductus arteriosus. During the repair, the surgeon takes special care to avoid injury to a closely related nerve. The surgeon is protecting which of the following nerves?
(A) Left vagus
(B) Left phrenic
(C) Left recurrent laryngeal
(D) Right recurrent laryngeal
(E) Right phrenic

44 A medical resident is preparing to insert a central venous line into the left brachiocephalic vein of her 10-year-old patient. Which of the following is a correct relation of the left brachiocephalic vein?
(A) The vein lies posterior to the arch of the aorta
(B) The brachiocephalic artery lies superficial to the vein
(C) The vein crosses the anterior aspect of the manubrium of the sternum
(D) The vein passes deep to the thymus gland
(E) The apex of the left lung lies superficial to the vein

45 A chest X-ray reveals lobar pneumonia located over the horizontal fissure of the lung. Which of the following lobes of the lung would be inflamed and full of fluid?
(A) Superior lobe of left lung
(B) Superior lobe of right lung
(C) Middle lobe of right lung
(D) Inferior lobe of right lung
(E) Inferior lobe of left lung

ANSWERS AND DISCUSSION

1   **The answer is D: Thoracic anterior roots.** Horner syndrome presents with ptosis (drooping) of the upper eyelid, miosis (constricted or "pin-point" pupil), anhydrosis (warm, flushed, dry skin), and enophthalmosis (sunken eye), and the presence of this syndrome suggests damage to the pathway of sympathetic fibers to the head. The thoracic anterior roots are the only listed structures that carry sympathetic fibers destined for the head. The presynaptic sympathetic cell bodies reside in the intermediolateral (IML) cell column in the lateral horn of the gray matter within the T1-L2 (or L3) spinal segmental levels. The sympathetic fibers destined for the head leave the spinal cord through thoracic anterior roots from T1 to T3. **Choice A** (Cervical anterior roots) is incorrect. The sympathetic nervous system is a thoracolumbar system, consisting of presynaptic cell bodies that reside in the IML cell column of spinal segmental levels of T1-L2 (or L3). The cervical anterior (ventral) roots is an incorrect answer because presynaptic sympathetic fibers ONLY reside in the anterior (ventral) roots of spinal nerves T1-L2 (or L3). Moreover, since the IML is somatotopically organized, the sympathetic fibers going to the head exist in the IML from T1 to T3 and ONLY run through the anterior (ventral) roots of these specific spinal nerves. The patient is exhibiting a loss of sympathetic innervation to the head, so damage to the cervical anterior roots would not result in Horner syndrome. **Choice B** (Thoracic posterior primary rami) is incorrect. Sympathetic fibers in the thoracic posterior (dorsal) primary rami have already synapsed in the sympathetic trunk and are not distributed to the head, so damage to these rami would not cause Horner syndrome. Postsynaptic sympathetic fibers pass through the thoracic posterior (dorsal) primary rami in order to vasoconstrict or vasodilate the vessels going to the areas supplied by these nerves, namely, the epaxial back muscles and the skin overlying these muscles. **Choice C** (Thoracic posterior roots) is incorrect. The autonomic nervous system is an entirely efferent (motor) system. The posterior (dorsal) roots contain only afferent (sensory) fibers, which eliminates these roots as a plausible choice. **Choice E** (Thoracic gray rami communicantes) is incorrect. The thoracic gray rami communicantes convey postsynaptic sympathetic fibers (which have already synapsed in the sympathetic trunk) to the spinal nerves at the vertebral level at which they synapsed. These fibers distribute to the body wall and limbs. Therefore, the sympathetic fibers located in the thoracic gray rami communicantes do not reach the head, and damage to these fibers would not cause Horner syndrome.

2   **The answer is E: Pericardium.** Due to the location of the stab wound, the pericardial sac and the right ventricle of the heart (the most anterior chamber of the heart) are most likely damaged. The pericardium is a fibrous, unyielding sac that surrounds the heart. Lesion of the right ventricle would cause blood to spill out of the heart into the pericardial space, causing a pericardial effusion (blood accumulation within the pericardial sac). Compression of the heart (cardiac tamponade) would result. These events make it impossible for the heart to fill completely, which limits the blood it can receive. Patients with cardiac tamponade present with engorged veins of the face and neck due the backup of blood. A pericardial effusion can be drained via a procedure known as pericardiocentesis, which temporarily relieves the patient's problem until the heart wall is repaired. However, time is critical because cardiac tamponade compresses the heart and may result in a quick death. **Choice A** (Left lung) is incorrect. The left lung, and the pleural sac in which it resides, are pushed laterally away from the sternum due to the position of the heart, which resides primarily on the left side of the body. Due to the location of the knife wound in this patient, the pericardium and right ventricle would be damaged, not the left lung. **Choice B** (Pulmonary trunk) is incorrect. The pulmonary trunk is the outflow tract of the right ventricle. The pulmonary trunk resides left of the sternum at approximately the 2nd intercostal space, which is located above the entry point of the knife in this patient. **Choice C** (Left bronchus) is incorrect. The bifurcation of the trachea occurs at the 4th thoracic vertebral level. The wound location is at the 7th or 8th thoracic vertebral level, or the 5th intercostal space of the anterior thoracic wall. Therefore, the left main stem bronchus is located above the damaged area. Furthermore, the left bronchus resides deep to the heart, and the depth of the stab wound (~4 cm) would not reach the left bronchus. **Choice D** (Stomach) is incorrect. The stomach resides inferior to the location of the knife wound. Also, due to its posterior positioning and the depth of the wound, the stomach would not be damaged in this patient.

3   **The answer is A: Anterior two thirds of interventricular septum.** The artery that anatomists entitle the anterior interventricular branch of the left coronary artery is often called the LAD artery by physicians in the clinic. This nomenclature is important because this artery represents the most commonly occluded coronary artery in myocardial infarctions (heart attacks). As its anatomical name implies, it supplies the anterior two thirds of the interventricular septum, so this portion of the heart would most likely be damaged following an ischemic event due to a 90% stenosis of the LAD. **Choice B** (Posterior one third of interventricular septum) is incorrect. The posterior one third of the interventricular (IV) septum is usually supplied by the posterior IV branch of the right coronary artery, so this part of the heart would most likely not be damaged in this patient. **Choice C** (Atrioventricular [AV] node) is incorrect. The right coronary artery gives off the AV nodal branch in most cases, so this part of the conducting system of the heart would not be damaged in this patient. **Choice D** (Diaphragmatic surface of left ventricle) is incorrect. The diaphragmatic surface of the left ventricle is usually supplied by the posterior IV branch of the right coronary artery, so this part of the heart would most likely not be damaged in this patient. **Choice E** (Right atrium) is incorrect. The right atrium is supplied by the right coronary artery, so this part of the heart would not be damaged due to the location of the blockage in the LAD.

4   **The answer is D: Pulmonary infundibular stenosis.** An abnormally narrowed right ventricular outflow tract (pulmonary infundibular stenosis) is one of the four components of TOF. This syndrome is the most common malformation complex resulting from unequal division of the conus cordis and truncus arteriosus by the spiraling conotruncal septum. This septum contributes significantly to the formation of the ventricular outflow tracts and the proximal parts of the aorta and pulmonary trunk. Anterior displacement of the developing conotruncal septum results in a narrow right ventricular outflow (pulmonary infundibular stenosis), plus an overriding aorta, ventricular septal defect (VSD), and hypertrophied right ventricle. The four classic characteristics of TOF are pictured in the given figure. Children with TOF are typically cyanotic due to the mixing of right and left side blood through the VSD and the overriding aorta. Also, the systolic heart murmur is typical due to the VSD. **Choice A** (Transposition of the great vessels) is incorrect. Failure of the conotruncal septum to follow its normal spiral course results in transposition of the great vessels. When the septum runs directly downward through the conotruncal region instead of spiraling, the aorta originates from the right ventricle and the pulmonary trunk arises from the left ventricle. **Choice B** (Hypertrophy of the left ventricle) is incorrect. In TOF, the combination of back-pressure from the infundibular stenosis and systemic pressure needs from the overriding aorta and VSD results in hypertrophy of the right ventricle. **Choice C** (Interatrial septal defect) is incorrect. The conotruncal septum contributes to the formation of the upper (membranous) part of the interventricular septum. Thus, malformation of the conus septum commonly results in a membranous VSD, not an atrial septal defect. **Choice E** (Aortic valvular atresia) is incorrect. In this condition, the valvular orifice into the aorta is absent, and the aorta and left side chambers are underdeveloped. In TOF, the conotruncal septum is displaced, resulting in an open, overriding aorta.

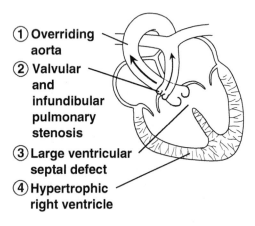

① **Overriding aorta**
② **Valvular and infundibular pulmonary stenosis**
③ **Large ventricular septal defect**
④ **Hypertrophic right ventricle**

5 **The answer is B: Midaxillary line—9th intercostal space.**   Secondary to her metastatic breast cancer, the patient is suffering from a pleural effusion (accumulation of excess fluid in the pleural cavity surrounding the lung). The effusion causes the difficulty in breathing due to limiting the expansion of the lungs during inspiration. A thoracentesis is an invasive procedure to remove the excess fluid from the pleural sac. In the midaxillary line, the lung resides at the 8th rib and the parietal pleura would reside at the 10th rib. The space between the parietal pleura and the lung is the costodiaphragmatic recess, and it gives space for the lung to inflate within the pleural cavity. To drain the pleural effusion, a doctor must place the cannula (hollow needle) in a location where the lung and parietal pleura are separated. The 9th intercostal space at the midaxillary line is the ideal location to perform a thoracentesis because here the pleural effusion can be drained without damaging the lung itself. **Choice A** (Midaxillary line—6th intercostal space) is incorrect. Performing a thoracentesis at this location would likely damage the lung, which extends to the 8th rib in the midaxillary line. However, this location (6th intercostal space at the midaxillary line) is often used for

placement of a chest tube, which is often inserted to remove air or fluids from the pleural space after the lung has collapsed due to a pneumothorax. Therefore, the lung tissue is no longer extending down to the 8th rib at the midaxillary line, so the drainage of the lung can occur at a higher level. **Choice C** (Parasternal line—6th intercostal space) is incorrect. Due to the majority of the heart residing on the left side of the thorax, the lung and parietal pleural are shifted away from the midline at this location. Therefore, a pleural effusion could not be drained at this location due to no access to the pleural cavity. At this location, a pericardiocentesis could be performed to drain fluid from the fibrous pericardium. **Choice D** (Parasternal line—2nd intercostal space) is incorrect. At the 2nd intercostal space immediately to the left of the sternum, no space exists between the parietal pleura and the lung. Therefore, this location is not ideal to drain a pleural effusion. This location, however, is often used for auscultation of the pulmonary valve of the heart with a stethoscope. **Choice E** (Midclavicular line—5th intercostal space) is incorrect. At the fifth intercostal space at the midclavicular line on the left side, no space exists between the parietal pleura and the lung. Therefore, this location is not ideal to drain a pleural effusion. This location, however, is often used for auscultation of the mitral (or bicuspid) valve of the heart with a stethoscope.

6 **The answer is C: Splanchnic mesoderm.**   Cardiac progenitor cells migrate from the epiblast into the cranial portion of the splanchnic layer of the lateral plate mesoderm. In the mesoderm, the progenitor cells ultimately form paired cardiac primordia, that is, the endocardial tubes. Subsequent lateral and cephalocaudal folding of the embryo causes merging of the paired endocardial tubes plus caudal shifting of the primitive heart tube and pericardial cavity. **Choice A** (Paraxial mesoderm) is incorrect. The paraxial mesoderm segments into somites along the long axis of the body wall. Each somite ultimately differentiates into three portions: sclerotome, myotome, and dermatome. **Choice B** (Intermediate mesoderm) is incorrect. The intermediate mesoderm is the small portion of mesoderm that connects the paraxial and lateral plate mesodermal areas. It differentiates into urogenital organs. **Choice D** (Parietal mesoderm) is incorrect. The lateral plate mesoderm splits into parietal (somatic) and visceral (splanchnic) parts, separated by the intraembryonic body cavity. The parietal layer becomes associated with the overlying ectoderm to form the lateral body wall folds. **Choice E** (Extraembryonic mesoderm) is incorrect. This cell population appears outside the embryonic body proper. It forms a loose connective tissue zone that eventually results in the chorionic cavity.

7 **The answer is A: Sinus venosus.**   The given diagram represents the primitive five-division heart in the 4th week of development. The caudal (venous) pole of the heart is formed by the sinus venosus (structure A). The sinus venosus receives venous blood through its two extensions, the right and left sinus horns. As the heart develops further, most of the left sinus horn is obliterated. Its major remnant forms the coronary sinus, which receives most of the cardiac venous return. The right sinus horn persists to a greater degree and forms the smooth part of the right atrium (sinus venarum) and the roots of the venae cavae. **Choice B** (Primitive atrium) is incorrect. The primitive common atrium undergoes septation and merges with the remnants of the sinus venosus to form the definitive right and left atria and auricles. The primitive right atrium forms the right auricle. The primitive left atrium forms the smooth part of the left atrium and the left auricle. **Choice C** (Primitive ventricle) is incorrect. The ventricle and the bulbus cordis of the primitive heart tube interact with each other in a complex septation process that produces the definitive right and left ventricles. The primitive ventricle forms most of the left ventricle. **Choice D** (Bulbus cordis) is incorrect. The bulbus cordis undergoes a complex spiral septation in close coordination with the septation of the ventricle and the truncus arteriosus. Ultimately, the bulbus forms most of the definitive right ventricle plus the right and left ventricular outflow channels. **Choice E** (Truncus arteriosus) is incorrect. The truncus arteriosus is the cranial third of the bulbus cordis. It undergoes a spiral septation and forms the proximal parts of the pulmonary trunk and the aorta.

8 **The answer is D: Vagus nerves.** The vagus nerves provide parasympathetic input to the thoracic viscera and to the abdominal viscera as far as the left colic (splenic) flexure. Cardiac branches of the vagi arise in the neck and descend into the thorax to supply the heart. Multiple additional branches arise in the thorax and supply the other thoracic viscera. Thus, parasympathetic input to the thorax is widespread from a great extent of the vagus nerves. **Choice A** (Cervical paravertebral ganglia) is incorrect. The paravertebral ganglia are the sympathetic ganglia. The cervical ganglia give rise to cardiac branches that provide much of the sympathetic supply to the thoracic viscera. **Choice B** (Greater splanchnic nerves) is incorrect. These nerves are branches of the thoracic sympathetic trunk ganglia. They convey sympathetic fibers to the upper abdomen. **Choice C** (Gray rami communicantes) is incorrect. Gray and white rami communicantes are short connections between individual spinal nerves and the sympathetic trunk. The gray rami carry mainly postsynaptic sympathetic fibers. The white rami convey mainly presynaptic fibers. **Choice E** (Intercostal nerves) is incorrect. There is no parasympathetic innervation in the body wall and limbs. Thus, the intercostal nerves (supplying the thoracic and abdominal walls) do not carry parasympathetic fibers.

9 **The answer is C: Tricuspid valve.** The ideal placement of the stethoscope for auscultation of the tricuspid valve is at the 5th intercostal space slightly to the left of the sternal border, identified by the letter "C" in the photo. The tricuspid valve separates the right atrium and the right ventricle. **Choice A** (Aortic valve) is incorrect. The ideal placement of the stethoscope for auscultation of the aortic valve is at the right second intercostal space slightly lateral to the sternal border, identified by the letter "A" in the photo. The aortic valve is the only heart valve best heard by placing the stethoscope to the right of the midline of a patient. **Choice B** (Pulmonary valve) is incorrect. Auscultation of the pulmonary valve would be best heard by placing the stethoscope over the left 2nd intercostal space slightly to the left of the sternal border. This location is marked by the letter "B" in the photo. To listen to the tricuspid valve, the stethoscope needs to be placed more inferiorly at the fifth intercostal space slightly to the left of the sternal border. **Choice D** (Mitral valve) is incorrect. The ideal placement of the stethoscope for auscultation of the mitral (bicuspid) valve is at the left 5th intercostal space in the midclavicular line, which is located near the nipple. This location corresponds

to the left ventricular area near the apex of the heart, identified in the photo by the letter "D". **Choice E** (Left sternal border of heart) is incorrect. The location for auscultation of the left sternal border of the heart is identified by the letter "E" in the photo. To listen to the tricuspid valve, the stethoscope needs to be placed more inferiorly at the fifth intercostal space slightly to the left of the sternal border.

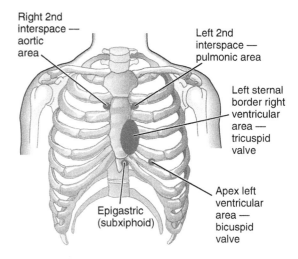

10 **The answer is B: Transposition of the great vessels.** The conus cordis and truncus arteriosus normally undergo an internal spiral partitioning (septation) that results in formation of the ventricular outflow tracts, pulmonary trunk, and ascending aorta. Failure of the conotruncal septum to follow its normal spiral course results in transposition of the great vessels. In this case, the septum runs directly downward through the conotruncal region instead of spiraling, causing the aorta to originate from the right ventricle and the pulmonary trunk to arise from the left ventricle. Alternately, displacement of the developing spiral septum causes unequal division of the conotruncal region, resulting in a narrow right ventricular outflow plus an overriding aorta. This condition is different from transposition of the great vessels and forms the basis for tetralogy of Fallot. **Choice A** (Double aortic arch) is incorrect. A double aortic arch is the result of the persistent right dorsal aorta connecting with the seventh intersegmental artery and the left dorsal aorta. This arrangement produces a vascular ring that surrounds both the trachea and esophagus. **Choice C** (Patent foramen ovale) is incorrect. A patent foramen ovale is a persistent opening in the atrial septum, resulting from failure of fusion of the septum secundum with the remnant of the septum primum. This defect allows postnatal exchange of blood between the two atria. **Choice D** (Ventricular septal defect) is incorrect. VSDs are gaps in the ventricular septum resulting from failure of fusion of the muscular walls of the primitive ventricles and/or failure of growth of tissue from the endocardial cushions. In either case, blood may be exchanged between the ventricles. VSDs are commonly closely associated with other defects that result from mistakes in partitioning of the conotruncal region. However, they are not directly derived from such defects. **Choice E** (Ectopia cordis) is incorrect. In this rare malformation, the heart lies on the surface of the chest, which results from failure of the lateral body wall folds to meet and fuse in the anterior midline of the thorax.

11 **The answer is C: Right subclavian artery.** The right subclavian artery arises off the brachiocephalic trunk (a direct branch off of the arch of the aorta) and runs to the lateral border of the first rib. At this location, the subclavian artery becomes the axillary artery, which continues on to supply the upper limb. The right cervical rib (C7), depicted on the given X-ray, extends inferiorly in close relationship to the first rib. The subclavian artery typically passes over the cervical rib, causing the vessel to take a steeper route. When the shoulder is depressed (e.g., when carrying a heavy load), the subclavian artery may be compressed against the cervical rib, leading to the symptoms present in the patient and resulting in thoracic outlet syndrome. Thoracic outlet syndrome causes pain, numbness, and paresthesia (tingling) in the neck and shoulder as well as the fingers of the hand. Moreover, the poor circulation in the right upper limb, due to the compression of the right subclavian artery, is causing the weakness (paresis) of the muscles of the hand. **Choice A** (Right common carotid artery) is incorrect. The right common carotid artery arises off the brachiocephalic trunk, which is a direct branch off of the arch of the aorta. The right common carotid artery ascends into the neck to split into the internal and external carotid arteries at the fourth cervical vertebra (C4). However, the common carotid is not closely associated with the first rib, so it will not be compromised by the presence of the right cervical rib (C7). Furthermore, compression of the right common carotid artery would lead to symptoms in the head and neck as well as affect the anterior circulation of the brain. However, the symptoms of this patient were localized to the right upper limb, so the right common carotid artery was not affected. **Choice B** (Brachiocephalic trunk) is incorrect. The brachiocephalic trunk, a direct branch off the arch of the aorta, gives rise to the right subclavian and common carotid arteries. If this artery were compressed by the right cervical rib (C7), the symptoms of the patient would include head and neck effects due to the involvement of the right common carotid artery. **Choice D** (Vertebral artery) is incorrect. The vertebral artery is the first branch off the subclavian artery, but this artery ascends through the cervical vertebral column to supply the posterior circulation of the brain. Compression of this artery would not explain the right upper limb symptoms, or the thoracic outlet syndrome, seen in this patient. **Choice E** (Right brachiocephalic vein) is incorrect. Compression of the right brachiocephalic vein would cause the superficial veins of the neck to become engorged due to the backflow of venous return to the heart. This sign is often seen in patients with congestive heart failure. However, compression of the right brachiocephalic vein would not explain the thoracic outlet syndrome seen in this patient because the right upper limb would still be receiving its arterial supply. Therefore, blockage of this vein would not cause the symptoms seen in this patient.

12 **The answer is D: Right coronary.** The right coronary artery gives off arterial branches that usually supply both the SA and AV nodes. The SA node is usually supplied by the SA nodal artery, which branches off the proximal aspect of the right coronary artery. The AV nodal branch, which usually branches off the posterior interventricular branch of the right coronary artery, supplies the AV node. Iatrogenic injury to the right coronary artery would compromise the conduction system of the heart and lead to a heart block, as seen in this patient. **Choice A** (Anterior interventricular) is incorrect. The anterior interventricular artery, which is often called the left anterior descending (LAD) artery by clinicians, arises off the left coronary artery to supply the anterior aspects of both ventricles as it runs within the interventricular groove. In rare cases, its branches supply the AV bundle of the conduction system. **Choice B** (Left marginal) is incorrect. The left marginal artery branches off the circumflex branch of the left coronary artery to supply the left ventricle. This artery follows the left margin of the heart; however, iatrogenic injury to this artery would not cause the heart block seen in this patient. **Choice C** (Left coronary) is incorrect. The left coronary artery supplies the left atrium, most of the left ventricle, and some of the right ventricle. In rare cases, its branches supply the AV node of the conduction system, but the AV node is usually supplied by branches of the right coronary artery. **Choice E** (Circumflex branch) is incorrect. The circumflex branch of the left coronary artery follows the coronary sulcus around the left border of the heart to reach its posterior surface. This artery usually does not supply the conduction system of the heart, though it occasionally supplies blood to the SA node. However, the SA node is more commonly supplied by the sinuatrial node artery of the right coronary artery.

13 **The answer is A: Coarctation of the aorta.** A coarctation of the aorta is a significant narrowing of the aorta distal to the origin of the left subclavian artery, as depicted on the given sagittal MRI. In coarctation of the aorta, blood flow into the descending aorta is diminished or blocked. However, arterial flow into the distal aorta is usually maintained via expansion of collateral circulation through the internal thoracic and intercostal arteries. The pressure dynamics in this patient, including hypertension in the upper limbs and diminished pressure in the lower limbs, represent the classic clinical signs of coarctation of the aorta. Many patients with coarctation of the aorta remain asymptomatic because of a persistent ductus arteriosus. When coarctation of the aorta is detected in newborns, the child is often given prostaglandin agonists (PGE-1) to keep the ductus arteriosus patent until this defect can be fixed. **Choice B** (Tetralogy of Fallot) is incorrect. In tetralogy of Fallot, the right ventricular outflow experiences stenosis due to unequal division of the conus cordis and truncus arteriosus by the conotruncal septum. This anomaly presents with the following four characteristics: (1) overriding aorta, (2) valvular and infundibular pulmonary stenosis, (3) large VSD, and (4) hypertrophied right ventricle. However, this sagittal MRI depicts a narrowing of the aorta, which is not indicative of tetralogy of Fallot. **Choice C** (Ventricular septal defect [VSD]) is incorrect. A VSD is an abnormal opening in the septum between the right and left ventricles and would be seen by the cardiologist on the echocardiogram. However, the given MRI depicts a coarctation of the aorta, which is also consistent with the symptoms of the patient, including diminished pressure and inability to detect a pulse in the lower limbs. **Choice D** (Atrial septal defect [ASD]) is incorrect. An ASD is an abnormal opening in the septum between the right atrium and the left atrium, and this defect would be seen by the cardiologist on the echocardiogram. However, the given MRI depicts a coarctation of the aorta, which is also consistent with the symptoms of the patient, which are hypertension in the upper limbs and diminished pressure in the lower limbs. **Choice E** (Transposition of the great vessels) is incorrect. Transposition of the aorta and pulmonary trunk is the result of failure of normal partitioning of the conus cordis and truncus arteriosus by the conotruncal septum. In this anomaly, the aorta originates from the right ventricle and the pulmonary trunk arises from the left ventricle; therefore, these major arteries are transposed from their normal positions. However, this sagittal MRI depicts a narrowing of the aorta distal to the left subclavian artery, or coarctation of the aorta.

14 **The answer is D: Terminal sac period.** The simple cuboidal epithelium within the terminal sacs differentiates into pneumocytes within the terminal sac period. The rapidly proliferating capillary network makes intimate contact with the terminal sacs, and the blood-air barrier is established with Type I pneumocytes (or alveolar epithelial cells). These events take place in the terminal sac period, which runs from embryonic week 24 until birth and are crucial for the survival of an infant born prematurely. Administration of steroids to the infant in utero can promote lung maturation by increasing the proliferation of Type II pneumocytes (or alveolar epithelial cells), which secrete surfactant, a fluid capable of decreasing the surface tension at the air-alveolar interface. Due to the terminal sac period of lung maturation, a premature infant's survival rate will increase considerably from week 24 to 28 as the blood-air barrier continues to be established. **Choice A** (Embryonic period) is incorrect. At approximately 4 weeks of gestation, the respiratory diverticulum, or lung bud, begins to arise from the ventral wall of the foregut. Two longitudinal tracheoesophageal ridges fuse in the midline to form the tracheoesophageal septum, which separates the lung bud away from the foregut, specifically the esophagus, forming the trachea. The distal end of the trachea divides into two lateral bronchial buds. At the beginning of week 5, the bronchial buds elongate to form the primary (left and right main stem) bronchi, which further divide into the secondary bronchi. **Choice B** (Pseudoglandular period) is incorrect. The pseudoglandular period occurs from week 5 to 16 of gestation. During this period of lung maturation, the terminal bronchioles, which were established in the embryonic period of lung development, continue to divide to establish respiratory bronchioles and alveolar ducts. The vascular supply to the lungs also increases; however, respiration is not possible until there are enough capillaries within the lungs to enable sufficient gas exchange. Adequate gas exchange is not possible until the terminal sac period is reached at approximately the seventh month of gestation. **Choice C** (Canalicular period) is incorrect. The canalicular period of lung maturation occurs from week 16 to 26 of gestation. During this period of lung development, the terminal sacs (primitive alveoli) form, and capillaries within the lung tissue begins to establish close contact with the primitive alveoli. However, respiration is not possible until the terminal sac period when an adequate supply of capillaries exist to enable sufficient gas exchange. Adequate gas exchange is not possible until the seventh month of gestation. **Choice E** (Alveolar period) is incorrect. The alveolar period of lung maturation continues from month 8 of gestation and/ or birth until well into childhood. During this period of lung development, the number of mature alveoli within the lungs continues to increase in number and the blood-air barrier is now well established. However, it is during the terminal sac period of lung development (week 26–birth) when adequate gas exchange is established, making respiration possible in a premature infant.

15 **The answer is E: Esophageal atresia.** Esophageal atresia is a congenital disorder in which the esophagus ends in a blind-ending pouch and is not connected to the stomach. In the given chest film, the catheter is resting in the blind-ending esophagus. The absence of air in the stomach also indicates an esophageal atresia. These malformations are detected during the infant's first feeding due to choking, coughing, and even sneezing. Excessive salivation may also be noted due to inability to swallow this secretion. In prenatal examinations, esophageal atresia is often associated with polyhydramnios in the third trimester. Also, an esophageal atresia can present with or without a tracheoesophageal fistula. The latter scenario is more probable due to the appearance of normal lungs on X-ray. **Choice A** (Pyloric stenosis) is incorrect. Due to the location of the catheter on the X-ray, which is located within the esophagus, a pyloric stenosis (narrowing of the pyloric end of the stomach) is not probable. Infants usually do not present with symptoms of pyloric stenosis until approximately 2 to 3 weeks after birth when they feed normally, but follow each feeding with nonbilious, projectile vomiting and a ravenous desire to continue to feed. Pyloric stenosis is usually detected with abdominal ultrasound and is prevalent in first-born Caucasian boys. **Choice B** (Tracheoesophageal fistula [TEF]) is incorrect. A TEF is an abnormal connection between the trachea and the esophagus due to incomplete development of the tracheoesophageal septum, which normally separates the developing trachea from the esophageal portion of the foregut. TEFs are often seen with esophageal atresia; however, in these cases, the baby would usually aspirate fluids into the lungs. In the given X-ray, there is no evidence of fluid accumulation in the lungs (pneumonia) secondary to the esophageal atresia. Normal lungs rule out the possibility of a TEF. **Choice C** (Large bowel obstruction) is incorrect. Large bowel obstruction would not explain the location of the catheter, which is stuck in the esophagus. Also, babies with large bowel obstruction would be able to feed; however, they would present with bilious, projectile vomiting a few hours after feeding. This patient exhibited feeding problems immediately, which rules out large bowel obstruction. **Choice D** (Respiratory distress syndrome [RDS]) is incorrect. RDS is common in babies of diabetic mothers and premature infants (born before 34 weeks of gestation). This patient is not exhibiting symptoms of RDS, which would include rapid breathing and shortness of breath. RDS rarely occurs in full-term infants.

16 **The answer is B: Membranous ventricular septal defect (VSD).** The developing endocardial cushions constitute a tissue mass in the center of the heart that can be envisioned schematically as a cross-like formation. The crossbar (horizontal part) forms the atrioventricular canals and valves. The post (vertical part) forms portions of the atrial and ventricular septa. The lower limb of the vertical part forms the membranous part of the ventricular septum. Thus, defects in outgrowth of this component result in membranous VSDs. VSDs as a whole are the most common congenital cardiac malformations. **Choice A** (Atrial septal defect) is incorrect. The upper limb of the vertical part of the endocardial cushion cross contributes to formation of the septum primum in the common atrium. Extensions of the endocardial cushions here help to close the foramen (ostium) primum.

Defects in this component result in primum type atrial septal defects. **Choice C** (Transposition of the great vessels) is incorrect. This malformation is the result of failure of normal partitioning of the conus cordis and truncus arteriosus. When the conotruncal septum runs directly downward through the conotruncal region instead of spiraling, the aorta originates from the right ventricle and the pulmonary trunk arises from the left ventricle. Thus, these major arteries are transposed from their normal positions. **Choice D** (Tricuspid atresia) is incorrect. In tricuspid atresia, the tricuspid valve is absent or fused and the right atrioventricular orifice is obliterated. The horizontal part of the endocardial cushion cross forms the atrioventricular canals and valves. Thus, defective formation of the right limb of the endocardial cushion crossbar may produce tricuspid atresia. **Choice E** (Muscular ventricular septal defect) is incorrect. The medial walls of the two primitive ventricles merge to form the muscular part of the ventricular septum. This fuses with the lower limb of the endocardial cushions to form the complete ventricular septum. Muscular VSDs are more common than membranous VSDs, and most of these defects resolve during normal growth.

17 **The answer is C: Left main bronchus.** The trachea, bronchi, and lungs appear as radiolucent (black) structures because of their air content. Left and right are differentiated by remembering that the conventional view of CT scans is from below, as if standing at the foot of the patient's bed and looking to the supine person's head. Also, the left main (primary) bronchus is more horizontally aligned, whereas the right main bronchus is more vertically aligned. Thus, the left main bronchus offers a more oblong profile in cross-sectional (axial) scans, while the right main bronchus is more circular. **Choice A** is incorrect. The ascending aorta is identified. Note the position of this structure relative to the left ventricle. **Choice B** is incorrect. The right main bronchus is identified. Note the differentiating features outlined previously. **Choice D** is incorrect. The azygos vein is identified. Note the size and position of the azygos vein slightly offset to the right

anterior aspect of the vertebral body. **Choice E** is incorrect. The descending aorta is identified. Note the size and position of the aorta slightly offset to the left anterior aspect of the vertebral body.

18 **The answer is B: Left atrium.** The left atrium forms most of the base (posterior aspect) of the heart. The esophagus passes immediately posterior to the left atrium, forming its major posterior relation. This relationship is readily seen in radiographs, especially following a barium swallow. Mitral valve stenosis restricts blood flow out of the left atrium, leading to dilation of this chamber. This dilation of the left atrium can compress the esophagus and impede swallowing. Heart valve damage is one possible outcome of rheumatic fever and occurs more often in young girls. The given figure shows a barium swallow of a normal esophagus (right) demonstrating narrowing of the lumen at the sites of constriction, including the aortic arch, left main stem bronchus, left atrium, and the diaphragmatic hiatus. **Choice A** (Right atrium) is incorrect. The right atrium contributes to a small portion of the base of the heart. However, it is not related to the esophagus. The right atrium forms the right border and right pulmonary surface of the heart. **Choice C** (Arch of the aorta) is incorrect. The esophagus passes posterior and to the right of the arch of the aorta. The aortic arch makes one of three normal thoracic impressions (constrictions) on the thoracic part of the esophagus and may compress the esophagus. This close relationship is readily observed in PA chest radiographs following a barium swallow. However, this patient's mitral valve stenosis makes compression by the left atrium a more likely condition. **Choice D** (Pulmonary trunk) is incorrect. The pulmonary trunk arises from the right ventricle, on the anterior (sternocostal) surface of the heart. This vessel does not have a relation to the esophagus. **Choice E** (Superior vena cava) is incorrect. The superior vena cava lies immediately above the right border of the heart and empties into the right atrium. This large vessel does not have a relation to the esophagus.

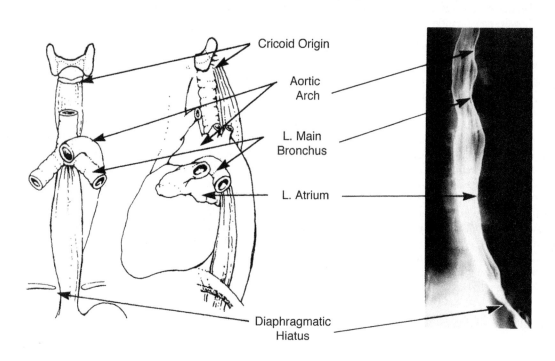

Cricoid Origin

Aortic Arch

L. Main Bronchus

L. Atrium

Diaphragmatic Hiatus

19 The answer is D: Septum secundum. The septum secundum is the second fold of tissue that forms across the common atrium. However, it never forms a complete wall between the right and left atria. The opening left by the incomplete septum secundum, through which blood flows from the right atrium to the left atrium, is the foramen ovale. Ultimately, the septum secundum fuses with the remnant of the septum primum (the valve of the foramen ovale) to close the foramen ovale and form a complete atrial septum. Thus, a patent foramen ovale is the result of failure of fusion (to greater or lesser degrees) of the septum secundum with the remnant of the septum primum. **Choice A** (Endocardial cushions) is incorrect. Four endocardial cushions form and fuse together in the atrioventricular and conotruncal regions. They contribute to the formation of the atrial and ventricular septa, the atrioventricular canals and valves, and the ventricular outflow tracts. Extensions of the endocardial cushions do contribute somewhat to the septum primum. However, the cushions have marginal contributions to the septum secundum. **Choice B** (Valve of the coronary sinus) is incorrect. This structure is not related to the atrial septum. The coronary sinus is derived from the left horn of the sinus venosus. The tissue flap that forms the valve of the coronary sinus is a derivative of the right sinus horn. **Choice C** (Ostium primum) is incorrect. The ostium primum is the opening between the septum primum and the endocardial cushions. It closes completely and does not contribute to the foramen ovale. **Choice E** (Septum spurium) is incorrect. This structure is not related to the foramen ovale. The septum spurium is a tissue ridge that forms at the junction of the right horn of the sinus venosus with the primitive atrium.

20 The answer is B: Lymph nodes. Enlarged lymph nodes are the most likely cause of the widened mediastinum in this patient due to his inhalation of anthrax, which presents with the described flu-like symptoms. A widened mediastinum is seen in bacterial infections (as in this case), lymphoma, a soft tissue mass, and aortic aneurysm usually associated with trauma. **Choice A** (Aorta aneurysm rupture) is incorrect. The patient came to the ER due to flu-like symptoms resulting from inhalation of anthrax, so a rupture of an aortic aneurysm is not likely because there was no reported trauma. During traumatic blows to the chest, the thoracic aorta can be ruptured, usually in the vicinity of the ligamentum arteriosum. A widened mediastinum would be seen on X-ray in a patient experiencing this type of trauma due to the blood collecting in the mediastinum. **Choice C** (Thymus) is incorrect. The thymus, a primary lymphatic organ, is located in the anterior mediastinum, and it reaches its height of growth in children approximately 8 years of age due to the maturation of the lymphatic system. After approximately age 12, the thymus regresses in size through a process known as accretion, in which the lymphatic tissue is slowly replaced with adipose fat. The thymus would not cause the abnormally wide space between the lungs seen in this patient because it rests in the anterior mediastinum. **Choice D** (Respiratory bronchioles) is incorrect. Respiratory bronchioles are located within the lungs and are continuous with alveolar ducts. Respiratory bronchioles can be identified by the presence of alveoli, which interrupt the epithelium. However, the lungs are located within the pulmonary cavity, so enlargement of the respiratory bronchioles would not cause a widened

mediastinum. **Choice E** (Heart) is incorrect. An enlarged heart is often seen in patients with a history of heart disease, and this condition would cause an abnormally wide space between the lungs. However, there is no history of heart disease. Thus, the mediastinum widening in this patient is most likely due to the inhalation anthrax diagnosis, which causes enlarged lymph nodes.

21 The answer is B: Secretion of epinephrine. The lesions in question will disrupt right-side sympathetic outflow below the T5 level. The greater and lesser splanchnic nerves arise from the T5 to T11 segments of the sympathetic trunk. These nerves descend into the abdomen and distribute to upper abdominal viscera via their postsynaptic connections. One specific target is the adrenal (suprarenal) medulla, where sympathetic stimuli produce secretion of epinephrine. **Choice A** (Ability to produce cardiac deceleration) is incorrect. Cardiac deceleration is modulated by parasympathetic input supplied by cardiac branches of the vagus nerves. The cardiac nerves typically originate in the neck and descend into the thorax. Thus, the sympathetic trunk lesions described would not directly influence cardiac deceleration. **Choice C** (Secretion of gastric juices) is incorrect. Secretion of gastric juices is controlled by parasympathetic input supplied by both the anterior and posterior vagus nerves in the abdomen. Sympathetic trunk lesions would not compromise this pathway. **Choice D** (Ability to produce bronchoconstriction) is incorrect. Bronchoconstriction is another parasympathetic function controlled by the vagus nerves. Again, sympathetic trunk lesions would not compromise this pathway. **Choice E** (Vasodilation of the coronary arteries) is incorrect. Vasodilation of the coronary arteries is a result of sympathetic stimulation. However, the sympathetic supply to the heart is derived from cardiac branches off the cervical sympathetic trunk and visceral branches off the T1 to T4 segments of the sympathetic trunk. These nerves pass into the thorax and distribute to the heart via the cardiac plexus. Thus, the sympathetic fibers destined for the coronary artery originate above the lesions and would not be affected by this condition.

22 The answer is D: Cardiac nerve branches of the cervical sympathetic ganglia. This question asks which structure contains postsynaptic autonomic axons. Presynaptic sympathetic neurons that stimulate thoracic viscera synapse in the cervical and upper thoracic (T1 to T4) sympathetic trunk ganglia. Postsynaptic fibers leave the sympathetic trunk via the cardiac branches of the cervical ganglia and visceral branches of the T1 to T4 ganglia to enter the thoracic cavity. **Choice A** (Greater splanchnic nerves) is incorrect. These nerves branch from the T5 to T9 sympathetic trunk ganglia. They carry presynaptic sympathetic fibers to the celiac and other upper abdominal plexuses. **Choice B** (Lumbar splanchnic nerves) is incorrect. These nerves branch from the L1 to L3 sympathetic chain ganglia. They convey presynaptic sympathetic fibers to preaortic ganglia in the abdomen and the hypogastric plexuses in the pelvis. **Choice C** (Pelvic splanchnic nerves) is incorrect. Pelvic splanchnic nerves are branches of the S2 to S4 ventral primary rami. They carry presynaptic parasympathetic fibers into the pelvic cavity for further distribution to the pelvis, perineum, and lower GI tract. **Choice E** (Cardiac nerve branches of the vagus nerve) is incorrect. The cardiac branches of the vagus nerves convey presynaptic parasympathetic axons into the thoracic cavity for distribution primarily to the heart.

23 **The answer is D: Left ventricle.** The left ventricle is the structure labeled "X" in the question and "D" on the given axial CT scan. Note the position of this chamber relative to the apex of the heart, which is pointing to the left. The left ventricle forms the left border of the heart, and its distinguishing feature is its thick walls, needed to pump blood into the systemic circulation. **Choice A** (Ventricular septum) is incorrect. The ventricular septum is labeled "A" on the given axial CT scan. Note the position of the septum between the right and left ventricles and its oblique anterolateral orientation to the left at approximately a 45-degree angle. **Choice B** (Right ventricle) is incorrect. The right ventricle is labeled "B" on the given axial CT scan. Note the position of this chamber on the anterior (sternocostal) aspect of the heart. It is the most anterior chamber of the heart, which makes it susceptible to damage following penetration wounds to the anterior chest. **Choice C** (Right atrium) is incorrect. The right atrium is labeled "C" on the given axial CT scan. Note its posterolateral position relative to the right ventricle. The right atrium forms the right border of the heart. **Choice E** (Left atrium) is incorrect. The left atrium is labeled "E" on the given axial CT scan. It is located posteromedial to the left ventricle and is the most posterior chamber of the heart.

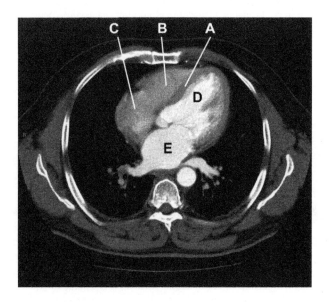

24 **The answer is D: It gives rise to the posterior interventricular (IV) artery.** Coronary dominance refers to which coronary artery gives rise to the posterior IV artery, which is often termed the posterior descending artery by clinicians. When the right coronary artery gives rise to the posterior IV, the condition is right coronary dominance, which is the usual pattern in approximately 66% of the population. When the circumflex branch of the left coronary artery gives rise to the posterior IV, the condition is left coronary dominance, which occurs in approximately 15% of human hearts. Other patterns, including codominance, also occur. The posterior IV supplies neighboring aspects of both ventricles, including part of the ventricular septum. Thus, coronary dominance is important in determining the roles of each of the coronary arteries in supplying specific areas of the heart. **Choice A** (It gives rise to the anterior interventricular artery) is incorrect. The anterior IV and the circumflex branch are the terminal branches of the left coronary artery. The anterior IV supplies both ventricles and most of the ventricular septum. It usually anastomoses with the posterior IV across the inferior border of the heart. **Choice B** (It is derived from the left 6th aortic arch) is incorrect. The coronary arteries are derived from both local epicardial tissue and migrating angioblasts. They are not related to the aortic arches. The left sixth aortic arch does give rise to the left pulmonary artery and the ductus arteriosus. **Choice C** (It supplies the right border of the heart) is incorrect. The right (acute) border of the heart is formed mainly by the right atrium, which is supplied by the right coronary artery. Coronary dominance is not related to supply to this area. **Choice E** (It supplies the margin of the heart) is incorrect. The margin (inferior border) of the heart is the nearly horizontal edge between the anterior (sternocostal) and inferior (diaphragmatic) surfaces of the heart. It is formed primarily by the right ventricle and is supplied largely by the marginal branch of the right coronary artery. Coronary dominance is not defined by the supply to this area.

25 **The answer is C: Endocardial cushions.** The ventricular septum is composed of two parts: (1) an upper, smaller, thinner (membranous) part and (2) a lower, larger, thicker (muscular) part. The position of this defect at the upper end of the ventricular septum indicates it is located in the membranous part. The membranous portion of the septum is formed from outgrowths of the endocardial cushions. The endocardial cushion tissue fuses with the upper end of the muscular ventricular septum to close the interventricular foramen and form the complete ventricular septum. **Choice A** (Septum secundum) is incorrect. The septum secundum is the partition that forms most of the final atrial septum. It does not extend beyond the endocardial cushions into the ventricle. **Choice B** (Bulbus cordis) is incorrect. The bulbus cordis gives rise to the primitive right ventricle and to the ventricular outflow tracts. Its walls contribute to the muscular part of the ventricular septum but not to the membranous part. **Choice D** (Truncus arteriosus) is incorrect. The truncus arteriosus is the cranial end of the primitive heart tube. This structure forms the ascending aorta and the pulmonary trunk via its internal spiral septation. **Choice E** (Sinus venosus) is incorrect. The sinus venosus forms the caudal end of the primitive heart tube. It gives rise to structures related to the right atrium, including the smooth part of that chamber, the roots of the venae cavae, and the coronary sinus.

26 **The answer is A: Diaphragm flattens.** The diaphragm is the primary muscle of respiration. It contracts during inspiration and relaxes during expiration. When the diaphragm contracts, its two domes descend and flatten. Descent of the diaphragm increases the vertical dimension (height) of the thoracic cavity, resulting in increased intrathoracic volume, decreased intrathoracic pressure, and increased intra-abdominal pressure. These essential actions occur during both quiet and forced respiration. **Choice B** (Intercostal muscles relax) is incorrect. The actions of the individual intercostal muscles have been debated without clear resolution for many years. It appears that the external intercostals are most active during forced inspiration, whereas the internal and innermost intercostals are most active during forced expiration. However, the main role of all the intercostals appears to be that of maintaining the spacing and rigidity of the intercostal spaces during all degrees (quiet and forced) and phases (inspiration and expiration) of respiration so that the rib cage moves as a complete unit in a coordinated fashion. Thus, we may consider the proposal that the external intercostals are most active in maintaining the intercostal spaces during inspiration, and the internal and innermost intercostals are most active in maintaining these spaces during expiration. **Choice C** (Ribs lower) is incorrect. The ribs are elevated during inspiration, especially in forced inspiration. Thus, the rib cage expands in upward and outward directions, resulting in increased anteroposterior and transverse dimensions, which, in turn, contributes to the increased intrathoracic volume and decreased intrathoracic pressure characteristic of inspiration. **Choice D** (Abdominal wall muscles contract) is incorrect. The three abdominal oblique muscles (external oblique, internal oblique, transversus abdominis) that form the anterolateral abdominal wall relax during inspiration and contract during expiration. Contraction of the diaphragm compresses the abdomen and increases intra-abdominal pressure. Simultaneous relaxation of the abdominal muscles assists in accommodating these changes. Subsequent contraction of these muscles during expiration increases intra-abdominal pressure and elevates the relaxed diaphragm. **Choice E** (Horizontal dimension of the rib cage decreases) is incorrect. The ribs are elevated during inspiration, causing expansion of the rib cage in upward and outward directions. This expansion results in increased horizontal (transverse) and anteroposterior dimensions of the thoracic cavity.

27 **The answer is C: Septum primum and the fused endocardial cushions.** Closure of the foramen primum (ostium primum) occurs when the free edge of the septum primum fuses with the endocardial cushions. While foramen secundum defects constitute the majority of atrial septal defects, foramen primum defects (primum atrial septal defects) do occur and often result in more severe conditions. The ventricular septal defects, seen on the given echocardiogram, are often associated with Down syndrome and fetal alcohol syndrome. **Choice A** (Septum secundum and the septum primum) is incorrect. Because the foramen primum closes before the septum secundum appears, the septum secundum does not play any role in closure of the foramen primum. **Choice B** (Septum secundum and the fused endocardial cushions) is incorrect. During normal development, the foramen primum closes via fusion of the septum primum with the endocardial cushions. This event occurs before the septum secundum appears. Thus, the septum secundum plays no role in closure of the foramen primum. **Choice D** (Septum primum and the septum spurium) is incorrect. The septum spurium is a fold in the right atrium formed by the right venous valve. It plays no role in partitioning of the atria. Thus, it plays no role in closure of the foramen primum. **Choice E** (Left inferior and right superior truncus swellings) is incorrect. The aorticopulmonary septum, which divides the truncus arteriosus into the ascending aorta and pulmonary trunk, is formed by these two truncus swellings. They play no role in atrial septation.

28 **The answer is E: Alveoli.** The lower respiratory tract (larynx, trachea, bronchi, lungs) develops from a single ventral outgrowth (respiratory diverticulum; lung bud) off the floor of the foregut. Thus, the epithelial lining of these structures, including the alveoli, is entirely derived from endoderm. The surrounding cartilage, muscle, and connective tissues are derived from the neighboring splanchnic mesoderm. **Choice A** (Nasal epithelium) is incorrect. The nasal cavities are derived from the nasal placodes, which are thickenings of surface ectoderm. Thus, the nasal epithelium is of ectodermal origin rather than endodermal origin. **Choice B** (Intrinsic laryngeal muscles) is incorrect. Intrinsic laryngeal muscles are all skeletal muscles derived from the 4th and 6th pharyngeal arches and of mesodermal origin. Due to their pharyngeal arch origins, these muscles are all innervated by the vagus nerve. **Choice C** (Bronchial cartilages) is incorrect. The bronchial cartilages that support the respiratory tree are derived from splanchnic mesoderm. **Choice D** (Trachealis muscle) is incorrect. The smooth trachealis muscle is derived from surrounding splanchnic mesoderm.

29 **The answer is E: Middle lobe of the lung.** The right lung is composed of three lobes: superior, middle, and inferior. The lobes are separated by two fissures: oblique and horizontal. The oblique fissure extends from the level of approximately T2 posterior to the sixth costal cartilage anterior. The horizontal fissure runs anterior from the oblique fissure along the fourth rib and costal cartilage. This stab wound is located in the anterior chest wall between the oblique and horizontal fissures. Therefore the middle lobe of the lung is most likely pierced. Because of the angulations of the ribs and the fissures, the damaged lobe will vary depending on the longitude of the wound (e.g., depending on an entry point in the midclavicular, midaxillary, or scapular line). **Choice A** (Superior lobe of the lung) is incorrect. The superior lobe extends down to the horizontal fissure, at approximately the 4th rib and costal cartilage. Thus, it is above the wound in question. However, if this wound were on the left side, it would pierce the superior lobe because the left lung has only superior and inferior lobes. **Choice B** (Lingula of the lung) is incorrect. The lingula is a feature of only the left lung. It is a thin, tongue-like projection of the anteroinferior margin of the superior lobe of the lung and is formed by the cardiac notch. **Choice C** (Inferior lobe of the lung) is incorrect. In the midclavicular line, the inferior lobe reaches as high as approximately the 6th rib and costal cartilage. Thus, it is below this wound point. **Choice D** (Apex of the lung) is incorrect. The apex is the rounded superior end of the lung. It extends into the root of the neck, above the level of the first rib.

30 **The answer is B: Right atrium.** The structures forming the cardiovascular shadow (mediastinal silhouette) comprise one of the most fundamental radiographic images seen in clinical studies. In PA radiographs such as seen here, the cardiovascular shadow presents right and left borders composed of major vessels and chambers of the heart. The right atrium forms the convex border that makes up most of the lower half of the right side of the silhouette. **Choice A** (Superior vena cava) is incorrect. The superior vena cava makes up the right border immediately above the right atrium. **Choice C** (Inferior vena cava) is incorrect. The inferior vena cava appears as a small concavity on the right border between the right atrium and the diaphragm. **Choice D** (Arch of the aorta) is incorrect. The arch of the aorta (aortic knuckle; aortic knob) appears as a distinct rounded prominence at the upper end of the left border. **Choice E** (Left ventricle) is incorrect. The left ventricle forms the large, slightly convex, lower part of the left border.

31 **The answer is A: Opening of the coronary sinus.** The coronary sinus is a large vein that receives most of the venous drainage of the heart. It empties into the right atrium, between the opening of the inferior vena cava and the right atrioventricular opening. The coronary sinus possesses a ridge-like valve at its aperture. **Choice B** (Openings of the pulmonary veins) is incorrect. The four pulmonary veins, carrying oxygenated blood from the lungs, open into the left atrium. The left atrium is the most posterior of the four heart chambers. **Choice C** (Septomarginal trabecula) is incorrect. The septomarginal trabecula (moderator band) is a segment of trabeculae carneae located in the right ventricle. It runs from the ventricular septum to the base of the anterior papillary muscle (located on the anterior marginal wall of the ventricle). It prevents ("moderates") overdistension of the right ventricle. Furthermore, it conveys the right limb of the atrioventricular bundle (Purkinje fibers) from the ventricular septum to the anterior wall of the ventricle. **Choice D** (Openings of the coronary arteries) is incorrect. The two coronary arteries arise from the ascending aorta, in the sinuses of the aortic valve. The right coronary arises from the right aortic sinus, whereas the left coronary arises from the left sinus. **Choice E** (Trabeculae carneae) is incorrect. These structures are located in both the right and left ventricles. They are a network of elevated ridges of myocardium that present a trabecular appearing surface within the ventricles.

32 **The answer is E: Increase heart rate.** Stimulation of parasympathetic neurons normally results in deceleration of the heart rate. However, by blocking parasympathetic stimulation, atropine negates normal parasympathetic function and allows the sympathetic system to exert its functional effects (such as increasing heart rate) without balanced regulation. **Choice A** (Paralyze the diaphragm) is incorrect. The diaphragm is composed of skeletal muscle. Autonomic neurons act on smooth and cardiac muscle and glands. Thus, the diaphragm is not affected by parasympathetic action or lack thereof. **Choice B** (Stimulate bronchoconstriction) is incorrect. Parasympathetic activity normally stimulates bronchoconstriction. However, blocking parasympathetic input allows unopposed sympathetic action to cause the bronchi to dilate beyond their normal caliber, resulting in bronchodilatation. **Choice C** (Increase sweat gland secretions) is incorrect. Sweat glands do not receive parasympathetic supply. Thus, they are not affected by blocking parasympathetic stimulation. **Choice D** (Paralyze the intercostal muscles) is incorrect. All the intercostal muscles are composed of skeletal muscle. They are not affected by parasympathetic action or lack thereof.

33 **The answer is A: Right 2nd intercostal space at the right parasternal line.** This location is optimal for listening to the aortic valve with a stethoscope. Auscultatory areas are those locations where the sounds of each heart valve can be best differentiated from the others. Because the sound of each valve tends to be carried in the direction that blood flows through it, the optimal auscultation point is over the location where blood

flows after passing through each valve, and removed from a bony covering. Thus, the auscultation points are not the same as the anatomical surface projections of each valve. **Choice B** (Left 2nd intercostal space at the parasternal line) is incorrect. This location is optimal for listening to the pulmonary valve with a stethoscope. **Choice C** (Left 4th intercostal space at the parasternal line) is incorrect. This location is optimal for listening to the tricuspid valve with a stethoscope. **Choice D** (Left 5th intercostal space at the midclavicular line) is incorrect. This location is optimal for listening to the mitral (bicuspid) valve with a stethoscope. **Choice E** (Subxiphoid point) is incorrect. This location is not an auscultation point for any of the heart valves; however, it is the location for auscultation of epigastric sounds.

34 **The answer is A: Double aortic arch.** A double aortic arch results when the right dorsal aorta persists with a connection between the seventh intersegmental artery and the left dorsal aorta. This arrangement produces a vascular ring that surrounds both the trachea and esophagus. The ring compresses these tubes and causes difficulty with breathing and swallowing. **Choice B** (Persistent right 2nd aortic arch) is incorrect. Both the right and left second aortic arches mostly disappear during development, with small remnants forming the stapedial arteries in the head. A persistent second arch (either right or left) would be well removed from the trachea and esophagus and would not cause the compression seen here. **Choice C** (Coarctation of the aorta) is incorrect. Coarctation (significant narrowing) of the aorta, in either preductal or postductal forms, occurs distal to the origin of the left subclavian artery. Thus, this malformation is well removed from the trachea and esophagus. Even if the aortic arch were distended due to the coarctation, this dilatation of the aorta would not cause notable compression of the trachea or esophagus. **Choice D** (Patent ductus arteriosus) is incorrect. The ductus arteriosus lies in a similar position as a coarctation of the aorta. Patency here is far enough from the trachea and esophagus to not cause compression of these structures. **Choice E** (Persistent left fourth aortic arch) is incorrect. The left 4th aortic arch normally persists and forms a large part of the arch of the aorta. Thus, this condition is not a congenital malformation and does not compress the trachea or esophagus.

35 **The answer is D: Right main bronchus.** The main (primary) bronchi are the first branches of the trachea. They supply the right and left lungs. Because of the position of the heart, the main bronchi have different orientations in their routes to the lungs. The right main bronchus is shorter, wider, and more vertical. Thus, aspirated foreign bodies are more likely to drop into and become lodged in this tube. The given chest film shows air trapped within the right lung during expiration due to the presence of the peanut within the right main bronchus. The right inferior lobar bronchus, a secondary bronchus that supplies the inferior lobe of the lung, is another common site for foreign objects to reside following accidental inhalation. **Choice A** (Larynx) is incorrect. The larynx is the compound chamber at the upper end of the lower respiratory tree, proximal to the trachea. Aspirated items may become lodged in the rima glottidis (the space between the true vocal folds). In such cases, the obstruction can usually be dislodged by using the Valsalva maneuver (i.e., by forcefully compressing the abdomen to rapidly expel air from the lungs). However, in this patient's case, the aspirated peanut is located in the thorax. If it were in the larynx, radiographs would show the peanut located in the neck. **Choice B** (Carina of the trachea) is incorrect. The carina is a small ridge at the inferior end of the trachea that separates the openings of the right and left main bronchi. Its mucosal covering is highly sensitive, and contact by an aspirated object stimulates the cough reflex. However, objects do not normally lodge at the carina of the trachea. Instead, they usually fall into the right main bronchus. **Choice C** (Left main bronchus) is incorrect. Because the left main bronchus must extend past the heart, it is longer, more narrow, and more horizontal than the right main bronchus. Thus, aspirated objects usually fall into the right main bronchus rather the left. **Choice E** (Right upper lobar bronchus) is incorrect. The right main bronchus divides into three lobar (secondary) bronchi, one to each lobe of the lung. The right superior lobar bronchus turns superiorly from the end of the main bronchus to enter the superior lobe. Thus, it is very difficult for an aspirated object to enter this tube. Instead, objects that pass beyond the main bronchus usually fall into the inferior lobar bronchus, which takes a more vertical descent.

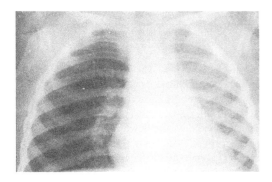

36   **The answer is E: Right ventricle.**   Due to the entry location of the ice pick, the right ventricle would be the most likely listed structure that is damaged. The right ventricle is the most anterior chamber of the heart, which makes it the most susceptible heart chamber during penetration wounds to the anterior chest. Based upon the wound site and the patient's symptoms, the fibrous pericardium, an unyielding sac that surrounds the heart, would also be damaged. Damage to the wall of the right ventricle would lead to a pericardial effusion (blood accumulation in the pericardial sac). Because the pericardial sac is filling with blood and the fibrous pericardium is unyielding, the heart is being constricted and is unable to fill completely. This condition, known as cardiac tamponade, leads to the engorgement of veins of the face and neck because the pressure has limited the heart's intake. Fortunately, blood can be drained from the pericardial cavity via a pericardiocentesis, which will relieve the patient's symptoms temporarily until the heart wall is repaired surgically. If a pericardiocentesis does not occur, blood will continue to constrict the heart until it is unable to fill, and death will occur. **Choice A** (Right atrium) is incorrect. Due to the location of the wound to the left of the sternum at the 5th intercostal space, the right atrium, which forms the right margin of the heart, is not likely to be injured. **Choice B** (Left atrium) is incorrect. The left atrium is the most posterior heart chamber, so it is the least likely option to be damaged by this penetration wound on the anterior chest wall. **Choice C** (Aortic arch) is incorrect. The aortic arch is located

above the 5th intercostal space, so it would not be damaged in this patient. Within the heart, the aorta is central in location, so even if the stab wound were at a higher level within the heart, the aorta could not be damaged without penetration through the right ventricle. **Choice D** (Left ventricle) is incorrect. Due to the location of the wound at the left parasternal border of the 5th intercostal space, the left ventricle may seem to be a likely answer. However, the ventricular septum, which separates the left and right ventricles, runs obliquely in an anterolateral direction at approximately a 45-degree angle. The position of this septum, as well as the deviation of the heart to the left side, causes the right ventricle to be the most anterior chamber of the heart. Damage to the left ventricle, without involvement of the right ventricle, would only occur if the wound were located toward the apex of the heart, which runs laterally toward the midclavicular line.

37   **The answer is C: Superior mediastinum.**   The superior mediastinum is the large interpleural space above the plane running from the sternal angle to the T4 intervertebral disc. The symptoms seen in this patient suggest obstructed venous return from the head and neck, upper limbs, and thoracic walls. Venous drainage from these regions flows through the brachiocephalic veins and the azygos vein to converge in the superior vena cava (SVC). The SVC enters the right atrium through the right aspect of the superior mediastinum. Thus, the tumor in the right lung is most likely located in the superior lobe of the lung and is compressing the SVC in the superior mediastinum. **Choice A** (Anterior mediastinum) is incorrect. The anterior mediastinum is the small interpleural space between the sternum and the pericardial sac. The right internal thoracic vein (which collects the small anterior intercostal veins) lies along the parasternal line inside the thoracic wall and could be compressed by an anterior lung tumor. However, such a condition would obstruct only a small portion of the thoracic wall drainage and would not produce the neck and upper limb effects seen here. **Choice B** (Posterior mediastinum) is incorrect. The posterior mediastinum is the large interpleural space posterior to the pericardial sac. The azygos vein ascends through roughly the right aspect of the posterior mediastinum and then curls through the superior mediastinum to join the SVC. A right lung tumor could compress the azygos vein and notably obstruct venous drainage from the thoracic walls. However, collateral connections with the anterior intercostal veins could help relieve such obstruction. Further, obstruction of the azygos vein would not influence the neck and upper limb drainage and would not account for the full condition in this patient. **Choice D** (Hilum of the lung) is incorrect. The hilum is the slight concavity on the medial aspect of the lung where the root of the lung is attached. The root of the lung is the pleura-invested bundle of structures that enter and leave the lung at the hilum. These structures include the bronchi, pulmonary and bronchial vessels, lymphatics, and nerves. Compression of the root of the lung at the hilum would obstruct pulmonary functions, but would not produce any of the conditions noted in this patient. **Choice E** (Vena caval foramen of the diaphragm) is incorrect. The inferior vena cava (IVC) passes through the venal caval foramen of the diaphragm and immediately enters the right atrium. Compression of the IVC at this, or any other, point would not produce the effects seen in this patient.

38 **The answer is C: Sinus venosus.** The right horn of the embryonic sinus venosus gives rise to the smooth part of the right atrium (the sinus venarum). In addition, it forms the roots of the superior and inferior vena cavae. Most of the left sinus horn is obliterated during development. Its major remnant forms the coronary sinus. **Choice A** (Pulmonary trunk) is incorrect. The pulmonary trunk and the ascending aorta are formed via the internal spiral septation of the truncus arteriosus. Thus, the pulmonary trunk is a derivative of an embryonic component rather than a source of other structures. **Choice B** (Conus cordis) is incorrect. The conus cordis is a derivative of the bulbus cordis. The conus cordis undergoes a complex spiral septation in close coordination with the septation of the ventricle and the truncus arteriosus. Ultimately, the conus cordis forms the right and left ventricular outflow channels. **Choice D** (Truncus arteriosus) is incorrect. The truncus arteriosus is the cranial third of the bulbus cordis. It undergoes a spiral septation and forms the proximal parts of the pulmonary trunk and the aorta. **Choice E** (Ascending aorta) is incorrect. As noted previously, the ascending aorta and the pulmonary trunk are formed via the internal spiral septation of the truncus arteriosus. Neither gives rise to the left or right atrium.

39 **The answer is D: Phrenic nerve.** The phrenic nerve supplies innervation to the diaphragm and the diaphragmatic parietal peritoneum closely associated with the superior surface of the liver. Irritation of the diaphragm, due to the large hepatic (liver) abscess seen on the MRI, would cause the phrenic nerve to carry visceral sensory (pain) sensation back to its level of origin. The phrenic nerve is derived from cervical spinal nerves C3 to C5, and visceral pain can be interpreted as cutaneous pain along the dermatomes of C3 to C5. Therefore, the patient would experience referred pain in the upper right shoulder and neck regions due to irritation of the diaphragm and subsequent involvement of the phrenic nerve. **Choice A** (Greater splanchnic nerve) is incorrect. The greater splanchnic nerve carries presynaptic sympathetic nerve fibers derived from the T5 to T9 vertebral levels. Visceral sensory fibers, associated with the greater splanchnic nerve and traveling retrograde with these visceral motor fibers, would refer pain to the T5 to T9 dermatomes, which corresponds to the anterolateral chest wall. Therefore, this nerve would not carry visceral sensory fibers that would refer pain to the right shoulder region. **Choice B** (Lesser splanchnic nerve) is incorrect. The lesser splanchnic nerve carries presynaptic sympathetic nerve fibers derived from the T10 to T11 vertebral levels. Visceral afferent fibers traveling along with the lesser splanchnic nerve would refer pain to the T10 to T11 dermatomes, which is located at the umbilicus, well below the right shoulder region. **Choice C** (Least splanchnic nerve) is incorrect. The least splanchnic nerve carries presynaptic sympathetic nerve fibers derived from the T12 vertebral level. Visceral afferent fibers traveling along with the least splanchnic nerve would refer pain to the T12 dermatome, which is located well below the right shoulder region. **Choice E** (Vagus nerve) is incorrect. The vagus nerve conveys presynaptic parasympathetic nerve fibers to supply the gastrointestinal tract up to the splenic flexure of the colon. It also conveys visceral afferent fibers, but these fibers are mainly for unconscious sensations associated with reflexes. Therefore, these fibers would not be responsible for pain radiating to the shoulder region of this patient.

40 **The answer is B: Closed ductus arteriosus.** Significant narrowing of the aorta distal to the origin of the left subclavian artery is termed a coarctation of the aorta. If the constriction of the aorta is proximal to the ductus arteriosus, which connects the pulmonary trunk to the arch of the aorta in fetal circulation, the condition is termed a preductal coarctation. If the constriction is distal to the ductus arteriosus, the condition is denoted as a postductal coarctation. In postductal coarctation (more common than the preductal form), the ductus arteriosus is normally closed and forms the ligamentum arteriosum. In this condition, blood flow into the descending aorta is blocked. However, arterial flow into the distal aorta is usually maintained via expansion of collateral circulation through the internal thoracic and intercostal arteries. The pressure dynamics in this situation account for the classic clinical signs of hypertension in the upper limbs (especially the right side) and diminished pulse and pressure in the lower limbs. **Choice A** (Patent ductus arteriosus) is incorrect. A patent ductus arteriosus is characteristic of preductal coarctation of the aorta. In this case, the collateral circulatory expansions are not required because blood flows into the distal aorta through the patent ductus arteriosus. However, blood oxygenation levels are altered due to persistence of this shunt. Interestingly, patients with preductal coarctation often appear healthy (asymptomatic). However, closure of the ductus arteriosus can be life threatening. **Choice C** (Patent ductus venosus) is incorrect. The ductus venosus is a fetal shunt between the umbilical vein and the inferior vena cava that allows blood from the placenta to mostly bypass the liver. It obliterates after birth and forms the ligamentum venosum. Because blood does not flow through this channel after birth, neither form of coarctation of the aorta affects this structure. **Choice D** (Patent foramen ovale) is incorrect. Arterial flow to the distal aorta is maintained in both forms of coarctation of the aorta. The pressure dynamics in each case are not sufficient to force persistence of a patent foramen ovale. If patency occurs, it is due to other factors. **Choice E** (Stenotic aortic valve) is incorrect. Formation of the aortic and pulmonary (semilunar) valves is related to septation of the conotruncal region. The mechanics behind constriction of the aorta are not the same as those related to failure of conotruncal septation. Thus, stenosis of the semilunar valves is not a feature of coarctation of the aorta.

41 **The answer is C: Right vagus passes posterior to the root of the lung.** The root of the lung is the pleura-invested bundle of structures that enter and leave the lung at the hilum, which includes the bronchi, pulmonary and bronchial vessels, lymphatics, and nerves. Both the right and left vagus nerves descend in the thorax posterior to the root of each lung. At this depth, they are well positioned to contribute to the pulmonary and esophageal plexuses, and to follow the esophagus into the abdomen. **Choice A** (Right vagus passes onto the anterior aspect of the esophagus to become the anterior vagus) is incorrect. Due to the developmental clockwise rotation of the stomach, the lower esophagus also rotates, carrying the right vagus onto its posterior aspect, where the nerve becomes the posterior vagus. In the same way, the left vagus shifts to the anterior aspect of the esophagus and becomes the anterior vagus. **Choice B** (Left vagus passes through the anterior mediastinum) is incorrect. Both the left and right vagus nerves descend in the thorax posterior to the pericardial sac, that is, in the posterior mediastinum. **Choice D** (Left vagus passes across the posterior side of the aortic arch) is incorrect. The left vagus nerve crosses the anterolateral aspect of the aortic arch in passing from the superior to posterior mediastinum. The right vagus has no relationship to the aortic arch. **Choice E** (Right vagus passes through the middle mediastinum) is incorrect. Both the left and right vagus nerves descend in the thorax posterior to the pericardial sac, that is, in the posterior mediastinum. However, both the phrenic nerves and the pericardiacophrenic vessels are held in the pericardial sac and pass through the middle mediastinum.

42 **The answer is C: Diaphragmatic hernia.** The traumatic force on the abdomen is sufficiently great to result in a tear of the right hemidiaphragm, allowing passage of the intra-abdominal organs into the thorax. In this patient, the presence of bowel sounds within the left thorax is the cardinal sign of a diaphragmatic hernia. The herniation of abdominal organs into the thoracic cavity would also account for the radiopacity seen on the chest film, the absence of audible breath sounds on the left side due to compression of the left lung, and the mediastinal shift due to increase in intrathoracic pressure on the left side. **Choice A** (Tension pneumothorax) is incorrect. A tension pneumothorax is a medical emergency in which air accumulates in the pleural cavity with each respiration, usually resulting in a collapsed lung. This damage to the parietal pleura causes an increase in intrathoracic pressure, which pushes the contents of the mediastinum (a mediastinal shift) to the contralateral side and puts additional pressure on the unaffected lung, which was noted in this patient. A patient with a pneumothorax would exhibit respiratory distress; however, the diagnosis of a pneumothorax does not explain the radiopacity in the left lower lung or the bowel sounds heard by the physician within the left thoracic cavity. **Choice B** (Hemopneumothorax) is incorrect. A hemopneumothorax is an accumulation of blood within in the pleural cavity. The presence of blood in the pleural cavity could lead to respiratory distress, radiopacity in the area of the blood accumulation, and a mediastinal shift. However, this diagnosis does not explain the presence of bowel sounds in the left thoracic cavity. **Choice D** (Emphysema) is incorrect. Emphysema is a lung disease characterized by continual enlargement of air spaces within the lungs due to the destruction of lung tissue. This disease can lead to difficulty in breathing, but it can be ruled out as a diagnosis in this patient due to the presence of trauma and a localized radiopacity on the chest film. Radiologic evidence for emphysema would be diffuse and would appear as radiolucent areas throughout the lungs. Emphysema would also not present with bowel sounds in the left thorax. **Choice E** (Left lower lobe pneumonia) is incorrect. Left lower lobe pneumonia would also present with radiopacity in the left lower lung on a chest film and difficulty in breathing. However, this diagnosis could not explain the bowel sounds in the left thorax or the sudden onset of the symptoms following the accident.

43 **The answer is C: Left recurrent laryngeal.** The ductus arteriosus is a fetal shunt that connects the root of the left pulmonary artery to the inferior side of the arch of the aorta. It normally closes soon after birth, leaving a fibrous remnant, the ligamentum arteriosum. The left recurrent laryngeal nerve is a branch of the left vagus nerve. The recurrent laryngeal originates at the inferior edge of the arch of the aorta, just lateral to the ductus arteriosus, curves under the aortic arch behind the ductus, and ascends into the neck. Thus, the left recurrent laryngeal nerve has an intimate relationship to the ductus arteriosus that must be cared for in surgery in this area. Lesion of the nerve has major consequences, as it ultimately supplies motor fibers to most of the left side intrinsic laryngeal muscles and sensory fibers to much of the left side of the larynx. **Choice A** (Left vagus) is incorrect. The left vagus nerve crosses the lateral aspect of the arch of the aorta, descends posterior to the root of the lung, and continues along the esophagus. Although it passes near the ductus arteriosus, the left vagus does not have as close a relation as its recurrent laryngeal branch. **Choice B** (Left phrenic) is incorrect. This nerve crosses the left surface of the arch of the aorta, descends anterior to the root of the lung in the wall of the pericardial sac, and continues to the diaphragm. It is not closely related to the ductus arteriosus. **Choice D** (Right recurrent laryngeal) is incorrect. The right recurrent laryngeal nerve takes a very different path from its left mate. It branches from the right vagus anterior to the right subclavian artery, curves under the right subclavian artery, and ascends into the neck between the trachea and esophagus. It is far removed from the ductus arteriosus. **Choice E** (Right phrenic) is incorrect. This nerve descends along the lateral (right) side of the right brachiocephalic vein, superior vena cava, and pericardial sac. It is far removed from the ductus arteriosus.

44 **The answer is D: The vein passes deep to the thymus gland.** The left brachiocephalic vein runs obliquely across the superior mediastinum from its origin posterior to the left sternoclavicular joint to its termination posterior to the right first costal cartilage. Due to its course from the left side to right side of the chest, it is approximately twice the length of the right brachiocephalic vein. The left brachiocephalic vein passes deep (posterior) to the thymus gland in its course toward the superior vena cava. The thymus is a major lymphoid organ situated in the anterior root of the neck, anterior part of the superior mediastinum, and anterior mediastinum. It achieves maximum size during puberty, then undergoes involution, and is replaced by fatty connective tissue. **Choice A** (The vein lies posterior to the arch of the aorta) is incorrect. In its path across the superior mediastinum, the left brachiocephalic vein runs just above the arch of the aorta, anterior to the roots of the three major branches of the arch of the aorta (brachiocephalic artery, left common carotid artery, left subclavian artery). **Choice B** (The brachiocephalic artery lies superficial to the vein) is incorrect. As it approaches its termination at the superior vena cava, the left brachiocephalic vein runs anterior to the brachiocephalic artery. **Choice C** (The vein crosses the anterior aspect of the manubrium of the sternum) is incorrect. The left brachiocephalic vein is contained within the superior mediastinum. It crosses the posterior aspect of the manubrium of the sternum in its course from the left to the right side. **Choice E** (The apex of the left lung lies superficial to the vein) is incorrect. The apex is the superior end of the lung. It extends into the root of the neck, above the level of the first rib. The apex is superior and deep to the left brachiocephalic vein.

45 **The answer is B: Superior lobe of right lung.** The horizontal fissure separates the superior and middle lobes of the right lung. This fissure is located in the right lung only, and its location corresponds to the position of the right 4th rib and costal cartilage on the anterior chest wall. Therefore, a lobar pneumonia located above the horizontal fissure would indicate involvement of the superior lobe of the right lung. Remember, the right lung is composed of three lobes: superior, middle, and inferior. The lobes are separated by two fissures: oblique and horizontal. The oblique fissure separates the lower lobe from the superior and middle lobes of the right lung, and it extends from the level of approximately T2 posterior to the sixth costal cartilage anterior. The given chest radiograph shows an upper right lobar pneumonia, and the inferior extent of the inflammation and fluid accumulation is demarcated by the horizontal fissure of the right lung. **Choice A** (Superior lobe of left lung) is incorrect. The left lung does not contain a horizontal fissure, so a lobar pneumonia located above the horizontal fissure would have to reside in the right lung. **Choice C** (Middle lobe of right lung) is incorrect. The horizontal fissure separates the superior and middle lobes of the right lung. This fissure is located in the right lung only, and its location corresponds to the position of the right fourth rib and costal cartilage on the anterior chest wall. A lobar pneumonia located above the horizontal fissure would indicate involvement of the superior lobe of the right lung, so the middle lobe of the lung would not be involved due to its position below the horizontal fissure. **Choice D** (Inferior lobe of right lung) is incorrect. The oblique fissure separates the lower lobe from the superior and middle lobes of the right lung, and this fissure extends from the level of approximately T2 posterior to the sixth costal cartilage anterior. Because the horizontal fissure separates the superior and middle lobes of the right lung, a lobar pneumonia located above the horizontal fissure would indicate involvement of the superior lobe of the right lung. **Choice E** (Inferior lobe of left lung) is incorrect. The left lung does not contain a horizontal fissure, so a lobar pneumonia located above the horizontal fissure would have to reside in the right lung.

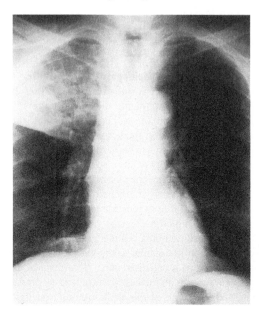

Chapter 4

Abdomen

QUESTIONS

Select the single best answer.

1 The given T1-weighted gradient echo of the abdomen demonstrates a malignant pancreatic islet cell tumor of the pancreas near the junction of the pancreatic body and tail. The pancreatic islet cells involved with this tumor are derived from which of the following embryonic sources?

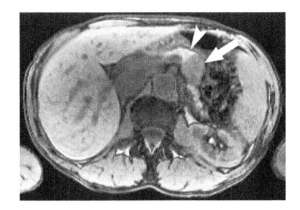

(A) Ectoderm
(B) Endoderm
(C) Somatic mesoderm
(D) Visceral mesoderm
(E) Neural crest

2 Following involvement in a car crash, a 20-year-old undergoes a splenectomy due to a lacerated spleen secondary to blunt abdominal trauma. During the procedure, the surgeon ligates the blood supply of the spleen at its hilum. Improper placement of the ligature may lead to damage to the arterial supply of which of the following structures?

(A) Fundic portion of the stomach
(B) Kidney
(C) Pyloric portion of stomach
(D) Head of pancreas
(E) Splenic flexure of colon

3 After moving heavy equipment at a construction site, a 42-year-old man goes to his family physician with a bulge in his left groin that does not descend into the scrotum.

The patient reports the bulge becomes more prominent when he is standing up, defecating, and coughing. On examination, the doctor places his finger in the location of the bulge and notes that his finger feels like it can pass into the abdominal cavity. Given his presentation and history, what is the most likely diagnosis?

(A) Direct inguinal hernia
(B) Indirect inguinal hernia
(C) Femoral hernia
(D) Lymphadenitis of superficial inguinal nodes
(E) Hydrocele testis

4 A 67-year-old woman comes to the ER after experiencing 2 days of red blood in her feces. She reports no vomiting of blood (hematemesis). The given arteriogram shows a stain of contrast material, indicated by the white arrow, at a bleeding diverticulum. What artery gives off direct branches to supply the bleeding portion of the gastrointestinal (GI) tract?

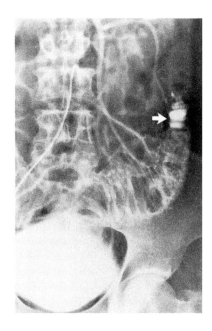

(A) Abdominal aorta
(B) Celiac trunk
(C) Superior mesenteric
(D) Inferior mesenteric
(E) External iliac

5 Which of the following structures is a remnant of the embryonic ventral mesentery?
(A) Sigmoid mesocolon
(B) Mesentery of the small intestine
(C) Greater omentum
(D) Falciform ligament
(E) Transverse mesocolon

6 A 13-year-old girl is brought to the ER after falling from a horse onto her left side. Her pulse is 120/min, blood pressure is 90/60 mm Hg, and respirations are 30/min. Physical examination reveals cold and clammy skin, bruising, and fractured 9th and 10th ribs on her left side at the posterior axillary line. Which of the following organs is most likely damaged in this patient?
(A) Stomach
(B) Kidney
(C) Lung
(D) Liver
(E) Spleen

7 A 2-year-old boy is brought to the emergency room with cramping abdominal pain, fever, and vomiting. His parents say these symptoms began 12 hours ago and have progressively worsened. Abdominal radiology indicates a bowel obstruction that appears related to an abnormal intestinal outpocketing connected to the anterior abdominal wall. The consulting surgeon makes a diagnosis of Meckel diverticulitis and recommends surgery to resolve the problem. At which of the following sites does the surgeon expect to find the diverticulum responsible for this condition?
(A) Lower duodenum
(B) Middle jejunum
(C) Lower ileum
(D) Cecum
(E) Transverse colon

8 A 58-year-old woman presents with pain in her side that radiates to the suprapubic (hypogastric) region of her abdomen, hematuria (blood in urine), and a reported history of urinary tract infections. The given axial CT scan verifies advanced polycystic kidney disease. Which of the following nerves would convey visceral sensory fibers from the stretched renal capsule and cause referred pain to the skin of the suprapubic region of her abdomen?

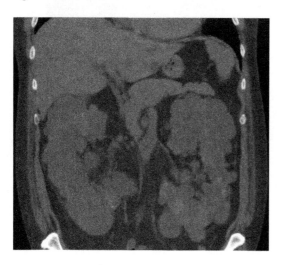

(A) Greater splanchnic
(B) Lesser splanchnic
(C) Least splanchnic
(D) Pelvic splanchnic
(E) Vagus

9 A breastfeeding 22-day-old infant was suddenly unable to hold down any milk after 3 weeks of normal feeding. In the pediatrician's office, the baby is obviously famished, presents with abdominal pain, appears slightly dehydrated, and has loose, watery stools. His mother nurses him in the office, and approximately 20 minutes later, the infant projectile vomits. The doctor notes the nonbilious and nonbloody vomitus. What is the most likely diagnosis for this infant?
(A) Esophageal atresia
(B) Pyloric stenosis
(C) Upper gastrointestinal (GI) bleed
(D) Lower GI bleed
(E) Intestinal obstruction

10 A 27-year-old woman comes to the hospital in the early stages of labor. She is 37 weeks pregnant in her first pregnancy, which has been normal. She has no notable past medical history, does not smoke or drink, and is not taking any medications. The examination in the labor and delivery unit is normal, and all appears well with the fetus. At this time, which of the following fetal vessels is carrying the highest concentration of oxygen?
(A) Abdominal aorta
(B) Umbilical arteries
(C) Pulmonary artery
(D) Umbilical vein
(E) Pulmonary veins

11 A woman brings her 4-year-old daughter to the pediatrician because of continuing problems with vomiting, constipation, and abdominal distension. Extensive examination results in a diagnosis of an aganglionic colon. The girl has a deficiency in which of the following neural cell types?
(A) Pseudounipolar sensory neurons
(B) Presynaptic sympathetic neurons
(C) Presynaptic parasympathetic neurons
(D) Postsynaptic sympathetic neurons
(E) Postsynaptic parasympathetic neurons

12 A 12-year-old boy is brought to the emergency room with a fever, nausea, and pain in his abdomen. Acute appendicitis is the preliminary diagnosis due to his symptoms and an elevated white blood cell count (leukocytosis). The given axial CT reveals an inflamed radiodense appendix in the retrocecal position, exhibiting a thickened wall and surrounding edema. The boy is taken to the operating room for a laparoscopic appendectomy. Branches of what artery will need to be ligated during the procedure to alleviate excessive bleeding?

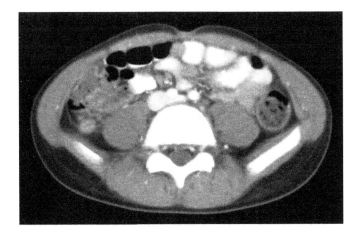

(A) Celiac
(B) Superior epigastric
(C) Superior mesenteric
(D) Inferior epigastric
(E) Inferior mesenteric

13 Failure of differentiation of the individual organs derived from the embryonic foregut would cause malformation of which of the following organs?
(A) Spleen
(B) Gall bladder
(C) Ascending colon
(D) Ileum
(E) Descending colon

14 An infant is born with a large defect in the central tendon of the diaphragm. This condition is most likely the result of malformation of which of the following structures?
(A) Dorsal mesentery of the esophagus
(B) Ventral mesentery of the gut tube
(C) Pleuroperitoneal folds
(D) Septum transversum
(E) Cervical somites

15 The given coronal MR arteriogram, taken after an appropriate time lapse, demonstrates abdominal venous anatomy. Which of the indicated veins drains the embryonic midgut?

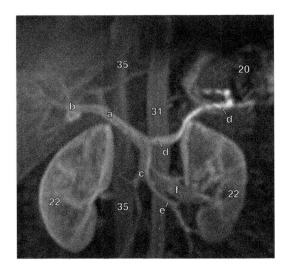

16 A 35-year-old man suffers sharp abdominal pain accompanied by hematemesis (vomiting of blood) for 2 days. He dies without seeking medical help. Autopsy findings reveal a perforated ulcer in the posterior wall of the first part of the duodenum, which damaged the artery in close proximity. Which of the following arteries was most likely ruptured?
(A) Short gastric
(B) Left gastroomental
(C) Gastroduodenal
(D) Splenic
(E) Left gastric

17 A 24-year-old man is brought to the ER with a knife wound located in the 9th intercostal space at the right midaxillary line. Given the location of the penetration wound, what structure is most likely damaged?
(A) Stomach
(B) Kidney
(C) Lung
(D) Liver
(E) Spleen

18 A 45-year-old man presents with pain in his left lower abdomen and proximal medial thigh, but the pain also radiates to his left shoulder. Physical examination of the left shoulder reveals no structural abnormalities or paresis (weakness). The given plain abdominal film reveals a left renal and perirenal abscess. Which of the following organs is irritated by the abscess, resulting in the radiating pain to the left shoulder?

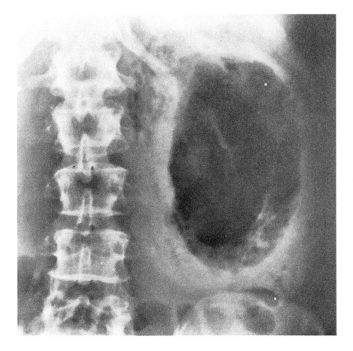

(A) Transverse colon
(B) Diaphragm
(C) Pancreas
(D) Duodenum
(E) Liver

19 A 25-year-old woman visits her obstetrician one year after a normal pregnancy and vaginal delivery of healthy twins. Following a physical examination, the physician informs the woman she is in good health and that all postnatal conditions are occurring as they should. At this time, the medial umbilical folds contain which of the following structures?
(A) Obliterated umbilical vein
(B) Obliterated urachus
(C) Obliterated umbilical arteries
(D) Obliterated ductus venosus
(E) Obliterated inferior epigastric vessels

20 A 58-year-old woman with a history of hypercholesterolemia came to the ER with severe abdominal pain, nausea, and vomiting. She is diagnosed with advanced atherosclerosis after radiologic imaging reveals atherosclerotic plaque narrowing the blood vessel supplying the embryonic foregut and its derivatives. What blood vessel is most likely affected?
(A) Celiac artery
(B) Superior mesenteric artery
(C) Inferior mesenteric artery
(D) Portal vein
(E) Umbilical vein

21 A fetal ultrasound examination of a 28-year-old pregnant woman reveals a defect in the anterior abdominal wall of the fetus. Further radiologic tests are ordered. The given sagittal T2-weight MRI demonstrates a midline defect involving the umbilical cord, which contains intestinal loops and part of the liver within a membranous sac. What developmental defect is depicted in this MRI?

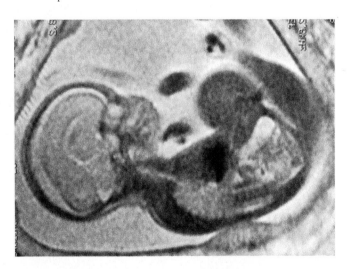

(A) Gastroschisis
(B) Congenital umbilical hernia
(C) Ileal diverticulum
(D) Omphalocele
(E) Prune belly syndrome

22 Familial dysautonomia is a rare genetic disorder of the autonomic nervous system. Problems include difficulty in feeding and respiration, vasomotor instability, insensitivity to pain, and ataxia (an unsteady gait). Patients with this syndrome have low numbers of autonomic neurons, probably related to defects in production and/or survival of the neural crest precursors of these neurons. Which of the following structures would not be affected by this disorder?
(A) Pyloric sphincter
(B) Abdominal aorta
(C) Teniae coli
(D) Diaphragm
(E) Hepatopancreatic sphincter

23 Following a radical mastectomy, a plastic surgeon uses a pedicled myocutaneous flap of the suprapubic portion of the rectus abdominis muscle to reconstruct the breast. What artery, supplying blood to the myocutaneous flap, needs to be isolated, transected, and later grafted to the reconstruction site?
(A) Superficial epigastric artery
(B) Superior epigastric artery
(C) Inferior epigastric artery
(D) Inferior mesenteric artery
(E) Musculophrenic artery

24 During inspections of a secret government biological warfare laboratory, a team of investigators discovers a genetically engineered virus that selectively attacks the cells bodies of postsynaptic parasympathetic neurons. In which of the following locations would this virus be found in the highest density if it were introduced into the body?
(A) Celiac plexus
(B) Paravertebral ganglia
(C) Myenteric plexus
(D) Hypogastric plexuses
(E) Gray matter of sacral spinal cord segments

25 A 47-year-old woman has lost 15 lb over the last 2 months and presents with upper abdominal pain that radiates to the middle and upper back. During physical examination, the doctor notes the sclera of her eyes are icteric (yellow in color), as seen on the given photo. An abdominal CT reveals a tumor within the head of the pancreas. The exocrine secretions of which of the following organs is being blocked leading directly to icteric sclera in this patient?

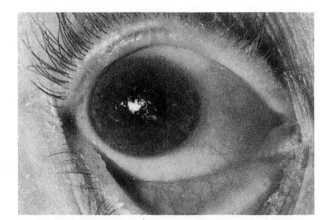

(A) Duodenum
(B) Liver
(C) Gall bladder
(D) Pancreas
(E) Stomach

26 A 60-year-old man is diagnosed with a posterior abdominal wall tumor that is causing lesions in the superior mesenteric plexus. Which of the following pathways is most likely affected?

(A) Parasympathetic supply to the posterior aspect of the stomach
(B) Sympathetic supply to the ascending colon
(C) Lymph drainage from the liver
(D) Venous drainage from the transverse colon
(E) Visceral afferents from the proximal duodenum

27 In anticipation for a medical school swimming party, a 60-year-old male professor squeezes into last year's bikini bathing suit despite gaining 25 lb over the winter. Following a day of "impressing" his students and colleagues, he notices numbness, tingling, and a burning sensation in the lateral aspect of his left upper thigh. His symptoms are exacerbated by applying pressure near the left anterior superior iliac spine. What nerve is most likely affected?

(A) Lateral femoral cutaneous nerve
(B) Femoral branch of genitofemoral nerve
(C) Anterior cutaneous branches of femoral nerve
(D) Ilioinguinal nerve
(E) Iliohypogastric nerve

28 A 62-year-old woman undergoes a Nissen fundoplication, in which the fundus of the stomach is completely sutured around the gastroesophageal junction, to treat a severe case of gastroesophageal reflux disease (GERD). During the procedure, the surgeon accidentally damages the right (posterior) vagal trunk while inserting staples into the stomach. Which of the following organs is most likely affected?

(A) Esophagus
(B) Urinary bladder
(C) Descending colon
(D) Prostate gland
(E) Second part of the duodenum

29 A 65-year-old woman is injured in an automobile accident. Examination indicates she suffers fractures of left ribs 8 to 10 and profuse internal bleeding. Which of the structures indicated in the given CT scan of the abdomen will likely need to be surgically removed?

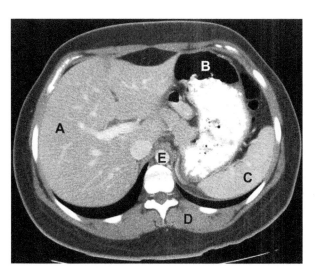

30 Which of the following functional outcomes could result from failure of synaptic transmission in the celiac ganglion?

(A) Decreased secretions from the gastric glands on the anterior wall of the stomach
(B) Reduced secretion of epinephrine from the adrenal (suprarenal) medulla
(C) Permanent relaxation of the pyloric sphincter
(D) Increased motility in the wall of the descending colon
(E) Paralysis of the quadratus lumborum muscle

31 During a splenectomy, a surgeon carefully dissects the peritoneal ligament containing the splenic vessels at the hilum of the spleen. Which of the following peritoneal ligaments is being dissected by the surgeon?

(A) Hepatoduodenal ligament
(B) Coronary ligament
(C) Transverse mesocolon
(D) Lienorenal ligament
(E) Gastrolienal ligament

32 A 52-year-old woman presents with severe upper right quadrant abdominal pain. She is jaundiced, obese, and has a history of gallstones. Further examination indicates acute cholecystitis, and she undergoes an open abdominal cholecystectomy (removal of gall bladder). During the surgery, the doctor inserts her index finger into the omental (epiploic) foramen to palpate the structures in the hepatoduodenal ligament. Which of the following structures lies immediately posterior to her finger?

(A) Bile duct
(B) Liver
(C) Inferior vena cava (IVC)
(D) Abdominal aorta
(E) Head of the pancreas

33 A 58-year-old man with a history of alcoholism arrives at the ER vomiting blood. The given endoscopy reveals esophageal varices, secondary to portal hypertension. Which of the following surgical venous anastomoses could relieve this patient's symptoms of portal hypertension in the short term?

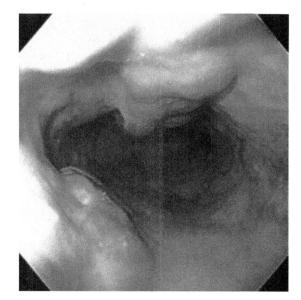

(A) Inferior mesenteric to superior mesenteric
(B) Left gastric to splenic
(C) Superior mesenteric to right renal
(D) Right gastric to left gastric
(E) Right testicular to right renal

34 An 18-year-old boy is brought to the ER after suffering a gun-shot wound to his back. Radiographic imaging reveals extensive damage to the neural arches of the L1 and L2 vertebrae, with bone and bullet fragments lodged in the vertebral canal at these levels. Comprehensive neurologic examination indicates destruction of the sacral segments of the spinal cord. Which of the following functional outcomes is most likely present?
(A) Reduced sweat gland secretion in the abdominal wall
(B) Decreased motility in the duodenum
(C) Increased motility in the ileum
(D) Paralysis of the psoas major muscle
(E) Relaxation of the teniae coli in the descending colon

35 During surgery to remove the gallbladder (cholecystectomy), a surgery resident damages the cystic artery before a clamp is properly placed. The attending physician applies pressure to the free edge of the hepatoduodenal ligament of the lesser omentum to control the bleeding until the damaged artery is clamped and ligated. Which of the following arteries was compressed by the attending physician?
(A) Celiac
(B) Splenic
(C) Gastroduodenal
(D) Common hepatic
(E) Proper hepatic

36 An axial CT of a 52-year-old man reveals a cancerous lesion in the middle aspect of the transverse colon compressing the lumen of the otherwise radiolucent colon. Based upon the location of the tumor, which of the following lymph node groups would first receive metastasizing cells from this cancerous lesion?

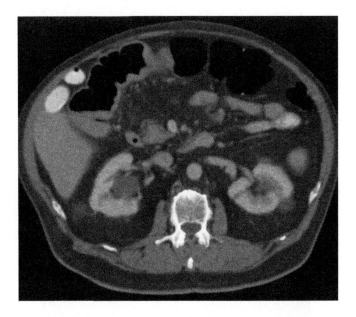

(A) Ileocolic
(B) Superior mesenteric
(C) Celiac
(D) Internal iliac
(E) Inferior mesenteric

37 Which of the following organs may be directly affected by malrotation of the caudal limb of the primary intestinal loop?
(A) Descending colon
(B) Stomach
(C) Spleen
(D) Fourth part of the duodenum
(E) Ascending colon

38 Which of the following structures is indicated with the letter "X" in this coronal CT?

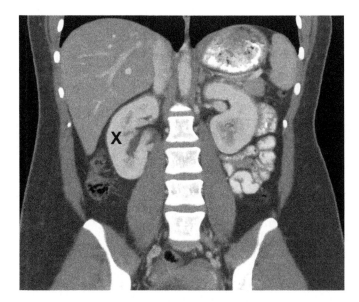

(A) Right kidney
(B) Liver
(C) Stomach
(D) Spleen
(E) Psoas major

39 During a physical examination of a 35-year-old man with a spinal cord injury, the neurologist lightly strokes the right upper medial side of the thigh to test the integrity of the L1-2 spinal cord segments. He notes the cremasteric reflex is absent. Which of the following nerves carries the efferent limb of this reflex arc?
(A) Iliohypogastric
(B) Genital branch of the genitofemoral
(C) Femoral branch of the genitofemoral
(D) Femoral
(E) Ilioinguinal

40 The given contrast radiograph of the small intestine shows a barium-filled diverticulum of the ileum identified by the white arrow. Branches of what artery will need to be ligated during surgical removal of this diverticulum?

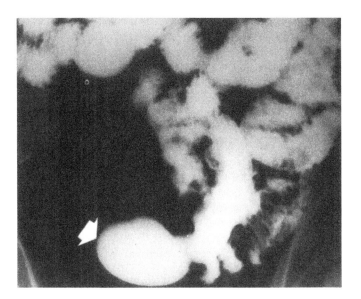

(A) Celiac
(B) Renal
(C) Superior mesenteric
(D) Inferior mesenteric
(E) Umbilical

41 The anterior abdominal wall of a 21-year-old woman impacts the steering wheel during a head-on car collision. The blunt trauma resulted in a lacerated pancreas with digestive enzyme spilling anterior. Which of the following locations would initially receive the contents of the lacerated pancreas?
(A) Supracolic part of greater peritoneal sac
(B) Infracolic part of greater peritoneal sac
(C) Subhepatic space
(D) Omental bursa
(E) Subphrenic space

42 The given photo shows a large left bulge in the inguinal canal and a swelling of the left scrotum in a newborn male. Ultrasound examination reveals a portion of the small intestine within the scrotal swelling. What is the deepest layer of the abdominal wall involved with this herniated bowel?

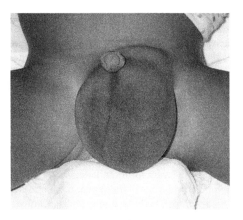

(A) Transverse abdominal muscle
(B) External oblique muscle
(C) Internal oblique muscle
(D) Rectus abdominis muscle
(E) Transversalis fascia

43 A 55-year-old woman develops a hiatal hernia in which the fundus of the stomach protrudes through the esophageal hiatus of the diaphragm into the thorax. Which of the following structures is/are at greatest risk of injury during surgical repair of this hernia?
(A) Thoracic duct
(B) Azygos vein
(C) Vagus nerves
(D) Sympathetic chains
(E) Superior epigastric vessels

ANSWERS AND DISCUSSION

1   **The answer is B: Endoderm.**   The primitive gut tube extends from the oropharyngeal membrane cranially to the cloacal membrane caudally. It is divided into three main parts: foregut, midgut, and hindgut. The epithelial lining of the entire primitive gut tube and its derivatives, including specific glandular cells (e.g., the endocrine and exocrine cells of the pancreas), is derived from endoderm. **Choice A** (Ectoderm) is incorrect. The primitive oral cavity (stomodeum) and the primitive lower anal canal (proctodeum) are formed from surface invaginations and are lined with ectoderm. With breakdown of the oropharyngeal and cloacal membranes, these areas become continuous with the foregut and hindgut, respectively. **Choice C** (Somatic mesoderm) is incorrect. The somatic (parietal) mesoderm lines the intraembryonic body cavity. It assumes a close relation with the overlying ectoderm, and together, these layers form the lateral body folds. The mesoderm forms the dermis of the skin and the bones and connective tissues in the body wall and limbs. **Choice D** (Visceral mesoderm) is incorrect. The visceral (splanchnic) mesoderm lines the organs formed within the intraembryonic body cavity (e.g., the gut tube and its derivatives). It joins closely with the endoderm to form the wall of the gut tube. The mesoderm forms the muscle, connective tissues, peritoneal layer, and the stroma of the glands in the gut wall. **Choice E** (Neural crest) is incorrect. Neural crest cells migrate into the primitive gut tube, where they form the parasympathetic ganglia in the wall of the gut. Thus, they form major components of the enteric nervous system. Neural crest cells also form the sympathetic chain, preaortic ganglia, and the adrenal medullary cells.

2   **The answer is A: Fundic portion of the stomach.**   Improper placement of a ligature on the splenic artery near the hilum of the spleen can compromise the blood supply in two additional arteries, the short gastric and left gastroomental, which branch off the splenic artery at this location. The short gastric artery leaves the hilum of the spleen, travels within the gastrosplenic ligament, and ultimately supplies the fundic portion of the stomach. The left gastroomental artery leaves the hilum of the spleen, travels within the gastrosplenic ligament, and supplies the left portion of the greater curvature of the stomach. Therefore, improper placement of a ligature during a splenectomy could damage the fundus and left greater curvature of the stomach by compromising the blood supply to these areas. **Choice B** (Kidney) is incorrect. The kidney is supplied by the renal arteries, which branch directly off the abdominal aorta. An improper placement of the ligature at the hilum of the spleen would not affect blood supply to the kidney. **Choice C** (Pyloric portion of the stomach) is incorrect. The pyloric portion of the stomach is supplied by branches of the gastroduodenal artery. Because of its blood supply and its location on the right side of the abdomen, the pyloric portion of the stomach would not be affected by improper ligature placement at the hilum of the spleen. **Choice D** (Head of the pancreas) is incorrect. The head of the pancreas is supplied by the superior and inferior pancreaticoduodenal arteries, which arise off the gastroduodenal and superior mesenteric arteries, respectively. Because of its blood supply and its location on the right side of the abdomen, the head of the pancreas would not be affected. **Choice E** (Splenic flexure of the colon) is incorrect. The splenic (left) flexure of the colon is

supplied by the marginal artery of the colon, which is formed by an anastomosis between the right and middle colic arteries. Though this portion of the large intestine is closely related to the spleen, it does not receive blood supply from the arteries originating from the hilum of the spleen. Therefore, the blood supply of the splenic flexure of the colon would not be affected by improper ligature placement at the hilum of the spleen.

3   **The answer is A: Direct inguinal hernia.**   A direct inguinal hernia is an acquired hernia that results when abdominal cavity contents herniate through a weakness in the anterior abdominal wall in the inguinal (Hesselbach) triangle. The borders of the inguinal triangle are the inferior epigastric artery located laterally, semilunar line of the rectus sheath medially, and the inguinal ligament inferiorly. A direct inguinal hernia exits through the superficial inguinal ring, but it does not usually descend into the scrotum, as seen in an indirect inguinal hernia. When comparing the direct inguinal hernia to an indirect inguinal hernia, remember that a direct inguinal hernia rarely descends into the scrotum, passes medial to the inferior epigastric artery, is not covered by the internal spermatic fascia, and is usually an acquired (not congenital) hernia. Groin hernias are 25 times more likely in men. **Choice B** (Indirect inguinal hernia) is incorrect. Indirect inguinal hernias are usually congenital herniae that result when abdominal cavity contents herniate through a patent processus vaginalis, or in an adult, the inguinal canal. An indirect inguinal hernia passes through the deep and superficial inguinal rings to descend into the scrotum of males. Indirect inguinal hernias are two to three times more common than direct inguinal hernias, but the location of the hernia (not descended into the scrotum) and the palpated weakness within the anterior abdominal wall would make a direct inguinal hernia more likely in this patient. **Choice C** (Femoral hernia) is incorrect. Femoral hernias enter into the femoral canal and often contain abdominal viscera. This type of hernia is more common in females due to their wider pelves. A femoral hernia is also more susceptible to strangulation (interruption of the blood supply of the herniated abdominal viscera) due to the sharp boundaries of the femoral ring, particularly the lacunar ligament. Strangulation can lead to ischemia, sharp pain, and necrosis of impinged tissue, which is not reported in this patient. Because this patient is male and no symptoms of bowel obstruction are reported, a femoral hernia is unlikely. It should be noted that the location of the globular mass of a femoral hernia would be hard to distinguish between an indirect or direct inguinal hernia. However, several studies suggest CT imaging can differentiate between these hernia types. **Choice D** (Lymphadenitis of superficial inguinal nodes) is incorrect. Lymphadenitis (swollen lymph nodes) of the superficial inguinal nodes could be responsible for a bulge in the groin. However, a recent bacterial or viral infection, which would cause these lymph nodes to be tender and swollen, is not reported in this patient. Moreover, the location of the weakness in the anterior abdominal wall reported by the doctor rules out this option. **Choice E** (Hydrocele testis) is incorrect. A hydrocele testis is a pathological accumulation of serous fluids around the testis. It is due to serous secretions from a remnant piece of peritoneum (tunica vaginalis) or a direct communication between the scrotum and the abdomen (persistent processus vaginalis). Patients with a hydrocele testis present with a painless, swollen testis that feels like a water balloon. A hydrocele testis can be drained by aspiration with a hollow needle (cannula) or surgery. However, in this patient, the groin bulge did not descend into the scrotum, which rules out this diagnosis.

4 **The answer is D: Inferior mesenteric.** A catheter is passed into the origin of the inferior mesenteric artery (IMA) to produce the given arteriogram. This plain film shows a bleeding diverticulum, stained by contrast material, in the descending colon. This finding leads to the lower GI bleed and associated symptoms in this patient. Lower GI bleeds lead to blood in the fecal matter of the patient and do not present with vomiting of blood (hematemesis), which is indicative of an upper GI bleed. The origin of the IMA is off the abdominal aorta at the third lumbar (L3) vertebral level, which is identified by the catheter in this arteriogram. The IMA supplies blood to the embryonic hindgut from the distal portion of the transverse colon to the superior aspect of the rectum. Branches off the IMA, specifically the left colic artery, supply the perforated descending colon in this patient. **Choice A** (Abdominal aorta) is incorrect. The abdominal aorta gives rise to the IMA at the third lumbar (L3) vertebral level. Because this question asks for direct branches of the artery involved with the bleeding diverticulum in the descending colon, the IMA is the best answer. **Choice B** (Celiac trunk) is incorrect. The celiac trunk arises from the abdominal aorta immediately after this artery traverses the diaphragm at the 12th thoracic (T12) vertebral level. The celiac artery supplies blood to the embryonic foregut extending between the lower esophagus and the second part of the duodenum. It does not supply blood to the descending colon, so it is not responsible for the lower GI bleed in this patient. Furthermore, damage to the celiac trunk would cause an upper GI bleed, which presents with hematemesis and melena (thick, black stool with a tar-like consistency due to the presence of altered blood), which is not reported in this patient. **Choice C** (Superior mesenteric) is incorrect. The superior mesenteric artery (SMA) arises from the abdominal aorta at the first lumbar (L1) vertebral level to supply the midgut extending from the second part of the duodenum to the distal portion of the transverse colon. Because it does not supply direct branches to the descending colon, the SMA is not the direct source of the lower GI bleed in this patient. **Choice E** (External iliac) is incorrect. The external iliac artery supplies blood to the iliac region and the anterior abdominal wall. This artery becomes the femoral artery, a major lower limb artery, after it passes under the inguinal ligament. Because it does not supply direct branches to the descending colon, the external iliac artery is not the source of the lower GI bleed in this patient.

5 **The answer is D: Falciform ligament.** The primitive gut tube is suspended from the dorsal and ventral walls of the embryonic peritoneal cavity (intraembryonic body cavity) by dorsal and ventral mesenteries, which give rise to all the adult mesenteries. The ventral mesentery is relatively short in that it extends only along part of the foregut. Growth of the liver subdivides the ventral mesentery into the falciform ligament, lesser omentum, and the coronary and triangular ligaments of the liver. The umbilical vein traverses the free margin of the falciform ligament to pass from the umbilicus to the liver. Its postnatal remnant, the round ligament of the liver (ligamentum teres hepatis), can be readily located in this position. **Choice A** (Sigmoid mesocolon) is incorrect. The sigmoid

mesocolon is derived from the dorsal mesentery. Initially, the dorsal mesentery extends most of the length of the primitive gut tube, attaching it to the dorsal (posterior) body wall. Later, it narrows somewhat but remains quite extensive. **Choice B** (Mesentery of the small intestine) is incorrect. The mesentery of the small intestine is derived from the dorsal mesentery. **Choice C** (Greater omentum) is incorrect. The greater omentum is derived from the dorsal mesentery. **Choice E** (Transverse mesocolon) is incorrect. The transverse mesocolon is derived from the dorsal mesentery.

6 **The answer is E: Spleen.** Though it is afforded the protection of the ninth through eleventh ribs on the left side of the flank, the spleen is the most frequently injured organ in the abdomen. The given axial CT reveals a splenic laceration, indicated by the white arrow, in proximity to the reported left 9th and 10th rib fractures. In addition to the location of the injury, the low blood pressure suggests blood loss within the systemic arterial circulation. The increased pulse and the rapid respiration rate are secondary to the pain that the patient is experiencing. A mnemonic for the spleen is the odd numbers "1, 3, 5, 7, 9, 11", which corresponds to various features of the spleen, including its size as 1 × 3 × 5 in., its weight as approximately 7 lb, and its relation with ribs 9 to 11. Note the relationship of the 9th through 11th ribs to the spleen in the CT. **Choice A** (Stomach) is incorrect. Due to the location of the injury on the left flank at the posterior axillary line, the stomach is not likely damaged because it resides anterior to this location. In the given axial CT scan, the radiodense appearance of the stomach is located anterior to the lacerated spleen. Unless a major artery was damaged, a laceration of the stomach would not account for the low blood pressure seen in this patient. **Choice B** (Kidney) is incorrect. Due to the damage to the left 9th and 10th ribs, the kidney is not likely damaged. As seen in the given axial CT scan, the superior pole of the left kidney is closely related to the 11th and 12th ribs. Because it resides below the injured area, the left kidney is not likely damaged. Encapsulated by a substantial amount of pararenal and perirenal fat, the kidneys are also afforded additional insulation from injury, when compared to the spleen. **Choice C** (Lung) is incorrect. The inferior border of the left lung usually resides at the 8th rib in the midaxillary line, so it is located above the injured area and is not likely to be damaged. **Choice D** (Liver) is incorrect. The liver resides on the right side of the body, so it is not likely damaged due to location of the damage being on the left side of the body.

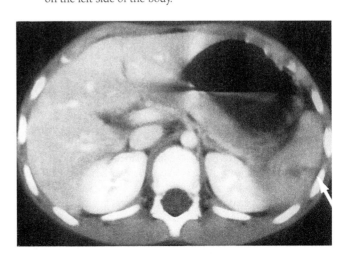

7 **The answer is C: Lower ileum.** Meckel (ileal) diverticulum is a persistent remnant of the embryonic vitelline duct (yolk stalk). The vitelline duct is the connection between the apex of the primary intestinal loop of the midgut and the yolk sac. The primary intestinal loop is the highly elongated embryonic midgut. When present, an ileal diverticulum is an outpocketing located on the antimesenteric border of the distal ileum, usually 2 ft proximal to the ileocecal junction in children. The diverticulum may be short or long (2 to 15 cm), and it may be free or connected to the umbilicus via a fibrous cord or fistula. There may be heterotrophic gastric or pancreatic mucosa in the diverticulum that can lead to ulceration, perforation, obstruction, or other abdominal problems that resemble acute appendicitis. A mnemonic for an ileal diverticulum is the "rule of 2," which says this type of diverticulum is 2 in. long, found 2 ft proximal to the ileocecal valve, and is present in approximately 2% of the population, with males more frequently experiencing symptoms. Of the 2% of the population with an ileal diverticulum, only 2% become symptomatic. So, remember the "rule of 2" mnemonic when discussing an ileal diverticulum.

Choice A (Lower duodenum) is incorrect. The duodenum is formed from the terminal end of the foregut and the cranial end of the midgut. The vitelline duct is located at the apex of the primary intestinal loop. Thus, the lower (distal) duodenum is well removed from the structure that produces the ileal diverticulum. **Choice B** (Middle jejunum) is incorrect. Due to its length, the primary intestinal loop folds into cranial and caudal limbs, with the vitelline duct at the apical bend between the two. The cranial limb of the loop gives rise to the lower duodenum, entire jejunum, and upper ileum. Thus, the middle jejunum is well removed from the vitelline duct. **Choice D** (Cecum) is incorrect. The cecum forms from the caudal limb of the primary intestinal loop, along with the lower (distal) ileum, appendix, ascending colon, and proximal 2/3 of the transverse colon. The cecum is well removed from the vitelline duct, so it is not positioned to produce a Meckel diverticulum. **Choice E** (Transverse colon) is incorrect. The transverse colon is formed from the distal end of the midgut and the proximal end of the hindgut. As with the duodenum, it is far removed from the apex of the primary intestinal loop and the site of the vitelline duct.

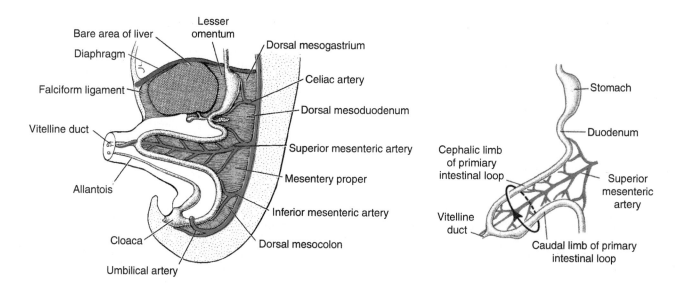

8 **The answer is C: Least splanchnic.** The least splanchnic nerve carries presynaptic sympathetic nerve fibers derived from the T12 spinal level. Visceral afferent fibers traveling along with the least splanchnic nerve refer pain to the T12 dermatome, which is located in the suprapubic region of the abdomen and is consistent with the presentation of this patient. Furthermore, the renal nerve plexus is supplied primarily from the least splanchnic nerve, with contributions from the lumbar splanchnic nerves derived from L1 and L2. Therefore, visceral sensory fibers conveying pain from the distension of the renal capsule, secondary to the polycystic kidney disease, would follow sympathetic nerves retrograde to the spinal ganglia at the T12-L2 vertebral levels. **Choice A** (Greater splanchnic nerve) is incorrect. The greater splanchnic nerve carries presynaptic sympathetic nerve fibers derived from the T5-9 spinal levels. Visceral sensory fibers, associated with the greater splanchnic nerve and traveling retrograde with these visceral motor fibers, refer pain to the T5-9 dermatomes, which corresponds to the anterolateral chest wall and epigastric region of the anterior abdominal wall. **Choice B** (Lesser splanchnic

nerve) is incorrect. The lesser splanchnic nerve carries presynaptic sympathetic nerve fibers derived from the T10-11 spinal levels. Visceral afferent fibers traveling along with the lesser splanchnic nerve refer pain to the T10-11 dermatomes. These dermatomes correspond to the umbilical region of the anterior abdominal wall, which is slightly higher than the reported level of pain in this patient. **Choice D** (Pelvic splanchnic) is incorrect. The pelvic splanchnic nerves carry presynaptic parasympathetic fibers derived from the S2-4 spinal levels. Visceral sensory fibers traveling along with the pelvic splanchnic nerve refer pain to the S2-4 dermatomes, which is located well below the suprapubic region of the abdomen. The pelvic splanchnic nerves receive visceral sensory fibers from pelvic organs located below the peritoneum. **Choice E** (Vagus nerve) is incorrect. The vagus nerve conveys presynaptic parasympathetic nerve fibers to supply the gastrointestinal tract down to the distal transverse colon. It also conveys visceral afferent fibers, but these fibers are mainly for unconscious sensations associated with reflexes. Therefore, these fibers are not responsible for pain radiating to the suprapubic region of the abdomen.

9 **The answer is B: Pyloric stenosis.** Pyloric stenosis is a thickening of the pyloric sphincter, which prevents the contents of the stomach from emptying into the duodenum. Children with pyloric stenosis usually present with the listed symptoms approximately 2 to 3 weeks after birth. The key to the diagnosis in this patient is the appearance of the vomitus. Nonbilious vomitus implies the milk did not reach the second part of the duodenum where the biliary tract empties bile into the duodenum. Nonbloody vomitus rules out the possibility of a GI bleed. Pediatricians have noted a tendency for pyloric stenosis to occur in first-born Caucasian boys. Because this newborn is healthy until the onset of the projective vomiting 2 to 3 weeks after birth, pyloric stenosis is the most likely diagnosis. Confirmation of pyloric stenosis can be achieved with an abdominal ultrasound, a blood chemistry panel to look for an electrolyte imbalance, and a barium X-ray (see the given figure), which reveals an abnormally dilated stomach and narrowed pylorus. Surgical intervention to rectify a pyloric stenosis is called pyloromyotomy. In this procedure, the overdeveloped pyloric sphincter muscles are split to allow food passage into the duodenum. **Choice A** (Esophageal atresia) is incorrect. Esophageal atresia is a congenital disorder in which the esophagus ends in a blind-ending pouch and is not connected to the stomach. A baby with esophageal atresia is unable to swallow food, so this defect is often detected during the first attempted feeding. Due to the late onset (21 to 22 days) of the symptoms and the time that elapsed between the feeding in the office and the projectile vomiting (~20 minutes), esophageal atresia is highly unlikely. **Choice C** (Upper gastrointestinal [GI] bleed) is incorrect. An upper GI bleed presents with hematemesis (vomiting blood) and melena (thick, black stool with a tar-like consistency due to the presence of altered blood), which were not reported in this patient. The nonbloody vomitus rules out the possibility of a GI bleed, and the nonbilious vomitus implies the milk never reached the second part of the duodenum. Therefore, an upper GI bleed is unlikely in this infant. **Choice D** (Lower GI bleed) is incorrect. A lower GI bleed presents with blood in the fecal matter, but this infant emits loose, watery stools. Furthermore, the nonbilious vomitus implies the milk never reached the second part of the duodenum, so a lower GI bleed is unlikely. **Choice E** (Intestinal obstruction) is incorrect. The bile, produced by the liver, is emptied into the second portion of the duodenum by the biliary system. Due to the nonbilious vomitus, the obstruction is located proximal to the second part of the duodenum. Therefore, an intestinal obstruction is highly unlikely.

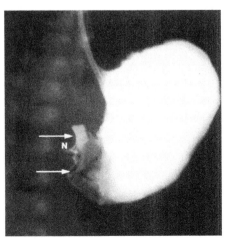

10 **The answer is D: Umbilical vein.** The umbilical vein runs from the placenta, through the umbilicus, and to the liver. Prenatally, this vessel carries blood with the highest oxygen saturation (~80%) in the fetal circulation, as it is the direct line from the placenta. Most of the blood in the umbilical vein is shunted around the liver through the ductus venosus into the inferior vena cava. Postnatally, both the umbilical vein and the ductus venosus are obliterated. The umbilical vein, located in the free margin of the falciform ligament, forms the round ligament of the liver (ligamentum teres hepatis). The ductus venosus forms the ligamentum venosum. **Choice A** (Abdominal aorta) is incorrect. Prenatally, blood in the abdominal aorta has low oxygen saturation. This artery carries blood distal to all the fetal circulatory shunts, except one (the umbilical arteries). Its flow has been mixed with deoxygenated blood in the liver, right atrium, left atrium, and distal arch of the aorta (at the junction with the ductus arteriosus). **Choice B** (Umbilical arteries) is incorrect. The paired umbilical arteries carry blood from the internal iliac arteries, through the umbilicus, and to the placenta. Because they are the exit routes from the fetal circulation to the placenta, these arteries carry blood with the lowest oxygen saturation (~58%) in the fetus. Postnatally, the proximal parts of the umbilical arteries remain patent and form the superior vesical arteries to the urinary bladder. The distal parts of the vessels gradually obliterate and form fibrous strands in the medial umbilical folds of the anterior abdominal wall. **Choice C** (Pulmonary artery) is incorrect. The pulmonary artery carries blood out of the right ventricle into the pulmonary circuit. Blood in the right ventricle has been mixed with deoxygenated blood in the liver, inferior vena cava, and right atrium. Thus, this flow is desaturated. Most of the blood in the pulmonary artery is shunted around the lungs through the ductus arteriosus and into the distal arch of the aorta. Postnatally, the ductus arteriosus obliterates and forms the ligamentum arteriosum. **Choice E** (Pulmonary veins) is incorrect. The pulmonary veins carry blood from the lungs into the left atrium. Because the prenatal pulmonary circuit carries a low volume of mixed blood, these veins carry a desaturated flow.

11 **The answer is E: Postsynaptic parasympathetic neurons.** Congenital megacolon (Hirschsprung disease) is the congenital absence of enteric ganglia in the colon (usually the distal portion) due to failure of neural crest cell migration into the colon to form the myenteric (Auerbach) plexus. The myenteric (intrinsic) ganglia are normally composed of postsynaptic (postganglionic) parasympathetic neurons that regulate gut motility. In this condition, the affected gut segment is aganglionic and inactive, causing the functioning proximal segment to dilate, sometimes into a severe megacolon. Classic symptoms include constipation, vomiting, poor appetite and weight gain, and abdominal distension. The usual treatment is surgical removal of the affected segment and connection of the normal proximal gut to the rectum or anus. **Choice A** (Pseudounipolar sensory neurons) is incorrect. Pseudounipolar sensory neurons carry information (touch, pain, temperature, etc.) to the central nervous system, composed of the brain and spinal cord. These neurons include general and visceral sensory (afferent) neurons. The general sensory neurons carry information from the body wall and limbs. Visceral sensory neurons carry visceral sensations from the gut tube and other internal organs. The latter neurons travel in close company with visceral motor (autonomic) neurons. **Choice B** (Presynaptic sympathetic neurons) is incorrect. The presynaptic sympathetic neurons that supply the gut tube run from the spinal cord to a series of prevertebral (preaortic) ganglia, where they synapse with postsynaptic neurons. Sympathetic neurons are not part of the enteric nervous system. **Choice C** (Presynaptic parasympathetic neurons) is incorrect. These neurons feed into the enteric ganglia but are not components of the enteric nervous system. The neural crest insufficiency in Hirschsprung disease typically results in absence of the enteric ganglia, with the presynaptic elements intact. **Choice D** (Postsynaptic sympathetic neurons) is incorrect. Sympathetic neurons are not components of the enteric ganglia or the enteric nervous system. Thus, they are not involved in an aganglionic colon.

12   **The answer is C: Superior mesenteric artery.** The superior mesenteric artery arises from the abdominal aorta at the first lumbar (L1) vertebral level, and it supplies the midgut from the second part of the duodenum to the distal portion of the transverse colon. The appendix is an outpocketing of the embryonic midgut connected to the cecum, located in the lower right quadrant of the abdomen in proximity to the ileocecal junction. Because the vermiform appendix is derived from the midgut, its blood supply arises from a branch of the superior mesenteric artery, specifically the appendicular artery arising off the ileocolic artery. The appendicular artery would need to be ligated to alleviate excessive bleeding during a laparoscopic appendectomy. The given photo shows a laparoscopic view of the appendix. **Choice A** (Celiac) is incorrect. The celiac artery (trunk) arises from the abdominal aorta immediately after this artery traverses the diaphragm at the 12th thoracic (T12) vertebral level. The celiac artery supplies blood to the embryonic foregut from approximately the lower esophagus to the second part of the duodenum. It does not supply blood to the appendix and is not ligated in a laparoscopic appendectomy. **Choice B** (Superior epigastric artery) is incorrect. The superior epigastric artery arises from the internal thoracic artery at approximately the 6th intercostal space and courses inferior to supply the rectus sheath and its contents. It anastomoses with the inferior epigastric artery near the umbilicus. It does not supply blood to the appendix, so it is not ligated in a laparoscopic appendectomy. **Choice D** (Inferior mesenteric) is incorrect. The inferior mesenteric artery arises from the abdominal aorta at the third lumbar (L3) vertebral level and supplies blood to the embryonic hindgut from approximately the distal portion of the transverse colon to the superior aspect of the rectum. It does not supply blood to the appendix, so it is not ligated in a laparoscopic appendectomy. **Choice E** (Inferior epigastric artery) is incorrect. The inferior epigastric artery arises from the external iliac artery just superior to the inguinal ligament and courses toward the rectus sheath to supply it and its contents. Once within the rectus sheath, the inferior epigastric artery ascends posterior to the rectus abdominis muscle to anastomose with the superior epigastric artery near the umbilicus.

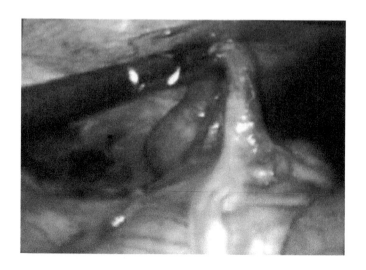

13   **The answer is B: Gall bladder.** The primitive gut tube extends from the oropharyngeal membrane cranially to the cloacal membrane caudally. It is divided into three main parts: foregut, midgut, and hindgut. The foregut gives rise to the esophagus, stomach, proximal duodenum, liver, gall bladder, biliary ducts, and pancreas. **Choice A** (Spleen) is incorrect. The spleen is not a derivative of the gut tube. It is a large, highly vascular lymphoid organ located in close association with the organs derived from the foregut. **Choice C** (Ascending colon) is incorrect. The ascending colon is derived from the midgut. Other derivatives of the midgut include the distal duodenum, jejunum, ileum, cecum, appendix, and proximal 2/3 of the transverse colon. **Choice D** (Ileum) is incorrect. The ileum is derived from the midgut. Other derivatives of the midgut include the distal duodenum, jejunum, cecum, appendix, ascending colon, and proximal 2/3 of the transverse colon. **Choice E** (Descending colon) is incorrect. The descending colon is derived from the hindgut. Other hindgut derivatives include the distal 1/3 of the transverse colon, sigmoid colon, rectum, and upper anal canal.

14   **The answer is D: Septum transversum.** The central tendon of the diaphragm is the expansive tendinous area into which the diaphragmatic muscle inserts and acts upon to produce respiratory movements. Also, it provides passage of the inferior vena cava, which traverses the diaphragm at the 8th thoracic (T8) vertebral level. The central tendon is formed from the embryonic septum transversum. The initial intraembryonic coelom is a single continuous area spanning the length of the trunk. Formation of the diaphragm separates the thoracic and peritoneal cavities. The diaphragm forms from fusion of tissues that originate from four different sources: septum transversum, paired pleuroperitoneal membranes, dorsal mesentery of the esophagus, and cervical somites. The septum transversum is a mesodermal wall that forms between the primitive heart tube and developing liver. It forms most of the diaphragm. **Choice A** (Dorsal mesentery of the esophagus) is incorrect. This portion of the dorsal mesentery of the gut tube forms the crura of the diaphragm. These muscular legs attach the diaphragm to the vertebral column and form the margins of the aortic hiatus. Additionally, the right crus forms the esophageal hiatus. **Choice B** (Ventral mesentery of the gut tube) is incorrect. The ventral mesentery of the gut tube is not related to formation of the diaphragm. It gives rise to the lesser omentum, falciform ligament, and the coronary and triangular ligaments of the liver. **Choice C** (Pleuroperitoneal folds) is incorrect. The paired pleuroperitoneal folds are extensions from the posterolateral body wall. They form much of the posterolateral aspect of the diaphragm that is not derived from the septum transversum or the dorsal esophageal mesentery. **Choice E** (Cervical somites) is incorrect. The septum transversum is initially located along cervical somites and spinal cord segments C3-5. Differential rates of body growth between the trunk and internal organs cause shifting and repositioning of the diaphragm to its final thoracolumbar position. However, myoblasts from the cervical somites invade the initial diaphragmatic folds and form the muscular parts of the diaphragm. Further, the cervical spinal cord segments give rise to the phrenic nerves that provide motor innervation to the diaphragm.

15 **The answer is C: Superior mesenteric vein.** The hepatic portal system collects blood from the abdominal gut tube and spleen and directs that flow into the liver. The superior mesenteric vein collects the venous flow from the embryonic midgut and empties it into the portal vein. Therefore, the distal duodenum, jejunum, ileum, cecum, appendix, ascending colon, and proximal 2/3 of the transverse colon drain via this route. **Choice A** (Hepatic portal vein) is incorrect. The hepatic portal vein (portal vein) receives the blood flow from the entire hepatic portal system and directs that blood into the liver. The portal vein is formed by the union of the splenic and superior mesenteric veins posterior to the neck of the pancreas. **Choice B** (Branches of the portal vein) is incorrect. At or close to the porta hepatis, the portal vein divides into right and left primary branches that supply the right and left lobes of the liver. These branches quickly divide further to supply the finer divisions of the liver. **Choice D** (Splenic vein) is incorrect. The splenic vein receives blood from the spleen and much of the foregut. The left gastric vein also collects blood from the foregut but typically empties directly into the portal vein. **Choice E** (Inferior mesenteric vein) is incorrect. The inferior mesenteric vein collects blood from the hindgut. This vessel usually drains into the splenic vein. However, it may end in the superior mesenteric vein or at the junction of the splenic and superior mesenteric veins.

16 **The answer is C: Gastroduodenal.** The gastroduodenal artery is one of the terminal branches of the common hepatic artery (the proper hepatic artery is the other). It descends immediately posterior to the first part of the duodenum, gives branches to the duodenum, and terminates by splitting into two branches: right gastroomental (gastroepiploic) and superior pancreaticoduodenal. Its close relation to the second part of the duodenum makes this vessel susceptible to lesions such as the perforating ulcer described in this case. **Choice A** (Short gastric) is incorrect. The short gastric arteries are branches of the distal part of the splenic artery. These vessels supply the fundus of the stomach on its greater curvature aspect. **Choice B** (Left gastroomental) is incorrect. The left gastroomental (gastroepiploic) artery is a large branch of

the distal part of the splenic artery. It passes along the greater curvature of the stomach and forms an anastomotic arc with the right gastroomental artery. **Choice D** (Splenic) is incorrect. The splenic artery is the largest branch of the celiac trunk. It weaves along the superior border of the pancreas, giving branches to the pancreas, fundus and greater curvature of the stomach, and greater omentum before terminating in the spleen. **Choice E** (Left gastric) is incorrect. The left gastric artery is the smallest branch of the celiac trunk. It ascends to the left (superior) aspect of the lesser curvature of the stomach and then follows along the lesser curvature. This vessel forms an anastomotic arc with the right gastric artery along the lesser curvature of the stomach.

17 **The answer is D: Liver.** The liver resides on the right side of the body, and its entire surface is afforded the protection of the thoracic cage in healthy individuals. The liver is the most likely damaged organ due to the location of the knife wound in the right 9th intercostal space. In fact, the liver can extend superior to approximately the level of the nipple, depending on the inflation state of the right lung. The given axial CT shows the damaged liver below the level of the entry wound. **Choice A** (Stomach) is incorrect. The stomach is seen on the given CT scan, and due to gut rotation, it resides on the left side of the body. Therefore, the stomach is not likely damaged by the knife wound in the right 9th intercostal space. **Choice B** (Kidney) is incorrect. The right kidney is located below the entry wound in this patient because the superior pole of the right kidney is closely related to the 12th rib. The kidney also lies deep to the liver, so the liver is more likely to be damaged in this patient. **Choice C** (Lung) is incorrect. The inferior border of the right lung would reside approximately at the 8th rib in the midaxillary line. The parietal pleura of the lung, which lines the pulmonary cavity, extends inferiorly to the tenth rib in the midaxillary line, but the lung itself would not descend to this level unless it was completely inflated at the time of the injury. Therefore, the liver is more likely to be injured in this patient, especially because breathing difficulties are not reported in this patient. **Choice E** (Spleen) is incorrect. The spleen resides on the left side of the body. Due to penetration wound being located on the right, the spleen is not damaged.

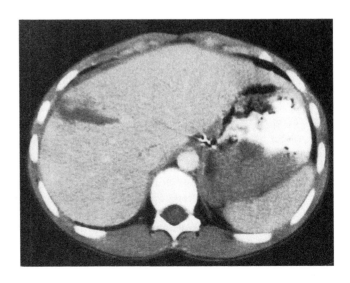

18 The answer is B: Diaphragm. Spread of the abscess superior would cause visceral pain derived from the diaphragm because the diaphragm is closely related to the superior pole of the left kidney. The visceral sensory fibers conveying pain from the kidney are derived from the T12-L1 vertebral levels, which leads to referred pain in the lower abdomen and proximal medial thigh. Remember, visceral pain is often perceived as cutaneous pain in an area supplied by the same spinal cord level as the affected abdominal organ. Involvement of the diaphragm would refer pain to the left lower cervical and shoulder regions because the phrenic nerve, derived from vertebral levels C3-5, innervates the diaphragm. **Choice A** (Transverse colon) is incorrect. The lesser splanchnic nerve, derived from spinal levels T10-11, innervates the transverse colon. Therefore, visceral sensory fibers extending from the transverse colon cause pain within the T10-11 dermatomes, which does not explain the pain specific to the left shoulder region. Furthermore, the transverse colon is located well anterior to the left kidney in the abdomen, so its involvement is unlikely based upon the given radiograph. **Choice C** (Pancreas) is incorrect. The greater splanchnic nerve, derived from spinal levels T5-9, innervates the pancreas. Therefore, visceral sensory fibers, extending from the pancreas, cause pain within the T5-9 dermatomes, which does not explain the pain specific to the left shoulder region. The body of the pancreas is located anterior to the left kidney, so spread of the abscess could affect the pancreas; however, this involvement would not explain the pain in the left shoulder. **Choice D** (Duodenum) is incorrect. The greater splanchnic nerve, derived from spinal levels T5-9, innervates the duodenum. Therefore, visceral sensory fibers extending from the duodenum cause pain within the T5-9 dermatomes, which does not account for the pain specific to the left shoulder region. Furthermore, the duodenum is located primarily on the right side of the body where it envelopes the head of the pancreas, so this abscess of the left kidney would not involve the duodenum. **Choice E** (Liver) is incorrect. The liver receives sensory innervation from the greater splanchnic nerve derived from the T5-9 nerves, so pain associated with the liver is referred to the T5-9 dermatomes and would not be localized in the right shoulder region. Furthermore, the liver is located primarily on the right side, far from the left kidney.

19 The answer is C: Obliterated umbilical arteries. The internal surface of the anterior abdominal wall presents fivefolds of peritoneum that run from the pelvic region to the umbilicus: a single, midline median umbilical fold, paired medial umbilical folds, and paired lateral umbilical folds. The medial umbilical folds lie lateral to the median umbilical fold and cover the obliterated distal portions of the umbilical arteries. The proximal parts of the umbilical arteries (branches of the internal iliac arteries) remain patent and form the superior vesicle arteries, which supply part of the urinary bladder. **Choice A** (Obliterated umbilical vein) is incorrect. The obliterated umbilical vein is the round ligament of the liver (ligamentum teres hepatis). This structure is located in the free margin of the falciform ligament, running from the umbilicus to the liver. **Choice B** (Obliterated urachus) is incorrect. The urachus is the remnant of the embryonic allantois. It is contained in the median umbilical fold, running superiorly in the midline from the apex of the bladder to the umbilicus. **Choice D** (Obliterated ductus venosus) is incorrect. The ductus venosus

is the fetal shunt from the umbilical vein to the inferior vena cava, thus bypassing the liver. Its remnant, the ligamentum venosum, may be found near the porta hepatis, in the umbilical (left sagittal) fissure on the visceral (posterior) surface of the liver. **Choice E** (Obliterated inferior epigastric vessels) is incorrect. The inferior epigastric vessels do not normally obliterate. Rather, they form significant vascular lines from the external iliac vessels upward into the anterior abdominal wall. These vessels are contained within the lateral umbilical folds, located lateral to the medial umbilical folds. Thus, the lateral umbilical folds are the only umbilical folds that bleed when cut. The lateral umbilical folds also mark the lateral boundary of the inguinal (Hesselbach) triangle and serve as a key landmark in differentiating direct from indirect inguinal hernias.

20 The answer is A: Celiac artery. The primitive gut tube extends from the oropharyngeal membrane, cranially, to the cloacal membrane, caudally. It is divided into three main parts: foregut, midgut, and hindgut. Each of these three segments is supplied by a single (unpaired) major arterial branch of the abdominal aorta. Most of the foregut is supplied by the celiac artery (trunk). Thus, occlusion of this vessel will obstruct blood flow to the lower esophagus, stomach, liver, gall bladder, pancreas, and proximal duodenum. Also, the celiac artery supplies the spleen, even though the spleen is not a derivative of the foregut. Most of the esophagus is located outside the abdomen and is supplied by local branches in the neck and thorax (e.g., esophageal branches of the thoracic aorta). Expansion of the anastomosis between the superior pancreaticoduodenal arteries (branches of the celiac axis) and the inferior pancreaticoduodenal arteries (branches of the superior mesenteric axis) in the head of the pancreas may help relieve some of the ischemia produced by occlusion of the celiac trunk. **Choice B** (Superior mesenteric artery) is incorrect. The superior mesenteric artery supplies the midgut. Occlusion here deprives the caudal duodenum, jejunum, ileum, cecum, appendix, ascending colon, and most of the transverse colon. Anastomoses occur between the superior mesenteric axis and both the celiac axis (see above) and inferior mesenteric axis. The anastomosis with the inferior mesenteric tract is via connections between the middle colic artery (superior mesenteric axis) and the left colic artery (inferior mesenteric axis), along the margin of the transverse and descending colon. **Choice C** (Inferior mesenteric artery) is incorrect. The inferior mesenteric artery supplies most of the hindgut. Occlusion here blocks flow to the distal transverse colon, descending colon, sigmoid colon, and upper rectum. The superior rectal branch of the inferior mesenteric artery anastomoses with middle rectal branches of the internal iliac arteries around the rectal walls. **Choice D** (Portal vein) is incorrect. The portal vein collects blood from all three portions of the gut tube and directs that flow into the liver. Thus, the hepatic portal system overlaps the three arterial axes but drains them rather than supplies them. **Choice E** (Umbilical vein) is incorrect. The umbilical vein carries blood from the placenta to the liver and into a liver bypass (the ductus venosus) in the fetus. It does not supply the gut tube.

21 The answer is D: Omphalocele. An omphalocele is a defect in the development of the muscles of the anterior abdominal wall in which intestinal loops and often parts of the liver remain outside the abdomen. The distinguishing characteristic of an omphalocele is a midline defect through the umbilicus in which the protruding organs (liver and intestine usually) remain in a sac composed of peritoneum, which can be appreciated in the given figure. In contrast to gastroschisis, the herniated organs in an omphalocele are surrounded by a membranous sac. **Choice A** (Gastroschisis) is incorrect. Gastroschisis is a defect of the anterior abdominal wall located off the midline, typically to the right of the umbilicus. Intestinal loops protrude through the defect into the amniotic cavity, where they float freely in the amniotic fluid. In gastroschisis, the umbilical cord is not involved and the protruding organs are not enclosed in a membranous sac composed of peritoneum. **Choice B** (Congenital umbilical hernia) is incorrect. Congenital umbilical hernia refers to a weakness in the umbilical region that allows abdominal contents to protrude through the abdominal wall. However, the abdominal contents are covered by skin, so the patient presents with a bulge in the umbilical region. **Choice C** (Ileal diverticulum) is incorrect. Ileal (Meckel) diverticulum is a persistent remnant of the embryonic vitelline duct (yolk stalk), which connects the apex of the primary intestinal loop of the midgut to the yolk sac. An ileal diverticulum is a remnant of the vitelline duct, and it is usually not detected by radiographic imaging in a fetus. **Choice E** (Prune belly syndrome) is incorrect. Prune belly syndrome is characterized by an extremely thin, distended abdominal wall due to an absence of abdominal musculature. Organs are often visible through the skin, but in Prune Belly syndrome, the abdominal wall defects do not allow protrusion of the liver out of the abdominal cavity.

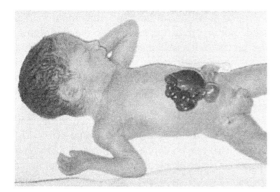

22 **The answer is D: Diaphragm.** The diaphragm is composed of skeletal muscle and is innervated by somatic nerves fibers in the phrenic nerves. It is not affected by autonomic dysfunction, so its function is spared in familial dysautonomia. **Choice A** (Pyloric sphincter) is incorrect. The pyloric sphincter is the smooth muscle sphincter at the gastroduodenal junction. It is supplied by both sympathetic and parasympathetic fibers, so its function could be affected by autonomic insufficiency. **Choice B** (Abdominal aorta) is incorrect. This large vessel has a distinct smooth muscle component. Therefore, it could be affected by autonomic insufficiency. **Choice C** (Teniae coli) is incorrect. The teniae coli are the three narrow bands of longitudinal smooth muscle that run the length of the colon. They are distinguishing features of the exterior surface of the colon. The teniae coli could be affected by autonomic insufficiency. **Choice E** (Hepatopancreatic sphincter) is incorrect. This structure is the smooth muscle sphincter around the hepatopancreatic (greater duodenal) ampulla, at the point where the bile and pancreatic ducts join and empty

into the duodenum. Thus, it regulates the flow of bile and pancreatic juice into the duodenum and prevents reflux of duodenal contents into the ampulla. It also could be affected by autonomic insufficiency.

23 **The answer is C: Inferior epigastric artery.** The suprapubic aspect of the rectus abdominis muscle is supplied by the inferior epigastric artery. Therefore, this artery would need to be isolated, transected, and later grafted to the reconstruction site to ensure viable breast reconstruction. The inferior epigastric artery arises from the external iliac artery just superior to the inguinal ligament and courses toward the rectus sheath. During its course to the rectus sheath of the anterior abdominal wall, it lies along the inferomedial margin of the superficial inguinal ring. At this location, the inferior epigastric artery can be used to distinguish between direct and indirect inguinal hernias. If the inguinal hernia passes lateral to this artery, it is an indirect inguinal hernia, which traverses both the deep and superficial inguinal rings. Once within the rectus sheath, the inferior epigastric artery ascends posterior to the rectus abdominis muscle to anastomose with the superior epigastric artery near the umbilicus. **Choice A** (Superficial epigastric artery) is incorrect. The superficial epigastric artery arises from the femoral artery, below the inguinal ligament, and courses superior to supply the superficial inguinal lymph nodes and the superficial fascia and skin of the anterior abdominal wall. It may anastomose with the inferior epigastric artery, but the caliber of this artery is not adequate for blood supply to a myocutaneous flap. Furthermore, the superficial epigastric artery is not the main blood supply of the suprapubic aspect of the rectus abdominis muscle. **Choice B** (Superior epigastric artery) is incorrect. The superior epigastric artery arises from the internal thoracic artery at approximately the 6th intercostal space, and courses inferior to supply the rectus sheath, including the superior aspect of the rectus abdominis muscle. It anastomoses with the inferior epigastric artery near the umbilicus; however, the caliber of this artery is often considered inadequate for blood supply to a myocutaneous flap. Furthermore, the superior epigastric artery is not the main blood supply of the suprapubic aspect of the rectus abdominis muscle. **Choice D** (Inferior mesenteric) is incorrect. The inferior mesenteric artery arises from the abdominal aorta and supplies blood to the embryonic hindgut from approximately the distal portion of the transverse colon to the superior aspect of the rectum. It does not supply blood to the anterior abdominal wall, so it is not involved with a myocutaneous flap of the suprapubic portion of the rectus abdominis muscle. **Choice E** (Musculophrenic artery) is incorrect. The musculophrenic artery arises from the internal thoracic artery at approximately the 6th intercostal space and courses inferolateral along the superior aspect of the costal margin of the ribcage. It supplies blood to the anterior 7th to 9th intercostal spaces, the diaphragm, and the inferior aspect of the pericardium. Due to its location, it does not supply blood to the rectus sheath, so it is not involved with this myocutaneous flap.

24 **The answer is C: Myenteric plexus.** The cell bodies of postsynaptic (postganglionic) parasympathetic neurons populate the myenteric (Auerbach) plexus in the walls of the gut tube. These plexuses are located between the circular and longitudinal smooth muscle layers and regulate gut motility, including peristalsis. The myenteric plexus is a major component of the enteric nervous system. **Choice A** (Celiac plexus) is incorrect. The celiac plexus houses the cell bodies of postsynaptic sympathetic neurons. It is a preaortic plexus located around the base of the celiac trunk and serves as a synapse point in sympathetic distribution to the abdominal viscera. Presynaptic parasympathetic and visceral afferent fibers do pass through the preaortic ganglia but do not synapse within the celiac plexus. **Choice B** (Paravertebral ganglia) is incorrect. The paravertebral ganglia compose the sympathetic chain ganglia located on the sides of the vertebral column. They contain cell bodies of postsynaptic sympathetic neurons. **Choice D** (Hypogastric plexuses) is incorrect. The hypogastric plexuses are located on the posterior walls of the pelvic cavity. They mainly convey postsynaptic sympathetic fibers into the pelvis and presynaptic parasympathetic fibers out of the pelvis to the abdominal hindgut region. **Choice E** (Gray matter of sacral spinal cord segments) is incorrect. The gray matter of spinal cord segments S2-4 houses the cell bodies of presynaptic parasympathetic neurons that form the sacral parasympathetic outflow.

25 **The answer is B: Liver.**   The tumor within the head of the pancreas is leading to obstruction of the lower biliary tract, specifically the draining of the common bile duct. The common bile duct drains bile, produced in the liver, into the second part of the duodenum. This interruption of the biliary system by the pancreatic tumor blocks the flow of bile from the liver. One of the main components of bile is bilirubin, and as bilirubin levels increase within the liver due to the obstruction, the patient's sclera becomes icterus, a symptom of being jaundiced. The head of the pancreas is closely associated with the drainage site of the common bile duct, so this pancreatic tumor is causing posthepatic (or obstructive) jaundice, which is also called cholestasis. **Choice A** (Duodenum) is incorrect. The second part of the duodenum is the termination site of the common bile duct. It does not produce the bile, which when obstructed can ultimately lead to the icteric sclera and jaundiced appearance of this patient. **Choice C** (Gall bladder) is incorrect. The gall bladder stores and concentrates the bile produced in the liver. It does not produce its own secretory product. **Choice D** (Pancreas) is incorrect. Though the exocrine ducts of the pancreas may also be blocked by the presence of a tumor within the head of the pancreas, the obstruction of the secretory products of the pancreas would not lead to the patient's icteric sclera. **Choice E** (Stomach) is incorrect. The stomach is not involved with the biliary tract. Furthermore, blockage of the secretions of the stomach would not lead to the jaundiced appearance of this patient.

26 **The answer is B: Sympathetic supply to the ascending colon.**   The superior mesenteric plexus (ganglia) is an autonomic network around the base of the superior mesenteric artery. Presynaptic sympathetic fibers synapse at this location, and postsynaptic sympathetic fibers follow branches of this artery to distribute to the midgut organs, including the ascending colon. Presynaptic parasympathetic fibers from the vagus nerve and visceral afferents also pass through this plexus en route to and from the midgut. **Choice A** (Parasympathetic supply to the posterior aspect of the stomach)

is incorrect. Parasympathetic supply to the posterior stomach is derived directly from the posterior (right) vagus nerve as it descends from the esophagus. Further parasympathetic distribution to the foregut runs mainly from the posterior vagus through the celiac plexus and follows the celiac arterial axis. **Choice C** (Lymph drainage from the liver) is incorrect. Lymphatic drainage of the abdominopelvic organs mainly parallels the arterial supply to those organs, so lymphatic drainage of the liver flows toward the celiac nodes. Lymph drainage from the midgut organs flows to the superior mesenteric nodes, where it could be affected by a tumor invading this area. **Choice D** (Venous drainage from the transverse colon) is incorrect. The transverse colon is mostly related to midgut origins. However, venous drainage of the gut tube is primarily into the hepatic portal system rather than directly into systemic veins. Thus, most of the gut tube drains into the liver via the portal vein. **Choice E** (Visceral afferents from the proximal duodenum) is incorrect. The visceral afferents from the foregut and midgut regions mainly parallel the sympathetic supply to those organs. Thus, afferents from the proximal duodenum pass mainly through the celiac ganglia.

27 **The answer is A: Lateral femoral cutaneous nerve.**   This misguided professor presents with classic signs and symptoms of entrapment of the lateral femoral cutaneous nerve, which passes under the inguinal ligament in proximity to the anterior superior iliac spine, demonstrated in the given figure. Impingement of the lateral femoral cutaneous nerve is called meralgia paresthetica or bikini brief syndrome and results in abnormal sensations of burning, pain, and numbness in the lateral portion of the upper thigh. In the case of this progressive professor, his fashionable swimwear compressed the lateral femoral cutaneous nerve near the anterior superior iliac spine. Moreover, meralgia paresthetica is seen in individuals who have gained considerable weight (e.g., pregnancy) in a short period. **Choice B** (Femoral branch of the genitofemoral nerve) is incorrect. The femoral branch of the genitofemoral nerve is formed by the anterior rami of the L1-2 spinal nerves. This nerve supplies the upper medial aspects of the thigh. Due to the location of the patient's symptoms in the lateral aspect of his left upper thigh, this nerve is not involved. **Choice C** (Anterior cutaneous branches of femoral nerve) is incorrect. The anterior cutaneous branches of femoral nerve supply the upper medial aspect of the thigh. These nerves are derived from L2-4, and they are located too medial to elicit the symptoms in this fashion-conscious professor. **Choice D** (Ilioinguinal nerve) is incorrect. The ilioinguinal nerve arises from the lumbar plexus from the anterior ramus of the L1 spinal nerve. This nerve supplies the upper medial aspects of the thigh and gives off the anterior scrotal nerves involved in the afferent limb of the cremasteric reflex. Due to the location of the patient's symptoms in the lateral aspect of his left upper thigh, this nerve is not involved. **Choice E** (Iliohypogastric nerve) is incorrect. The iliohypogastric nerve arises primarily from the ventral ramus of L1, with possible contributions from T12. This nerve runs above the anterior superior iliac spine within the anterolateral muscular wall of the abdomen. However, if this nerve were involved, the abnormal sensations would have been located in the suprapubic region of the abdomen.

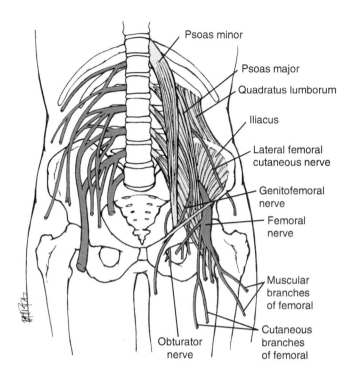

Psoas minor
Psoas major
Quadratus lumborum
Iliacus
Lateral femoral cutaneous nerve
Genitofemoral nerve
Femoral nerve
Muscular branches of femoral
Cutaneous branches of femoral
Obturator nerve

to repair. Therefore, it is usually removed in a splenectomy to prevent the patient from bleeding to death. Luckily, the spleen is not an essential organ, in that an individual can live without it. **Choice A** (Liver) is incorrect. The liver is the largest visceral organ, and it is highly vascularized. It is located mainly in the upper right quadrant of the abdomen, under the right dome of the diaphragm and deep to ribs 7 to 11. Thus, the liver is located on the opposite side of the body from the injury and is not likely the injured organ. The liver is an essential organ that cannot be removed in its entirety. **Choice B** (Stomach) is incorrect. The label is on an air space above contrast material in the stomach. The stomach is very mobile and distensible. Its base position is in the left upper quadrant of the abdomen, under the left dome of the diaphragm. However, it typically extends into the right upper quadrant. Because of its pliability, the stomach is rarely ruptured by fractured ribs. Also, it is not so vascular as to produce the level of internal bleeding seen in splenic injuries. **Choice D** (Erector spinae) is incorrect. The erector spinae is the largest component of the deep muscle layer in the back. It gives rise to three individual muscle columns: spinalis, longissimus, and iliocostalis. **Choice E** (Abdominal aorta) is incorrect. The abdominal aorta is slightly offset to the left anterior aspect of the vertebral body. It would not be damaged by fractured ribs. If ruptured in an automobile accident, as described here, the patient would likely have died before reaching the emergency room.

28 **The answer is E: Second part of the duodenum.** The vagus nerve conveys parasympathetic fibers to the gut tube and its derivatives as far distally as the left (splenic) flexure of the transverse colon. The second part of the duodenum is the only listed organ distal to the iatrogenic injury to the stomach but proximal to the left colic flexure. Thus, this organ would suffer loss of parasympathetic input. **Choice A** (Esophagus) is incorrect. Damaging the vagal trunk at the stomach would affect organs distal to the stomach but proximal to the left colic flexure, thus sparing the esophagus. **Choice B** (Urinary bladder) is incorrect. The urinary bladder is located below the level of supply of the vagus nerves. Therefore, it receives its parasympathetic innervation from nerves derived from sacral spinal cord outflow (S2-4) via the pelvic splanchnic nerves. **Choice C** (Descending colon) is incorrect. The descending colon is located distal to the supply of the vagus nerves. Therefore, it receives its parasympathetic innervation from nerves derived from sacral spinal cord outflow (S2-4) via the pelvic splanchnic nerves. **Choice D** (Prostate gland) is incorrect. The prostate is located below the level of supply of the vagus nerves. It also receives its parasympathetic innervation from the pelvic splanchnic nerves, derived from S2-4.

29 **The answer is C: Spleen.** The spleen is a large, highly vascular lymphatic organ located in the upper left quadrant of the abdomen, behind the stomach and deep to ribs 9 to 11. In its normal state, the spleen (as with the heart) is approximately the size of its owner's clenched fist on the handed side (e.g., right hand if right-handed). The spleen is frequently ruptured by fractured ribs or severe blows to the left upper quadrant of the abdomen, resulting in copious internal bleeding. Once ruptured, the spleen is very difficult

30 **The answer is C: Permanent relaxation of the pyloric sphincter.** The celiac ganglion (plexus) is the synapse point between presynaptic and postsynaptic sympathetic neurons that supply the celiac arterial axis (i.e., the foregut region). Sympathetic stimulation inhibits gut motility and glandular secretions and causes contraction of gut sphincters. Thus, disruption of synapses in the celiac ganglion will result in loss of sympathetic action, thus, relaxation of the pyloric sphincter. **Choice A** (Decreased secretions from the gastric glands on the anterior wall of the stomach) is incorrect. Gastric secretion is stimulated by parasympathetic input through the vagus nerves. Most of these fibers pass through the celiac plexus but synapse in the submucosal (terminal) plexuses in the walls of the stomach. The vagal branches to the anterior wall of the stomach descend from the anterior (left) vagus and do not run through the celiac plexus. Instead, they pass directly onto the stomach to synapse in the enteric plexuses there. **Choice B** (Reduced secretion of epinephrine from the adrenal [suprarenal] medulla) is incorrect. Secretion from the adrenal medulla is stimulated by sympathetic input. However, the sympathetic fibers to the adrenal medulla do not synapse in the celiac or other preaortic ganglia. Instead, they run into the medulla to synapse directly upon the adrenal medullary cells (chromaffin cells), which are modified postsynaptic sympathetic neurons. **Choice D** (Increased motility in the wall of the descending colon) is incorrect. Failure of sympathetic stimulation can result in increased gut motility, as this normally inhibits motility. However, the descending colon is derived from the embryonic hindgut. Its sympathetic input is through the inferior mesenteric plexus and would not be affected by disruption of the celiac plexus. **Choice E** (Paralysis of the quadratus lumborum muscle) is incorrect.

The quadratus lumborum lies in the posterior abdominal wall, connecting the 12th rib with the iliac crest. It is a skeletal muscle, innervated by somatic efferent neurons in spinal nerves T12–L3.

31 **The answer is D: Lienorenal ligament.** The lienorenal (splenorenal) ligament is the portion of the greater omentum that connects the hilum of the spleen with the left kidney. It conveys the splenic vessels and also contains the tail of the pancreas. The mesenteries are double layers of peritoneum that support the abdominopelvic viscera and transmit associated neurovascular structures. The splenic artery is the largest branch of the celiac trunk. It weaves along the superior border of the pancreas and enters the splenorenal ligament to reach the spleen. In its course, it gives branches to the pancreas, fundus and greater curvature of the stomach, and greater omentum. **Choice A** (Hepatoduodenal ligament) is incorrect. The hepatoduodenal ligament is the portion of the lesser omentum that attaches the porta hepatis of the liver to the first part of the duodenum. Its free margin forms the anterior wall of the epiploic foramen and conveys three significant structures: proper hepatic artery, bile duct, and portal vein. **Choice B** (Coronary ligament) is incorrect. The coronary ligament connects the diaphragmatic surface of the liver to the diaphragm. It defines the bare area of the liver but does not transmit any major neurovascular structures. **Choice C** (Transverse mesocolon) is incorrect. The transverse mesocolon attaches the transverse colon to the posterior abdominal wall. It transmits the middle colic vessels and associated nerves and lymphatics. **Choice E** (Gastrolienal ligament) is incorrect. The gastrolienal (gastrosplenic) ligament is the portion of the greater omentum that runs from the left part of the greater curvature of the stomach to the hilum of the spleen. It carries the short gastric and the left gastroomental (gastroepiploic) vessels.

32 **The answer is C: Inferior vena cava (IVC).** The omental (epiploic) foramen is the opening lying posterior to the hepatoduodenal ligament (the free edge of the lesser omentum). This passage connects the greater and lesser peritoneal sacs. The posterior boundary of the omental foramen is formed by the IVC and the right crus of the diaphragm, both of which lie retroperitoneally. Thus, pressure exerted posteriorly in the omental foramen can compress the IVC. **Choice A** (Bile duct) is incorrect. The anterior boundary of the omental foramen is formed by the hepatoduodenal ligament, which contains the bile duct, proper hepatic artery, and portal vein. These structures can be readily palpated and pinched between the index finger and the thumb when the index finger is inserted into the omental foramen. In Pringle's maneuver, the hepatoduodenal ligament is intermittently clamped to control hepatic bleeding during liver surgery. **Choice B** (Liver) is incorrect. The liver forms the superior boundary of the omental foramen. This opening can be located by tracing along the gall bladder until reaching the foramen. However, the gall bladder itself is not a boundary of the

omental foramen. **Choice D** (Abdominal aorta) is incorrect. The abdominal aorta lies to the left of the IVC. Thus, the aorta lies posterior to the lesser sac but not posterior to the omental foramen. **Choice E** (Head of the pancreas) is incorrect. The head of the pancreas lies cradled in the C-shaped concavity of the duodenum. The first part of the duodenum forms the inferior boundary of the omental foramen. Thus, the head of the pancreas is situated well below the omental foramen.

33 **The answer is C: Superior mesenteric to right renal.** To lower venous pressure within the portal system and temporarily alleviate symptoms secondary to portal hypertension, surgical venous anastomoses can connect a large caliber vein within the portal system to a similar vein within the systemic (caval) venous circulation. The portal vein drains blood from the gastrointestinal (GI) tract and the spleen, and it is formed by the union of the superior mesenteric and splenic veins posterior to the neck of the pancreas. A figure of the hepatic portal venous system is enclosed. Diseases of the liver, such as liver cirrhosis, can lead to a stenosis of the portal system, causing portal hypertension. Out of the listed choices, the only surgical venous anastomosis suggested which lowers the portal hypertension would be grafting the superior mesenteric vein to the right renal vein, creating an anastomosis between the portal and the systemic venous systems, respectively. **Choice A** (Inferior mesenteric to superior mesenteric) is incorrect. Surgical venous anastomoses between the inferior mesenteric and superior mesenteric veins, which are both components of the portal system, would not alleviate the signs and symptoms of portal hypertension. The inferior mesenteric vein usually drains into the splenic vein, but it has a common variation in which it drains directly into the superior mesenteric vein. To alleviate portal hypertension, surgical venous anastomoses must connect the portal system to the systemic (or caval) venous circulation. **Choice B** (Left gastric to splenic) is incorrect. As seen on the given figure, surgical venous anastomoses between the left gastric and splenic veins would not alleviate the signs and symptoms of portal hypertension because these veins are components of the portal venous system. To be effective, surgical venous anastomoses must connect the portal system to the systemic (or caval) venous circulation. **Choice D** (Right gastric to left gastric) is incorrect. As seen on the given figure, surgical venous anastomoses between the left gastric and gastric veins would not alleviate the signs and symptoms of portal hypertension because these veins are components of the portal venous system. Surgical venous anastomoses between the portal and systemic venous circulations need to be established. **Choice E** (Right testicular to right renal) is incorrect. Surgical venous anastomoses between the right testicular and right renal veins would not alleviate the signs and symptoms of portal hypertension because these veins are components of the systemic (caval) venous system. A surgical shunt between these veins would not alleviate the portal hypertension signs and symptoms.

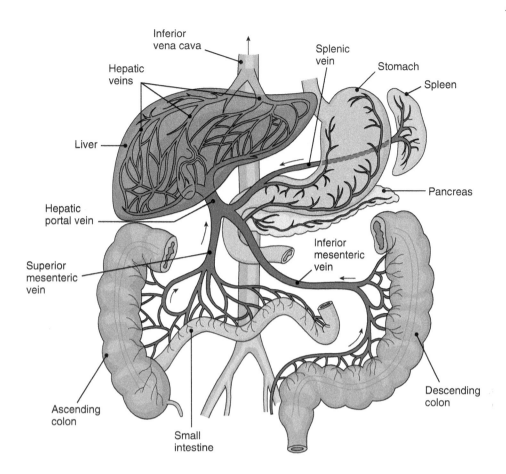

34 **The answer is E: Relaxation of the teniae coli in the descending colon.** Destruction of the sacral spinal cord will eliminate parasympathetic outflow to the hindgut, pelvic organs, and perineum as well as somatic innervation to much of the pelvis and lower limbs. Because it stimulates gut motility and tone, loss of parasympathetic input will result in relaxation and inactivity of the teniae coli in the descending colon. **Choice A** (Reduced sweat gland secretion in the abdominal wall) is incorrect. Sweat gland secretion is controlled by the sympathetic system, without parasympathetic balance. Sympathetic outflow is from the thoracolumbar spinal cord (T1-L2), and it would not be affected by loss of the sacral spinal cord segments. **Choice B** (Decreased motility in the duodenum) is incorrect. Decreased gut motility may be the result of loss of parasympathetic input. However, the duodenum is innervated by the vagus nerves, not the sacral spinal cord. **Choice C** (Increased motility in the ileum) is incorrect. Increased gut motility may result from the interruption of sympathetic input. However, the ileum receives its sympathetic input from the thoracolumbar spinal cord (T1-L2/3), not the sacral spinal cord. **Choice D** (Paralysis of the psoas major muscle) is incorrect. The psoas major is a large muscle in the posterior abdominal wall. It is a skeletal muscle supplied by somatic motor fibers via spinal nerves L2-3. Thus, the psoas major is not affected by loss of the sacral spinal cord segments.

35 **The answer is E: Proper hepatic.** The proper hepatic artery travels within the free edge of the hepatoduodenal ligament of the lesser omentum. Compression of this artery by an astute surgeon would reduce blood loss from the cut surface of the

cystic artery. The proper hepatic artery supplies the gallbladder, liver, and upper biliary tract. Within the hepatoduodenal ligament, it parallels the bile duct and the portal vein. These three structures, collectively termed the portal triad, are enveloped within the free edge of the lesser omentum, specifically its hepatoduodenal component. **Choice A** (Celiac) is incorrect. The celiac artery (trunk) arises from the abdominal aorta immediately after this artery traverses the diaphragm at the 12th thoracic (T12) vertebral level. The celiac artery supplies blood to the embryonic foregut from approximately the lower esophagus to the second part of the duodenum. While clamping this artery would reduce loss of blood from the cut edge of the cystic artery, this artery does not reside in the free edge of the hepatoduodenal ligament of the lesser omentum. Due to its deep origin from the aorta, compression of this artery is not feasible and would affect many organs, due to its extensive blood supply to the embryonic foregut. **Choice B** (Splenic) is incorrect. The splenic artery arises off the celiac trunk to supply the body of the pancreas, spleen, and greater curvature and fundic portion of the stomach. The splenic artery does not reside in free edge of the hepatoduodenal ligament of the lesser omentum, and compression of this artery would not limit bleeding from the cystic artery. **Choice C** (Gastroduodenal) is incorrect. The gastroduodenal artery arises off the common hepatic artery to supply the stomach, head of the pancreas, and first part of the duodenum. The gastroduodenal artery is not located in the hepatoduodenal ligament, and its compression would not control the bleeding of the cystic artery. **Choice D** (Common hepatic) is incorrect. Branches of the common hepatic artery do supply the gallbladder via the cystic artery. However, this artery is not located in the free edge of the hepatoduodenal ligament of the lesser omentum, so it was not the artery compressed by the attending surgeon.

36 **The answer is B: Superior mesenteric.**   Cancer cells from a lesion within the middle aspect of the transverse colon would likely metastasize in the superior mesenteric lymph nodes in advanced cancer staging. The superior mesenteric lymph nodes lie in the mesentery along the superior mesenteric artery and receive lymphatic drainage from the embryonic midgut. Because most lymphatic vessels supplying abdominal viscera follow arteries retrograde, lymph from the middle portion of the transverse colon, which receives arterial blood from the middle colic artery off the superior mesenteric artery, travels to the superior mesenteric nodes after traversing paracolic and middle colic lymph nodes. Therefore, cancer cells from a lesion of the middle aspect of the transverse colon may metastasize to the superior mesenteric nodes. Remember, when considering spread of cancer with abdominal visceral organs, it is crucial to remember the arterial supply of the organ in question. **Choice A** (Ileocolic) is incorrect. The ileocolic lymph nodes receive lymphatic drainage from the ascending colon and distal portion of the ileum of the small intestine and carry lymph to the superior mesenteric lymph nodes. Because these lymph nodes do not receive lymph from the middle aspect of the transverse colon, the ileocolic lymph nodes are not involved. **Choice C** (Celiac) is incorrect. The celiac lymph nodes are located along the celiac artery (trunk) and receive lymphatic drainage from the embryonic foregut, including the stomach, proximal duodenum, pancreas, spleen, gall bladder, and biliary tract. Because this cancerous lesion is located in a derivative of the embryonic midgut, the celiac lymph nodes are not involved. **Choice D** (Internal iliac) is incorrect. The internal iliac lymph nodes, which are located along the internal iliac artery and its branches, receive lymphatic drainage from the pelvic viscera, gluteal region, and deep parts of the perineum. Therefore, the internal iliac lymph nodes are not involved with the spread of cancer originating in the transverse colon. **Choice E** (Inferior mesenteric) is incorrect. The inferior mesenteric lymph nodes, which are located along the inferior mesenteric artery, receive lymphatic drainage from the descending colon, sigmoid colon, and superior aspect of the rectum. Therefore, the inferior mesenteric lymph nodes are not involved with the spread of cancer originating in the transverse colon.

37 **The answer is E: Ascending colon.**   The primary intestinal loop is the highly elongated, U-shaped embryonic midgut. The limbs of the "U" form cranial and caudal limbs in the midgut, with the vitelline duct residing at the apical bend. The caudal limb ultimately forms the lower (distal) ileum, cecum, appendix, ascending colon, and proximal 2/3 of the transverse colon. The cranial limb gives rise to the distal duodenum, jejunum, and upper (proximal) ileum. During its development, the primary intestinal loop undergoes a normal physiologic umbilical herniation through the umbilicus and into the extraembryonic coelom. As it returns to the fetal abdominal cavity, the loop rotates 270 degrees counterclockwise around the superior mesenteric artery and differentiates into its specific organ derivatives, which take their positions in the abdomen. Thus, malrotation of the reducing physiologic umbilical herniation can affect the proper formation and/or position of components of the midgut. **Choice A** (Descending colon) is incorrect. The descending colon is derived from the embryonic hindgut. It is not related to the primary intestinal loop or the physiologic umbilical herniation. **Choice B** (Stomach) is incorrect. The stomach is derived from the embryonic foregut. It is not related to the primary intestinal loop or the physiologic umbilical herniation. However, the stomach does undergo an important developmental rotation of 90 degrees clockwise about its longitudinal axis. This rotation affects the entire foregut and accounts for the placement of all its derived organs. **Choice C** (Spleen) is incorrect. The spleen is a lymphoid organ, which is not derived from any part of the gut tube. However, it is closely related to the foregut and is influenced by its rotation. **Choice D** (Fourth part of the duodenum) is incorrect. The duodenum is divided into four parts: superior (first) part, descending (second) part, horizontal (third) part, and ascending (fourth) part. The first two (upper or proximal) parts of the duodenum are derived from the foregut. The third and fourth (lower or distal) parts of the duodenum are derived from the midgut. The lower duodenum is derived from the cranial limb of the primary intestinal loop but is not affected by disorders of the caudal limb.

38 **The answer is A: Right kidney.**   The image is a coronal CT scan of the abdomen and pelvis. The kidneys lie retroperitoneally, against the posterior abdominal wall, extending from approximately vertebrae T12-L3. The right kidney is normally slightly lower than the left due to the superior position of the large liver. **Choice B** (Liver) is incorrect. The liver is the largest visceral organ. It is located mainly in the upper right quadrant of the abdomen, under the right dome of the diaphragm, underlying ribs 7 to 11. **Choice C** (Stomach) is incorrect. The stomach is very mobile and distensible. Its base position is in the left upper quadrant of the abdomen, under the left dome of the diaphragm. However, it typically extends into the right upper quadrant. **Choice D** (Spleen) is incorrect. The spleen is a large, highly vascular lymphoid organ. It is located deep to ribs 9 to 11 in the upper left quadrant of the abdomen, or lateral and posterior to the stomach. **Choice E** (Psoas major) is incorrect. The psoas major muscle lies against the posterior abdominal wall and runs from its origin at vertebrae T12-L5 to insert into the lesser trochanter of the femur. Together with the iliacus muscle, it forms the iliopsoas, the major flexor of the hip. This muscle is also important in flexing the trunk against the lower limb.

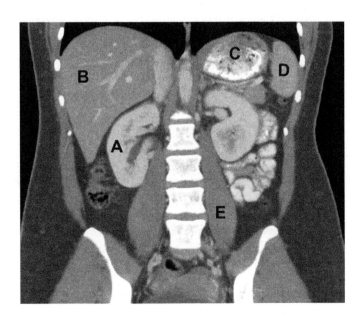

39 **The answer is B: Genital branch of the genitofemoral.** The genitofemoral nerve is a branch of the lumbar plexus, arising from the anterior rami of the L1-2 spinal nerves. Its genital branch runs through the inguinal canal within the spermatic cord to innervate the cremaster muscle and lateral aspect of the scrotum (or labium majus in women). The cremaster muscle is a thin layer of skeletal muscle surrounding the spermatic cord, which is derived from the internal abdominal oblique muscle. The cremaster contracts in response to cold temperature and cutaneous stimuli to raise the testicle upward, closer to the superficial inguinal ring. **Choice A** (Iliohypogastric) is incorrect. The iliohypogastric nerve originates from the lumbar plexus (L1). It supplies the internal oblique and transversus abdominis muscles in the anterolateral abdominal wall, and it has a cutaneous territory in the suprapubic (hypogastric) region of the anterior abdominal wall. **Choice C** (Femoral branch of the genitofemoral) is incorrect. The femoral branch of the genitofemoral nerve is formed by the anterior rami of the L1-2 spinal nerves. This nerve supplies the upper medial aspects of the thigh and the skin overlying the femoral triangle. **Choice D** (Femoral) is incorrect. The femoral nerve is a large branch of the lumbar plexus arising from the anterior rami of the L2-4 spinal nerves. It has extensive motor and cutaneous territories in the thigh and leg, but it is not responsible for the efferent limb of the cremasteric reflex. **Choice E** (Ilioinguinal) is incorrect. This nerve arises from the lumbar plexus from the anterior ramus of the L1 spinal nerve. It is the main route for the afferent limb of the cremasteric reflex. Its cutaneous territory is the upper medial thigh and anterior scrotum/labium majus.

40 **The answer is C: Superior mesenteric.** The superior mesenteric artery supplies the embryological midgut from the second part of the duodenum to the distal one third of the transverse colon. Branches of this artery, specifically ileal branches, need to be ligated before surgical repair of this diverticulum occurs. The ileal (Meckel) diverticulum depicted in this contrast radiograph is a true congenital diverticulum that is a vestigial remnant of the vitelline duct located in the distal ileum. **Choice A** (Celiac) is incorrect. The celiac artery supplies the embryological foregut from the distal portion of the esophagus to the second part of the duodenum. This artery does not supply blood to the distal ileum. **Choice B** (Renal) is incorrect. The renal arteries supply blood to the kidneys, the inferior aspects of the adrenal glands, and the proximal part of the ureters. Ligating this artery does not prevent bleeding of the distal ileum. **Choice D** (Inferior mesenteric) is incorrect. The inferior mesenteric artery supplies the embryological hindgut from the distal 1/3 of the transverse colon to the superior aspect of the rectum. Ligating this artery does not prevent bleeding in the distal ileum. **Choice E** (Umbilical) is incorrect. The umbilical arteries are usually not patent in adults and do not supply blood to the distal ileum.

41 **The answer is D: Omental bursa.** The omental bursa (or lesser peritoneal sac) is an isolated part of the peritoneal cavity, which lies posterior to the stomach and anterior to the pancreas. Because of its location, the omental bursa would receive digestive enzymes emanating from the lacerated section of the anterior pancreas. The only connection between the omental bursa and the remaining aspects of the peritoneal cavity is through the epiploic (omental) foramen. **Choice A** (Supracolic part of greater peritoneal sac) is incorrect. The supracolic part of greater peritoneal sac is located above the transverse mesocolon. Digestive enzymes emanating from a lacerated pancreas would only reach this space if the fluids traveled through the epiploic foramen. Remember, these fluids initially spill into the omental bursa. **Choice B** (Infracolic part of greater peritoneal sac) is incorrect. The infracolic part of greater peritoneal sac is located below the transverse mesocolon. Digestive enzymes emanating from a lacerated pancreas could only reach this space if the fluids traveled inferiorly via the right paracolic gutter to reach this lower aspect of the peritoneal cavity. However, these pancreatic enzymes would initially spill into the omental bursa. **Choice C** (Subhepatic space) is incorrect. The subhepatic space is a recess in the supracolic part of the greater peritoneal sac located between the visceral surface of the liver and the transverse colon. Digestive enzymes emanating from the anterior pancreas initially spill into the omental bursa. **Choice E** (Subphrenic space) is incorrect. The subphrenic space is a recess located in the anterior part of the liver and the diaphragm. Therefore, it is a component of the supracolic part of the greater peritoneal sac. Due to the superior location of the damaged organ, the subphrenic space is not a likely location to find the emitted pancreatic enzymes.

42 **The answer is E: Transversalis fascia.** The herniated small bowel would be covered by internal spermatic fascia, which is derived from the transversalis fascia of the abdominal wall. Therefore, the transversalis fascia is the deepest layer of the abdominal wall involved with this hernia. This baby boy presents with a congenital indirect inguinal hernia in which contents of the abdominal cavity, specifically the small intestine, herniate through a patent processus vaginalis to reside in the scrotum (see figure). The herniated bowel traverses the deep and superficial inguinal rings of the inguinal canal. **Choice A** (Transverse abdominal muscle) is incorrect. The transverse abdominal muscle is the deepest (of three) muscle of the anterolateral abdominal wall. Due to its position, the transverse abdominal muscle does not contribute a layer to the inguinal canal. **Choice B** (External oblique muscle) is incorrect. The external oblique muscle is the most superficial (of three) muscle of the anterolateral abdominal wall. As the testis descends into the scrotum, a derivative of this muscle called the external spermatic fascia forms a fascial layer of the spermatic cord. Due to its superficial location, the external oblique muscle is not the deepest layer of the abdominal wall associated with the herniated bowel. **Choice C** (Internal oblique muscle) is incorrect. The internal oblique muscle is the second (of three) muscle of the anterolateral abdominal wall. As the testicle descends into the scrotum, a derivative of this muscle called the cremasteric (or middle spermatic) fascia forms a fascial layer of the spermatic cord. Due to its intermediate location, the internal oblique muscle is not the deepest layer of the abdominal wall associated with the herniated bowel. **Choice D** (Rectus abdominis muscle) is incorrect. The rectus abdominis muscle is located within the rectus sheath, which is not associated with the inguinal canal. Therefore, this muscle does not contribute a derivative that would be involved with the herniated bowel.

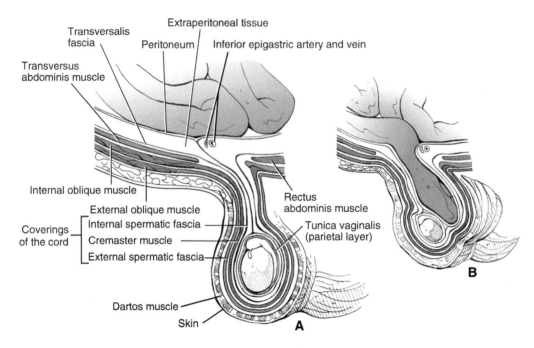

Extraperitoneal tissue

Transversalis fascia

Peritoneum   Inferior epigastric artery and vein

Transversus abdominis muscle

Internal oblique muscle

External oblique muscle

Coverings of the cord
- Internal spermatic fascia
- Cremaster muscle
- External spermatic fascia

Rectus abdominis muscle

Tunica vaginalis (parietal layer)

Dartos muscle

Skin

A

B

43 **The answer is C: Vagus nerves.** The vagus nerves are intimately wrapped around the esophagus and onto the stomach as they follow the gut tube into the abdomen. These nerves must be given close attention and care during repairs of the esophageal hiatus. **Choice A** (Thoracic duct) is incorrect. The thoracic duct passes through the aortic hiatus of the diaphragm, along the anterior aspect of the vertebral column, in its course from the abdomen into the thorax. **Choice B** (Azygos vein) is incorrect. The azygos vein passes through the aortic hiatus of the diaphragm, next to the thoracic duct, in its course from the abdomen into the thorax. **Choice D** (Sympathetic chains) is incorrect. The sympathetic chains pass behind the medial arcuate ligaments of the diaphragm, on the anterior surfaces of the psoas major muscles. **Choice E** (Superior epigastric vessels) is incorrect. The superior epigastric vessels pass through the sternocostal hiatus, at the anterior aspect of the diaphragm, in descending from the thorax into the abdomen.

Chapter 5

Pelvis and Perineum

QUESTIONS

Select the single best answer.

1 A pregnant woman in active labor receives an epidural anesthetic to relieve pain from her uterine contractions and cervical dilation in preparation for the birth of her child. Visceral sensory fibers project the pain derived from the dilation of the uterine cervix to what spinal cord level?

(A) T4
(B) L1
(C) L4
(D) S1
(E) S3

2 While performing a newborn checkup on a baby boy, a pediatrician discovers the external urethral orifice (urethral opening) is located on the ventral (bottom) surface of the penis, as depicted in the given illustration. What is the most likely diagnosis in this newborn?

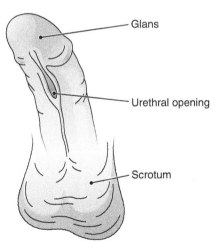

(A) Epispadias
(B) Hypospadias
(C) Micropenis
(D) Exstrophy of the bladder
(E) Cryptorchidism

3 A 72-year-old man comes to his urologist complaining of urinary frequency, urgency, weak urinary stream, hesitancy, and straining to void. A rectal examination and blood tests revealing normal prostate-specific antigen levels lead to a diagnosis of benign prostatic hyperplasia. The man undergoes a prostatectomy to remove the prostate gland. During the surgical procedure, the prostatic nerve plexus is damaged. What is the most likely complication of this surgery?

(A) Loss of sensation from the anus
(B) Fecal incontinence
(C) Erectile dysfunction
(D) Loss of sensation from the posterior scrotum
(E) Vasomotor dysfunction in the rectum

4 A 58-year-old postmenopausal mother (of four children) goes to her gynecologist complaining of discomfort and problems during micturition (emptying of the bladder). Physical examination reveals a herniation in the anterior aspect of the vaginal orifice, as illustrated below. What is the most likely diagnosis?

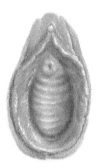

(A) Urinary tract infection
(B) Hydrocele
(C) Urethrocele
(D) Cystocele
(E) Rectocele

5 As part of a general pelvic examination, an obstetrician measures the diagonal conjugate diameter of the true pelvis in his 26-year-old pregnant patient. This measurement is taken between which of the following points?

(A) Ischial spine to the opposite ischial spine
(B) Sacral promontory to the inferior edge of the pubic symphysis
(C) Sacral promontory to the posterosuperior edge of the pubic symphysis
(D) Sacroiliac joint to the posterior side of the opposite side body of the pubis
(E) Tip of the coccyx to the pubic symphysis

6 A 24-year-old man comes to his family physician with an irregular scrotal swelling on his left, as seen in the given photo. He reports aching pain within the scrotum and a feeling of heaviness in his left testis. During the physical examination, the physician reports that the scrotal mass feels like a bag of worms. What is the most likely diagnosis?

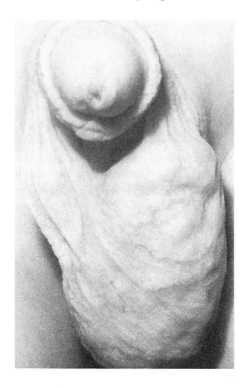

(A) Hydrocele
(B) Varicocele
(C) Testicular cancer
(D) Indirect inguinal hernia
(E) Spermatocele

7 A 72-year-old woman, who lost 50 lb (22.7 kg) of weight in the past year, visited her physician complaining of abdominal cramps, pain, and vomiting. Physical examination detected a distended abdomen with no visible or palpable masses in the groin and upper thigh area. She also described a sharp cutting pain in the medial aspect of her left thigh, which was exacerbated by the physician extending and medially rotating her left thigh at the hip joint. An abdominal CT revealed small bowel obstruction. What is the most likely cause of the obstruction?

(A) Direct inguinal hernia
(B) Indirect inguinal hernia
(C) Umbilical hernia
(D) Femoral hernia
(E) Obturator hernia

8 A 34-year-old woman presents with pain and discomfort related to an abscess in the posterior aspect of her left labium majus, as shown in the given photo. The abscess is determined to be derived from a greater vestibular (Bartholin) gland cyst. What group of lymph nodes should be checked first for lymphadenitis?

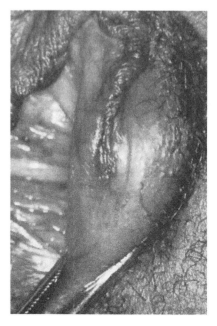

(A) Superficial inguinal
(B) Deep inguinal
(C) Lumbar
(D) External iliac
(E) Internal iliac

9 A genetic coding error during the 5th week of development causes a unilateral failure of development of the ureteric bud. This condition would directly affect the formation of which of the following structures?

(A) Proximal convoluted tubules
(B) Renal glomeruli
(C) Urinary bladder
(D) Uterine tube
(E) Ureter

10 A 25-year-old woman suffers a severe back injury in an automobile accident. Thorough examination in the ER reveals a fracture dislocation of T12 on L1 with a complete spinal cord transection that severes the sacral segments of the spinal cord, as noted by the black arrow on the given MRI. This patient will likely experience which of the following outcomes?

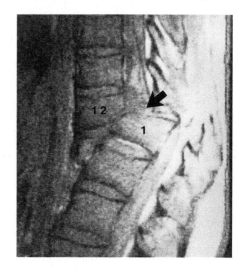

(A) Loss of voluntary control of defecation
(B) Intact ability to achieve erection of the clitoris
(C) Intact voluntary control of micturition
(D) Loss of ovulation
(E) Loss of sensation in the skin overlying the urinary bladder

11 A 20-year-old woman delivers a stillborn infant with bilateral agenesis of the kidneys. During the later stages of pregnancy, the fetus likely also had which of the following conditions?
(A) Polyhydramnios
(B) Oligohydramnios
(C) Renal hypoplasia
(D) Pelvic kidneys
(E) Polycystic kidneys

12 The given pelvic CT scan of a 65-year-old man who has been suffering from colon cancer reveals recurrent perirectal masses, indicated by the white arrows, which compress the pelvic splanchnic nerves. Damage to these nerves could affect the organs supplied by which of the following arteries?

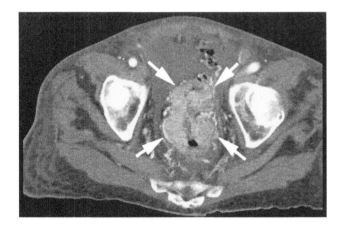

(A) Right colic artery
(B) Left colic artery
(C) Renal arteries
(D) Testicular arteries
(E) Lumbar arteries

13 A male infant is born with undescended testes that remain intra-abdominal 5 months later (cryptorchidism). Each testis possesses an elongate, distinctive gubernaculum testis running into the scrotum. Which of the following structures in female anatomy is homologous to the gubernaculum testis?
(A) Uterine tube
(B) Ureter
(C) Labium minus
(D) Round ligament of the uterus
(E) Vestibular bulb

14 A 52-year-old man riding his bicycle is struck by a passing car and thrown into a wall alongside the road. The given figure depicts the damage this man sustained to his pubic symphysis, anterior sacroiliac ligament, and sacrospinous ligament. Which of the following muscles is most likely damaged in company with the torn sacrospinous ligament?

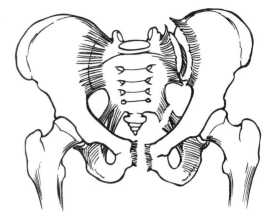

(A) Coccygeus
(B) External anal sphincter
(C) Iliococcygeus
(D) Pubococcygeus
(E) Puborectalis

15 A physician examining a 16-year-old girl for the first time notes that she is in good overall health and appears outwardly to have reached puberty. However, she explains that she has not yet had a menstrual period. Full physical and radiological examinations reveal a short, closed vaginal pouch, and no upper vagina, cervix, or uterus. Which of the following descriptions is the most likely cause of this condition?
(A) Atresia of the paramesonephric ducts
(B) Atresia of the mesonephric ducts
(C) Atresia of the urogenital sinus
(D) Imperforate hymen
(E) Agenesis of the ureteric bud

16 An obstetrician performs a median episiotomy to expand the birth canal during a childbirth, as shown in the photo. Which of the following structures is typically incised during this procedure?

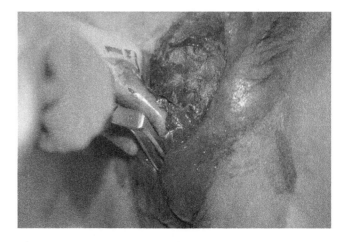

(A) Bulbospongiosus muscle
(B) Urethra
(C) Anal canal
(D) Ischiocavernosus muscle
(E) Perineal body

17 A medical resident is charged with catheterizing the urethra in a 68-year-old man in order to drain urine from the bladder. Which of the following sequence of structures correctly lists the order of the structures encountered when passing a catheter through the external urethral orifice to the urinary bladder?

(A) Navicular fossa, spongy urethra, membranous urethra, ductus deferens, prostatic urethra

(B) Navicular fossa, spongy urethra, membranous urethra, prostatic urethra, intramural urethra

(C) Spongy urethra, membranous urethra, prostatic urethra, intramural urethra, ureter

(D) Spongy urethra, membranous urethra, ejaculatory duct, ductus deferens, prostatic urethra

(E) Intramural urethra, prostatic urethra, membranous urethra, spongy urethra, navicular fossa

18 To reduce pain during her childbirth, an obstetrician performs a local nerve block on his 25-year-old patient while she is in the lithotomy position, as depicted in the given figure. Which of the following structures will remain fully sensitive following administration of this local anesthetic?

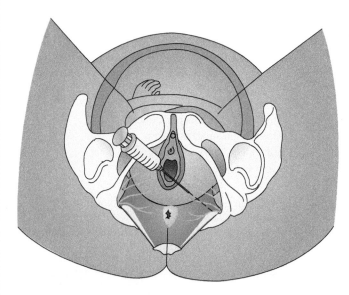

(A) Lower anal canal

(B) Rectum

(C) Perineal body

(D) Urogenital diaphragm

(E) Vulva

19 Development of the primitive gonads into testes or ovaries is induced by invasion of the genital ridges by the primordial germ cells. These cells migrate from which of the following locations?

(A) Paraxial mesoderm

(B) Intermediate mesoderm

(C) Lateral plate mesoderm

(D) Neural crest

(E) Yolk sac endoderm

20 The urinary system develops from which of the embryonic sources labeled in the given diagram?

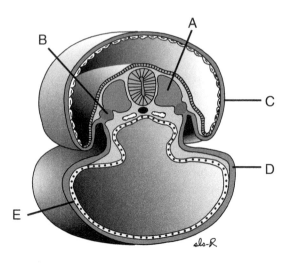

21 During micturition (urination), excitation of parasympathetic nerve fibers causes contraction of which of the following muscles?

(A) Pubococcygeus muscle

(B) Detrusor muscle

(C) Internal urethral sphincter

(D) Bulbospongiosus muscle

(E) External urethral sphincter

22 A 72-year-old man is brought to the ER after being struck by a car. Radiographic imaging reveals a rotationally unstable pubic ramus fracture, which is depicted in the given figure. Which of the following structures is most likely damaged specifically by the fracture of the superior pubic ramus?

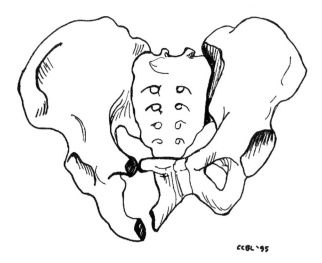

(A) Sympathetic chain

(B) Superior gluteal artery

(C) Ductus deferens

(D) Lumbosacral trunk

(E) Piriformis muscle

23 A 15-year-old girl delivering her first child at home with only her mother's help experiences a difficult birthing. As the baby's head passes through the birth canal, the perineum begins to tear. Which of the following muscles is the most likely to tear in this event?

(A) Coccygeus
(B) Ischiocavernosus
(C) Obturator internus
(D) Pubococcygeus
(E) External anal sphincter

24 A young boy has a chronic problem with urine dripping from abnormal openings on the underside (anterior or ventral side) of the glans and body of the penis, similar to those shown in the given photograph. Which of the following structures most likely did not fuse normally during development?

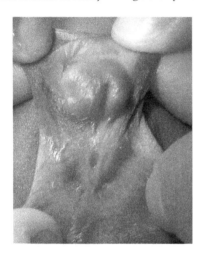

(A) Mesonephric ducts
(B) Paramesonephric ducts
(C) Urethral folds
(D) Scrotal swellings
(E) Genital tubercle

25 Familial dysautonomia is a rare genetic disorder characterized by abnormal functioning of the autonomic nervous system. Problems include difficulty in feeding and respiration, vasomotor instability, insensitivity to pain, and ataxia (an unsteady gait). Patients with this syndrome have low numbers of autonomic (visceral motor) neurons, probably related to defects in production and/or survival of the neural crest precursors of these neurons. Such a disorder could directly affect the innervation of the muscle cells in which of the following structures?

(A) Pelvic diaphragm
(B) External anal sphincter
(C) Urogenital diaphragm
(D) Internal urethral sphincter
(E) Levator ani

26 A 67-year-old man falls off his roof while cleaning his gutters. The impact of the landing causes a dislocation of his right hip joint and fractures his right superior and inferior pubic rami, as seen on the given X-ray. Which of the following structures is most likely damaged in company with this extensive trauma to the right lateral wall of the true pelvis?

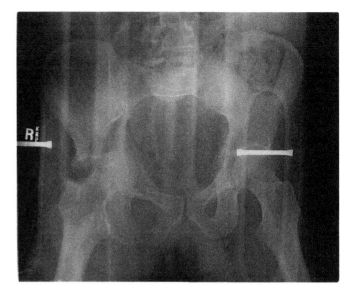

(A) Pubic symphysis
(B) Piriformis muscle
(C) Sacral promontory
(D) Obturator internus muscle
(E) Ganglion impar

27 Multiple tumors in the pelvic cavity cause widespread destruction through the hypogastric plexuses in a 67-year-old man. The nerve fibers that degenerate as a result of these lesions are mainly those of which of the following?

(A) Presynaptic sympathetic neurons
(B) Presynaptic parasympathetic neurons
(C) Postsynaptic parasympathetic neurons
(D) Somatic motor neurons
(E) General sensory neurons

28 The given sagittal MRI of a 45-year-old woman revealed severe uterine fibroids (noncancerous tumors) within the walls of the uterus. She underwent a complete hysterectomy, and the uterine artery was ligated near the junction of the uterus and vagina during the procedure. What structure would most likely be at risk during the ligation of the uterine artery?

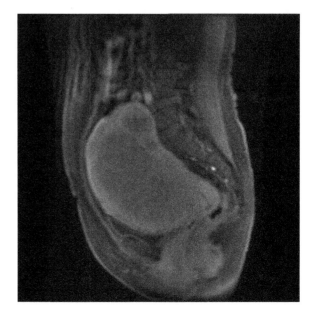

(A) Ureter
(B) Pudendal nerve
(C) Round ligament of the uterus
(D) Obturator artery
(E) Ovarian artery

29 A 65-year-old woman suffers chronic constipation. Which of the following events occurs when she strains heavily in attempting to pass her stool?
(A) Relaxation of the pubococcygeus
(B) Relaxation of the puborectalis
(C) Relaxation of the coccygeus
(D) Contraction of the external anal sphincter
(E) Contraction of the internal anal sphincter

30 After a blood test showed an elevated prostate-specific antigen level in a 65-year-old man, the given axial T2-weighted MRI of the prostate was obtained via an endorectal coil. The image shows abnormally low signal intensity within the right peripheral zone of the prostate, which is characteristic of an adenocarcinoma and is identified by the white arrowheads. A radical prostatectomy was scheduled. Before surgery, his physician wants to rule out possible metastases of the cancer. Which group of lymph nodes should be checked in the first instance to rule out metastases?

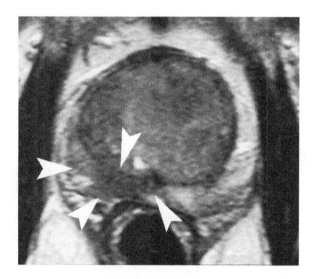

(A) Lumbar
(B) Deep inguinal
(C) Superficial inguinal
(D) Internal iliac
(E) External iliac

31 During dissection of deep pelvic lymph nodes in a 60-year-old man, the surgeon accidentally severs the internal pudendal artery at its origin. Which of the following structures will maintain its normal blood supply immediately following this lesion?
(A) Penis
(B) Urinary bladder
(C) Anal canal
(D) Scrotum
(E) Urogenital diaphragm

32 A 25-year-old man is admitted to the emergency room after a fall, complaining of lower back pain and paresthesia into the lower extremities. The given CT reveals a L2 burst fracture with a fracture fragment that is displaced posterior into the vertebral canal. A comprehensive neurologic examination indicates destruction of the sacral segments of the spinal cord. Which of the following functional outcomes is expected?

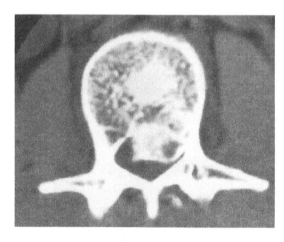

(A) Lowered sperm count
(B) Paralysis of the arrector pili muscles in the lower limbs
(C) Reduced sweat gland secretion in the lower limbs
(D) Inability to achieve erection
(E) Increased motility in the descending colon and rectum

33 A pregnant woman in active labor receives an epidural anesthetic to relieve pain from her uterine contractions and cervical dilation in preparation for the birth of her child. Pain derived from the labor contractions of the upper uterus is referred to what spinal cord level?
(A) T6
(B) T12
(C) L4
(D) S1
(E) S3

34 During the physical examination of a newborn male, a pediatrician noted a painless, tense, fluctuant scrotal mass on the left side. Shining a light toward the enlarged scrotal mass caused the left side of the scrotum to light up, as depicted in the given figure. What is the most likely diagnosis?

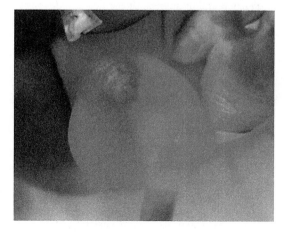

(A) Hydrocele
(B) Varicocele
(C) Indirect inguinal hernia
(D) Direct inguinal hernia
(E) Spermatocele

35 As part of a complete physical examination, an obstetrician conducts a digital vaginal examination of her 25-year-old patient. Which of the following structures is normally palpable through the posterior fornix?
(A) Urethra
(B) Ovaries
(C) Ischial spines
(D) Perineal body
(E) Ureters

36 A 31-year-old woman delivers her first child via natural childbirth, without anesthetics. During the delivery, she experiences painful spasms in the muscles in the medial part of her right thigh and paresthesia in the skin in the medial thigh. Following delivery, these conditions gradually dissipate. Which of the following nerves may have been compressed during this childbirth?
(A) Inferior gluteal nerve
(B) Pudendal nerve
(C) Obturator nerve
(D) Sciatic nerve
(E) Pelvic splanchnic nerves

37 A 24-year-old woman is the driver of a car in a head-on collision. She suffers bilateral fractures of the pubic rami and dislocation of the pubic symphysis as a result of anteroposterior compression of the pelvis, as shown in the given X-ray. Which of the following structures is most likely damaged in this patient?

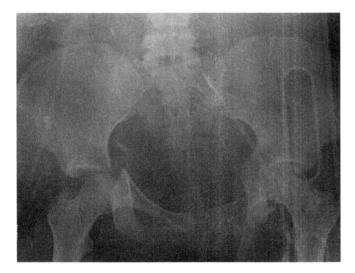

(A) Anal canal
(B) Piriformis muscles
(C) Urinary bladder
(D) Uterus
(E) Vagina

38 A 26-year-old medical student noticed a lump on his left testis, which was later diagnosed as testicular cancer. To rule out metastases of the testicular cancer, what group of lymph nodes should be checked in the first instance?
(A) Superficial inguinal
(B) Deep inguinal
(C) Lumbar
(D) External iliac
(E) Internal iliac

39 A forensic anthropologist is called to the basement of an abandoned house, where an intact human skeleton has been discovered in a shallow grave. Without the benefit of soft tissue, the gender of the body can still be established based upon the characteristics of the two unearthed coxal (hip) bones. Which of the following characteristics is indicative of the female pelvis?
(A) Subpubic angle less than 70 degrees
(B) Heart-shaped (android) pelvic inlet
(C) More inverted ischial tuberosities
(D) More everted alae of the ilia
(E) Ischial spines close together in the midline

40 The given axial T2-weighted MRI of the prostate of a 50-year-old man was obtained via an endorectal coil. The image shows prostate cancer with extracapsular spread, indicated by the black arrow, which damages the neighboring hypogastric plexuses. Lesions of these nerves are most likely to result in which of the following deficits?

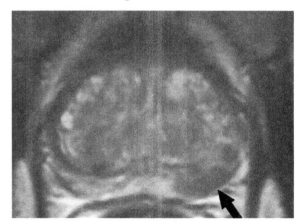

(A) Inability to control the detrusor muscle
(B) Inability to control the external anal sphincter
(C) Chronic increased motility in the sigmoid colon
(D) Reduced sensation on the glans penis
(E) Loss of vasomotor control in the lower limb

41 A 70-year-old patient with a history of hypercholesterolemia complains of severe cramps in his gluteal region despite no history of physical exertion in the past few days. An arteriogram shows atherosclerotic blockage leading to insufficient perfusion to the gluteal region. What artery is most likely occluded leading to his complications?
(A) External iliac
(B) Internal iliac
(C) Femoral
(D) Internal pudendal
(E) Abdominal aorta

42 An abscess is detected between the perineal membrane and the inferior fascia of the pelvic diaphragm in a 27-year-old man. Which of the following structures would most likely be affected by this abscess within the deep perineal space?

(A) Bulbourethral glands
(B) Perineal body
(C) Superficial transverse perineal muscles
(D) Bulbospongiosus muscles
(E) Ischiocavernosus muscles

43 A painful abscess is located in the ischioanal fossa of a 39-year-old man. The given CT reveals the abscess contains air, indicated by the arrows, and displaces the rectum to the right. Which of the following locations should the surgeon avoid during drainage of the abscess to prevent damage to the pudendal nerve and internal pudendal vessels?

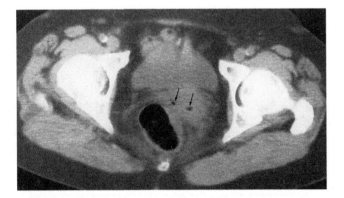

(A) Roof of the ischioanal fossa
(B) Lateral wall of the ischioanal fossa
(C) Medial wall of the ischioanal fossa
(D) Posterior recess of the ischioanal fossa
(E) Anterior recess of the ischioanal fossa

44 A 16-year-old boy, who was riding his skateboard down a stair railing, falls and impacts his perineum on the railing, causing a straddle injury. He presents in the ER with discoloration and swelling in the scrotum, penis, and anterior abdominal wall, which is characteristic of extravasation of urine. Which of the following structures is most likely compromised?

(A) Ureter
(B) Urinary bladder
(C) Prostatic urethra
(D) Intermediate urethra
(E) Spongy urethra

ANSWERS AND DISCUSSION

1 **The answer is E: S3.** Visceral sensory fibers relaying pain from the lower part of the uterus (cervix) and upper part of the vagina are referred to the S2-4 spinal cord levels, as these organs are located below the pelvic pain line, which generally corresponds to the lower limit of the peritoneum. Because visceral sensory fibers follow the visceral motor (autonomic) fibers retrograde, visceral pain from the uterine cervix will follow the presynaptic parasympathetic nerves of the pelvic splanchnic nerves retrograde to spinal cord levels S2-4. Conversely, pelvic and lower abdominal organs located above the pelvic pain line are, by definition, in contact with or located above the peritoneum, and their visceral sensory fibers follow the visceral motor fibers retrograde to refer pain to the lowest limits of the sympathetic (thoracolumbar) nervous system located at spinal cord levels T11-L2. Therefore, labor pains derived from the dilation of the uterine cervix will be referred by visceral sensory fibers to the S3 spinal cord level. **Choice A** (T4) is incorrect. Visceral sensory fibers associated with the T4 spinal cord level would be involved in conveying visceral pain associated with the heart and lungs, due to traveling retrograde with cardiopulmonary splanchnic nerves derived from postsynaptic sympathetic fibers from T1 to T6. **Choice B** (L1) is incorrect. The uterine cervix is located below the peritoneum, which implies it is below the pelvic pain line. Because visceral sensory fibers follow the visceral motor (autonomic) fibers retrograde, visceral pain from the uterine cervix will follow the presynaptic parasympathetic nerves of the pelvic splanchnic nerves retrograde to the spinal cord levels S2-4. However, pain derived from the labor contractions of the upper uterus, which is in contact with the peritoneum and thus located above the pelvic pain line, travel via visceral sensory fibers that follow the visceral motor fibers retrograde to refer pain to the lowest limits of the sympathetic (thoracolumbar) nervous system located at spinal cord levels T11-L2. Though pain derived from the labor contractions of the upper uterus refer to the L1 vertebral level, this question asked specifically about labor pains derived from the dilation of the uterine cervix, which would be referred to the S2-4 vertebral levels. **Choice C** (L4) is incorrect. Visceral sensory fibers carrying pain from visceral organs and involuntary (smooth or cardiac) muscle follow retrograde to the pathway of the visceral motor (autonomic) nerve fibers. There are no presynaptic autonomic nerve fibers that arise from L4, so there are no visceral sensory nerves associated with this spinal cord level. **Choice D** (S1) is incorrect. Visceral sensory fibers carrying pain from visceral organs and involuntary (smooth or cardiac) muscle follow retrograde to the pathway of the visceral motor (autonomic) nerve fibers. Because there are no presynaptic autonomic nerve fibers that arise from S1, there are no visceral sensory nerves associated with this spinal cord level.

2 **The answer is B: Hypospadias.** Hypospadias is a congenital defect of the external genitalia, in which the external urethral orifice is incompletely developed and located along the ventral (bottom) surface of the penis. This common anomaly of the external genitalia is seen in approximately 1:300 newborn males. It may be easy to detect due to the presence of a hooded foreskin, i.e., a foreskin that is developed normally on the dorsal (top) and sides of the glans penis but not the ventral

(bottom) surface, not appreciated in the figure. Though a hooded foreskin is common in newborns with hypospadias, the foreskin can be completely formed in approximately 5% of the cases. The severity of hypospadias can also vary greatly. The mildest form, glanular (first degree) hypospadias, occurs in approximately 60% of the cases. Penile (second degree) hypospadias occurs in approximately 25% of cases and is described as the external urethral orifice being located along the anterior shaft of the penis from the midshaft of the penis to the subcoronal region (ventral to the glans penis). Penile hypospadias is illustrated in the given drawing. Finally, perineal (third degree) hypospadias results in approximately 15% of cases. In this condition, the external urethral orifice is located in the perineum, midscrotum, or base of the penis. During development in males, the phallus elongates, and paired urogenital (urethral) folds come together in the midline and fuse to enclose the penile urethra. Hypospadias results when the urogenital folds fail to fuse completely along the midline. **Choice A** (Epispadias) is incorrect. Epispadias is a rare congenital defect of the external genitalia, seen in 1:120,000 newborn males. In this malformation, the external urethral orifice is located along the dorsal (top) surface of the penis between the pubic bones and the dorsal surface of the glans penis. Epispadias can result in a short, widened penis with an abnormal curvature, reflux nephropathy (backward flow of urine into the kidney), and urinary tract infections. Epispadias results when the primordium of the genital tubercle develops in the region of the urorectal septum, so when the urogenital membrane ruptures, clefts are formed on the dorsal aspect of the phallus. Epispadias is often associated with exstrophy of the bladder, in which the bladder is exposed due to a defect in the anterior abdominal wall. The etiology of these defects may be due to insufficient migration of mesodermal tissue to the area cranial to the genital tubercle. Due to the external urethral orifice being located on the ventral (bottom) surface of the penis in this patient, hypospadias is the correct diagnosis. **Choice C** (Micropenis) is incorrect. Micropenis is a penis with normal developmental features that is well below the normal size range for an infant. It is caused by lack of growth during development, often due to reduced androgen production. Treatment of micropenis in infancy can be achieved with injections of human chorionic gonadotropin or testosterone. **Choice D** (Exstrophy of the bladder) is incorrect. Exstrophy of the bladder is a rare congenital abnormality in which the bladder is everted through a midline defect in the lower anterior abdominal wall. It is thought to be caused by insufficient migration of mesodermal tissue to the lower portion of the abdominal wall, and it often presents with epispadias, widening of the pubic symphysis, and maldescent of the testes. **Choice E** (Cryptorchidism) is incorrect. Cryptorchidism is the absence of one or both of the testes within the scrotum due to maldescent of the testes. This finding was not noted in this patient.

3 **The answer is C: Erectile dysfunction.** The cavernous nerves of the penis supply parasympathetic (visceral motor; autonomic) fibers to erectile (cavernous) tissues of the penis, stimulating penile erection. These nerves arise from the prostatic portion of the pelvic nerve plexus, which surrounds the capsule of the prostate, and it is at this location that the cavernous nerves can be damaged during prostatectomy.

After enveloping the prostatic capsule, the cavernous nerves descend to penetrate the perineal membrane to reach erectile tissues of the penis, providing parasympathetic stimulation. This innervation causes the helicine arteries of the penis, the coiled terminal branches of the deep and dorsal arteries of the penis, to uncoil, enabling blood at arterial pressure to fill the cavernous tissue causing penile erection. Thus, damage to these nerves would most likely result in erectile dysfunction. **Choice A** (Loss of sensation from the anus) is incorrect. The sensation from the skin surrounding the anus is conveyed by the inferior anal (rectal) nerves, which are branches of the pudendal nerve. The pudendal nerve exits the pelvis via the greater sciatic notch and enters the perineum through the lesser sciatic notch to supply the external anal sphincter and its surrounding skin, the superficial and deep perineal compartments, and the external genitalia. Neither the inferior anal or pudendal nerves would be at risk during a prostatectomy due to their posterior locations. **Choice B** (Fecal incontinence) is incorrect. Fecal incontinence may be due to loss of innervation to the external anal sphincter, which is supplied by the inferior anal (rectal) nerves, which are branches from the pudendal nerve. Due to the posterior location of the pudendal nerve, it would not be at risk during a prostatectomy. **Choice D** (Loss of sensation from the posterior scrotum) is incorrect. The sensation from the posterior scrotum is supplied by the posterior scrotal nerve, which is a superficial perineal branch of the pudendal nerve. Due to the inferior and posterior locations of the posterior scrotal and pudendal nerves, they would not be at risk during a prostatectomy. **Choice E** (Vasomotor dysfunction in the rectum) is incorrect. The vasomotor functions of the rectum are supplied by the rectal plexus, which is derived from the inferior hypogastric plexus. The rectal plexus contains visceral motor (parasympathetic and sympathetic) fibers, but due to its proximity to the lateral sides of the rectum, it would be unlikely for it to be at risk during a prostatectomy.

4   **The answer is D: Cystocele.**   A cystocele is a herniation of the urinary bladder into the anterior aspect of the vagina through a tear in the pubocervical fascia, which separates the bladder from the vagina. This fascia is often torn during childbirth (parturition), creating a passage for the herniation of the bladder. A cystocele often causes discomfort or problems during micturition due to the change in the normal position of the bladder. Because estrogen strengthens the elastic tissues around the vagina, a cystocele may not occur until menopause, when levels of estrogen decrease. Therefore, a cystocele is the most likely diagnosis due to the patient being a postmenopausal mother (of four children) and the location of the herniated bladder in the anterior aspect of the vaginal orifice. **Choice A** (Urinary tract infection) is incorrect. Patients with urinary tract infections often present with dysuria, pain during voiding of urine, which is reported in this patient. However, this diagnosis does not account for the herniation in the vaginal orifice. **Choice B** (Hydrocele) is incorrect. A hydrocele testis is a pathological accumulation of serous fluids within the spermatic cord of the testis due to serous secretions from a remnant piece of peritoneum, termed the tunica vaginalis. This diagnosis can be easily eliminated in this female patient. **Choice C** (Urethrocele) is incorrect. A urethrocele is a prolapse of the urethra

into the vestibule of the vagina, in which the inner lining of the urethra sticks out through the external urethral orifice. A urethrocele may occur with a cystocele, but in these cases, a distinct groove is usually seen between the border of the prolapsed urethra and bladder, not seen in this illustration. Interestingly, a urethrocele may occur in prepubertal girls and presents as a small pink donut-shaped mass (with the external urethra orifice making the hole of the donut) in the vestibule of the vagina. This condition is often detected by a parent who finds a small amount of blood in the child's underwear, and it can be treated with an estrogen cream to strengthen the elastic fibers around the urethra. Anatomical knowledge of the location of the female urethra being anterior to the vagina rules out this diagnosis because the herniation was located in the anterior aspect of the vaginal orifice. **Choice E** (Rectocele) is incorrect. A rectocele is a herniation of rectal tissue through a tear in the rectovaginal septum, which separates the rectum from the vagina. It is detected in the posterior aspect of the vaginal orifice. A rectocele may be present in women following childbirth or hysterectomy, but this diagnosis can be ruled out by the location of the herniation in the anterior aspect of the vaginal orifice.

5   **The answer is B: Sacral promontory to the inferior edge of the pubic symphysis.**   The true (obstetrical) conjugate diameter of the true pelvis (see Discussion point C below) cannot be measured directly in a manual pelvic exam because of the presence of the urinary bladder. Therefore, the next best approximation of that, the diagonal conjugate, is measured instead (see the given figure). This measurement is taken by first palpating the sacral promontory with the tip of the middle finger of the gloved examining hand. Next, the other hand marks the position of the inferior edge of the pubic symphysis on the examining hand. Finally, after withdrawing the examining hand, the distance from the tip of the index finger to the marked point for the symphysis is measured to obtain an estimate of the true conjugate. This distance should be 11.5 cm or greater. The diameters of the true pelvis are important measurements in determining the capacity of the pelvic canal for childbirth. **Choice A** (Ischial spine to the opposite ischial spine) is incorrect. This measurement is the interspinous distance in the pelvis. Because the ischial spines project into the true pelvis and toward one another, this distance is normally the narrowest part of the pelvic (birth) canal. However, the interspinous length is not a fixed distance because of normal relaxation of pelvic ligaments and added joint mobility during pregnancy. **Choice C** (Sacral promontory to the posterosuperior edge of the pubic symphysis) is incorrect. This measurement is the true (obstetrical) conjugate of the true pelvis. It is the narrowest fixed distance (diameter) of the true pelvis and indicates the smallest anteroposterior space available for the fetal head to pass during vaginal delivery. **Choice D** (Sacroiliac joint to the posterior side of the opposite side body of the pubis) is incorrect. This distance is the oblique diameter of the true pelvis. It is a diameter that usually is noted via radiographic imaging rather than manual palpation. **Choice E** (Tip of the coccyx to the pubic symphysis) is incorrect. This distance indicates the anteroposterior diameter of the pelvic outlet. However, it is not a fixed distance because of enhanced pelvic mobility during pregnancy.

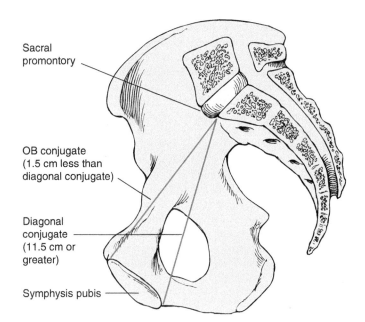

Sacral
promontory

OB conjugate
(1.5 cm less than
diagonal conjugate)

Diagonal
conjugate
(11.5 cm or
greater)

Symphysis pubis

6   **The answer is B: Varicocele.** A varicocele is an abnormal dilation of the pampiniform plexus of veins, which travels within the spermatic cord. This scrotal mass often resembles and feels like a "bag of worms" on physical examination, as seen in the photo. Idiopathic varicocele is usually caused by defective one-way valves within the pampiniform plexus, which cause dilatation of these veins near the testis. However, a secondary varicocele will be seen following compression of the venous drainage of the testis due to the presence of a pelvic or abdominal malignancy, and this possibility must be ruled out by the physician. Varicoceles are found in the left side in approximately 98% of cases, can develop in 15% to 20% of all males, and are most frequently diagnosed between 15 and 25 years of age. **Choice A** (Hydrocele) is incorrect. A hydrocele testis is a pathological accumulation of serous fluids within the spermatic cord due to serous secretions from a remnant piece of peritoneum, termed the tunica vaginalis. Patients with a hydrocele testis present with a painless swollen testis that feels like a water balloon, which may be corrected via drainage with a needle (aspiration) or surgery. To identify a hydrocele, a diagnostic technique called transillumination (shining a light through the enlarged portion of the scrotum) can be implemented. If the scrotum is full of clear fluid, the scrotum will light up. A hydrocele testis is not likely in this patient due to the irregular nature of the scrotal mass seen within the photo. **Choice C** (Testicular cancer) is incorrect. Testicular cancer presents with a lump on or hardening of the testis leading to unilateral enlargement of the affected testis, abnormal sensitivity within the testes, dull pain within the lower back, abdomen, or groin, loss of libido, and general weakness and tiredness. The extent of the scrotal mass and its irregular nature make the diagnosis of testicular cancer unlikely. If testicular cancer were present, it would not grow to this size without the patient noticing its presence. Moreover, the cardinal sign for testicular cancer is unilateral enlargement of the testis; however, in a varicocele, the testis is usually smaller on the affected side. **Choice D** (Indirect inguinal hernia) is incorrect. An indirect inguinal hernia is usually a congenital hernia that results when abdominal cavity contents herniate through a patent processus vaginalis, or in an adult, travel through the inguinal canal. The hernia traverses the deep and superficial inguinal

rings to descend into the scrotum in males. The hernia often presents as a visible or palpable lump underneath the skin in the groin region, which was seen in this patient. However, given the irregular nature of this scrotal mass and the physician's observation that the mass felt like a "bag of worms," a varicocele is more likely. **Choice E** (Spermatocele) is incorrect. A spermatocele is a cyst-like mass within the scrotum that develops in a tubule of the rete testis or the head of the epididymis. It usually contains a milky fluid and spermatozoa. These retention cysts are usually not painful and can be confirmed by an ultrasound of the scrotum. Given the irregular nature, size, and "bag of worms" description of the scrotal mass in this patient, a varicocele is the most likely diagnosis.

7   **The answer is E: Obturator hernia.** An obturator hernia can present with small bowel obstruction and lancinating (sharp cutting) pain in the medial thigh region. This type of hernia is most often seen in elderly females (over the age of 70), especially women who have recently lost a large amount of weight. It occurs when a portion of the small bowel is entrapped within the confines of the obturator canal, which compresses the obturator nerve and leads to sharp cutting pain within its distribution pattern. When a physician is able to exacerbate this pain by extension, medial rotation, and adduction of the thigh at the hip joint, it is called a positive Howship-Romberg sign, which is further suggestive of an obturator hernia. Remember that an obturator hernia does not present with visible lumps because the herniation is trapped under the muscles of the medial compartment of the thigh. **Choice A** (Direct inguinal hernia) is incorrect. A direct inguinal hernia is an acquired hernia that results when abdominal cavity contents herniate through a weakness in the anterior abdominal wall in the inguinal (Hesselbach) triangle. The hernia traverses the superficial inguinal ring and often presents as a visible or palpable lump underneath the skin overlying the superficial inguinal ring, which was not present in this patient. Moreover, direct inguinal hernias are rare in women; in fact, some references cite groin hernias are 25 times more likely to occur in men than women. **Choice B** (Indirect inguinal hernia) is incorrect. An indirect inguinal hernia is usually a congenital hernia that results when abdominal cavity contents herniate through a patent processus vaginalis, or in an adult, the inguinal canal. The hernia exits through the deep and superficial inguinal rings and descends into the labium majus of females or the scrotum of males. An indirect inguinal hernia often presents as a visible or palpable lump underneath the skin in the groin region, and this finding was not reported in this patient. **Choice C** (Umbilical hernia) is incorrect. Umbilical hernias are protrusions in the umbilical region that can be congenital (seen in newborns) or acquired (occurring later in life). These hernias present as a visible or palpable lump underneath the skin in the umbilical region, and this finding was not reported in this patient. **Choice D** (Femoral hernia) is incorrect. A femoral hernia is a protrusion through the femoral ring that extends into the femoral canal and compresses its contents (lymphatic vessels and connective tissue). Initially the hernia is contained in the femoral canal; however, it may extend inferiorly to the saphenous hiatus where it creates a bulge within the femoral triangle. The femoral ring is a weakened aspect in the anterior abdominal wall through which femoral hernias enter the femoral canal. These hernias are more common in females due to their wider pelves and often contain abdominal viscera. Moreover, femoral hernias are more susceptible to strangulation, wherein the blood supply to the herniated viscera can be interrupted due to the sharp boundaries of the femoral ring, particularly the lacunar ligament. Strangulation can lead to ischemia, sharp pain, and necrosis of the impinged tissue. However, a patient with a femoral hernia would not present with sharp cutting pain in the medial aspect of the thigh or a positive Howship-Romberg sign (exacerbation of this pain after extending and medially rotating the thigh at the hip joint).

8 **The answer is A: Superficial inguinal.** Superficial inguinal lymph nodes, which are located in the subcutaneous tissue near the termination of the great saphenous vein, receive lymphatic drainage from the lower abdominal wall, buttock, lower limb, and all of the perineum and external genitalia, except for the glans clitoris. Therefore, the superficial inguinal lymph nodes should be checked initially for lymphadenitis in the case of a cyst located on the labium majus. **Choice B** (Deep inguinal) is incorrect. Deep inguinal lymph nodes, which are located deep to the fascia lata and medial to the femoral vein, receive lymphatic drainage directly from the glans clitoris, deep structures of the lower limb, and indirect lymphatic drainage from the superficial inguinal lymph nodes. Because the lymphatic drainage of the posterior labium majus drains to the superficial inguinal lymph nodes initially, these nodes should be checked for lymphadenitis before the deep inguinal nodes. **Choice C** (Lumbar) is incorrect. Lumbar lymph nodes, which are located anterior to the lumbar vertebrae and surrounding the inferior vena cava and abdominal aorta, receive lymphatic drainage directly from the posterior abdominal wall, gonads (ovaries and testes), kidneys, ureters, uterus, and uterine tubes. Because the lymphatic drainage of the posterior labium majus drains to the superficial inguinal lymph nodes initially, these nodes should be checked for lymphadenitis before the lumbar nodes. **Choice D** (External iliac) is incorrect. The external iliac lymph nodes, which are associated with the external iliac vein, receive lymphatic drainage from pelvic organs in direct contact with the peritoneum, including the superior bladder and superior pelvic ureters. Because the lymphatic drainage of the posterior labium majus drains to the superficial inguinal lymph nodes initially, these nodes should be checked for lymphadenitis before the external iliac nodes. **Choice E** (Internal iliac) is incorrect. The internal iliac lymph nodes, which are located along the internal iliac artery and its branches, receive lymphatic drainage from the pelvic viscera, gluteal region, and deep parts of the perineum. Because the lymphatic drainage of the posterior labium majus drains to the superficial inguinal lymph nodes initially, these nodes should be checked for lymphadenitis before the internal iliac nodes.

9 **The answer is E: Ureter.** The permanent kidneys develop from two sources: (1) the ureteric bud and (2) the metanephric mesoderm. The ureteric bud is an outgrowth of the mesonephric duct near its junction with the cloaca. It forms the renal collecting ducts, including the ureter, renal pelvis, renal calyces, and collecting tubules. The ureteric bud invades the metanephric mesoderm, inducing it to form a metanephric cap over its distal end. The cap differentiates into the kidney parenchyma and the nephrons (i.e., the excretory and functional units in the kidney). **Choice A** (Proximal convoluted tubules) is incorrect. The metanephric mesoderm forms the nephrons in the kidney, including Bowman capsule, the proximal convoluted tubule, loop of Henle, and distal convoluted tubule. Nephrons are formed throughout prenatal development. **Choice B** (Renal glomeruli) is incorrect. Renal glomeruli are small capillary bundles that form in association with Bowman capsule. They are not derived from either the ureteric bud or the metanephric mesoderm. **Choice C** (Urinary bladder) is incorrect. The urinary bladder is derived from the cloaca. The cloaca divides into a urogenital sinus and an anal canal, which are located anterior and posterior, respectively. The urogenital sinus subsequently differentiates into the urinary bladder and urethra. **Choice D** (Uterine tube) is incorrect. The uterine tube is formed from the paramesonephric duct. More caudally, the paired paramesonephric ducts join together to form the uterus, cervix, and cranial third of the vagina.

10 **The answer is A: Loss of voluntary control of defecation.** The sacral part of the spinal cord (segments S2-4) gives rise to the pudendal nerve. This nerve leaves the pelvic cavity and passes into the perineum, where it has a wide distribution. The first major branch of the pudendal nerve is the inferior anal (rectal) nerve to the inferior end of the anal canal, external anal sphincter, and perianal skin. The external anal sphincter is the voluntary anal sphincter, controlled by somatic motor fibers. It acts to constrict the end of the anal canal, resisting defecation. Thus, loss of the sacral segments of the spinal cord results in loss of voluntary control of defecation, as well as loss of sensation in the anal canal inferior to the pectinate line and in the perianal skin. Involuntary control of defecation is governed by the internal anal sphincter, a thickening of the circular smooth muscle layer in the wall of the upper part of the anal canal, which is controlled by autonomic (visceral motor) fibers. **Choice B** (Intact ability to achieve erection of the clitoris) is incorrect. Erection of the clitoris (and penis) is controlled by parasympathetic outflow from the sacral segments of the spinal cord (S2-4). Thus, destruction of the sacral cord results in loss of erection rather than intact control. **Choice C** (Intact voluntary control of micturition) is incorrect. The pudendal nerve also controls the external sphincter muscle of the urethra, which is the voluntary sphincter that regulates urination (micturition), via its perineal branches. Thus, loss of the sacral spinal cord segments will cause loss of voluntary control of urination rather than intact voluntary control. **Choice D** (Loss of ovulation) is incorrect. Ovulation is not controlled by direct neural input. Thus, loss of the sacral spinal cord will not affect ovulation. **Choice E** (Loss of sensation in the skin overlying the urinary bladder) is incorrect. The skin overlying the urinary bladder is that of the pubic (suprapubic; hypogastric) region of the lower abdominal wall. Cutaneous sensation here is conveyed by the ilioinguinal and iliohypogastric nerves, both branches of the first lumbar segment of the spinal cord. Because only the sacral segments of the spinal cord were destroyed by the transection of the spinal cord, this sensation in the pubic region of the lower abdominal wall would remain intact. Remember, the medullary cone (conus medullaris) of the spinal cord typically lies within the T12-L3 vertebral levels, so only the sacral segments of the spinal cord were destroyed in this injury.

11 **The answer is B: Oligohydramnios.** Oligohydramnios is a diminution in the volume of amniotic fluid as a result of the fetus' failure to excrete urine into the amniotic sac, for example, as resulting from renal agenesis or urethral obstruction. Renal agenesis occurs when the ureteric bud fails to develop, thus preventing formation of the kidney. Normally, the fetus produces urine and excretes it into the amniotic cavity, where it mixes with the amniotic fluid. The fetus drinks amniotic fluid, which is absorbed into the bloodstream, filtered at the placenta, and excreted by the fetus. Thus, the prenatal kidneys are not necessary for waste exchange but are important in regulating the volume of amniotic fluid. In renal agenesis (no kidneys), urine is not produced and not secreted, thus reducing the volume of fluid in the amniotic sac (oligohydramnios). The given obstetric sonographic image, an ultrasound-based diagnostic imaging technique, depicts severe oligohydramnios associated with bilateral renal agenesis. In this image, the spine (Sp) of the infant is noted, and the shadow, which is highlighted by the black arrowheads, corresponds to the adrenal gland. The kidneys are absent. Bilateral renal agenesis is relatively rare, with a usual ultimate outcome of stillbirth or death soon after birth. Unilateral renal agenesis is relatively more common, often asymptomatic, and compatible with life, as the remaining kidney typically hypertrophies and produces an appropriate volume of urine. **Choice A** (Polyhydramnios) is incorrect. Polyhydramnios is an increased volume of amniotic fluid in the amniotic sac. In this case, the kidneys are normal, and urine is produced and excreted into the amniotic sac. However, obstruction (atresia) of the gut tube prevents the fetus from drinking and/or absorbing that fluid, resulting in accumulation of greater volume of fluid in the amniotic sac. **Choice C** (Renal hypoplasia) is incorrect. Renal hypoplasia is a condition of abnormally small kidneys. In renal agenesis, the kidneys are not formed. **Choice D** (Pelvic kidneys) is incorrect. In the case of pelvic kidneys, the kidneys are formed; however, one or both fail to ascend from their origination point in the pelvis. Thus, they are ectopic, located in the pelvis or lower lumbar region, and fully functional. **Choice E** (Polycystic kidneys) is incorrect. Here, the kidneys are formed. However, the collecting ducts and tubules are dilated, forming multiple, large fluid-filled cysts within the kidney parenchyma.

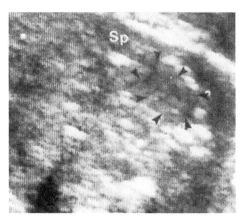

12 **The answer is B: Left colic artery.** The pelvic splanchnic nerves provide the sacral parasympathetic outflow that supplies the gut tube below the left colic flexure, the pelvic viscera, and the perineum. Part of the distribution route for the parasympathetic nerves to the descending colon, sigmoid colon,

and upper rectum (i.e., to most of the hindgut) is to hitch-hike along the arterial branches that supply those organs. Because the left colic artery is the parent vessel to those structures, damage to the pelvic splanchnic nerves would affect the organs supplied by the left colic artery. **Choice A** (Right colic artery) is incorrect. The right colic artery carries parasympathetic fibers derived from the vagus nerve to the ascending colon. This vessel/organ pairing is outside the pelvic splanchnic territory. **Choice C** (Renal arteries) is incorrect. These vessels supply the kidneys and suprarenal glands. Again, any parasympathetic supply to these organs is derived from vagal branches that travel with the renal arteries. **Choice D** (Testicular arteries) is incorrect. The gonads do not receive autonomic innervation. Thus, it is questionable if the gonadal vessels convey any parasympathetic fibers. **Choice E** (Lumbar arteries) is incorrect. The lumbar arteries supply structures in the posterior abdominal wall (e.g., psoas muscles, vertebral column). Parasympathetic nerves do not supply the body walls and limbs. Thus, the lumbar arteries do not convey parasympathetic fibers.

13 **The answer is D: Round ligament of the uterus.** Both the round ligament of the uterus and the ovarian ligament are the homologues of the gubernaculum testis. In males, the testes descend along a path formed by the caudal genital ligament and gubernaculum testis. In females, the same structures guide the ovaries in their descent. However, the upward growth of the reproductive tract and different hormonal influences disrupt full ovarian descent. When the ovaries settle into their final position in the lateral aspect of the true pelvis, the remnants of the caudal genital ligament and gubernaculum are retained as the ovarian ligament and round ligament of the uterus. The round ligament extends through the inguinal canal and into the labium majus, marking what would be the full descent pathway in males. **Choice A** (Uterine tube) is incorrect. The uterine tubes (and uterus, cervix, and superior third of the vagina) are derived from the embryonic paramesonephric ducts. In males, the paramesonephric ducts are suppressed, and the only remnant is the vestigial appendix of the testis. **Choice B** (Ureter) is incorrect. The ureter is formed from the ureteric bud, an outgrowth of the mesonephric duct. Overall, the ureteric bud gives rise to the renal collecting ducts, including the ureter, renal pelvis, renal calyces, and collecting tubules. **Choice C** (Labium minus) is incorrect. The labia minora are formed from the embryonic urethral (urogenital) folds. In males, these folds fuse in the midline to form the ventral (anterior) aspect of the penis enclosing the penile urethra. In females, the folds do not fuse, forming the separate labia minora. **Choice E** (Vestibular bulb) is incorrect. The vestibular bulbs are formed from the more posterior part of the embryonic phallus, which is continuous with the urethral folds. In males, this area fuses in the midline to form the corpus spongiosum and bulb of the penis. In females, the structures remain separate and form the bulbs of the vestibule, underlying the labia minora.

14 **The answer is A: Coccygeus.** The sacrospinous ligament runs from the pelvic surface of the lower sacrum to the ischial spine. It aids in resisting loading-induced sacral rotation that could disarticulate the sacroiliac joint. The coccygeus muscle, the most posterior component of the pelvic diaphragm, attaches to the ischial spine and sacrospinous ligament. Often, the muscle is so well intertwined with the ligament that it is difficult to differentiate the two. Thus, damage to the ligament typically also includes damage to the muscle. Developmentally, the epimysium of the coccygeus muscle modifies and thickens to form the sacrospinous ligament, which underscores the intimate relation between these two structures. **Choice B** (External anal sphincter) is incorrect. The external anal sphincter is a multilayered skeletal muscle bundle encircling the lower anal canal. It is entirely subcutaneous, having no bony or ligamentous attachments. **Choice C** (Iliococcygeus) is incorrect. This component of the pelvic diaphragm originates from the tendinous arch of the obturator fascia on the lateral wall of the true pelvis. In the fetus, the muscle originally attaches to the pelvic brim along the arcuate line of the ilium, explaining the *ilio*-part of its name. During development, it shifts downward onto the thickened obturator fascia to reach its final position. **Choice D** (Pubococcygeus) is incorrect. This anterior component of the pelvic diaphragm originates from the pelvic side of the pubic bone. It is at the opposite end of the pelvic diaphragm from the sacrospinous ligament. **Choice E** (Puborectalis) is incorrect. This part of the pelvic diaphragm originates from the pubic bone and forms a loop around the anorectal junction with its opposite side mate. It is not related to the sacrospinous ligament.

15 **The answer is A: Atresia of the paramesonephric ducts.** In females, the paired embryonic paramesonephric ducts form the uterine tubes, uterus, cervix, and superior third of the vagina. Thus, if the paramesonephric ducts are absent (atretic), these organs do not form. The lower 2/3 of the vagina develops from the sinovaginal bulbs, which are paired evaginations of the wall of the urogenital sinus. The two parts of the vagina (paramesonephric duct part and sinovaginal bulb part) canalize to form a single, complete vaginal canal. However, without the paramesonephric duct components, only a short vaginal pouch forms. Because the ovaries form from the indifferent embryonic gonads, they can still develop normally, providing the hormonal stimuli to puberty. **Choice B** (Atresia of the mesonephric ducts) is incorrect. In females, the mesonephric ducts are normally suppressed. Only small vestigial structures form in association with the reproductive tract. However, because the ureteric bud develops from the mesonephric duct, the renal collecting ducts would not form in case of atresia there. **Choice C** (Atresia of the urogenital sinus) is incorrect. The urogenital sinus gives rise to the urinary bladder and the urethra. In addition, in females, the sinovaginal bulbs evaginate from the wall of the urogenital sinus and form the lower 2/3 of the vagina. Thus, with atresia of the urogenital sinus, the lower part of the vagina would be absent or imperforate, whereas the upper vagina, cervix, uterus, and uterine tubes would be intact. Further, one would expect malformation of the urinary bladder and/or urethra. **Choice D** (Imperforate hymen) is incorrect. The hymen is the thin plate of tissue that separates the vestibule from the lumen of the vagina. Remember, the sinovaginal bulbs originate as solid tissue masses off the posterior wall of the urogenital sinus. When these sinovaginal bulbs canalize to form the vaginal lumen, the hymen remains at the junction of the urogenital sinus and vagina. It usually develops one or more small openings during postnatal life. **Choice E** (Agenesis of the ureteric bud) is incorrect. The ureteric bud is an outgrowth from the wall of the mesonephric duct. It forms the renal collecting ducts, including the ureter, renal pelvis, renal calyces, and collecting tubules. Additionally, it induces the formation of the metanephric cap that forms the kidney parenchyma and the nephrons (i.e., the excretory units in the kidney).

16 **The answer is E: Perineal body.** An episiotomy is a surgical incision from the posterior wall of the vagina into the perineum posterior to the vagina. This procedure is used to gain a controlled enlargement of the vaginal canal during childbirth. In a median episiotomy, the incision is made in the midline and extends through the perineal body (see diagram). The advantage of this procedure is that it may decrease excessive reduction of the perineal body and minimize trauma to the pelvic diaphragm and perineal muscles. An alternate procedure is the posterolateral episiotomy. In this protocol, the incision begins in the median line and then is directed laterally and posteriorly toward the ischial tuberosity. The advantage here is that the perineal body is spared. **Choice A** (Bulbospongiosus muscle) is incorrect. The bulbospongiosus is the skeletal muscle sheath surrounding the individual vestibular bulbs. The bulbs are located deep to the labia minora, lateral to the vaginal opening. Thus, the bulbs are anterior to the incision line in either type of episiotomy and are not cut. **Choice B** (Urethra) is incorrect. The urethra is anterior to the vagina. It is not in the line of incision in an episiotomy and is not cut. **Choice C** (Anal canal) is incorrect. The anal canal is directly in the line of incision in a median episiotomy. However, the incision normally stops short of the anal canal. It is undesirable to have a communication between the anal and vaginal canals because of the danger of anal material contacting the fetus during delivery. **Choice D** (Ischiocavernosus muscle) is incorrect. The ischiocavernosus is the thin skeletal muscle layer surrounding the crus of the clitoris. Each crus is attached to the ischiopubic ramus, lateral to the vagina and anterior to the ischial tuberosity. Thus, the crus of the clitoris would not be incised because it is located off the median sagittal plane.

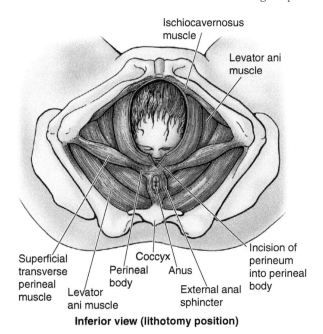

Ischiocavernosus muscle

Levator ani muscle

Superficial transverse perineal muscle

Levator ani muscle

Coccyx

Perineal body

Anus

External anal sphincter

Incision of perineum into perineal body

Inferior view (lithotomy position)

17 **The answer is B: Navicular fossa, spongy urethra, membranous urethra, prostatic urethra, intramural urethra.** The urethra is a continuous tube that can be divided into four main parts: (1) spongy urethra, (2) membranous (intermediate) urethra, (3) prostatic urethra, (4) intramural urethra, which can be seen in the given figure. The urethra terminates (or begins for catheter insertion) at the external urethral orifice. The spongy (penile) urethra is the longest part, running though the corpus spongiosum in the penis. The distal end of the spongy urethra is the expanded navicular fossa within the glans penis. The membranous (intermediate) urethra passes through the deep perineal compartment and is the narrowest segment of the urethra. The prostatic urethra, which is the widest and most distensible part of the urethra, traverses the prostate gland. The final segment, the intramural (preprostatic) urethra, extends through the neck of the urinary bladder. Because the urethral wall is thin, it can be ruptured easily by inserted instruments. Thus, understanding and properly navigating the curved pathway of the urethra are critical. **Choice A** (Navicular fossa, spongy urethra, membranous urethra, ductus deferens, prostatic urethra) is incorrect. The ductus (vas) deferens is not part of the urethral pathway to the urinary bladder. The ductus deferens empties into the prostatic urethra after joining the duct of the seminal

vesicle to form the ejaculatory duct. **Choice C** (Spongy urethra, membranous urethra, prostatic urethra, intramural urethra, ureter) is incorrect. The ureter is not part of the urethral pathway to the bladder. The paired ureters drain into the urinary bladder separately from the bladder drainage into the urethra. The two ureteric orifices plus the urethral orifice mark the angles of the trigone of the bladder. **Choice D** (Spongy urethra, membranous urethra, ejaculatory duct, ductus deferens, prostatic urethra) is incorrect. The ejaculatory duct and the ductus deferens are not parts of the urethral pathway to the urinary bladder. The ductus deferens joins with the duct of the seminal vesicle to form the ejaculatory duct, which empties into the prostatic urethra. **Choice E** (Intramural urethra, prostatic urethra, membranous urethra, spongy urethra, navicular fossa) is incorrect. This sequence is the correct order of urethral segments through which urine would leave the urinary bladder to exit the external urethral orifice, but the inverse order of structures encountered when inserting a catheter into the urinary bladder.

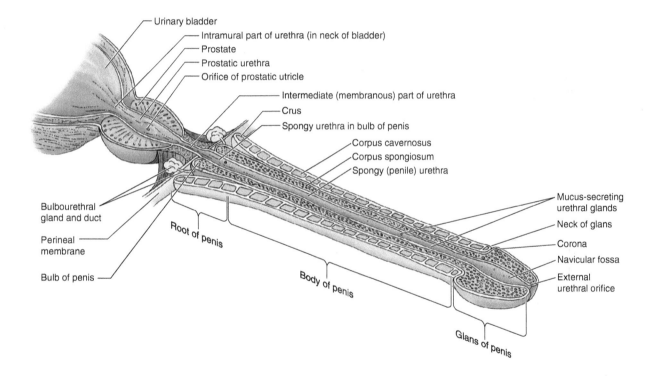

18 **The answer is B: Rectum.** The illustration shows a pudendal nerve block, which anesthetizes the area innervated by the pudendal nerve, that is, the majority of the perineum, including the lower vagina and lower anal canal. The rectum lies above the perineum and is supplied by visceral sensory fibers from the hypogastric plexuses rather than by the pudendal nerve. Thus, it retains visceral sensation following a pudendal block. The block is accomplished by injecting a local anesthetic into the tissues around the pudendal nerve where it crosses the sacrospinous ligament near the ischial spine. Achieving total anesthesia of the perineum additionally requires blocking the ilioinguinal nerve (covering the anterior perineum) and perhaps the posterior cutaneous nerve of the thigh (for the extreme posterior perineum). **Choice A** (Lower anal canal) is incorrect. The lower anal canal (i.e., the area below the pectinate line) receives general sensory innervation through the inferior anal (rectal) nerve, a branch of the pudendal nerve.

Thus, this area is anesthetized by a pudendal block. **Choice C** (Perineal body) is incorrect. The perineal body is a dense connective tissue mass in the center of the perineum. This area is innervated by branches of the pudendal nerve. **Choice D** (Urogenital diaphragm) is incorrect. The urogenital diaphragm is a musculofascial complex within the urogenital triangle of the perineum. Its major component is the external urethral sphincter. This area is supplied by the perineal branches of the pudendal nerve. Remember, the anatomical concept of the urogenital diaphragm has changed considerably in recent years. It is important to reference the most current texts for a proper understanding of the morphology here so as not to be confused by the traditional, inaccurate description. **Choice E** (Vulva) is incorrect. The vulva is the part of the perineum in females containing the external genitalia, which includes the mons pubis, labia majora and minora, vestibule of the vagina, clitoris, and bulbs of the vestibule. The vulva is innervated largely by the dorsal nerve of the clitoris and the perineal nerves, all branches of the pudendal nerve. However, of note, the anterior aspect of the vulva (especially the mons pubis and anterior labia majora) is mainly supplied by the ilioinguinal nerve. Thus, a pudendal nerve block greatly reduces sensation in the vulva but likely does not provide total anesthesia.

19 **The answer is E: Yolk sac endoderm.** The primordial germ cells originate in the epiblast and migrate to the caudal endodermal wall of the yolk sac, near the allantois. From there, they migrate along the dorsal mesentery of the gut tube to the genital ridges. Once they invade the genital ridges, they induce the primitive gonads to develop into either testes or ovaries. **Choice A** (Paraxial mesoderm) is incorrect. The paraxial mesoderm is the thickened portion of mesoderm closest to the midline and neural tube. It becomes segmented and forms somites, which further differentiate into myotome, dermatome, and sclerotome units that form skeletal muscles, dermis, and most of the vertebral column, respectively. **Choice B** (Intermediate mesoderm) is incorrect. The intermediate mesoderm is the small bridge of mesoderm that connects the paraxial mesoderm with the lateral plate mesoderm. It differentiates into urogenital structures, including the kidney parenchyma and nephrons and the gonads. Thus, the intermediate mesoderm is the target of the migrating primordial germ cells rather than their source. **Choice C** (Lateral plate mesoderm) is incorrect. The lateral plate mesoderm is a relatively flat, wide area, which divides into the parietal (somatic) mesoderm and visceral (splanchnic) mesoderm. The parietal part becomes associated with the wall of the amniotic sac, ultimately forming (along with the ectoderm) the lateral body wall folds. The visceral part joins with the endodermal lining of the yolk sac and forms the wall of the gut tube. **Choice D** (Neural crest) is incorrect. The neural crest forms at the free lips of the neural folds, dissociates from the neural tube, and spreads widely across the body. Crest cells form a diverse assortment of structures, including melanocytes, neural ganglia, craniofacial skeleton, and odontoblasts.

20 **The answer is B: Intermediate mesoderm.** The intermediate mesoderm is a small bridge of mesoderm that connects the paraxial mesoderm with the lateral plate mesoderm. It differentiates into urogenital structures, including the kidney parenchyma and nephrons, and the gonads. **Choice A** (Paraxial mesoderm) is incorrect. The paraxial mesoderm is the thickened portion of mesoderm closest to the midline and neural tube. It becomes segmented and forms somites, which further differentiate into myotome, dermatome, and sclerotome units that form skeletal muscles, dermis, and most of the vertebral column, respectively. **Choice C** (Parietal [somatic] mesoderm) is incorrect. This derivative of the lateral plate mesoderm becomes associated with the wall of the amniotic sac. Ultimately, it forms (along with the ectoderm) the lateral body wall folds and gives rise to the dermis plus the bones and connectives tissues in the body wall and limbs. **Choice D** (Visceral [splanchnic] mesoderm) is incorrect. The visceral (splanchnic) mesoderm is the other derivative of the splitting of the lateral plate mesoderm. It joins with the endodermal lining of the yolk sac and forms the wall of the gut tube. **Choice E** (Yolk sac endoderm) is incorrect. This germ layer becomes associated with the visceral mesoderm to form the wall of the gut tube. Specifically, it forms the lining of the gut tube.

21 **The answer is B: Detrusor muscle.** The smooth muscle walls of the urinary bladder are composed mainly of the detrusor muscle. Parasympathetic input during urination stimulates the detrusor to contract, thus emptying the bladder into the urethra. **Choice A** (Pubococcygeus muscle) is incorrect. The pubococcygeus muscle is a skeletal muscle that forms part of the levator ani in the pelvic diaphragm. It acts to support and lift the pelvic floor. Its contraction is evoked by somatic motor branches of the sacral plexus, including branches of the pudendal nerve. **Choice C** (Internal urethral sphincter) is incorrect. The internal urethral sphincter is a smooth muscle bundle located at the internal urethral orifice in the neck of the urinary bladder in males. During urination (in males), parasympathetic stimulation causes the internal urethral sphincter to relax, allowing urine to flow into the urethra. An organized internal urethral sphincter is not present in females. **Choice D** (Bulbospongiosus muscle) is incorrect. The bulbospongiosus is a skeletal muscle enveloping the bulb of the penis in males and the individual vestibular bulbs in females. During urination in males, contraction of the muscle squeezes the bulb, assisting in draining the penile urethra. However, the innervation of the bulbospongiosus muscle is via somatic motor fibers of the perineal nerves. **Choice E** (External urethral sphincter) is incorrect. The external urethral sphincter is composed of skeletal muscle and acts as the voluntary urethral sphincter to constrict the urethra and prevent urination. The innervation of the external urethral sphincter is controlled by somatic motor fibers in the perineal nerves.

22 **The answer is C: Ductus deferens.** The ductus (vas) deferens separates from the spermatic cord as the cord emerges from the deep inguinal ring. The ductus crosses over the external iliac vessels and enters the true pelvis over the pelvic brim at the superior pubic ramus. It then runs along the lateral pelvic wall and on to the posterolateral side of the urinary bladder. Thus, fractures of the lateral wall of the true pelvis, especially those at the superior pubic ramus, endanger the ductus deferens. **Choice A** (Sympathetic chain) is incorrect. The sympathetic chain crosses the pelvic brim at the ala of the sacrum to enter the true pelvis. It descends along the pelvic surface of the sacrum and finally terminates as the ganglion impar. Therefore, the sympathetic chain is situated in relation to the roof of the posterior wall of the true pelvis and is not in position to be affected by a lateral wall fracture. **Choice B** (Superior gluteal artery) is incorrect. The superior gluteal artery branches from the posterior division of the internal iliac artery, within the true pelvis. It immediately leaves the pelvis through the greater sciatic foramen at the upper margin of the piriformis muscle. This vessel does not cross the pelvic brim and is not in position to be affected by a fracture of the brim. **Choice D** (Lumbosacral trunk) is incorrect. The lumbosacral trunk is formed by the union of the L4 and L5 ventral primary rami as they descend into the true pelvis to merge with the sacral plexus. These nerves cross the ala of the sacrum and typically form the lumbosacral trunk below the pelvic brim, within the true pelvis. However, the junction may occur at a higher level. In either case, the lumbosacral trunk is related to the roof of the posterior wall of the true pelvis rather than to the lateral wall. **Choice E** (Piriformis muscle) is incorrect. The piriformis muscle originates from the pelvic surface of the superior part of the sacrum, lateral to the anterior sacral foramina, within the true pelvis. It exits the pelvis through the greater sciatic foramen to reach the greater trochanter of the femur. The piriformis does not cross the pelvic brim. It forms the postero-lateral wall of the true pelvis and is not affected by a fracture of the lateral wall.

23 **The answer is D: Pubococcygeus.** The pubococcygeus, the major component of the levator ani, is the muscle most often torn during childbirth. The pelvic diaphragm supports the fetal head during delivery. The pubococcygeus plays a key mechanical role in that it encircles the urethra, vagina, and anal canal and provides the main support for these organs during birthing. However, because of its proximity to the vagina, it also is subject to tearing if the perineum ruptures. Subsequent weakening of the muscle and associated pelvic fascia may cause changes in the positioning of the bladder and urethra that may lead to urinary stress incontinence. **Choice A** (Coccygeus) is incorrect. The coccygeus is the most posterior component of the pelvic diaphragm. However, it is not part of the levator ani portion of the pelvic diaphragm. Because of its relative distance from the birth canal, the coccygeus is less subject to the stresses applied to the pubococcygeus during delivery, therefore less subject to tearing. **Choice B** (Ischio-cavernosus) is incorrect. The ischiocavernosus is the thin skeletal muscle layer surrounding the crus of the clitoris. The crura are attached to the ischiopubic rami, well lateral to the birth canal. Thus, the levator ani will normally tear before that opening reaches the crus of the clitoris and the ischiocaverno-sus muscle, which envelops it. **Choice C** (Obturator internus) is incorrect. The obturator internus is applied to the internal lateral wall of the true pelvis and sends its tendon of insertion out of the lesser sciatic foramen into the gluteal region. This muscle is far removed from the birth canal, and it is highly unlikely to be damaged during childbirth. **Choice E** (External anal sphincter) is incorrect. The external anal sphincter surrounds the lower anal canal. It is not part of the pelvic diaphragm. Because of its proximity to the vagina, it may be damaged during extensive tearing of the perineum. However, the pubococcygeus normally tears before the external anal sphincter becomes involved.

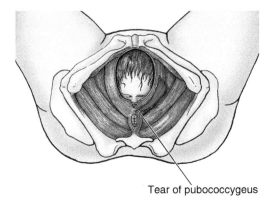

Tear of pubococcygeus

24 **The answer is C: Urethral folds.** In male fetuses, the urethral (urogenital) folds close over the urethral groove and fuse in the midline to form the ventral (anterior) aspect of the penis. This enclosure of the urethral groove forms the penile ure-thra. Incomplete fusion of the urethral folds results in abnor-mal openings of the penile urethra along the underside of the penis. This condition is termed hypospadias and may include one or more openings anywhere from the glans to the base of

the penis. In females, the urethral folds do not fuse but form the separate labia minora. The urethral groove remains open and forms the vestibule. **Choice A** (Mesonephric ducts) is incorrect. In males, the mesonephric ducts are stimulated but do not fuse with one another. They form the testicular drain-age ducts, including the efferent ductules, ductus epididymis, ductus deferens, and ejaculatory duct. The seminal vesicle forms from a secondary bud off the ductus deferens. In females, the mesonephric ducts are normally suppressed, leaving only small vestigial structures in association with the reproductive tract. **Choice B** (Paramesonephric ducts) is incorrect. These ducts are normally suppressed in male fetuses. The sole rem-nant is the small, vestigial appendix of the testis. In females, the paramesonephric ducts are stimulated and partly fused. They form the uterine tubes, uterus, cervix, and superior third of the vagina. **Choice D** (Scrotal swellings) is incorrect. The scrotal swellings arise from the genital swellings on the lateral sides of the urethral folds. They enlarge and fuse in the mid-line to form the scrotum. Rarely, hypospadias extends poste-rior into the scrotal raphe. In females, the genital swellings enlarge, but do not fuse, forming the labia majora. **Choice E** (Genital tubercle) is incorrect. The genital tubercle forms at the cranial junction of the cloacal folds and elongates to form the phallus, which in turn forms the glans penis, corpora cav-ernosa, and corpus spongiosum. In females, the phallus forms the glans clitoris, corpora cavernosa, and vestibular bulbs.

25 **The answer is D: Internal urethral sphincter.** Familial dysauto-nomia is an autonomic disorder that affects control of smooth muscle. The internal urethral sphincter is a thickening of the circular layer of smooth muscle at the internal urethral orifice. It is the involuntary sphincter that regulates urination (mictu-rition) and is the only smooth muscle structure of the choices provided. It is supplied by both sympathetic (for contraction) and parasympathetic (for relaxation) fibers through the hypo-gastric plexuses in the pelvis. **Choice A** (Pelvic diaphragm) is incorrect. The pelvic diaphragm is a musculofascial sheet that forms a large part of the pelvic floor. It is composed of two main parts: the levator ani and the coccygeus. Because it is composed of skeletal muscle, it is innervated by somatic motor fibers. These nerves branch directly off the sacral plexus and off the perineal branches of the pudendal nerve. **Choice B** (External anal sphincter) is incorrect. The exter-nal anal sphincter is the skeletal muscle complex surround-ing the lower anal canal that forms the voluntary sphincter, regulating defecation. It is innervated by somatic motor fibers of the inferior anal (rectal) nerves (branches of the pudendal nerves). **Choice C** (Urogenital diaphragm) is incorrect. Tra-ditionally, the urogenital diaphragm has been described as a three-layered, triangular structure that makes up the deep perineal pouch within the urogenital triangle. The middle layer is a skeletal muscle zone composed mainly of the exter-nal urethral sphincter (sphincter muscle of urethra) and the deep transverse perineal muscles. However, current concepts describe this area as a much more complex region, with the muscle and fascial components arranged in three-dimensional relations rather than in a flat sandwich-like manner. In either case, the muscles here receive somatic motor innervation from the perineal nerves, which are branches of the pudendal nerve. Readers are advised to reference the most current texts for a proper and better understanding of this region. **Choice E** (Levator ani) is incorrect. The levator ani is the larger of the two parts of the pelvic diaphragm. It is usually divided into three main subparts: puborectalis, pubococcygeus, and iliococcygeus. These muscles are supplied by somatic motor fibers of the perineal nerves.

26 The answer is D: Obturator internus muscle. The lateral wall of the true (lesser) pelvis is composed of the iliopubic ramus, ischiopubic ramus, body of the ischium, and the obturator foramen (mostly closed by the obturator membrane). The obturator internus muscle lies on the lateral wall of the true pelvis, surrounding and covering the obturator foramen. Fractures of the pubic and obturator areas are relatively common. In the case of a lateral wall fracture, the obturator internus muscle can easily be torn in association with disruption of the bony elements and/or the obturator membrane. **Choice A** (Pubic symphysis) is incorrect. Many students believe that the pubic symphysis forms the anterior border of the pelvis. However, the pelvis is tilted in its normal anatomical position such that the anterior superior iliac spines and the pubic tubercles are aligned in the same vertical plane. This orientation causes the bodies of the pubic bones and the symphysis to actually occupy the floor of the true pelvis, where they take on a weight-bearing function. **Choice B** (Piriformis muscle) is incorrect. The piriformis muscle originates from the pelvic surface of the superior part of the sacrum, lateral to the anterior sacral foramina. It exits the pelvis through the greater sciatic foramen to reach the greater trochanter of the femur. Because the piriformis fills a large extent of the greater sciatic foramen, it forms the posterolateral wall of the true pelvis. **Choice C** (Sacral promontory) is incorrect. The sacral promontory is the anterosuperior lip of the S1 element of the sacrum. It forms the posterior midline part of the bony edge that defines the pelvic inlet (pelvic brim; superior pelvic aperture) and separates the false (greater) pelvis from the true (lesser) pelvis. Due to the orientation of the pelvis in the anatomical position, the sacrum and coccyx form the roof of the posterior wall of the true pelvis. **Choice E** (Ganglion impar) is incorrect. The ganglion impar is the single, midline coccygeal ganglion that forms the inferior end of the sympathetic chain. It lies on the pelvic surface of the sacrum. Thus, it may be damaged in fractures of the posterior wall of the true pelvis.

27 The answer is B: Presynaptic parasympathetic neurons. The hypogastric plexuses are an extensive network of visceral motor (autonomic—both sympathetic and parasympathetic) and visceral sensory fibers within the pelvic cavity that supply the pelvic viscera and the perineum. The parasympathetic components are mainly presynaptic neurons derived from the pelvic splanchnic nerves, which synapse in the intramural ganglia of the target organs. The sympathetic components are mainly postsynaptic neurons derived from the aortic (intermesenteric) plexuses in the abdomen, where they synapsed with presynaptic elements. **Choice A** (Presynaptic sympathetic neurons) is incorrect. The presynaptic sympathetic neurons that signal to pelvic viscera originate in the low thoracic and upper lumbar segments of the spinal cord and send axonal processes through the lumbar splanchnic nerves to the aortic (intermesenteric) plexuses, where they synapse with postsynaptic elements. **Choice C** (Postsynaptic parasympathetic neurons) is incorrect. The pelvic splanchnic nerves send presynaptic fibers

through the hypogastric plexuses to the hindgut, pelvic viscera, and perineum. These neurons synapse with postsynaptic cells in the intramural (terminal) ganglia in the walls of the target organs. The postsynaptic neurons make up a large component of the enteric nervous system in the walls of the gut tube. **Choice D** (Somatic motor neurons) is incorrect. Somatic motor neurons supply skeletal muscles in the pelvic walls and floor and perineum. They are conveyed via the branches of the sacral plexus (e.g., pudendal nerve) which, strictly speaking, are not components of the hypogastric plexuses. **Choice E** (General sensory neurons) is incorrect. General sensory (general somatic afferent) neurons from the pelvic walls and floor as well as the perineum travel through the branches of the sacral plexus, in company with the somatic motor fibers to those areas. However, the visceral sensory fibers from pelvic viscera travel with visceral motor (autonomic) fibers through the hypogastric plexuses.

28 The answer is A: Ureter. As it descends into the pelvis, the ureter travels anterior to the external iliac artery just distal to the bifurcation of the common iliac vessels. It continues anterior and medial to pass inferior to the uterine artery, which is enveloped by the transverse cervical (cardinal) ligament, near the lateral aspect of the cervix. When ligating the uterine artery during a hysterectomy (surgical excision of the uterus), a surgeon must positively identify the ureter and exclude it from the ligature. To accomplish this task and avoid iatrogenic injury to the ureter, a surgeon will ligate the uterine artery as close to the cervix as possible. The relationship of the ureter to the uterine artery can be remembered with the mnemonic "The water runs under the bridge," in which the water equals urine traveling within the ureter and the bridge is the uterine artery as it travels horizontally toward the uterine cervix. **Choice B** (Pudendal nerve) is incorrect. The pudendal nerve is located inferior to the pelvic diaphragm where it innervates a majority of the perineum. It arises from the ventral primary rami of spinal levels S2-4 but quickly exits the true pelvic cavity via the greater sciatic foramen. It is not located in close proximity to the uterine artery, so it is unlikely the pudendal nerve would be damaged in this procedure. **Choice C** (Round ligament of the uterus) is incorrect. The round ligament of the uterus extends from the superior part of the body of the uterus (near the uterotubal junction) to the labium majus via the inguinal canal. It is not located in close proximity to the uterine artery, so it is unlikely the round ligament of the uterus would be damaged in this procedure. **Choice D** (Obturator artery) is incorrect. The obturator artery emerges from the anterior division of the internal iliac artery near the uterine artery; however, the paths of these arteries diverge as the arteries travel distally. The uterine artery travels medially toward the uterine cervix, whereas the obturator artery travels along the lateral pelvic wall toward the obturator foramen. Because the ligation of the uterine artery was located near the junction of the uterus and vagina, it is unlikely the obturator artery would be damaged. **Choice E** (Ovarian artery) is incorrect. The ovarian artery travels along the lateral wall of the pelvis within the infundibulopelvic (suspensory) ligament of the ovary. It splits into tubal and ovarian branches, which later coalesce and anastomose with the proper uterine artery at the junction of the uterine tube and the fundus of the uterus. This location is well above the ligated uterine artery, so it is unlikely the ovarian artery would be damaged.

29 **The answer is B: Relaxation of the puborectalis.** The puborectalis is the component of the levator ani that joins with its opposite side mate to form a U-shaped sling around the anorectal junction, as shown in the given figure. Tension of this muscle produces the anorectal angle (perineal flexure), which aids significantly in resisting fecal movement. Relaxation of the puborectalis sling causes the anorectal junction to straighten, thus allowing defecation to proceed. The other parts of the levator ani normally contract during defecation. This action raises the pelvic floor and assists the abdominal wall muscles in increasing intra-abdominal pressure and compressing the abdominopelvic contents, thus assisting in expelling feces during defecation. Thus, the complementary actions of relaxation of the puborectalis plus contraction of the remainder of the levator ani are important in voluntary control of defecation. **Choice A** (Relaxation of the pubococcygeus) is incorrect. The pubococcygeus is the major component of the levator ani. It contracts to raise the pelvic floor during defecation and other actions requiring increased intra-abdominal pressure (e.g., forced expiration, sneezing, vomiting, and urination). **Choice C** (Relaxation of the coccygeus) is incorrect. The coccygeus is the most posterior component of the pelvic diaphragm. However, it is not part of the levator ani portion of the pelvic diaphragm. Even so, it contracts in the same fashion as the levator ani during defecation to raise and tense the pelvic floor. **Choice D** (Contraction of the external anal sphincter) is incorrect. The external anal sphincter is the voluntary sphincter surrounding the lower anal canal. It must relax in order to allow dilation of the anal canal and passage of feces. **Choice E** (Contraction of the internal anal sphincter) is incorrect. The internal anal sphincter is the involuntary sphincter in the lower rectal wall. It relaxes during defecation to allow passage of feces into the anal canal.

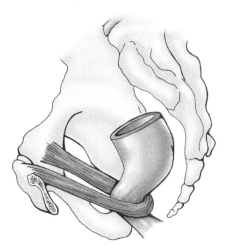

30 **The answer is D: Internal iliac.** Cancer cells from an adenocarcinoma within the posterior part of the prostate would most likely metastasize initially to the internal iliac lymph nodes, which lie along the internal iliac artery and receive lymph from the pelvic visceral and gluteal region. Because most lymphatic vessels supplying pelvic viscera follow arteries retrograde, lymph from the prostate gland, which receives arterial blood from the inferior vesical artery arising off the anterior division of the internal iliac artery, would terminate primarily in the internal iliac lymph nodes. Therefore, cancer cells from an adenocarcinoma within the posterior part of the prostate

would most likely metastasize to the internal iliac lymph nodes. The sacral lymph nodes may also receive lymphatic drainage from the prostate, so these nodes should also be checked for metastases. Remember, when considering spread of cancer from pelvic organs, it is crucial to remember the arterial supply of the organ in question. **Choice A** (Lumbar) is incorrect. Lumbar lymph nodes, which are located anterior to the lumbar vertebrae and surrounding the inferior vena cava and abdominal aorta, receive lymphatic drainage directly from the posterior abdominal wall, gonads (ovaries and testes), kidneys, ureters, uterus, and uterine tubes. Unless metastasis is in advanced stages by spreading through several sets of lymph nodes, the lumbar lymph nodes would not be affected because they do not directly receive lymphatic drainage from a prostatic adenocarcinoma. **Choice B** (Deep inguinal) is incorrect. Deep inguinal lymph nodes, which are located deep to the fascia lata and medial to the femoral vein, receive lymphatic drainage directly from the glans penis, the distal spongy urethra of the penis, and deep structures of the lower limb and indirect lymphatic drainage from the superficial inguinal lymph nodes. Since the prostate is a pelvic organ, it does not have lymphatic drainage to the deep inguinal lymph nodes. **Choice C** (Superficial inguinal) is incorrect. Superficial inguinal lymph nodes, which are located in the subcutaneous tissue near the termination of the great saphenous vein, receive lymphatic drainage from the lower abdominal wall, buttock, lower limb, and all of the perineum and external genitalia, except for the glans penis and its distal spongy urethra. Since the prostate is a pelvic organ, it does not have lymphatic drainage to the superficial inguinal lymph nodes. **Choice E** (External iliac) is incorrect. The external iliac lymph nodes, which are associated with the external iliac vein, receive lymphatic drainage from pelvic organs in direct contact with the peritoneum, including the superior bladder and superior pelvic ureters. Since the prostate is situated well below the peritoneum in the pelvis, it does not drain to the external iliac lymph nodes.

31 **The answer is B: Urinary bladder.** In males, the urinary bladder is supplied by the superior and inferior vesicle arteries, both of which usually are branches of the anterior division of the internal iliac artery. The internal pudendal artery is usually a terminal branch of the anterior division of the internal iliac artery. However, rather than supplying pelvic viscera, it exits the pelvis, enters the posterolateral aspect of the perineum, and provides the main supply to that entire region. Severing the internal pudendal artery usually does not alter blood flow to the bladder. However, remember that the internal iliac arterial tract is the most variable branching network of all the arteries. In this variation pattern, the internal pudendal artery may be closely related to the inferior vesicle artery, or, may be well removed from it. **Choice A** (Penis) is incorrect. The penis is supplied by terminal branches of the internal pudendal artery within the perineum. Thus, it will be deprived of blood in case of lesion at the origin of the internal pudendal artery. **Choice C** (Anal canal) is incorrect. The anal canal is supplied by the inferior anal (rectal) branches of the internal pudendal artery within the perineum. It will be deprived of blood in case of lesion at the origin of the internal pudendal artery. **Choice D** (Scrotum) is incorrect. The scrotum is supplied by posterior scrotal branches of the internal pudendal artery and anterior scrotal branches of the external pudendal artery (a branch of the femoral artery). Thus, lesion of the internal pudendal artery will reduce blood flow to the scrotum. **Choice E** (Urogenital diaphragm) is incorrect. The structures of the anatomically questionable urogenital diaphragm are supplied by the perineal branches of the internal pudendal artery. Thus, this area will be deprived of blood following lesion of the internal pudendal artery.

32 **The answer is D: Inability to achieve erection.** Destruction of the sacral segments of the spinal cord by a posterior fracture fragment of L2 would lead to pain within the lower back and paresthesia in the lower limbs. It would also eliminate the sacral parasympathetic outflow due to damage to the presynaptic parasympathetic cell bodies, which are located in the grey matter of spinal cord segments S2-4. The sacral parasympathetic outflow affects the gut tube below the left (splenic) flexure of the colon, the pelvic viscera, and the external genitalia. Parasympathetic stimulation produces genital erection, whereas sympathetic stimulation governs ejaculation. This pattern of innervation can be remembered by the mnemonic "Point" and "Shoot." Thus, this injury will result in inability to achieve erection. However, ejaculation can still occur, and such patients can impregnate a woman. **Choice A** (Lowered sperm count) is incorrect. Sperm production is not governed by the autonomic nervous system. This patient will continue to produce sperm and, as noted above, can still ejaculate and father a child. **Choice B** (Paralysis of the arrector pili muscles in the lower limbs) is incorrect. Parasympathetic fibers distribute to the body cavities and the external genitalia but not to the body wall and limbs. The innervation of arrector pili muscles in the lower limbs is governed by the sympathetic nervous system, which was not damaged in this patient. **Choice C** (Reduced sweat gland secretion in the lower limbs) is incorrect. Parasympathetic fibers distribute to the body cavities and the external genitalia but not to the body wall and limbs. The innervation of sweat glands in the lower limbs is governed by the sympathetic nervous system, which was not damaged in this patient. **Choice E** (Increased motility in the descending colon and rectum) is incorrect. The sacral parasympathetic outflow does govern the descending colon and rectum, with one normal effect being increased motility (peristalsis) in these regions. Therefore, loss of parasympathetic supply, combined with unopposed sympathetic input, would result in decreased motility here.

33 **The answer is B: T12.** Visceral sensory fibers relaying pain from the labor contractions of the upper uterus are referred to the T11-L2 spinal cord levels because these organs are located above the pelvic pain line, as defined by their being in contact with or above the peritoneum. Because visceral sensory fibers follow the visceral motor (autonomic) fibers retrograde, visceral pain from the contractions of the upper uterus follow the presynaptic sympathetic nerves of the abdominopelvic splanchnic nerves retrograde to spinal cord levels T11-L2. Conversely, pelvic organs located below the pelvic pain line are, by definition, located below, and not in contact with, the peritoneum. The visceral sensory fibers from these organs follow the presynaptic parasympathetic nerves of the pelvic splanchnic nerves retrograde to spinal cord levels S2-4. Therefore, labor pains derived from the contractions of the upper uterus will be referred by visceral sensory fibers to the T12 spinal cord level. **Choice A** (T6) is incorrect. Visceral sensory fibers associated with the T6 vertebral level would be involved with

conveying visceral pain associated with the heart and lungs, due to traveling retrograde with cardiopulmonary splanchnic nerves derived from postsynaptic sympathetic fibers from T1-6. **Choice C** (L4) is incorrect. Visceral sensory fibers carrying pain from visceral organs and involuntary (smooth or cardiac) muscle follow retrograde the pathway of the visceral motor (or autonomic) nerve fibers. There are no presynaptic autonomic nerve fibers that arise from the L4 vertebral level, so there are no visceral sensory nerves associated with this vertebral level. **Choice D** (S1) is incorrect. Visceral sensory fibers carrying pain from visceral organs and involuntary (smooth or cardiac) muscle follow retrograde the pathway of the visceral motor (or autonomic) nerve fibers. There are no presynaptic autonomic nerve fibers that arise from the S1 vertebral level, so there are no visceral sensory nerves associated with this vertebral level. **Choice E** (S3) is incorrect. Pain derived from labor contractions of the upper uterus would not refer to vertebral level S3, because the upper uterus is in contact with the peritoneum, which means it is located above the pelvic pain line. However, labor pains from the dilation of the uterine cervix, an important stage of labor, will follow the presynaptic parasympathetic nerves of the pelvic splanchnic nerves retrograde to the vertebral levels of S2-4. Therefore, the uterine cervix is a pelvic organ located below the pelvic pain line, which means it is located below, and not in contact with, the peritoneum. Therefore, the vertebral level of S3 would receive visceral sensory fibers conveying pain from labor due to the dilation of the uterine cervix; however, this question asked specifically about labor pains derived from the contractions of the upper uterus, which would be referred to the T11-L2 vertebral levels.

34 **The answer is A: Hydrocele.** A hydrocele testis is an accumulation of serous fluids within the spermatic cord of the testis. This pathology may be due to serous secretions from a remnant piece of peritoneum (tunica vaginalis), or due to communication with the abdomen via a persistent processus vaginalis. Patients with a hydrocele testis present with a painless swollen testis that feels like a water balloon, which may be corrected via drainage with a needle (aspiration) or surgery. Verification of a hydrocele can be accomplished by the diagnostic technique of transillumination, in which a light is placed near the enlarged portion of the scrotum. If the scrotum is full of clear fluid and a hydrocele testis is present, the scrotum will light up on the affected side, which was seen in this newborn. **Choice B** (Varicocele) is incorrect. A varicocele is an abnormal dilation of the pampiniform plexus of veins within the spermatic cord. This scrotal mass often resembles and feels like a "bag of worms" on physical examination (see photo in question 6). Idiopathic varicocele is usually caused by defective one-way valves within the pampiniform plexus, which cause dilatation of these veins near the testis. However, a secondary varicocele will be seen following compression of the venous drainage of the testis due to the presence of a pelvic or abdominal malignancy, and this possibility must be ruled out by the physician. Varicoceles are found in the left side in approximately 98% of cases, can develop in 15% to 20% of all males, and are most frequently diagnosed in males between 15 and 25 years of age. Due to the nature (tense and fluctuant) of this scrotal mass, the fact that the scrotum is transilluminated, and the age of this newborn, a hydrocele is the most likely diagnosis. **Choice C** (Indirect inguinal hernia) is incorrect. An indirect inguinal hernia is usually a congenital hernia that results when abdominal cavity contents herniate through a patent processus vaginalis (open communication between the abdomen and scrotum). The hernia traverses the deep and superficial inguinal rings to descend into the scrotum in males. An indirect inguinal hernia often presents as a soft, nontender, reducible bulge in the inguinal canal that can extend into the scrotum. It is located off the midline, especially at times of increased intra-abdominal pressure, and exists as a visible or palpable lump underneath the skin in the groin region, which was seen in this patient. Due to the nature (tense and fluctuant) of this scrotal mass and the fact that the scrotum is transilluminated by the light used by the physician, a hydrocele is the most likely diagnosis. It should be noted that indirect inguinal hernias may present with a hydrocele, so further diagnosis with an ultrasound can be utilized to rule out a herniation of abdominal contents into the scrotum. **Choice D** (Direct inguinal hernia) is incorrect. A direct inguinal hernia is an acquired hernia that results when abdominal cavity contents herniate through a weakness in the anterior abdominal wall in the inguinal (Hesselbach) triangle. The hernia exits through the superficial inguinal ring and often presents as a soft, nontender, reducible bulge underneath the skin overlying the superficial inguinal ring. Given the age of this patient and the presence of the mass that has descended into the scrotum, a direct inguinal hernia is not likely. **Choice E** (Spermatocele) is incorrect. A spermatocele is a cyst-like mass within the scrotum that develops in a tubule of the rete testis or the head of the epididymis. It usually contains a milky fluid and spermatozoa. These retention cysts are usually not painful and can be confirmed by an ultrasound of the scrotum. Given the size of this scrotal mass, the age of the patient, and the fact that the entire scrotum is transilluminated with the light used by the physician, a hydrocele is the most likely diagnosis.

35 **The answer is D: Perineal body.** The vaginal fornix is the recess that surrounds the cervix. It has anterior, lateral, and posterior parts. Because of the postural angles between the vagina, cervix, and uterine body, the posterior fornix is the deepest part, affording a wide palpation area plus direct access to the rectouterine pouch. The perineal body lies in the midline directly posterior to the vagina and can be readily palpated. Additionally, the rectum, anal canal, sacrum, and sacral promontory are available to palpation. **Choice A** (Urethra) is incorrect. The urethra and the base of the bladder lie against the anterior wall and fornix of the vagina. They can be palpated in that direction. **Choice B** (Ovaries) is incorrect. The ovaries, ischial spines, ureters, uterine tubes, and the uterine arteries can be palpated through the lateral fornices of the vagina. **Choice C** (Ischial spines) is incorrect. The ischial spines, ovaries, ureters, suterine tubes, and the uterine arteries can be palpated through the lateral fornices of the vagina. **Choice E** (Ureters) is incorrect. The ureters, ovaries, ischial spines, uterine tubes, and the uterine arteries can be palpated through the lateral fornices of the vagina.

36 **The answer is C: Obturator nerve.** The obturator nerve branches from the lumbar plexus in the false (greater) pelvis of the lower abdomen. It descends into the true pelvis, runs across the surface of the obturator internus muscle on the lateral pelvic wall, and passes through the obturator canal to enter the medial thigh. In the thigh, the obturator nerve supplies the

adductor muscles in the medial compartment of the thigh and also a cutaneous area in the medial thigh. During childbirth, the nerve may be compressed against the lateral wall of the pelvis by the passing baby. **Choice A** (Inferior gluteal nerve) is incorrect. The inferior gluteal nerve arises from the sacral plexus and immediately exits the pelvis through the greater sciatic foramen to reach the gluteal region. In the buttock, it supplies the gluteus maximus muscle. **Choice B** (Pudendal nerve) is incorrect. This nerve arises from the sacral plexus, leaves the pelvis through the greater sciatic foramen, curls around the ischial spine, and enters the perineum. It is the primary motor and sensory nerve to the perineum. **Choice D** (Sciatic nerve) is incorrect. The sciatic nerve is the largest nerve in the body. It originates from the sacral plexus, leaves the pelvis through the greater sciatic foramen, runs through the buttock, and into the posterior thigh. The sciatic nerve supplies the hip joint, the muscles in the posterior compartment of the thigh, all muscles below the knee, and considerable cutaneous areas below the knee. **Choice E** (Pelvic splanchnic nerves) is incorrect. These nerves are presynaptic parasympathetic fibers arising off the sacral plexus. They distribute through the hypogastric plexuses to the hindgut organs and the pelvic and perineal viscera. Parasympathetic nerves do not supply the body wall or limbs.

37 **The answer is C: Urinary bladder.** When empty (i.e., in the "resting" anatomical position), the adult urinary bladder is located in the true (lesser) pelvis, lying partly on the pubic bones and pubic symphysis. It is separated from these bones by only the thin, potential retropubic space. The bladder may be ruptured by fractures of the pubic bones or, especially when distended, by injuries to the anteroinferior abdominal wall. Rupture of the bladder wall may allow extravasation (passing out) of urine into extraperitoneal spaces or into the peritoneal cavity. **Choice A** (Anal canal) is incorrect. The anal canal is far posterior of the pubic bones, with other organs intervening. It is not normally directly affected by fracture of those bones. **Choice B** (Piriformis muscles) is incorrect. The piriformis muscles run from the pelvic surface of the sacrum through the greater sciatic foramina to the femur. They form part of the posterolateral wall of the true pelvis and so are on the opposite side of the true pelvis from the pubic bones. **Choice D** (Uterus) is incorrect. The uterus normally lays anteverted and anteflexed in the reproductive tract. Its anterior surface lies on the posterosuperior aspect of the urinary bladder. Thus, the bladder intervenes between the pubic bones and the uterus. **Choice E** (Vagina) is incorrect. The vagina lies posterior to the base of the urinary bladder and the urethra. Therefore, those organs would be directly affected in pubic fractures before the vagina.

38 **The answer is C: Lumbar.** The lymphatic drainage of the testes goes directly to the lumbar lymph nodes due to their developmental origin in the superoposterior abdominal wall. Lumbar lymph nodes, which are located anterior to the lumbar vertebrae and surrounding the inferior vena cava and abdominal aorta, also receive lymphatic drainage directly from the posterior abdominal wall, kidneys, ovaries, ureters, uterus, and uterine tubes. Because most lymphatic vessels supplying pelvic viscera follow arteries retrograde, lymph from the testes, which receive arterial blood from testicular artery arising off the abdominal aorta at vertebral level L1, terminates primarily in the lumbar lymph nodes. Therefore, the lumbar lymph nodes should be checked initially to rule out metastases in the case of testicular cancer. Remember, when considering spread of cancer from pelvic visceral organs, it is crucial to remember the arterial supply of the organ in question. **Choice A** (Superficial inguinal) is incorrect. Superficial inguinal lymph nodes, which are located in the subcutaneous tissue near the termination of the great saphenous vein, receive lymphatic drainage from the lower abdominal wall, buttock, lower limb, and all of the perineum and external genitalia, except for the glans penis and its distal spongy urethra. Despite the fact that the scrotum drains to the superficial inguinal lymph nodes, the testes drain to the lumbar nodes due to their descent from the posterior abdominal wall in development. **Choice B** (Deep inguinal) is incorrect. Deep inguinal lymph nodes, which are located deep to the fascia lata and medial to the femoral vein, receive lymphatic drainage directly from the glans penis, the distal spongy urethra of the penis, deep structures of the lower limb, and indirect lymphatic drainage from the superficial inguinal lymph nodes. Due to their descent from the posterior abdominal wall in development, the lymphatic drainage of the testes goes directly to the lumbar lymph nodes. **Choice D** (External iliac) is incorrect. The external iliac lymph nodes, which are associated with the external iliac vein, receive lymphatic drainage from pelvic organs in direct contact with the peritoneum, including the superior bladder and superior pelvic ureters. Even though the tunica vaginalis is a serous covering of the testes derived from the peritoneum, the lymphatic drainage of the testes goes directly to the lumbar lymph nodes due to their descent from the posterior abdominal wall in development. **Choice E** (Internal iliac) is incorrect. The internal iliac lymph nodes, which are located along the internal iliac artery and its branches, receive lymphatic drainage from the pelvic viscera, gluteal region, and deep parts of the perineum. The testes drain to the lumbar nodes due to their descent from the posterior abdominal wall in development and their arterial supply from the testicular artery arising off the abdominal aorta.

39   **The answer is D: More everted alae of the ilia.**   The greater pelvis (pelvis major; false pelvis) of a female is relatively shallow due to the everted wings (alae) of the iliac portions of the coxal (hip) bones. This shallow greater pelvis shortens the distance the head of a fetus needs to descend through the pelvic aperture during parturition. If the wings of the iliac portions of the coxal bones are more everted, then the unearthed coxal bones are most likely female. The rest of the characteristics listed within this question are more characteristic of a male pelvis. **Choice A** (Subpubic angle less than 70 degrees) is incorrect. A subpubic angle of less than 70 degrees is a characteristic of a male pelvis. This angle can be approximated by spreading the index and middle finger. In the female pelvis, this subpubic angle is wider (greater) than 80 degrees, which enables the head of a fetus more space to descend through the pelvic outlet (inferior pelvic aperture). The size of the female subpubic angle can be approximated by spreading the thumb and index finger. **Choice B** (Heart-shaped [android] pelvic inlet) is incorrect. A heart-shaped (android) pelvic inlet (superior pelvic aperture) is a characteristic of a male pelvis. In contrast, the female pelvis has an oval and rounded pelvic inlet, which is better adapted for parturition. **Choice C** (More inverted ischial tuberosities) is incorrect. Inverted ischial tuberosities are often seen in the male pelvis. This feature decreases the

diameter of the pelvic outlet (inferior pelvic aperture), which is not conducive to parturition. In contrast, the ischial tuberosities in the female pelvis are more everted, which increases the diameter of the pelvic outlet. **Choice E** (Ischial spines close together in the midline) is incorrect. A small interspinous distance, due to inverted ischial spines, is often seen in the male pelvis. This characteristic decreases the diameter of the pelvic outlet (or inferior pelvic aperture), which is not conducive to parturition. In contrast, the distance between the ischial spines in the female pelvis is wider, which increases the diameter of the pelvic outlet.

40   **The answer is A: Inability to control the detrusor muscle.**   The hypogastric plexuses are an extensive network of visceral motor (autonomic—both sympathetic and parasympathetic) and visceral sensory fibers across the true pelvis. The pelvic splanchnic nerves send presynaptic parasympathetic fibers through the inferior hypogastric plexus to the urinary bladder, where they supply the detrusor muscle in the wall of the bladder and the internal urethral sphincter in the neck of the bladder. The aortic (intermesenteric) plexus sends sympathetic fibers descending into the hypogastric plexuses and on to the bladder and internal urethral sphincter. Thus, damage within the lower part of the hypogastric plexuses will compromise autonomic control of urination. The axial T2-weighted MRI demonstrates a low signal intensity adenocarcinoma (indicated by the black arrow) arising in the normally high intensity peripheral zone of the prostate. The prostatic adenocarcinoma damages the hypogastric plexus and leads to an inability to control the detrusor muscle of the bladder. **Choice B** (Inability to control the external anal sphincter) is incorrect. The external anal sphincter is a skeletal muscle complex innervated by the inferior anal (rectal) branches of the pudendal nerve. The pudendal nerve originates within the pelvis from anterior primary rami of spinal nerves S2-4, and immediately exits the pelvis through the greater sciatic foramen. It is not a component of the hypogastric plexuses. **Choice C** (Chronic increased motility in the sigmoid colon) is incorrect. Parasympathetic fibers from the pelvic splanchnic nerves course through the inferior hypogastric plexus and ascend posterior to the peritoneum to reach the descending colon and sigmoid colon. Their normal function is to stimulate peristalsis in these organs. Thus, loss of parasympathetic input results in decreased motility here. **Choice D** (Reduced sensation on the glans penis) is incorrect. Sensation on the glans penis (and glans clitoris) is conveyed by general sensory fibers in the dorsal nerve of the penis (or clitoris), a terminal branch of the pudendal nerve. As noted above, the pudendal nerve is not related to the hypogastric plexuses. **Choice E** (Loss of vasomotor control in the lower limb) is incorrect. Sympathetic fibers that govern vasomotor function in the vessels of the lower limb originate in the sympathetic chain, pass into the sacral plexus, and run into the lower limb via the lower limb branches of the sacral plexus (e.g., sciatic nerve). This pathway is essentially separate from the hypogastric plexuses.

41   **The answer is B: Internal iliac.**   The blood supply to the gluteal region is supplied by the superior and inferior gluteal arteries, which arise off the internal iliac artery. The internal iliac artery is occluded in this patient, and his symptoms are due to lack of blood perfusion to the gluteal muscles and surrounding tissue, which causes ischemia and severe pain in the affected (gluteal) region. Remember that the internal iliac artery and its branches supply the gluteal region as well as contents of the pelvis and the medial thigh. **Choice A** (External iliac) is incorrect. The external iliac artery supplies blood to the iliac region and the anterior abdominal wall. This artery becomes the femoral artery, the major lower limb artery, after it passes under the inguinal ligament. Atherosclerotic blockage of the external iliac would affect arterial supply to the hip and lower limb, not the gluteal region. **Choice C** (Femoral artery) is incorrect. The femoral artery is the continuation of the external iliac artery, which changes its name to the femoral artery after passing under the inguinal ligament. Atherosclerotic blockage of the femoral artery would affect the blood supply to the lower limb, except for the gluteal region. **Choice D** (Internal pudendal) is incorrect. The internal pudendal artery is a branch of the anterior division of the internal iliac artery, which supplies the anal and urogenital triangles of the perineum with its three major branches: inferior anal, perineal, and dorsal artery of the penis. Blockage of this artery would not be responsible for poor blood perfusion to the gluteal region; however, blockage of the internal iliac artery would lead to similar signs and symptoms in the arterial distribution of the internal pudendal artery. **Choice E** (Abdominal aorta) is incorrect. Atherosclerotic blockage of the abdominal aorta would lead to more widespread complications than simply pain in the gluteal region.

42   **The answer is A: Bulbourethral glands.** Bulbourethral (Cowper) glands secrete nonviscous material into the urethra before and during ejaculation to mix with sperm, seminal vesicle fluid, and prostatic fluid to form semen. The bulbourethral glands are found deep to the perineal membrane within the deep perineal compartment, so they are the most likely structures to be affected by the described abscess within the deep perineal compartment. **Choice B** (Perineal body) is incorrect. The perineal body is located at the central point of the perineum where the perineal muscles converge. This unique structure serves as an anchoring point for the perineum and contains collagen and elastic fibers as well as skeletal and smooth muscles. Due to its location between the anal and urogenital triangles of the perineum, it is generally not considered part of the superficial or deep perineal compartments. Therefore, it would not be the most likely structure on this list affected by the described abscess. **Choice C** (Superficial transverse perineal muscles) is incorrect. The superficial transverse perineal muscles attach to the ischial tuberosities and help to support and stabilize the superficial perineal region. The muscles are, however, located in the superficial perineal space, which is inferior to the perineal membrane, so they would most likely not be affected by this abscess in the deep perineal space. **Choice D** (Bulbospongiosus muscles) is incorrect. The bulbospongiosus muscles envelop and compress the bulb of the penis and corpus spongiosum to aid in penile erection by increasing pressure on erectile tissue in the root of the penis. These muscles also support and fix the male pelvic floor and play an important role in emptying the penile (spongy) urethra of residual urine or semen. However, these muscles are located in the superficial perineal space, which is inferior to the perineal membrane, so the bulbospongiosus muscles would most likely not be affected by this abscess in the deep perineal space. **Choice E** (Ischiocavernosus muscles) is incorrect. The ischiocavernosus muscles are paired muscles covering the crura of the penis and the associated erectile tissue, the corpora cavernosa. These muscles force blood

within the crura into the distal parts of the corpora cavernosa and compress venous outflow via the deep dorsal vein of the penis. Both of these actions increase the turgidity (firm distension) of the penis during erection. However, these muscles are located in the superficial perineal space, which is inferior to the perineal membrane, so the ischiocavernosus muscles would most likely not be affected by this abscess in the deep perineal space.

43   **The answer is B: Lateral wall of the ischioanal fossa.** The lateral wall of the ischioanal fossa is formed by the ischium and the overlying inferior part of the obturator internus muscle. The pudendal (Alcock) canal is a shallow depression on the surface of the obturator internus muscle formed by the investing fascia of this muscle. The pudendal canal contains the pudendal nerve and the internal pudendal vessels along their entry into the ischioanal fossa. When draining an ischioanal abscess, a surgeon must avoid damage to the pudendal canal and its contents by avoiding the lateral wall of the ischioanal fossa. Remember that the ischioanal fossa is a large wedge-shaped space on each side of the anal canal located between the skin of the anal region and the pelvic diaphragm. This fascia-filled fossa supports the anal canal while simultaneously providing a space that accommodates the expansion of the anal canal during defecation. **Choice A** (Roof of the ischioanal fossa) is incorrect. The roof of the ischioanal fossa is formed by the levator ani muscle, which ascends laterally to the point where this muscular component of the pelvic diaphragm arises from the investing fascia of the obturator internus. The surgeon draining the ischioanal abscess should avoid the lateral wall, not the roof, of the ischioanal fossa to avoid damage to the pudendal nerve and the internal pudendal vessels. **Choice C** (Medial wall of the ischioanal fossa) is incorrect. The medial wall of the ischioanal fossa is also formed by the levator ani muscle and the external anal sphincter, which merge to form this medial wall. An incision in the vicinity of the medial wall of the ischioanal wall would not damage the pudendal nerve and the internal pudendal vessels specifically. However, it may damage the inferior anal (rectal) nerve and inferior rectal artery, which branch off of this neurovascular bundle. **Choice D** (Posterior recess of the ischioanal fossa) is incorrect. The posterior recess of the ischioanal fossa extends posterior to the sacrotuberous ligament and gluteus maximus muscle. A surgeon can avoid damage to the pudendal nerve and the internal pudendal vessels by avoiding the medial wall of this posterior recess. **Choice E** (Anterior recess of the ischioanal fossa) is incorrect. The anterior recess of the ischioanal fossa extends into the urogenital triangle of the perineum superior to the perineal membrane. When draining an ischioanal recess, a surgeon can avoid damage to the pudendal nerve and the internal pudendal vessels by avoiding the medial wall of this anterior recess.

44   **The answer is E: Spongy urethra.** In men, a straddle injury may rupture the spongy urethra, which courses through the corpus spongiosum of the penis. Damage to the spongy urethra causes extravasation of urine, in which the urine leaves the spongy urethra and spills out into the surrounding tissue. This extravasation of urine would be confined by the superficial layer of perineal fascia, which is continuous with the superficial (dartos) fascia of the scrotum, the superficial fascia of the penis, and the membranous layer of subcutaneous tissue of the lower abdomen (Scarpa fascia). Therefore, urine (and blood, due to the trauma and the discoloration noted in this presentation) will spread into the scrotum, penis, and lower anterior abdominal wall, as noted in this patient. Because the superficial layer of perineal fascia blends with the posterior edge of the perineal membrane and adheres onto the ischiopubic rami laterally, urine will not spread into the anal triangle of the perineum or the thighs, respectively. Damage to the spongy urethra can also occur following an incorrect insertion of a catheter to drain the urinary bladder. **Choice A** (Ureter) is incorrect. The ureters descend posterior to the peritoneum of the abdomen to connect the kidneys to the urinary bladder. Due to their location, the ureters would not be at risk during a straddle injury to the perineum. Furthermore, rupture of the ureters would cause extravasation of urine in the abdomen or pelvis, but not the perineum, as noted in this patient. **Choice B** (Urinary bladder) is incorrect. The urinary bladder is located in the true pelvis (or pelvis minor), and due to its position above the perineal membrane and the pelvic diaphragm, it would not be at risk during a straddle injury to the perineum. Furthermore, rupture of the urinary bladder would cause extravasation of urine into extraperitoneal spaces or into the peritoneal cavity, which was not seen in this patient. **Choice C** (Prostatic urethra) is incorrect. The prostatic urethra is the portion of the male urethra that traverses the prostate gland. Because it is not located within the perineum, prostatic urethra damage would result in extravasation of urine in the true pelvis (or pelvis minor). **Choice D** (Intermediate urethra) is incorrect. The intermediate (membranous) urethra passes through the deep perineal compartment. This portion of the male urethra is the narrowest urethral segment. Due to its location within the deep perineal compartment, extravasation of urine from the intermediate urethra would reside between the inferior fascia of the pelvic diaphragm and the perineal membrane. So, damage to the intermediate urethra would not cause discoloration and swelling in the scrotum, penis, and anterior abdominal wall, which was noted in this patient.

Chapter 6

Back

QUESTIONS

Select the single best answer.

1 A 55-year-old man experiences severe lower back pain for 4 days after moving heavy furniture. After a thorough back evaluation and review of associated radiological imaging, a surgeon removes the herniated portion of the L3-4 intervertebral (IV) disc. What type of cartilage most likely gives the tensile strength of the disc extracted from this patient?

(A) Hyaline
(B) Elastic
(C) Fibrous
(D) Epiphysial
(E) Anular

2 A 45-year-old man goes to his family physician complaining of lower back pain after spending a weekend clearing trees off his property. During examination, the doctor notes a tuft of hair and a dimple on the skin of the patient's lower back. A plain film reveals a congenital defect in his L5 vertebra, indicated by the black arrow in the given X-ray. No other structural abnormalities are noted. Based on these findings, what is the most likely diagnosis for this patient?

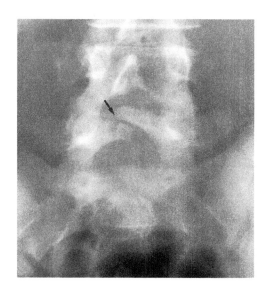

(A) Meningocele
(B) Anencephaly
(C) Spina bifida occulta
(D) Spina bifida cystica
(E) Spina bifida with myeloschisis

3 A developmental biologist studying the derivatives of the somites and somitomeres treats the epimeres in a mouse embryo with a toxin that kills all of their cells. If the mouse develops to full term, which of the following muscles is most likely to be absent?

(A) Trapezius
(B) Latissimus dorsi
(C) Rhomboid major
(D) Longissimus
(E) Levator scapulae

4 A lesion of which of the indicated structures would cause loss of sensation in the skin overlying the trapezius muscle?

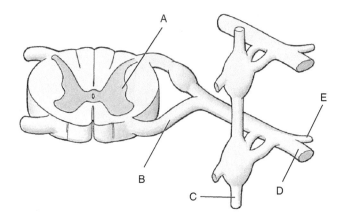

5 An infant suffers a vertebral malformation in which the nucleus pulposus component of multiple intervertebral discs is hypertrophied. From what embryonic structure is the hypertrophied structure derived?

(A) Notochord
(B) Dermatome
(C) Myotome
(D) Sclerotome
(E) Neural crest

6 Idling at a stoplight in his vintage car without headrests, a 71-year-old-man's car is struck from behind by a truck going approximately 30 mph (48 kph). The man is brought to the ER suffering from a severe hyperextension neck injury due to the crash. The given T2-weighted MRI shows a rupture of the anterior anulus of the C4-5 intervertebral disc, inflammation of that disc (the white appearance), and a prevertebral hematoma, which compromised his airway and required intubation. Which of the following ligaments is disrupted in this injury?

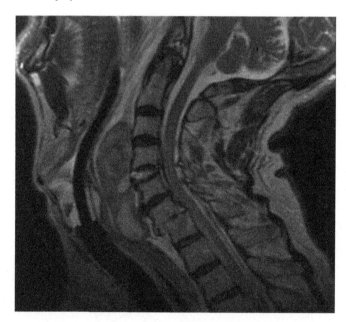

(A) Anterior longitudinal ligament
(B) Posterior longitudinal ligament
(C) Ligamentum flavum
(D) Interspinous ligament
(E) Intertransverse ligament

7 Amyotrophic lateral sclerosis (ALS; Lou Gehrig's disease) is a progressive, fatal neurodegenerative disease caused by degeneration of the motor neurons controlling skeletal (voluntary) muscle movement. Postmortem analysis of which of the following structures would show the cell bodies of neurons affected by this disease?

(A) Anterior gray horn of the spinal cord
(B) Lateral gray horn of the spinal cord
(C) Posterior gray horn of the spinal cord
(D) Spinal ganglia
(E) Lateral column of spinal cord white matter

8 A 19-year-old girl gives birth to a baby girl diagnosed with a meningomyelocele, as seen in the given midsagittal MRI. The mother lived in a rural area and did not have prenatal visits with her obstetrician. Which of the following drugs, if taken in the proper doses during the periconceptional period, would have greatly reduced the chances of her fetus having a neural tube defect (NTD)?

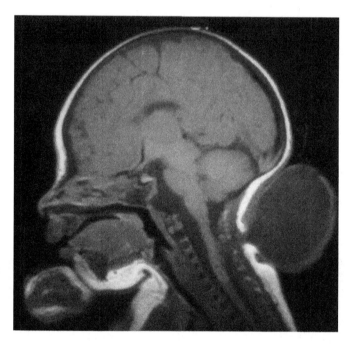

(A) Valproic acid (Depakote)
(B) Folic acid (Folacin)
(C) Cephalexin (Keflex)
(D) Acetaminophen (Tylenol)
(E) Famotidine (Pepcid)

9 An internal medicine attending physician asks a medical student to place the bell of her stethoscope on the triangle of auscultation to hear a patient's breathing sounds. Which of the following structures make up the boundaries of this triangle?

(A) Deltoid, latissimus dorsi, scapula
(B) Trapezius, scapula, latissimus dorsi
(C) Latissimus dorsi, ilium, external abdominal oblique
(D) Rhomboids, levator scapulae, splenius capitis
(E) Longissimus, rhomboids, vertebral spinous processes

10 A 34-year-old man fell 25 ft out of a barn loft, landing on his back. He was found unconscious and taken to the ER. The given sagittal CT reformat image reveals a T9 spinal fracture dislocation, as noted by the black arrow. The patient had unequivocal clinical findings indicating spinal cord transection. Given the results of this CT image and the clinical information, what deficits will the patient incur?

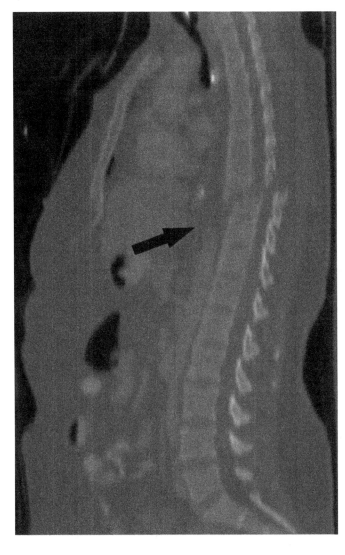

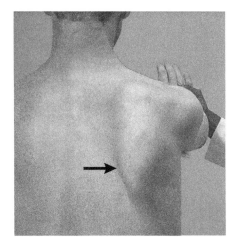

(A) Axillary nerve
(B) Thoracodorsal nerve
(C) Long thoracic nerve
(D) Dorsal scapular nerve
(E) Suboccipital nerve

13 An 81-year-old woman visits her family physician for an annual physical examination and complains of weakness and loss of sensation in her legs. Radiological studies show bony spurs (osteophytes) narrowing the intervertebral foramina at levels T12-L3. Which of the following structures is most likely to be impinged in this condition?
(A) Posterior primary rami of spinal nerves
(B) Spinal ganglia
(C) Ganglia of the sympathetic trunk
(D) Anterior primary rami of spinal nerves
(E) Anterior rootlets of spinal nerves

14 A 16-year-old male soccer player was brought to the ER because of the acute lower back pain he experienced after performing a high-velocity kick of the ball. The given right posterior oblique X-ray reveals pathology within the L5 vertebra that has the appearance of a "headless Scottie Dog" when outlined. Based upon the X-ray results, which of the following diagnoses is the most likely cause of his lower back pain?

(A) Quadriplegia and incontinence
(B) Paraplegia and incontinence
(C) Incontinence only
(D) Loss of only sensory information below the lesion
(E) Loss of only motor function below the lesion

11 A 35-year-old woman suffers intractable pain in her left forearm. Neurosurgical consultation leads to a decision to conduct a rhizotomy to relieve the condition. At which of the following locations is the rhizotomy best performed to relieve the patient's pain?
(A) Posterior (dorsal) roots
(B) Posterior (dorsal) primary rami
(C) Spinal nerves
(D) Anterior (ventral) roots
(E) Anterior (ventral) primary rami

12 An 18-year-old soldier presents with shrapnel wounds in the lateral wall of his right chest following an explosion of a landmine. After several months of recovery, his physical therapist observes that his scapula moves away from the thoracic wall when he leans on his right hand, as noted by the black arrow in the given photo. Which of the following nerves is likely damaged?

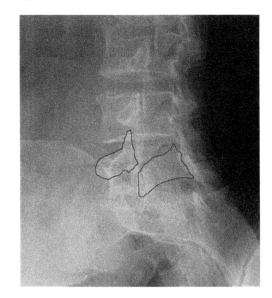

(A) Ankylosing spondylitis
(B) High-grade spondylolisthesis
(C) Spondyloptosis
(D) Spondylolysis
(E) Spondylosis

15   A physician orders a lumbar puncture (spinal tap) for his 43-year-old female patient in order to obtain a sample of cerebrospinal fluid (CSF). He explains to her that this procedure will be done in the lower back, between the spinous processes of the L3 and L4 vertebrae. What is the best reason for performing the lumbar puncture at this location?
(A) The medullary cone ends at or above the L3 level
(B) The subarachnoid space ends at the L3 level
(C) The intervertebral foramina at L3-4 are large and easy to penetrate
(D) No vertebral venous plexuses exist below the L3 level
(E) The ligamenta flava are absent below the L3 level

16   A 22-year-old man is brought to the ER with severe back pain and lower limb weakness after falling off the top of a 16-ft ladder and landing on his feet. The ER physician orders a CT scan, and the given midsagittal CT directs the physician toward making which of the following diagnoses?

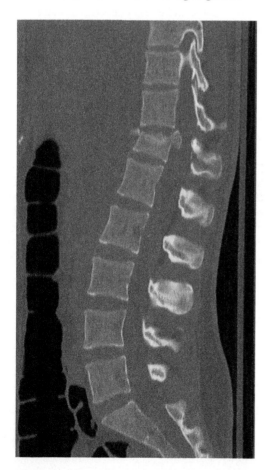

(A) Herniated intervertebral disc
(B) Burst fracture of T12 vertebral body
(C) Lumbar spinal stenosis
(D) Spondylolisthesis of L5-S1 articulation
(E) Excessive lumbar lordosis

17   After several months of engaging in a vigorous exercise program, a 28-year-old woman experiences periodic pain and muscle spasms in her left upper limb. Thorough physical and radiographic examinations by her primary care physician and a consulting surgeon determine that she suffers a posterolateral herniation of the C5-6 intervertebral disc. Which of the following structures is this herniation most likely impinging?
(A) C5 spinal nerve roots
(B) C5 anterior primary ramus
(C) C6 spinal nerve roots
(D) C6 posterior primary ramus
(E) C7 posterior horn segment of the spinal cord

18   During a head-on motor vehicular accident (MVA), the upper cervical vertebrae of a 34-year-old woman are flexed violently forward until her head impacts the steering wheel and is thrown into hyperextension and slight rotation. She is immobilized and brought to an ER. The given sagittal CT of her upper cervical vertebrae is viewed by a radiologist and reveals which of the following diagnoses?

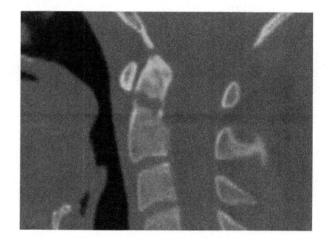

(A) Traumatic spondylolisthesis of C2
(B) Fracture of dens axis (odontoid process)
(C) Atlanto-axial subluxation
(D) Ruptured intervertebral disc between C1 and C2
(E) No pathology is apparent on the CT scan

19   As a result of multiple vertebral fractures incurred in an automobile crash, an 8-year-old girl suffers a series of torn posterior primary rami of spinal nerves C1-6. Which of the following muscles will be paralyzed as a result?
(A) Trapezius
(B) Latissimus dorsi
(C) Levator scapulae
(D) Rhomboid major
(E) Splenius capitus

20   A 73-year-old man comes to his physician complaining of a tingling numbness within the fourth and fifth digits of his right hand. These symptoms are exacerbated when he looks up at the ceiling. The given sagittal T2-weighted MRI reveals degenerative changes in his cervical vertebrae. Which of the following diagnoses is confirmed by the MRI and would result in the symptoms of this patient?

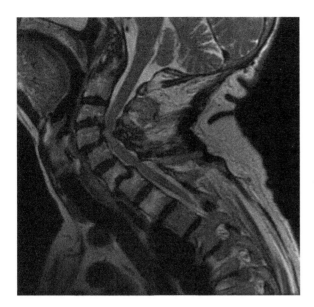

(A) Burst fracture of C3 vertebral body
(B) Ruptured anterior longitudinal ligament
(C) Transection of the cervical spinal cord
(D) Cervical spinal stenosis
(E) Traumatic spondylolisthesis of C5

21 A 17-year-old gymnast grips a high bar with his arms outstretched and begins to pull himself straight upward to the level of the bar, as in doing a chin-up. Which of the following muscles is the prime agonist in this action?
(A) Serratus posterior superior
(B) Rhomboid major
(C) Levator scapulae
(D) Latissimus dorsi
(E) Longissimus

22 A 77-year-old man presents with shingles on his anterolateral abdomen and umbilicus, as shown in the figure. Shingles (or herpes zoster) is caused by the varicella zoster virus, which resides latent in sensory ganglia in the body for many years. When a patient is immunocompromised, this virus can cause a painful skin rash called shingles, which usually presents unilaterally along the infected nerve's dermatome distribution. Given the location of the rash, what ganglion is most likely affected in this patient?

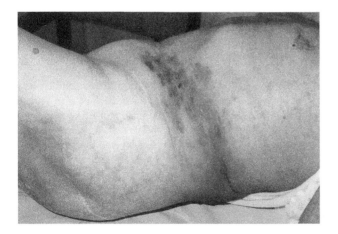

(A) Paravertebral ganglion
(B) Prevertebral ganglion
(C) Lumbar ganglion
(D) Spinal ganglion of T10
(E) Spinal ganglion of L2

23 A 35-year-old man presents with pain radiating from his lower back into his left lower limb, periodic sensory loss and paresthesia in that limb, and associated motor weakness. His physician suspects unilateral entrapment of lumbar nerve roots secondary to a herniated lumbar intervertebral disc. In examining the patient, the physician conducts a straight-leg raising test. Which of the following best describes a positive straight-leg raising sign (Lasèque's sign) for this condition in this patient?
(A) Walking while keeping the left leg in a straight position (i.e., the knee is kept straight) relieves the pain in the back and limb
(B) Flexing the hip by raising the straightened left leg (i.e., the knee is kept straight) with the patient lying in the supine position relieves the pain in the back and leg
(C) Abducting the hip by raising the straightened left leg with the patient lying on his right side relieves the pain in the back and leg
(D) Flexing the hip by raising the straightened left leg with the patient lying in the supine position increases pain in the back with radiation down the left leg
(E) Extending the hip by raising the straightened left leg with the patient lying in the prone position increases pain in the back with radiation down the left leg

24 A helmet-less 24-year-old man was riding an all-terrain vehicle (ATV or quad bike) when a thin, unseen, horizontal clothes line impacted the man's neck under his chin, knocking him backward off the ATV. Due to his forward momentum at the time of impact, his head was hyperextended on his neck. Emergency medical technicians (EMTs) established his airway, stabilized his neck, and brought him to the emergency room. A lateral cervical X-ray revealed pathology within the cervical vertebrae. Based upon the nature of the accident and the evidence of the given X-ray, which of the following diagnoses is most probable?

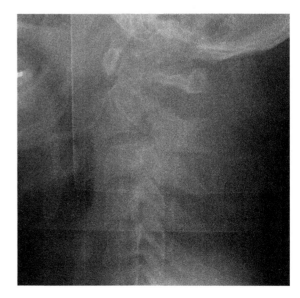

(A) Ruptured anterior longitudinal ligament
(B) Jefferson (burst) fracture of C1
(C) Traumatic spondylolysis of C2
(D) Fracture of the dens axis (odontoid process)
(E) Atlanto-axial subluxation

25 An anesthesiologist administers epidural anesthestic immediately lateral to the spinous processes of vertebrae L3 and L4 of a pregnant woman in labor. During this procedure, what would be the last ligament perforated by the needle in order to access the epidural space?

(A) Ligamentum flavum
(B) Anterior longitudinal ligament
(C) Posterior longitudinal ligament
(D) Interspinous ligament
(E) Intertransverse ligament

26 During a routine prenatal examination of a pregnant 16-year-old woman entering her second trimester (15 weeks of gestation), elevated maternal serum alpha-fetoprotein (AFP) levels were detected and later confirmed by amniocentesis. A follow-up diagnostic ultrasound examination reveals defects in the lower back of the fetus. In the given longitudinal ultrasound scan, open arrows indicate the bases of the vertebrae, and solid arrows point to a cyst-like sac containing protruding neural tissue. Which of the following terms best describes this neural tube defect?

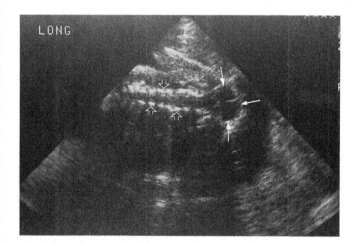

(A) Meningocele
(B) Anencephaly
(C) Spina bifida occulta
(D) Meningomyelocele
(E) Rachischisis

27 A 25-year-old medical student feels a sharp pain in his lower back while helping his landlady move a piano. After 3 days, the pain does not subside, so he receives a comprehensive examination from his physician that reveals a compression of the left side L3 spinal nerve. Which of the following is the most likely cause of this condition?

(A) The pedicles of L2 and L3 are compressed together
(B) The pedicles of L3 and L4 are compressed together
(C) The laminae of L2 and L3 are compressed together
(D) The laminae of L3 and L4 are compressed together
(E) The spinous processes of L3 and L4 are compressed together

28 A 46-year-old supervisor was reading a work order on a construction site when a 60 lb bag of concrete mix was accidentally dropped on the apex of his head. He was immobilized and brought to the ER where he presented with upper neck pain but no neurological signs. Based upon the given axial CT scan and the patient's presentation, which of the following diagnoses is most likely?

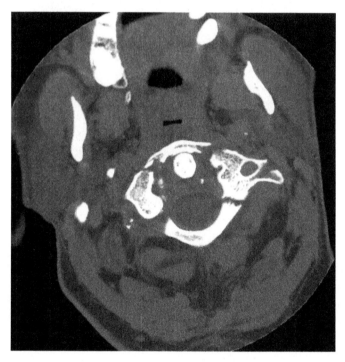

(A) Damage to the cervical spinal cord
(B) No pathology is apparent on the CT scan
(C) Jefferson (burst) fracture of C1
(D) Fracture of the dens axis (odontoid process)
(E) Atlanto-axial subluxation

29 A 12-year-old girl is examined by a school nurse who notices the girl's right scapula is more prominent than the left, her head is not centered directly over the pelvis, and her right hip is raised and more prominent. When the girl is asked to bend forward at the waist, the nurse observes asymmetry of the trunk. Which of the following diagnoses is most likely?

(A) Scoliosis
(B) Lordosis
(C) Kyphosis
(D) Osteoporosis
(E) Osteoarthritis

30 After moving his parents' heavy furniture out of their house, a 38-year-old man experiences lower back pain and presents to his doctor with tingling numbness radiating down his right lower limb to the lateral part of his foot. A thorough physical examination reveals weakness when standing on the toes of his right foot. A T1-weighted MRI revealed an intervertebral disc herniation, as indicated by the white arrow. Which of the following structures is most likely impinged by this disc herniation?

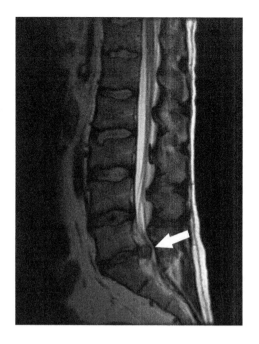

(A) S1 spinal nerve roots
(B) S1 anterior primary ramus
(C) L5 spinal nerve roots
(D) L5 posterior primary ramus
(E) L5 anterior primary ramus

31 Attempting to do a backflip with his bicycle off a high ramp at the finish line of a race, a 24-year-old professional BMX rider fell from a height of 20 ft and attempted to land on his feet. A sagittal CT reveals a burst fracture of the L1 vertebral body with a posterior displaced fracture fragment compressing the medullary cone (conus medullaris). Which of the following spinal cord segments would most likely be impinged by the bone fragment in this injury?

(A) T7
(B) T9
(C) T11
(D) L2
(E) S2

ANSWERS AND DISCUSSION

1 **The answer is C: Fibrous.** Fibrous cartilage, or fibrocartilage, is one of the three types of cartilage composed of chondrocytes that secrete, and are surrounded by, an extensive extracellular matrix composed of collagen fibers, elastin fibers, and a plethora of ground substance rich in proteoglycan. Fibrocartilage is a very tough, white material that provides high tensile strength to the anulus fibrosus of the IV discs, which would have ruptured in this patient. The fibrocartilage of the anulus fibrosus is composed of a dense network of Type I collagen, but it can tear due to sudden hyperflexion in older individuals (such as when lowering heavy objects), which pushes the gelatinous nucleus pulposus of the IV disc posterior toward the thinnest part of the anulus fibrosus. When the fibrocartilage of the anulus fibrosus is compromised, the nucleus pulposus may herniate into the vertebral canal and compress spinal nerve roots or the spinal cord, leading to back pain. Fibrocartilage, or fibrous cartilage, provides the tensile strength of the IV discs. **Choice A** (Hyaline) is incorrect. Hyaline cartilage is one of the three types of cartilage composed of chondrocytes that secrete, and are surrounded by, an extensive extracellular matrix composed of collagen fibers, elastin fibers, and a plethora of ground substance rich in proteoglycan. Hyaline cartilage is a translucent, hard material rich in Type II collagen fibers and proteoglycan. Covering the articular surfaces of bones, it is found in many joints. Hyaline cartilage is also found in the tracheal rings, larynx, and costal cartilages. In endochondral ossification, bone is formed from a hyaline cartilage intermediate. It is also found in maturing long bones within the epiphysial (or growth) plates. Hyaline cartilage does not provide the tensile strength of the IV discs. **Choice B** (Elastic) is incorrect. Elastic cartilage is one of the three types of cartilage composed of chondrocytes that secrete, and are surrounded by, an extensive extracellular matrix composed of collagen fibers, elastin fibers, and a plethora of ground substance rich in proteoglycan. It is composed of large amounts of elastic fibers and Type II collagen, and it is found in the external ear (auricle), pharyngotympanic (auditory) tube, and epiglottis, where it provides a rigid but elastic framework. Elastic cartilage does not provide the tensile strength of the IV discs. **Choice D** (Epiphysial) is incorrect. In endochondral ossification, bone is formed from a hyaline cartilage intermediate. It is also found in maturing long bones and is called epiphysial cartilage, located within the epiphysial (growth) plates of bone. This new type of cartilage forms the resting zone of chondrocytes located on the epiphysial (distal) side of the zone of growing cartilage, which unites the epiphysis with the shaft of the long bone. Because the patient is 55 years old, the presence of epiphysial cartilage is unlikely. Moreover, fibrocartilage provides the tensile strength of the IV discs. **Choice E** (Anular) is incorrect. Anular cartilage is a synonym for the cricoid cartilage, the lowest portion of the laryngeal skeleton. Because the cricoid cartilage is shaped like a signet ring, with its arch located anterior and its widened lamina posterior, it is sometimes referred to as the anular cartilage. Because the anular cartilage is not a type of cartilage, it is unable to provide tensile strength to the IV disc and can easily be eliminated as a possible answer. Fibrocartilage provides the tensile strength of the IV discs.

2 **The answer is C: Spina bifida occulta.** Spina bifida occulta is the mildest form of spina bifida (*L:* split spine). In this developmental disorder, the left and right neural arch elements fail to fuse completely in the dorsal midline. However, the split in the vertebra is so small that the meninges and elements of the spinal cord do not protrude through the defect. In the given plain film, the black arrow indicates a failure of fusion of the laminae of L5, producing a cleft. Individuals with spina bifida occulta may possess a tuft of hair and/or dimple in the skin overlying the affected vertebral levels, as noted in this patient. Other individuals with this condition may have no visible evidence, a lipoma, or even a birthmark in the overlying skin of the affected region. Some studies suggest approximately 10% of the general population have this mildest form of spina bifida. In this case, the X-ray verifies the diagnosis of spina bifida occulta. Because this condition is normally clinically asymptomatic and unnoticed, it is seemingly "hidden" (occult). In fact, most research suggests no relationship between spina bifida occulta and back pain. **Choice A** (Meningocele) is incorrect. The least common form of spina bifida is a posterior meningocele (or meningeal cyst). In this developmental disorder, the bilateral neural arch elements fail to fuse completely in the dorsal midline but the meninges protrude through the defect into a sac or cyst. Therefore, multiple vertebral defects are present, accompanied with the presence of a cyst, which contains cerebrospinal fluid (CSF). In a meningocele, the spinal cord and nerve roots are typically in normal position, not protruding into the cyst, and there are usually no long-term effects on the individuals. Without the presence of a meningeal cyst in the lower back of this man, a meningocele can be easily eliminated. **Choice B** (Anencephaly) is incorrect. Anencephaly is a severe neural tube defect in which the cephalic (head) end of the neural tube fails to close in the embryo. This birth defect is lethal with the baby being born without a forebrain, skullcap (calvaria), and scalp, leaving the remaining portions of the brain exposed. If proper prenatal care is available, most cases of anencephaly are detected by elevated maternal serum alpha-fetoprotein (AFP) levels and ultrasound examinations during prenatal examinations. Elevated AFP levels are often correlated with neural tube defects. The addition of folic acid to the diet of women in their childbearing years has been shown to reduce the incidence of neural tube anomalies. A patient with anencephaly would not reach 45 years of age. **Choice D** (Spina bifida cystica) is incorrect. Spina bifida cystica is a severe form of spina bifida and receives its name because of the characteristic presence of a cyst-like sac protruding from the defective area. The membranous walls of the sac are composed of very thin skin plus dura and arachnoid components. In these neural tube defects, the unfused neural arches of multiple vertebrae allow the meninges (and potentially the spinal cord) to protrude through the structural defect. The inclusion of a displaced portion of the spinal cord and nerve roots in the malformation designate this neural tube defect as a meningomyelocele, which is the most common form of spina bifida cystica. That is, the defect involves the meninges (meningo-), the spinal cord (myelo-) and the membranous sac (-cele). Because of the severity of this type of spina bifida, this 45-year-old man would not have this condition. **Choice E** (Spina bifida with myeloschisis) is incorrect. Spina bifida with myeloschisis, or rachischisis, involves the same signs and symptoms as the most common form of spina bifida cystica, a meningomyelocele; however, the protruded portions of the spinal cord are not afforded the enveloping protection of the meninges. Physical examination would reveal a flattened mass of nervous tissue with no associated membranes, which makes the patient more prone to life-threatening infections. Because of the severity of spina bifida with myeloschisis, this 45-year-old man would not have this condition.

3 The answer is D: Longissimus. Destruction of the embryonic epimeres will result in loss of the deep group of back muscles, including the longissimus muscle, one of three erector spinae muscles (along with the iliocostalis and spinalis muscles). Muscles derived from the epimeres are the proper muscles of the back, which are innervated by the posterior (dorsal) primary rami of spinal nerves. These deep muscles of the back include the previously mentioned erector spinae group, splenius capitis and cervicis muscles, suboccipital muscles, transversospinales muscles (including the semispinalis, multifidus, and rotatores muscles), and other small muscles. Remember, each embryonic somite differentiates into three components: myotome, dermatome, and sclerotome. Each myotome splits into two parts: epimere and hypomere. The epimere develops dorsal to the incipient vertebral column, and the longissimus muscle is the only listed muscle which is derived from the embryonic epimere. The muscles derived from the epimeres form the deep group of muscles in the back and are often termed the intrinsic back muscles or epaxial muscles. **Choice A** (Trapezius) is incorrect. The trapezius is a member of the superficial extrinsic layer of back muscles, which connect the upper limbs to the trunk. When these muscles contract (or shorten), they produce movements of the upper limb. However, the trapezius muscle does not originate from either the epimere or hypomere, as evidenced by its innervation via the spinal accessory nerve (CN XI). Instead, it is likely related to postbranchial origins, along with its mate, sternocleidomastoid. Thus, destruction of epimeres will not directly affect the formation of the trapezius. **Choice B** (Latissimus dorsi) is incorrect. The latissimus dorsi (*L:* widest muscle of back) is a member of the superficial extrinsic layer of back muscles, which connect the upper limbs to the trunk. When these muscles contract, they produce movements of the upper limb. The latissimus dorsi muscle is derived from hypomeres, which develop lateral and anterior to the vertebral axis, and it migrates secondarily into the back. All of the muscles derived from hypomeres are innervated by the anterior (ventral) primary rami of spinal nerves. The latissimus dorsi muscle is innervated by the thoracodorsal (middle subscapular) nerve and acts on the upper limb. Due to being derived from the embryonic hypomeres, the latissimus dorsi muscle would not be affected by the toxin injected into the epimeres within this mouse embryo. **Choice C** (Rhomboid major) is incorrect. The rhomboid major muscle is a member of the superficial extrinsic layer of back muscles, which connect the upper limbs to the trunk. When these muscles contract, they produce movements of the upper limb. The rhomboid major muscle is derived from hypomeres, which develop lateral and anterior to the vertebral axis. All of the muscles derived from hypomeres are innervated by the anterior (ventral) primary rami of spinal nerves. Due to being derived from the embryonic hypomeres, the rhomboid major muscle would not be affected by the toxin injected into the epimeres within this mouse embryo. **Choice E** (Levator scapulae) is incorrect. The levator scapulae muscle is a member of the superficial

extrinsic layer of back muscles, which connect the upper limbs to the trunk. When these muscles contract, they produce movements of the upper limb. The levator scapulae muscle is derived from hypomeres, which develop lateral and anterior to the vertebral axis. All of the muscles derived from hypomeres are innervated by the anterior (ventral) primary rami of spinal nerves. Due to being derived from the embryonic hypomeres, the levator scapulae muscle would not be affected by the toxin injected into the epimeres within this mouse embryo.

4 The answer is E: Posterior (dorsal) primary ramus. Sensory receptors in the skin overlying the trapezius muscle project through general sensory (general somatic afferent) neurons to the spinal cord via the posterior (dorsal) primary rami of spinal nerves (marked "E" in this diagram), traverse the mixed spinal nerves, travel within posterior (dorsal) roots of spinal nerves, and reach the posterior (dorsal) gray horn of the spinal cord. Cutting the posterior rami of spinal nerves would cause degeneration of the distal axonal processes of the general sensory fibers and lead to loss of sensation in the skin of the back. Additionally, the distal axonal processes of somatic motor (general somatic efferent or GSE) neurons and visceral motor (general visceral efferent or GVE) neurons contained within the posterior primary rami would be damaged as well, causing motor and autonomic deficits in the back, respectively. Remember that the trapezius muscle is a component of the superficial extrinsic layer of back muscles, which connect the upper limbs to the trunk. These muscles are innervated by anterior primary rami of spinal nerves, except for the trapezius, which is supplied by the accessory nerve (CN XI). However, the skin overlying the trapezius muscle is innervated by the posterior (dorsal) primary rami of spinal nerves. **Choice A** (Lateral gray horn of spinal cord) is incorrect. The lateral gray horn of the spinal cord is the location of the intermediolateral cell column (IML), which contains the cell bodies of presynaptic (preganglionic) sympathetic neurons of the autonomic nervous system (ANS). The IML only exists within the lateral gray horn between spinal segmental levels T1-L2 (or L3), which is the reason the sympathetic division of the ANS is also called the thoracolumbar division of the ANS. A lesion of the lateral gray horn of the spinal cord would cause autonomic deficits; however, it would not affect the general sensory fibers supplying cutaneous innervation to the skin overlying the trapezius muscle. **Choice B** (Anterior root of spinal nerve) is incorrect. The anterior (ventral) roots of spinal nerves convey the axonal processes of somatic and visceral motor neurons into the periphery. Damage to the anterior roots of spinal nerves would not affect the general sensory fibers supplying cutaneous innervation to the skin overlying the trapezius muscle. However, damage to the anterior roots of spinal nerves would affect muscles in the superficial layer of the back, except for the trapezius muscle, which is innervated by the accessory nerve (CN XI). **Choice C** (Sympathetic trunk) is incorrect. The sympathetic trunk carries both presynaptic and postsynaptic (postganglionic) sympathetic neurons as well as visceral sensory (general visceral afferent or GVA) neurons. The visceral sensory neurons within the sympathetic trunk convey pain from organs of the body cavities and are not involved with cutaneous innervation to the skin overlying the trapezius muscle. **Choice D** (Anterior primary ramus) is incorrect. The anterior (ventral) primary rami of spinal nerves contain general sensory, somatic motor, and visceral motor fibers. However, the general sensory fibers in the anterior primary rami are bringing sensory information from the lateral and anterior parts of the body wall, including the limbs. Therefore, cutting the anterior primary rami would not affect innervation to the skin overlying the trapezius muscle. It would, however, affect the proprioceptive (general sensory) fibers leaving the trapezius muscle, which are carried by the anterior primary rami of C3 and C4.

5 **The answer is A: Notochord.** The nucleus pulposus is the sole remnant of the embryonic notochord, the initial longitudinal skeletal axis of the body. The developing bodies and intervertebral discs of the vertebral column replace the notochord, except for the nucleus pulposus. Remember that each intervertebral disc is composed of two parts: the central nucleus pulposus and the peripheral anulus fibrosus. **Choice B** (Dermatome) is incorrect. Each embryonic somite differentiates into three components: dermatome, myotome, and sclerotome. The dermatome contributes to the formation of the dermis, most of which is derived from the somatic layer of the lateral plate mesoderm. The nucleus pulposus component of an intervertebral disc is derived from the notochord, not the dermatome. **Choice C** (Myotome) is incorrect. Each embryonic somite differentiates into three components: myotome, dermatome, and sclerotome. The myotomes represent the muscle generating components of the somites. Remember, each myotome splits into two parts: epimere and hypomere. The epimere gives rise to the deep group of muscles in the back (intrinsic back muscles or epaxial muscles), which develop dorsal to the incipient vertebral column and are innervated by the posterior (dorsal) primary rami. The hypomere gives rise to muscles located lateral and anterior to the vertebral axis, which are innervated by the anterior (ventral) primary rami of spinal nerves. The nucleus pulposus component of an intervertebral disc is derived from the notochord, not the myotome. **Choice D** (Sclerotome) is incorrect. The sclerotomes give rise to most of the vertebral column, including the vertebrae, part of the occipital bone, and the anulus fibrosus portion of the intervertebral discs. The nucleus pulposus component of an intervertebral disc is derived from the notochord, not the sclerotome. **Choice E** (Neural crest) is incorrect. Most of the vertebral column and immediately surrounding tissues are derived from mesoderm. However, neural crest cells do migrate into this area, where they form spinal (dorsal root) ganglia and autonomic ganglia. The nucleus pulposus component of an intervertebral disc is derived from the notochord, not the neural crest cells.

6 **The answer is A: Anterior longitudinal ligament.** The anterior longitudinal ligament is a vertical connective tissue band that attaches along the anterior aspects of the vertebral bodies. Its peripheral fibers have strong attachments to the intervertebral discs. The anterior longitudinal ligament resists hyperextension of the vertebral column. However, in this patient, the extreme forces involved with the hyperextension of the neck overpowers the resistance of this ligament, rupturing it as well as displacing part of the C4-5 intervertebral disc. In the given T2-weighted MRI, the anterior longitudinal ligament is represented by a hypointense (dark band) signal located anterior to the vertebral column. However, the locations where the anterior longitudinal ligament is interrupted appear as an abnormal hyperintense (white) signal, which is evident anterior to the

C5 vertebral body. **Choice B** (Posterior longitudinal ligament) is incorrect. The posterior longitudinal ligament runs vertically along the posterior aspect of the vertebral column, mirroring the position of the anterior longitudinal ligament located along the anterior aspect of the vertebral column. The posterior longitudinal ligament resists flexion of the vertebral column. Posterolateral herniation of the gelatinous nucleus pulposus through the anulus fibrosus of an intervertebral disc most often projects lateral to the strong attachment sites of the posterior longitudinal ligament. If the herniated disc compresses spinal nerve roots, then neck, back, and/or limb pain may be present. The T2-weighted MRI clearly shows disruption of the anterior longitudinal ligament, evident by the abnormal hyperintense (white) signal located anterior to the C5 vertebral body. **Choice C** (Ligamentum flavum) is incorrect. The ligamenta flava (*L:* yellow ligament) are paired ligaments of yellow elastic fibrous tissue, which bind together the laminae of adjoining vertebrae and form the posterior wall of the vertebral canal. Because these ligaments resist flexion of the vertebral column, it is unlikely the ligamenta flava were damaged in this hyperextension injury of the neck. **Choice D** (Interspinous ligament) is incorrect. The interspinous ligament is composed of fibrous bands that connect the spinous processes of adjacent vertebrae. Because these ligaments resist flexion of the vertebral column, it is unlikely the interspinous ligaments were damaged in this hyperextension injury of the neck. **Choice E** (Intertransverse ligament) is incorrect. The intertransverse ligament is one ligament that connects the transverse processes of adjacent vertebrae. Because the intertransverse ligaments resist contralateral bending (abduction; lateral flexion) of the vertebrae, it is unlikely the intertransverse ligaments were damaged in this hyperextension injury of the neck.

7 **The answer is A: Anterior gray horn of the spinal cord.** Cell bodies of somatic motor neurons (α-motor neurons) innervating skeletal muscle are located within the anterior (ventral) gray horn of the spinal cord, at all segmental levels throughout the entire length of the spinal cord. The innervation of the skeletal muscles affected by ALS is through somatic motor (general somatic efferent or GSE) neurons and branchial motor (special visceral efferent or SVE) neurons (neurons that supply the embryonic pharyngeal arches). In ALS patients, postmortem analysis of the anterior gray horn of the spinal cord would show significant degeneration. In the given diagram, the anterior gray horn of the spinal cord is labeled as "A." The locations for all five possible choices for this question are also indicated in this figure. **Choice B** (Lateral gray horn of the spinal cord) is incorrect. The lateral gray horn of the spinal cord is the location of the intermediolateral cell column (IML), which contains the cell bodies of presynaptic (preganglionic) sympathetic neurons of the autonomic nervous system (ANS). The IML only exists within the lateral gray horn between spinal segmental levels T1-L2 (or L3), which is the reason the sympathetic division of the ANS is also called the thoracolumbar division of the ANS. Degeneration in the lateral gray horn of the spinal cord would cause autonomic deficits but would not include the somatic motor neurons involved in ALS. **Choice C** (Posterior gray horn of the spinal cord) is incorrect. The posterior (dorsal) gray horn, located along the entire length of the spinal cord, contains cell bodies of spinal interneurons. The central process of each pseudounipolar sensory neuron conveys general sensory (afferent) fibers through the posterior (dorsal) nerve root and synapses within the posterior horn of the spinal cord. Degeneration within the posterior gray horn of the spinal cord would cause sensory deficits but would not include the somatic motor neurons involved in ALS. **Choice D** (Spinal ganglia) is incorrect. The spinal (dorsal root) ganglia, located at the distal ends of the posterior (dorsal) roots of spinal nerves, contain cell bodies of the general sensory (afferent) neurons. Degeneration within the spinal ganglia would result in sensory deficits but would not include the somatic motor neurons involved in ALS. **Choice E** (Lateral column of spinal cord white matter) is incorrect. All columns within the spinal cord white matter contain neuronal processes and supporting glial cells. Degeneration within the lateral column of the spinal cord would not include the somatic motor neurons involved in ALS.

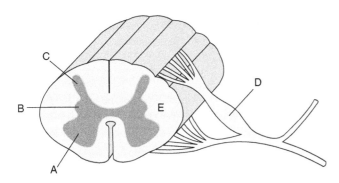

8 **The answer is B: Folic Acid (Folacin).** Supplementing a diet with folic acid (vitamin B_9 or folacin) has been shown to reduce the incidence of NTDs up to 70%. Neural tube closure occurs within the first 28 days after conception, and at this time in the pregnancy, many mothers do not realize they are pregnant. Women anticipating getting pregnant should take 400 mg of folic acid daily beginning 3 months prior to conception and continue the folic acid supplement throughout their pregnancy. NTD prevention is best achieved by adequate daily folic acid intake throughout the reproductive years. In this neonate, the sagittal MRI revealed a neural tube defect called a meningomyelocele, so the defect in the cervical region involves the meninges (meningo-), the spinal cord (myelo-) and the membranous sac (-cele). A meningomyelocele is the most common form of spina bifida cystica. **Choice A** (Valproic acid [Depakote]) is incorrect. Valproic acid (brand name Depakote) is an anticonvulsant and mood-stabilizing drug used in the treatment of bipolar disorder, depression, and epilepsy. Exposure to Valproic acid, during the first month of pregnancy, has been shown to have a teratogenic effect on the fetus, including increasing the incidence of neural tube defects. **Choice C** (Cephalexin [Keflex]) is incorrect. Cephalexin (brand name Keflex) is an antibiotic used to fight bacterial infections, including upper respiratory, ear, skin, and urinary tract infections. Exposure to Cephalexin, during the first month of pregnancy, has been shown to have a teratogenic effect on the fetus, including increasing the incidence of neural tube defects. **Choice D** (Acetaminophen [Tylenol]) is incorrect. Acetaminophen (brand name Tylenol) is an analgesic (or pain reliever) and antipyretic (or fever reducer). Exposure to Acetaminophen, during the first month of pregnancy, has been shown to have a teratogenic effect on the fetus, including increasing the incidence of neural tube defects. **Choice E**

(Famotidine [Pepcid]) is incorrect. Famotidine (brand name Pepcid) is a histamine H_2-receptor antagonist that inhibits stomach acid production, and it is often used to treat gastroesophageal reflux disease (GERD). Exposure to Famotidine, during the first month of pregnancy, has been shown to have a teratogenic effect on the fetus, including increasing the incidence of neural tube defects.

9 **The answer is B: Trapezius, scapula, latissimus dorsi.** The triangle of auscultation is a space in the back bounded by the lateral edge of the trapezius muscle, medial border of the scapula, and upper edge of the latissimus dorsi muscle. Placing a stethoscope within the triangle of auscultation enables the medical student to hear breathing sounds because (1) this site offers a gap between layers of bone and muscle, and (2) the location lies directly over the midposterior chest wall and the lung, which is ideal for auscultation. **Choice A** (Deltoid, latissimus dorsi, scapula) is incorrect. A triangle marked by these boundaries is located over the posterior aspect of the axilla. A medical student would be unable to hear breathing sounds of the lungs at this location. **Choice C** (Latissimus dorsi, ilium, external abdominal oblique) is incorrect. The lumbar triangle is the space bounded by the lower edge of the latissimus dorsi muscle, the iliac crest of the coxal (hip) bone, and the posterior border of the external abdominal oblique muscle. An abdominal hernia may protrude through the lumbar triangle, a weak spot in the abdominal wall. The lumbar triangle also offers a surgical pathway through the back for access to the kidney. **Choice D** (Rhomboids, levator scapulae, splenius capitis) is incorrect. The intermuscular space marked by these muscles is located at the base of the neck. A medical student would be unable to hear breathing sounds of the lungs at this location. **Choice E** (Longissimus, rhomboids, vertebral spinous processes) is incorrect. These boundaries form a site just off the dorsal midline. Listening for breathing sounds of the lungs at this site is not optimal.

10 **The answer is B: Paraplegia and incontinence.** Transection of the spinal cord results in loss of all motor and sensory functions movements that emerge from the cord inferior to the site of the lesion. General sensory, somatic motor, and visceral motor fibers for the pelvis and lower limbs would be lost inferior to the level of T9 due to the transection of the spinal cord. Also, parasympathetic outflow to the pelvis and perineum would be eliminated due to the origin of these nerve fibers from S2-4. The CT image reveals a T9 spinal fracture dislocation, and the clinical findings indicate a spinal cord transection. Therefore, this patient would present with paraplegia (or paralysis of both lower limbs), fecal and urinary incontinence, impotence, and loss of motor functions and sensation below the level of the T9 lesion, which is right above the level of the umbilicus (supplied by T10). **Choice A** (Quadriplegia and incontinence) is incorrect. A transection of the spinal cord at the level of T9 would spare the upper limbs from sensory and motor deficits because the upper limbs are supplied by the anterior rami of C5-T1. This patient would present with paraplegia (or paralysis of both lower limbs), fecal and urinary incontinence, impotence, and loss of motor functions and sensory input below the level of the T9 lesion. **Choice C** (Incontinence only) is incorrect. A transection of the spinal cord at the level of T9 would result in paraplegia (or paralysis of both lower limbs), fecal and urinary incontinence, impotence, and loss of motor functions and sensory input below the level of the T9 lesion. Though incontinence would result from this spinal cord transection at T9, this deficit would be accompanied by additional signs and symptoms due to the severity and location of this spinal cord injury. **Choice D** (Loss of only sensory information below the lesion) is incorrect. Transection of the spinal cord at T9 would result in the loss of all sensation and voluntary movements inferior to T9. Therefore, loss of only sensory information is not a viable option. **Choice E** (Loss of only motor function below the lesion) is incorrect. Transection of the spinal cord at T9 would result in the loss of all sensation and voluntary movements inferior to T9. Therefore, loss of only motor function is not a viable option in this patient.

11 **The answer is A: Posterior (dorsal) roots.**   A rhizotomy is a neurosurgical procedure that selectively severs problematic spinal nerve roots to relieve pain or spastic paralysis (e.g., as often seen in cerebral palsy patients). The posterior roots are the only site where afferent (sensory) fibers are segregated from efferent (motor) fibers. In selective dorsal rhizotomy (SDR), severing the left C6-8 posterior roots could relieve the pain symptoms in the left forearm of this patient because they carry only sensory information. **Choice B** (Posterior [dorsal] primary rami) is incorrect. Cutting the posterior primary rami of spinal nerves would cause degeneration of the distal axonal processes of the general sensory (afferent) fibers as well as fibers to the intrinsic back muscles. However, the general sensory fibers contained within the posterior primary rami only supply innervation to the skin over the back, so the patient's pain within the left forearm would remain. Because they do not convey pain fibers from the left forearm, selective rhizotomy of the posterior primary rami would not relieve this patient's pain. **Choice C** (Spinal nerves) is incorrect. Cutting the spinal nerves would cause loss of sensory, motor, and (depending on the vertebral level) autonomic deficits. Because spinal nerves convey both sensory and motor fibers, this location is inappropriate for selective rhizotomy to relieve pain in the left forearm. **Choice D** (Anterior [ventral] roots) is incorrect. The anterior roots of the spinal nerve are the only site where motor fibers are segregated from sensory fibers. So, selective rhizotomy at the anterior roots would cause motor deficits but would not relieve the patient's pain. **Choice E** (Anterior [ventral] primary rami) is incorrect. Cutting the appropriate anterior primary rami of spinal nerves, which supply the left forearm, would cause degeneration of the distal axonal processes of the general sensory (afferent) fibers and relieve pain symptoms in this patient. However, the anterior primary rami also contain somatic motor (general somatic efferent or GSE) fibers, so a selective rhizotomy at this location would also cause motor deficits. Because they convey both sensory and motor fibers, the anterior primary rami are inappropriate for selective rhizotomy to afford relief from pain.

12 **The answer is C: Long thoracic nerve.**   The photo demonstrates a case of "winged scapula," indicative of lesion of the long thoracic nerve and subsequent paralysis of the serratus anterior muscle. The nerve is located on the lateral thoracic wall, on the superficial aspect of the serratus anterior, where it is not afforded the protection of the muscle it innervates (like most motor nerves), especially when the limb is elevated. In this patient, shrapnel wounds to the lateral thoracic wall caused damage to the long thoracic nerve and subsequent loss of

innervation to the serratus anterior muscle. When the affected limb is protracted, the medial border and inferior angle of the scapula pull away from the posterior chest wall, giving the scapula a wing-like appearance. Additionally, the affected arm cannot be abducted above the horizontal plane because the serratus anterior is not available to superiorly rotate the glenoid cavity of the scapula to allow full abduction. Following damage to the long thoracic nerve, it takes several weeks for a winged scapula to the develop because the trapezius muscle, which attaches to the spine of the scapula, must stretch before winging is apparent. **Choice A** (Axillary nerve) is incorrect. This nerve passes deeply through the axilla, around the surgical neck of the humerus, to supply the teres minor and deltoid muscles. A lesion of this nerve results in significant weakness in abduction of the arm and wasting of the rounded contour of the shoulder, which is not reported in this patient. **Choice B** (Thoracodorsal nerve) is incorrect. This nerve runs downward through the axilla to supply the latissimus dorsi muscle. Loss of the nerve would result in weakness in extension and medial rotation of the arm, plus wasting of the posterior axillary fold. These signs and symptoms were not reported in this patient. **Choice D** (Dorsal scapular nerve) is incorrect. This nerve courses into the upper, medial part of the back and the lower neck to supply the levator scapulae and rhomboid muscles. Paralysis of these muscles would result in weakness in elevation and retraction of the scapula, and perhaps wasting of the contour of the back under the trapezius muscle, which was not reported in this patient. **Choice E** (Suboccipital nerve) is incorrect. The suboccipital nerve is also the posterior (dorsal) ramus of the first cervical nerve (C1), which passes through the suboccipital triangle to innervate the rectus capitis posterior major and minor, obliquus capitis superior and inferior, rectus capitis lateralis, and semispinalis muscles. It is generally believed that the suboccipital nerve contains only motor fibers, but it may receive afferent (sensory) fibers related to proprioception. Damage to the suboccipital nerve would result in weakness extending and rotating the head on the C1 and C2 vertebrae, which was not reported in this patient.

13 **The answer is B: Spinal ganglia.**   The posterior (dorsal) and anterior (ventral) roots of spinal nerves typically merge within the intervertebral foramina to form individual spinal nerves. Because the spinal (dorsal root) ganglia are located at the distal ends of the posterior roots, they are also normally found within the intervertebral foramina. Thus, narrowing (stenosis) or compression of the intervertebral foramina may cause impingement of the posterior and anterior roots, spinal nerves, and spinal ganglia due to the presence of bony spurs (osteophytes) in this patient. **Choice A** (Posterior primary rami of spinal nerves) is incorrect. Each spinal nerve divides into its first branches (primary rami) immediately after exiting the intervertebral foramen. Because the primary rami are located distal to the intervertebral foramina, the posterior primary rami would not be compressed by stenosis of the intervertebral foramina due to the presence of osteophytes in this patient. Remember that the posterior primary rami extend into the epaxial tissues to innervate the deep (intrinsic; epaxial) muscles of the back. **Choice C** (Ganglia of the sympathetic trunk) is incorrect. The sympathetic trunk lies along the lateral side of the vertebral column, outside the intervertebral foramina. Thus, the ganglia of the sympathetic trunk would not be impinged by the osteophytes found in this patient. **Choice D** (Anterior primary rami of spinal nerves) is incorrect. Each spinal nerve divides into its first branches (primary rami) immediately after exiting the intervertebral foramen. Because the primary rami are located distal to the intervertebral foramina, the anterior primary rami would not be compressed by stenosis of the intervertebral foramina. Remember, the anterior (ventral) primary rami extend into the hypaxial tissues to innervate the superficial and intermediate (extrinsic; hypaxial) muscles of the back. **Choice E** (Anterior rootlets of spinal nerves) is incorrect. The anterior (ventral) rootlets of spinal nerves are located proximal to the intervertebral foramina, close to the spinal cord, and would not be impinged by a stenosis of the intervertebral foramina due to the presence of osteophytes.

14 **The answer is D: Spondylolysis.** Spondylolysis refers to a defect in the pars interarticularis of the affected vertebra (or L5 in this patient). Its meaning is derived from the Greek words "*spondylos*" (**G**: vertebra) and "*lysis*" (**G**: loosening). The given right posterior oblique X-ray reveals a fracture in the isthmus (or neck) of the pars interarticularis or the bony column formed by the superior and inferior articular processes of L5. This fracture has the appearance of a "headless Scottie Dog" in this image. To visualize the Scottie Dog, look at the intact L4 vertebra, and remember that the ear is formed by the superior articular process, the head is formed by the transverse process, its eye is the radiopaque pedicle, its foreleg is the inferior articular process, its body is represented by the lamina and spinous process, and the hind leg of the dog is the opposite inferior articular process. Because there is a fracture within the isthmus (or neck) of the pars interarticularis of L5, spondylolysis of L5 is the proper diagnosis. **Choice A** (Ankylosing spondylitis) is incorrect. Ankylosing spondylitis is arthritis of the spine, which presents with inflammation, stiffening of the joint, and potentially bony ankylosis (synostosis) due to ossification of the posterior and anterior longitudinal ligaments. Ankylosing spondylitis is derived from the Greek words "*ankylosis*" (**G**: stiffening of the joint), "*spondylos*" (**G**: vertebra), and "*itis*" (**G**: inflammation). Ankylosing spondylitis, a degenerative joint disease of the spine, with an autoimmune component. However, this diagnosis is not supported by the given lumbar spine X-ray. **Choice B** (High-grade spondylolisthesis) is incorrect. Spondylolisthesis describes the anterior displacement of a vertebra in relation to the vertebra below it. Its meaning is derived from the Greek words "*spondylos*" (**G**: vertebra) and "*olisthesis*" (**G**: slipping and falling). A high-grade (III or IV) spondylolisthesis implies the anteriorly displaced posterior edge of the L5 vertebral body is located anterior to the center of the S1 vertebral body. A high-grade spondylolisthesis means the vertebral body of L5 is displaced anteriorly by the width of more than half of the vertebral body of S1. The given lumbar spine X-ray does not support this diagnosis. **Choice C** (Spondyloptosis) is incorrect. Spondyloptosis is the most extreme type of spondylolisthesis in which the posterior edge of the L5 vertebra is dislocated anterior to the entire S1 vertebral body, so it would fall off the vertebral column. "Spondyloptosis" is derived from the Greek words "*spondylos*" (**G**: vertebra) and "*ptosis*" (**G**: falling). This extreme form of spondylolisthesis was not supported by the given lumbar spine X-ray. **Choice E** (Spondylosis) is incorrect. Spondylosis is a term that implies stiffening of the spine (ankylosis) due to any lesion of the spine of a degenerative nature. Due to the young age of this male athlete,

a degenerative joint disease of the spine described by the word "spondylosis" is highly unlikely. Furthermore, this diagnosis is not supported by the given lumbar spine X-ray.

15 **The answer is A: The medullary cone ends at or above the L3 level.** The objective of a lumbar puncture is to enter (tap) the subarachnoid space and access the CSF. This procedure is performed using a long spinal needle. For several reasons, this procedure is best performed in the low lumbar region, between the spinous processes of the L3 and L4 (sometimes L4 and L5) vertebrae. The medullary cone (or conus medullaris) is the tapered terminal end of the spinal cord. In adults, the medullary cone is normally located within the T12-L3 vertebral levels. Thus, penetrating the vertebral canal and subarachnoid space below L3 is the "safe" place to go, in that the spinal needle should not penetrate the spinal cord. **Choice B** (The subarachnoid space ends at the L3 level) is incorrect. The subarachnoid space is the CSF-filled space between the arachnoid and pia mater layers of the meninges. The dura-arachnoid layers line the vertebral canal and end at the S2 level. The pia mater lines the exterior surface of the neural tube and continues distally to envelope the spinal nerve rootlets and roots. Because the spinal cord ends at approximately the L1 level, there is a large separation between the dura and arachnoid mater layers of the meninges and the pia mater below L1. Thus, the subarachnoid space is quite large below the medullary cone (conus medullaris), providing a significant pool (the lumbar cistern) of CSF. **Choice C** (The intervertebral foramina at L3-4 are large and easy to penetrate) is incorrect. The intervertebral foramina in the lumbar region are large openings; however, the lumbar puncture does not occur at these locations. During a spinal tap, the spinal needle is inserted through an interlaminar space, on the posterior side of the vertebral column. These spaces are largest in the low lumbar spine, thus affording a relatively open path to the vertebral canal. Before a spinal tap is administered, the patient is often bent forward into the fetal position by flexing the spine, which expands the interlaminar spaces during the lumbar puncture. **Choice D** (No vertebral venous plexuses exist below the L3 level) is incorrect. The vertebral venous plexuses are an extensive network of valveless, interconnecting vessels running the entire length of the vertebral column. The external vertebral venous plexus lies on the anterior aspect of the vertebral column and the posterior side of the vertebral arch. The internal vertebral venous plexus is a major constituent of the epidural space within the vertebral canal. A lumbar puncture must traverse both the external and internal plexuses to reach the subarachnoid space. **Choice E** (The ligamenta flava are absent below the L3 level) is incorrect. The ligamenta flava are short ligaments that connect the anterior sides of adjacent vertebral laminae along the entire length of the vertebral column. The spinal needle must pierce a ligamentum flavum in order to enter the vertebral canal.

16 **The answer is B: Burst fracture of T12 vertebral body.** The sagittal CT clearly shows a burst (crush or compression) fracture of the 12th thoracic vertebral body (T12). This T12 burst fracture also presents with a fracture fragment that is displaced posterior into the vertebral canal where it would compress the terminal end of the spinal cord, the medullary cone (conus medullaris), which typically lies within the T12-L3 vertebral levels. Compression of the spinal cord would lead to pain within the lower back that would likely extend into the lower limbs. This injury might also result in incontinence, loss of sensation, and paraplegia or paraparesis (loss of motor function). Remember that a CT scan is a valuable means of viewing "blood and bone," and this type of radiological imaging is the standard way to view injuries resulting from trauma, as seen in this patient. With this patient falling off the ladder and landing on his feet, the downward force from the high fall and the upward force from the impact on the ground have crushed the body of the T12 vertebra, resulting in the burst fracture of the T12 vertebral body seen on this sagittal CT. **Choice A** (Herniated intervertebral disc) is incorrect. The intervertebral discs in a young person are usually so strong that the vertebrae often fracture before the discs rupture, and in this 22-year-old man, this scenario is confirmed by the sagittal CT scan. A herniated nucleus pulposus of the intervertebral disc can cause lower back pain that extends into the lower limbs, as seen in this patient. However, in this CT scan, the spaces occupied by the discs, located between the vertebral bodies, are relatively uniform in both the lumbar and lower thoracic regions, which would also rule out a herniated intervertebral disc. A CT scan is valuable in assessing bone injuries while a MRI would be the best means to view damage to the intervertebral discs, the spinal cord and its nerve roots, and the ligaments of the spine. **Choice C** (Lumbar spinal stenosis) is incorrect. Lumbar spinal stenosis describes a narrowing of the vertebral foramen or canal that is normally seen in older individuals with a genetic disposition toward this condition. In the given CT, the vertebral canal, which houses the spinal cord, is relatively uniform throughout the lumbar region. The fracture fragment from the T12 vertebral body does enter the spinal canal and impinges the spinal cord and its nerve roots. However, lumbar spinal stenosis is usually due to degeneration of the intervertebral discs, which narrows the vertebral canal and potentially impinges the spinal cord and its nerve roots. Due to the age of the patient and the traumatic nature of his injury, lumbar spinal stenosis is not likely, especially with the visual evidence of a wide vertebral canal on the given CT scan. **Choice D** (Spondylolisthesis of L5-S1 articulation) is incorrect. Spondylolisthesis of the L5-S1 articulation is defined by the forward displacement of the vertebral body of L5 relative to the upper part of the sacrum (S1). The given CT does not show spondylolisthesis of the L5-S1 articulation, so this choice can be eliminated. **Choice E** (Excessive lumbar lordosis) is incorrect. The natural curvature of the lumbar portion of the vertebral column is concave posterior, or lordosis. The secondary curvature of the lumbar spine to lordosis occurs when an infant begins to assume the upright position during standing or walking. The given CT does not show excessive lumbar lordosis (sway back or hollow back), which is often associated with weakened anterolateral abdominal musculature, which is unlikely in this 22-year-old man.

17 **The answer is C: C6 spinal nerve roots.** Classic posterolateral herniation of the nucleus pulposus of the intervertebral disc occurs most often within the C4-5 and L4-5 intervertebral discs. A herniated nucleus pulposus may displace or disrupt the posterior longitudinal ligament and extend into the vertebral canal and impinge upon spinal nerve roots either within the vertebral canal or as they traverse the intervertebral foramen (or both). When dealing with such cases in the cervical and lower lumbar regions, remember the formula "$N+1$." That is, N = the number of the intervertebral disc; +1 = the number

of the spinal nerve roots primarily contacted by the herniation. Thus, the herniated C5-6 disc will most likely impinge upon the C6 spinal nerve roots. In the cervical region, this formula works because there are eight pairs of cervical spinal nerves but only seven cervical vertebrae. Each numbered spinal nerve exits above the matching numbered vertebra. Thus, the C6 cervical spinal nerve exits the intervertebral foramen formed by the C5 and C6 vertebrae, where it may be impinged. The formula also works in the low lumbar region because of the acute angles the nerve roots take in entering the intervertebral foramina. Here, the numbered spinal nerves exit below the matching vertebra, so the L4 nerve roots enter the intervertebral foramen between the L4 and L5 vertebrae. Because these lumbar nerve roots take a very acute turn to enter that opening, they are typically held against the upper pedicle and are superior to the level of the intervertebral disc. Thus, the L4 roots would not be impinged by a bulging L4-5 disc. Therefore, the L4-5 intervertebral disc would, instead, push primarily against the L5 roots as they align to enter the intervertebral foramen formed by the L5 and S1 vertebrae. **Choice A** (C5 spinal nerve roots) is incorrect. Because of the "extra" pair of cervical spinal nerves (compared to the number of vertebrae), the cervical nerves exit the vertebral canal superior to their matching numbered vertebra. Thus, the C5 spinal nerve roots pass into the intervertebral foramen formed by the C4 and C5 vertebrae and would not be impinged by the bulging C5-6 intervertebral disc. Remember the $N+1$ rule. **Choice B** (C5 anterior primary ramus) is incorrect. The anterior (ventral) and posterior (dorsal) primary rami are the first branches of the spinal nerves, located outside the vertebral canal. Regardless of the spinal segmental level, these structures are not impinged by a herniation of the nucleus pulposus of the intervertebral disc. **Choice D** (C6 posterior primary ramus) is incorrect. The posterior (dorsal) and anterior (ventral) primary rami are the first branches of the spinal nerves, located outside the vertebral canal. Regardless of the spinal segmental level, these structures are not impinged by a herniation of the nucleus pulposus of the intervertebral disc. **Choice E** (C7 posterior horn segment of the spinal cord) is incorrect. The C7 posterior horn segment is inferior to the level of the herniated disc. Also, this structure is located on the opposite side of the spinal cord from the disc and would not be directly contacted by a herniation of the nucleus pulposus of the intervertebral disc.

18 **The answer is B: Fracture of the dens axis (odontoid process).** The sagittal CT clearly shows a Type II dens axis (odontoid process) fracture, which is the most common type of fracture (approximately 60% of cases) involving the dens. This fracture occurs at the base of the dens where it extends superiorly from the axis (or second cervical vertebra). The precise mechanism for odontoid fractures is unknown, but it most likely includes a combination of flexion, extension, and rotation. In this case, the patient's cervical spine was forced into a flexed position by the impact of the crash and then a hyperextended position with slight rotation due to the impact of her head on the steering wheel. The forces involved fractured the odontoid process at its base, but luckily, the fractured dens axis does not extend posterior to impinge upon the spinal cord. Patients with this type of odontoid fracture are placed in halo immobilization or undergo internal fixation (or odontoid screw fixation) to reattach the fractured axis dens to the body of the axis. Remember Steele's

Rule of Thirds, which states one third of the atlas (C1) ring is occupied by the dens axis, one third by the spinal cord, and one third by the fluid-filled space and surrounding tissues of the cord. This extra space within the atlas ring explains why people with odontoid fractures may not have spinal cord injuries, but they will often feel unstable when they move their head suddenly. The incidence of odontoid fractures approaches 15% of all cervical spine fractures. **Choice A** (Traumatic spondylolisthesis of C2) is incorrect. Spondylolisthesis describes the anterior displacement of a vertebra in relation to the vertebra below it. Its meaning is derived from the Greek words "*spondyl*" (**G**: vertebrae) and "*olisthesis*" (**G**: slip). One of the most common injuries of the cervical vertebrae involves the fracture of the vertebral arch of the axis (or 2nd cervical vertebra). The fracture usually occurs in the pars interarticularis or the bony column formed by the superior and inferior articular processes of the axis, and it is called a traumatic spondylolisthesis (or defect in the pars interarticularis) of C2 or hangman fracture. The precise mechanism for traumatic spondylolisthesis of C2 is the hyperextension of the head on the neck, not the combination of hyperflexion, rotation, and hyperextension of the head and neck seen in this MVA. It receives its alternative name, hangman fracture, because it is often seen in criminals executed by hanging due to the hyperextension of the head due to the placement of the noose under their chin. A sagittal CT would not be the best means to view a hangman fracture because the vertebral arch of the axis is not seen. A lateral cervical X-ray would be a better imaging technique to visualize a traumatic spondylolisthesis of C2 (or hangman fracture). **Choice C** (Atlanto-axial subluxation) is incorrect. Atlanto-axial subluxation, or the incomplete dislocation of the median atlanto-axial joint, occurs following the rupture of the transverse ligament of the atlas, which holds the dens axis (odontoid process) in place. Losing the integrity of the transverse ligament of the atlas can result in compression of the upper cervical spinal cord, leading to quadriplegia (paralysis of all four limbs) and even death (if the medulla of the brainstem is compressed). Atlanto-axial subluxation is prevalent in patients with Down syndrome (trisomy 21) but it can occur with other connective tissue disorders. In this patient, a fracture at the base of the odontoid process of the axis was noted on the sagittal CT scan. This fracture fragment is held in place by an intact transverse ligament of the atlas, so atlanto-axial subluxation did not occur in this patient. **Choice D** (Ruptured intervertebral disc between C1 and C2) is incorrect. A ruptured intervertebral disc between C1 and C2 is not possible because no disc exists between these two vertebrae. The given sagittal CT clearly shows a dens axis (odontoid process) fracture. The space between the fractured odontoid process and the body of the axis could be misinterpreted as a translucent space for an intervertebral disc. Knowledge of the proper anatomy of the atlanto-axial joint would eliminate this option. Remember that a CT scan is valuable in assessing bone injuries, so a herniated disc would be better seen with an MRI. An MRI would be the best means to view damage to the intervertebral discs, the spinal cord and its nerve roots, and the ligaments of the spine. **Choice E** (No pathology is apparent on the CT scan) is incorrect. The given sagittal CT clearly shows a dens axis (odontoid process) fracture. The space between the fractured odontoid process and the body of the axis could be misinterpreted as a translucent space for an intervertebral disc; however, no disc exists in the atlanto-axial joint. Knowledge

of the proper anatomy of the atlanto-axial joint would enable easy elimination of this option.

19 **The answer is E: Splenius capitis.** The posterior (dorsal) primary rami of spinal nerves innervate the embryonic epimere and all the skeletal muscles derived from it. The derivatives of the epimere constitute the deep (intrinsic) muscles of the back (or epaxial muscles), including the splenius capitis and cervicis muscles, suboccipital muscles, transversospinales muscles (including the semispinalis, multifidus, and rotatores muscles), and several other small muscles. Thus, damage to the cervical posterior (dorsal) primary rami, specifically C2-6, would result in paralysis of the splenius capitis muscle. **Choice A** (Trapezius) is incorrect. The trapezius is a member of the superficial extrinsic layer of back muscles, which connect the upper limbs to the trunk. When these muscles contract, movements result in the upper limb. However, the trapezius muscle does not originate from either the epimere or hypomere, as evidenced by its innervation via the spinal accessory nerve (CN XI). Instead, it is likely related to postbranchial origins, along with the sternocleidomastoid. Thus, destruction of the cervical posterior (dorsal) primary rami will not directly affect the innervation of the trapezius muscle. **Choice B** (Latissimus dorsi) is incorrect. The latissimus dorsi (**L**: widest muscle of back) is a member of the superficial extrinsic layer of back muscles, which connect the upper limbs to the trunk. When these muscles contract, movements result in the upper limb. The latissimus dorsi muscle is derived from hypomeres, which develop lateral and anterior to the vertebral axis. All of the muscles derived from hypomeres are innervated by the anterior (ventral) primary rami of spinal nerves. The latissimus dorsi muscle acts on the upper limb, and it migrates secondarily into the back. Due to being innervated by the anterior (ventral) primary rami, the latissimus dorsi muscle would not be affected by destruction of the cervical posterior (dorsal) primary rami seen in this patient. **Choice C** (Levator scapulae) is incorrect. The levator scapulae muscle is a member of the superficial extrinsic layer of back muscles, which connect the upper limbs to the trunk. When these muscles contract, movements result in the upper limb. The levator scapulae muscle is derived from hypomeres, which develop lateral and anterior to the vertebral axis. All of the muscles derived from hypomeres are innervated by the anterior (ventral) primary rami of spinal nerves. Due to being innervated by the anterior (ventral) primary rami, the levator scapulae muscle would not be affected by destruction of the cervical posterior (dorsal) primary rami seen in this patient. **Choice D** (Rhomboid major) is incorrect. The rhomboid major muscle is a member of the superficial extrinsic layer of back muscles, which connect the upper limbs to the trunk. When these muscles contract, movements result in the upper limb. The rhomboid major muscle is derived from hypomeres, which develop lateral and anterior to the vertebral axis. All of the muscles derived from hypomeres are innervated by the anterior (ventral) primary rami of spinal nerves. Due to being innervated by the anterior (ventral) primary rami, the levator scapulae muscle would not be affected by destruction of the cervical posterior (dorsal) primary rami seen in this patient.

20 **The answer is D: Cervical Spinal Stenosis.** Cervical spinal stenosis describes a narrowing of the vertebral canal that is typically seen in older individuals with degenerative changes in the cervical spine. In the given MRI, the vertebral canal, which houses the spinal cord, is impinged by intervertebral disc degeneration in the midcervical region, which results in no cerebral spinal fluid (CSF), which appears as a hyperintense (white) signal in this MRI, being visible anterior or posterior to the spinal cord. CSF can be seen surrounding the spinal cord above and below the midcervical region. In this patient, the tingling numbness of the fourth and fifth digits within his right hand is exacerbated by hyperextension of the cervical vertebrae (or looking up), which implies the spinal cord is further compressed by hyperextension of the neck leading to myelopathy (damage to the spinal cord itself). Due to the age of the patient, the degenerative nature of the cervical vertebrae, and the absence of trauma, spinal cord stenosis is the most likely diagnosis, and this condition was confirmed with the given T2-weighted MRI. **Choice A** (Burst fracture of C3 vertebral body) is incorrect. A burst (crush or compression) fracture of the vertebral body of the 3rd cervical vertebra (C3) would likely result from trauma, and no trauma has been reported in this patient. Moreover, the given MRI does not confirm a burst fracture of C3, though degenerative changes can be seen within this vertebra. A burst fracture of C3 could lead to compression of the spinal cord due to a displaced posterior fracture fragment; however, the given MRI does not confirm this type of injury. **Choice B** (Ruptured anterior longitudinal ligament) is incorrect. The anterior longitudinal ligament is a vertically running band that attaches along the anterior sides of the vertebral bodies, which resists hyperextension of the vertebral column. Damage to the anterior longitudinal ligament can occur following traumatic hyperextension of the head on the neck, which was not reported in this patient. Moreover, damage to (or interruption of) the anterior longitudinal ligament would appear as a hyperintense (white) signal located anterior to the vertebral column at the location of the damage to this ligament, and this evidence is not apparent on this T2-weighted MRI. **Choice C** (Transection of the spinal cord) is incorrect. Transection of the spinal cord would result in the loss of all sensation and voluntary movements inferior to the site of the lesion. Visual evidence of a transection of the cervical spinal cord is not apparent on this MRI, and because the patient only reported a tingling numbness of the fourth and fifth digits within his right hand, this diagnosis is not possible. **Choice E** (Traumatic spondylolisthesis of C5) is incorrect. Traumatic spondylolisthesis of C5 describes the anterior displacement of the C5 vertebral body in relation to the C6 vertebra located below it. In this patient, spondylolisthesis of C5 is apparent on the sagittal MRI. However, due to the absence of trauma, the anterior displacement of C5 is probably due to degenerative changes (such as facet arthritis, disc degeneration, and the presence of osteophytes, or bone spurs) within the cervical vertebrae. This radiologic evidence would imply degenerative spondylolisthesis, not traumatic spondylolisthesis, of C5 as the reason for the anterior displacement of C5.

21 **The answer is D: Latissimus dorsi.** The latissimus dorsi (*L*: widest muscle of back) is a large, fan-shaped muscle and a member of the superficial extrinsic layer of back muscles, which connect the upper limbs to the trunk. The chin-up movement described includes lifting the body toward the upper limb, which is a powerful extension action. In conjunction with the pectoralis major muscle, the latissimus

dorsi muscle raises the trunk to the arm, which is crucial in performing chin-ups or climbing a tree. Remember that the superficial layer of back muscles is composed of upper limb muscles that take large bases of origin in the back. Athletes who make heavy use of extension and medial rotation of the arm (as in chin-ups or climbing in conditional exercises) typically have well-developed "lats" that give the classic "V" shape to the back. **Choice A** (Serratus posterior superior) is incorrect. The serratus posterior superior muscle is a member of the intermediate layer of back muscles that lies deep to the rhomboid muscles. Due to its insertion into the superior borders of the 2nd to 5th ribs, it is said to elevate the ribs to increase the diameter of the thorax, acting as an accessory muscle of respiration. Due to its small size and lack of attachment to the appendicular skeleton, it would not be the primary muscle involved with performing chin-ups. **Choice B** (Rhomboid major) is incorrect. The rhomboid major and minor muscles act to retract (adduct) the scapula. In the chin-up movement, the trunk of the body is lifting toward the upper limb, and the rhomboids are important in stabilization of the scapula to allow the latissimus dorsi muscle to raise the trunk toward the upper limb. However, these muscles are not the prime agonist in this climbing movement. **Choice C** (Levator scapulae) is incorrect. The levator scapulae muscle acts mainly to elevate the scapula. During the chin-up movement, the levator scapulae muscle also aids in downward rotation of the scapula, which would aid the latissimus dorsi muscle in raising the trunk toward the upper limb. However, the levator scapulae muscle is not the prime agonist in this climbing movement. **Choice E** (Longissimus) is incorrect. The longissimus muscle is one of the three components of the erector spinae group of deep back muscles. Its primary action is to extend the back. Because it does not attach or originate within the upper limb, the longissimus muscle is unable to lift the trunk toward the upper limb, which is what defines a chin-up.

22 **The answer is D: Spinal ganglion of T10.** In this patient, herpes zoster, or shingles, is a painful skin rash affecting the dermatome distribution pattern of the left 10th thoracic (T10) nerve, as evidenced by the involvement of the umbilicus. Shingles is seen in patients who have had previous exposure to the varicella zoster virus, which causes chickenpox in children or young adults. After the initial exposure to chickenpox, this virus can reside latent in ganglia of an individual for years. If this individual becomes immunocompromised, the skin (or dermatomes supplied by the infected ganglia) can develop shingles, a painful skin rash, which blisters, breaks open, crusts over, and then disappears. In this patient, the herpetic lesions were found in the sensory distribution of the left T10 nerve, which means the virus resides in this nerve's sensory ganglion, or the spinal ganglion of T10. Remember that two types of ganglia exist: sensory (afferent) and autonomic. The sensory ganglia, which are most often affected by shingles, are equivalent to the spinal (dorsal root) ganglia of spinal nerves in that they house typical pseudounipolar cell bodies of afferent neurons and do not contain synapses. If a spinal ganglion were infected by the varicella zoster virus, shingles may present in its dermatome distribution patterns when the patient is immunocompromised. **Choice A** (Paravertebral ganglion) is incorrect. The paravertebral (sympathetic) ganglia are located within the sympathetic trunk. They receive efferent fibers from the presynaptic (preganglionic) sympathetic neurons originating in the intermediolateral (IML) cell column of the thoracic and upper lumbar segments (T1-L2). Due to their location, these sympathetic ganglia are called paravertebral ganglia. Before it causes shingles (or herpes zoster), the varicella zoster virus resides latent in sensory ganglia for many years. Because the paravertebral ganglia are autonomic ganglia, it is unlikely they would be responsible for the skin rash in this patient. **Choice B** (Prevertebral ganglion) is incorrect. The prevertebral ganglia are sympathetic ganglia that receive their name as they are located anterior to the vertebral column, as distinguished from the ganglia of the sympathetic trunk (paravertebral ganglia). Prevertebral ganglia exist near major branches of the abdominal aorta in the abdominopelvic cavity. These ganglia send postsynaptic (postganglionic) sympathetic fibers to the abdominopelvic organs with periarterial plexuses. Before it causes shingles (or herpes zoster), the varicella zoster virus resides latent in sensory ganglia for many years. Because the prevertebral ganglia are autonomic ganglia, it is unlikely they would be responsible for the skin rash in this patient. **Choice C** (Lumbar ganglion) is incorrect. The lumbar ganglia are paravertebral ganglia located in the abdominopelvic part of the sympathetic trunk. Before it causes shingles (or herpes zoster), the varicella zoster virus resides latent in sensory ganglia for many years. Because the lumbar ganglia are autonomic ganglia, it is unlikely they would be responsible for the skin rash in this patient. **Choice E** (Spinal ganglion of L2) is incorrect. The spinal (posterior root) ganglion is a sensory ganglion, so it could be infected by the varicella zoster virus and present with a painful, skin rash along its dermatome distribution pattern. The sensory distribution of L2 would extend along the back, hip, and extend into the anterior and medial aspects of the thigh. Because this patient presents with a skin rash at the level of the umbilicus, the spinal ganglion of T10 would be the source of this painful skin rash.

23 **The answer is D: Flexing the hip by raising the straightened left leg with the patient lying in the supine position increases pain in the back with radiation down the left leg.** The straight-leg raising test is designed to stretch the lower back and apply tension to the lumbar spinal nerves and roots. Thus, a positive test will stress compromised nerves and elicit pain and/or spasticity in the areas supplied by the affected nerves. If the diagnosis of left side lumbar nerve entrapment secondary to a herniated lumbar disc is correct, raising the left leg (i.e., flexing the hip) with the knee straight (extended) from the supine position (lying on the back) will apply traction to the entrapped nerve roots and elicit pain in the affected areas. Conducting the same maneuver on the right side will not elicit a pain reaction. Lasèque sign is a medical maneuver that involves raising a straight leg to exacerbate pain and is useful in diagnosing lumbar disc disorders and tension of the sciatic nerve. **Choice A** (Walking while keeping the left leg in a straight position [i.e., the knee is kept straight] relieves the pain in the back and limb) is incorrect. The forward swing of the straight left leg during walking is essentially the same maneuver as raising the straight leg from the supine position. Traction is applied to the entrapped nerve roots during flexion of the hip, with pain stimulated rather than relieved. **Choice B** (Flexing the hip by raising the straightened left leg [i.e., the knee is kept straight] with the patient lying in the supine position relieves the pain in the back and leg) is incorrect. This maneuver is basically the same as the one explained in

Choice A. Again, pain should be elicited rather than relieved in a positive test. **Choice C** (Abducting the hip by raising the straightened left leg with the patient lying on his right side relieves the pain in the back and leg) is incorrect. Raising (abducting) the limb toward the affected side will again apply traction to the affected nerve roots, resulting in stimulating pain rather than relieving pain. **Choice E** (Extending the hip by raising the straightened left leg with the patient lying in the prone position increases pain in the back with radiation down the left leg) is incorrect. From the prone position, raising the left limb means extending the limb. This maneuver will not produce as great an excursion of the limb as flexing the straightened limb at the hip from the supine position. Therefore, this maneuver will reduce traction on the affected nerve roots and relieve pain rather than increase pain.

24 **The answer is C: Traumatic spondylolysis of C2.** Spondylolysis means a defect in the pars interarticularis of the affected vertebra (or C2 in this patient). The lateral cervical X-ray of this patient reveals a bilateral fracture of the axis (or C2) in the pars interarticularis or the bony column formed by the superior and inferior articular processes of C2. This type of cervical fracture is often seen after hyperextension of the head in relationship to the neck, and it is called a traumatic spondylolysis of C2 or hangman fracture. It receives its alternative name, hangman fracture, because it is often seen in criminals executed by hanging due to the hyperextension of the head due to the placement of the noose under their chin. This lateral cervical film also reveals a traumatic spondylolisthesis of C2, which is sometimes evident following an acute fracture of the pars interarticularis of C2. Spondylolisthesis describes the anterior displacement of a vertebra in relation to the vertebra below it, and its meaning is derived from the Greek words "*spondyl*" (**G**: vertebrae) and "*olisthesis*" (**G**: slip). In the given X-ray, the vertebral body of C2 is displaced anterior in relationship to C3, which confirms the traumatic spondylolisthesis of C2. Therefore, the X-ray clearly shows a bilateral fracture of the pars interarticularis of C2 (or traumatic spondylolysis of C2 [hangman fracture]) and spondylolisthesis, anterior displacement, of C2 in relationship to the vertebral body of C3. This specific fracture was classified in 1981 by Effendi into a subtype called "forward dislocation, axial arch fracture, Effendi Type II." **Choice A** (Ruptured anterior longitudinal ligament) is incorrect. The anterior longitudinal ligament is a vertically running band that attaches along the anterior sides of the vertebral bodies. Its peripheral fibers have strong attachments to the intervertebral discs. This ligament resists hyperextension of the vertebral column, and in this patient who experienced hyperextension of the head on the neck, the extreme forces involved with the impact of the clothes line on the patient's neck may have damaged the anterior longitudinal ligament, particularly due to the spondylolisthesis of C2. However, a ruptured anterior longitudinal ligament is not apparent on this lateral cervical X-ray, so the integrity of this ligament is unknown. The anterior longitudinal ligament would be better viewed with a T2-weighted MRI, which would show this ligament as a hypointense (dark black) band located anterior to the vertebral column. If damaged, the hypointense anterior longitudinal ligament will be interrupted by abnormal hyperintense (white) signal. **Choice B** (Jefferson [burst] fracture of C1) is incorrect. The C1 vertebra, or atlas, is a closed ring with no vertebral body. Excessive vertical, or downward, force on the top of the head can fracture the anterior and posterior arches of C1 in multiple places, leading to a Jefferson (or burst) fracture of C1. Jefferson fractures of C1 often occur with axial loading force when the top of the head is impacted by a hard or heavy object. The downward force of the impact drives the lateral masses of the atlas lateral and fractures the anterior and posterior arches of C1. Because of the nature of this hyperextension injury and lack of visual evidence on the lateral cervical film of damage to C1, a Jefferson (or burst) fracture of C1 is not the diagnosis. **Choice D** (Fracture of the dens axis [odontoid process]) is incorrect. In the given lateral cervical X-ray, there is no apparent fracture of the dens (odontoid process) of the axis, or second cervical vertebra (C2). Because odontoid fractures are likely due to a combination of excessive flexion, extension, and some rotation within the cervical vertebrae, this patient, whose injury was caused by hyperextension of the head on the neck, is unlikely to have an odontoid fracture. The lateral cervical film confirms the presence of traumatic spondylolysis of C2, or a hangman fracture, and traumatic spondylolisthesis of C2. **Choice E** (Atlanto-axial subluxation) is incorrect. Atlanto-axial subluxation, or the incomplete dislocation of the median atlanto-axial joint, occurs following the rupture of the transverse ligament of the atlas, which holds the dens axis (odontoid process) in place. Losing the integrity of the transverse ligament of the atlas can result in compression of the upper cervical spinal cord, leading to quadriplegia (paralysis of all four limbs) and even death (if the medulla of the brainstem is compressed). Atlanto-axial subluxation is prevalent in patients with Down syndrome (trisomy 21), but it can also occur with other connective tissue disorders. In this lateral cervical film, a bilateral fracture of the pars interarticularis of C2 is apparent, and the odontoid process of C2 is in its normal position, which implies an intact transverse ligament of the atlas. Therefore, atlanto-axial subluxation did not occur in this patient.

25 **The answer is A: Ligamentum flavum.** The ligamentum flavum (**L:** yellow ligament) consists of yellow elastic fibrous tissue, which binds together the laminae of adjoining vertebrae and forms the posterior wall of the vertebral canal. During proper administration of an epidural anesthetic, the needle will pass (in order) through the supraspinous ligament overlying the spinous processes of the lumbar vertebrae, the interspinous ligament connecting the spinous processes of adjacent vertebrae, and finally the ligamentum flavum, which stretches between the laminae of adjacent vertebrae. Due to its high elastic fiber content and the usual placement of the pregnant woman into the fetal position, the anesthesiologist will feel substantial resistance before the needle passes through the ligamentum flavum and potentially an audible "pop" when it is penetrated. In the given diagram, the epidural space resides between the ligamentum flavum and the posterior longitudinal ligament. Remember that the ligamentum flavum is the last ligament the needle penetrates during administration of an epidural anesthetic. **Choice B** (Anterior longitudinal ligament) is incorrect. The anterior longitudinal ligament is a vertical connective tissue band that attaches along the anterior sides of the vertebral bodies, as noted in the given figure. During proper administration of an epidural anesthetic, the needle will pass (in order) through the supraspinous ligament, the interspinous ligament, and finally the ligamentum flavum. Due to its position residing anterior to the vertebral bodies,

the anterior longitudinal ligament will not be penetrated by the needle during proper administration of an epidural anesthetic. **Choice C** (Posterior longitudinal ligament) is incorrect. The posterior longitudinal ligament runs vertically along the posterior aspect of the vertebral column, as noted in the given figure. Due to its position residing posterior to the vertebral bodies, the posterior longitudinal ligament will not be penetrated during proper administration of an epidural anesthetic. **Choice D** (Interspinous ligament) is incorrect. The interspinous ligament is composed of fibrous bands that connect the spinous processes of adjacent vertebrae, as noted in the given figure. This ligament is penetrated by the needle during proper administration of an epidural anesthetic; however, the ligamentum flavum is the last ligament penetrated by the needle to reach the epidural space. **Choice E** (Intertransverse ligament) is incorrect. The intertransverse ligament is one ligament that connects the transverse processes of adjacent vertebrae. Because the intertransverse ligaments do not lie in the median sagittal plane, these ligaments would not be penetrated by the needle during administration of an epidural anesthetic and cannot be appreciated on the given figure.

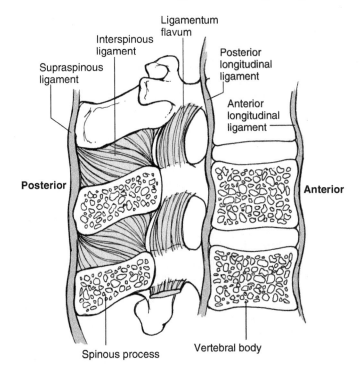

26 **The answer is D: Meningomyelocele.** A meningomyelocele is the most common form of spina bifida cystica. In this developmental disorder, the unfused portion of the vertebral column allows the meninges and the spinal cord to protrude through the structural defect, as noted in this longitudinal ultrasound scan. The protruded portion of the spinal cord is damaged (or not completed developed), and this defect may result in paralysis and loss of sensation below the level of the spinal cord defect. This condition is termed spina bifida cystica because of the characteristic presence of a cyst-like sac, composed of meninges and very thin skin, protruding from the defective area. The inclusion of a displaced portion of the spinal cord and nerve roots in the malformation designate this defect as a meningomyelocele. That is, the defect involves the meninges (meningo-), the spinal cord (myelo-), and the membranous sac (-cele). If it reaches full-term, this fetus will likely be paralyzed below the level of the meningomyelocele. In prenatal tests, elevated levels of AFP in the amniotic fluid and maternal blood are strongly associated with the more severe forms of spina bifida, and an ultrasound scan is ordered to confirm the presence of a neural tube defect. **Choice A** (Meningocele) is incorrect. The least common form of spina bifida is a posterior meningocele (or meningeal cyst). In this developmental disorder, the bilateral neural arch elements fail to fuse completely in the dorsal midline, but the meninges protrude through the defect into a sac or cyst. Therefore, the multiple vertebral defects are accompanied with the presence of a cyst, which contains cerebrospinal fluid (CSF). In a meningocele, the spinal cord and nerve roots are typically in normal position, not protruding into the cyst, and there are usually no long-term effects on the individuals. In this fetus, the ultrasound scan showed a protruding cyst-like sac containing neural tissue, which would rule out a meningocele. **Choice B** (Anencephaly) is incorrect. Anencephaly is a severe neural tube defect in which the cephalic (head) end of the neural tube fails to close in the embryo. This birth defect is lethal with the baby being born without a forebrain, calvaria, and scalp, leaving the remaining portions of the brain exposed. If proper prenatal care is available, most cases of anencephaly are detected by elevated maternal serum AFP levels and ultrasound scans during prenatal examinations. Elevated AFP levels are often correlated with neural tube defects, and the addition of folic acid to the diet of women in their childbearing years has been shown to reduce the incidence of neural tube defects. Because the given ultrasound scan localized the neural tube defect in the lower back, anencephaly can be eliminated as a valid answer. **Choice C** (Spina bifida occulta) is incorrect. Spina bifida occulta is the mildest form of spina bifida (**L:** split spine). In this developmental disorder, the bilateral neural arch elements fail to fuse completely in the dorsal midline; however, the split in the vertebrae is so small that the meninges and elements of the spinal cord do not protrude through the defect. Because spina bifida occulta is such a mild defect, maternal serum AFP levels are usually not elevated during pregnancy. In fact, full-term babies with spina bifida occulta may be asymptomatic, and most individuals with this condition are unaware of having this mild developmental birth defect. Individuals with spina bifida occulta may possess a tuft of hair, dimple, lipoma, or even a birthmark in the overlying skin of the affected region. Some research suggests that approximately 10% of the general population have this mildest form of spina bifida. Because maternal serum AFP levels would not be elevated in the case of spina bifida occulta, this defect can be eliminated as a valid answer. **Choice E** (Rachischisis) is incorrect. Rachischisis, or spina bifida with myeloschisis, is the most severe form of spina bifida. In rachischisis, the protruded portions of the spinal cord are not afforded the enveloping protection of the meninges, so no cyst-like sac would be present. A physician would see a flattened mass of nervous tissue with no associated membranes, which makes the patient more prone to life-threatening infections. Because the presence of a cyst-like sac was noted in the ultrasound scan, rachischisis can be eliminated as a valid answer.

27 **The answer is B: The pedicles of L3 and L4 are compressed together.** Spinal nerves exit the vertebral canal through the intervertebral foramina on the lateral sides of the vertebral column. Each intervertebral foramen is formed by the juxtaposing of the pedicles of successive articulated vertebrae. Thus, if the pedicles are compressed together, the intervertebral foramen is narrowed and a spinal nerve may be compressed ("pinched") as it traverses the intervertebral foramen. In the thoracic, lumbar, and sacral regions, each numbered segmental nerve passes through the intervertebral foramen below the matched numbered vertebra. Thus, the L3 spinal nerve traverses the intervertebral foramen below the L3 vertebra, between the L3 and L4 vertebrae. Because there is one more cervical spinal nerve (N = 8) than cervical vertebrae (N = 7), the cervical nerves exit the intervertebral foramina above the matching numbered vertebrae. Thus, the C3 spinal nerve passes through the opening between vertebrae C2 and C3. In this patient, the damage to the L3 spinal nerve on the left side is due to narrowing the intervertebral foramen caused by the compression of the pedicles of L2 and L3. **Choice A** (The pedicles of L2 and L3 are compressed together) is incorrect. When the pedicles of L2 and L3 are compressed together, the result is stenosis of the L2 intervertebral foramen. This narrowing would damage the ipsilateral L2 spinal nerve, resulting in lower back pain and potentially lower limb deficits. In this patient, damage to the L3 spinal nerve on the left side was reported, so compression of the L2 and L3 pedicles is not likely. **Choice C** (The laminae of L2 and L3 are compressed together) is incorrect. Compression of the interlaminar spaces would not affect the spinal nerves, as they do not pass through these openings. In fact, such compression would cause a lever arm reaction that would expand the intervertebral foramina. **Choice D** (The laminae of L3 and L4 are compressed together) is incorrect. Compression of the interlaminar spaces would not affect the spinal nerves, as they do not pass through these openings. In fact, such compression would cause a lever arm reaction that would expand the intervertebral foramina. **Choice E** (The spinous processes of L3 and L4 are compressed together) is incorrect. Compression of the spinous processes does not affect the spinal nerves because they do not pass through these gaps. Again, a compression of the L3 and L4 spinous processes would expand the intervertebral foramina because of a lever arm reaction.

28 **The answer is C: Jefferson (burst) fracture of C1.** The C1 vertebra, or atlas, is normally a closed ring with no vertebral body. Excessive vertical, or downward, force on the top of the head can fracture the anterior and posterior arches of C1 in multiple places, leading to a Jefferson (burst) fracture of C1. Due to the vertical force of the concrete mix striking the top of the man's head, the lateral masses of C1 are driven laterally due to the oblique articulation between the occipital condyles and the superior articular processes of the lateral masses of C1. This vertical compression force fractures the anterior and posterior arches of C1 bilaterally, as confirmed by the axial CT scan. Jefferson fractures of C1 often occur with axial loading force when the top of the head is impacted by a hard or heavy object. Because the fractures within the bony ring of the atlas actually increase its dimension, this type of fracture does not usually result in spinal cord injury; however, upper neck pain would be present. The axial CT scan confirms the diagnosis of a Jefferson (burst) fracture of C1. **Choice A** (Damage to the cervical spinal cord) is incorrect. Damage of the cervical spinal cord is highly unlikely due to the lack of neurological signs reported in this patient. The axial CT scan depicts bilateral fractures within the anterior and posterior arches of C1, and none of these fracture fragments are in close approximation to the spinal cord. **Choice B** (No pathology is apparent on the CT scan) is incorrect. The axial CT scan depicts bilateral fractures within the anterior and posterior arches of C1. Knowledge of the anatomy of the atlas (C1) would eliminate this diagnosis as a likely option. **Choice D** (Fracture of the dens axis [odontoid process]) is incorrect. In the given axial CT scan of the C1 arch, it would be hard to detect a fracture of the dens axis (odontoid process). Moreover, odontoid fractures have been reported to occur following a combination of excessive flexion, extension, and some rotation within the cervical vertebrae, so the nature of this traumatic injury would not suggest an odontoid fracture. A sagittal CT scan would give more information concerning the integrity of the odontoid process. **Choice E** (Atlanto-axial subluxation) is incorrect. Atlanto-axial subluxation, or the incomplete dislocation of the median atlanto-axial joint, occurs following the rupture of the transverse ligament of the atlas, which holds the dens axis (odontoid process) in place. Losing the integrity of the transverse ligament of the atlas can result in compression of the upper cervical spinal cord, leading to quadriplegia (paralysis of all four limbs) and even death (if the medulla of the brainstem is compressed). In this axial CT scan, the odontoid process (dens axis) of C2 is in its normal position, which implies an intact transverse ligament of the atlas. Therefore, atlanto-axial subluxation did not occur in this patient.

29 **The answer is A: Scoliosis.** Scoliosis (*G*: crookedness) is abnormal lateral and rotational curvature of the spine that may present with uneven hips, shoulders, and rib cage, a head that is not centered over the pelvis, the entire body leaning to one side, back pain, and/or fatigue. The given Anterior-Posterior (AP) X-ray shows an S-shaped curvature of the spine or vertebral column in this patient. In this X-ray, no apparent vertebral anomaly is apparent, so the diagnosis is most likely adolescent idiopathic scoliosis, which has an onset of 10 to 18 years of age and has no known cause. Most cases of adolescent idiopathic scoliosis (with curvatures of less than 20 degrees) require no treatment; however, if the curvature goes above 25 degrees, a back brace can be implemented to slow the progression of scoliosis. **Choice B** (Lordosis) is incorrect. Lordosis (*G*: bending backward) is an anteriorly convex curvature of the vertebral column (spine). The cervical and lumbar vertebral curvatures are normally lordotic; however, excessive lordotic curvature (also called hollow back, swayback, and saddleback) can be caused by tight lower back muscles, excessive abdominal fat, and pregnancy. Excessive lordosis can lead to lower back pain and can be treated with strengthening of the abdominal muscles and hamstrings. **Choice C** (Kyphosis) is incorrect. Kyphosis (*G*: hump-back) is an anteriorly concave curvature of the vertebral column (spine). The thoracic and sacral vertebral curvatures are normally kyphotic; however, deformities of the spine, due to degenerative arthritis, osteoporosis with compression fractures of the vertebrae, trauma, and developmental problems, can lead to excessive kyphotic curvature (or hunchback). Excessive kyphosis can cause pain and breathing difficulties. The given lateral X-ray shows an example of abnormal kyphotic curvature of the lumbar spine due to benign compression fractures of the L1 and L3 vertebrae secondary to osteoporosis. This disease is characterized by compromised bone strength and decreased bone mass.

The affected L1 and L3 vertebrae depict an anterior wedging deformity, which would cause the patient to appear shorter (lose height). **Choice D** (Osteoporosis) is incorrect. Osteoporosis is a disease characterized by compromised bone strength and decreased bone mass, which can lead to an increased rate of fracture in the vertebral column, the mid-forearm, and more frequently the proximal femur resulting in hip fractures. Women are four times more likely to receive the prognosis of osteoporosis, with approximately 25% of women between 65 and 85 years old being diagnosed with osteoporosis. Due to the age of this 14-year-old patient and the findings of the nurse, osteoporosis is not likely. **Choice E** (Osteoarthritis) is incorrect. Osteoarthritis (or degenerative arthritis) erodes the articular cartilage in primarily weight-bearing joints. Because this type of arthritis is found in older populations, this diagnosis is not likely in this 14-year-old patient, especially due to the symptoms noted by the nurse.

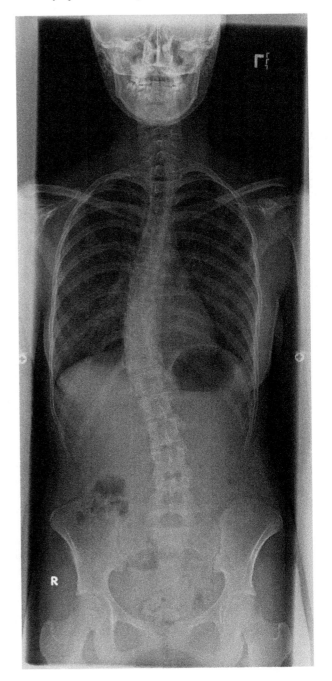

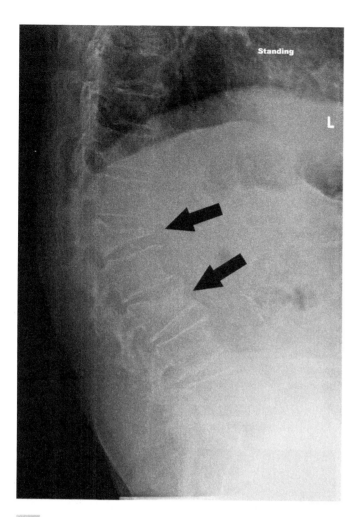

Standing

L

30 **The answer is A: S1 spinal nerve roots.** Approximately 90% of intervertebral disc herniations occur toward the bottom of the spine at the L4-5 or L5-S1 segments. This T1-weighted MRI reveals posterolateral herniation of the nucleus pulposus of the L5-S1 intervertebral disc, as indicated by the white arrow. Remember that a herniated nucleus pulposus may displace or disrupt the posterior longitudinal ligament and extend into the vertebral canal and impinge upon spinal nerve roots either within the vertebral canal or as they traverse the intervertebral foramen (or both). When dealing with such cases in the lower lumbar regions, remember the formula "N+1." That is, N = the number of the intervertebral disc; +1 = the number of the spinal nerve roots primarily contacted by the herniation. Thus, the herniated L5-S1 intervertebral disc would impinge the S1 nerve roots, which resulted in the lower back pain, tingling numbness radiating down his right lower limb to the lateral part of his foot, and weakness when standing on the toes of his right foot. **Choice B** (S1 anterior primary ramus) is incorrect. The anterior (ventral) and posterior (dorsal) primary rami are the first branches of the spinal nerves, located outside the vertebral canal. Regardless of the spinal segmental level, these structures are not impinged by a herniation of the nucleus pulposus of the intervertebral disc. **Choice C** (L5 spinal nerve roots) is incorrect. Because of the acute angles that the lower lumbar nerve roots take in exiting the vertebral canal via the intervertebral foramina, the L5 spinal nerve roots would typically be held against the upper pedicle of L5, above the level of the L5-S1 disc. Thus, the L5 roots would not be impinged by a bulging L5-S1 disc. Therefore,

impingement of the S1 nerve roots is a more likely scenario. **Choice D** (L5 posterior primary ramus) is incorrect. The anterior (ventral) and posterior (dorsal) primary rami are the first branches of the spinal nerves, located outside the vertebral canal. Regardless of the spinal segmental level, these structures are not impinged by a herniation of the nucleus pulposus of the intervertebral disc. **Choice E** (L5 anterior primary ramus) is incorrect. The anterior (ventral) and posterior (dorsal) primary rami are the first branches of the spinal nerves, located outside the vertebral canal. Regardless of the spinal segmental level, these structures are not impinged by a herniation of the nucleus pulposus of the intervertebral disc.

31 **The answer is E: S2.** The medullary cone (conus medullaris) is the tapered terminal end of the spinal cord, composed of the sacral and coccygeal segments. In adults, the conus medullaris typically lies within the T12-L3 vertebral levels, but it generally ends at approximately L2. Thus, displacement fractures of these vertebrae are likely to affect one or more of the sacral-coccygeal spinal cord segments. In this case, given the statistical range of variation for the medullary cone, the displaced fracture fragment of the L1 vertebral body is more likely to impinge the lower lumbar and upper sacral segments of the medullary cone. S2 is the only choice from this region. When thinking of the spinal cord, remember the "rule of 2," which states the conus medullaris usually ends at the second lumbar vertebra (L2); the subarachnoid space ends at the second sacral vertebra (S2); and the terminal filum (filum terminale), a long connective tissue (pia mater) strand extending from the end of the medullary cone that anchors the inferior aspect of the spinal cord, usually attaches to the second coccygeal vertebra (Co2). Due to the location of the displaced fracture fragment of the L2 vertebral body, the higher sacral segments of the spinal cord related to the medullary cone are more likely to be damaged. **Choice A** (T7) is incorrect. The normal range of variation for the location of the conus medullaris in adults is the T12-L3 vertebral levels. The seventh thoracic (T7) spinal cord segment lies posterior to the vertebral bodies of the T6 and T7 vertebrae. Therefore, the T7 spinal cord segment is located well above the displaced posterior fracture fragment of the L1 vertebral body and the medullary cone, and it would not be damaged in this patient. **Choice B** (T9) is incorrect. The ninth thoracic (T9) spinal cord segment lies posterior to the vertebral bodies of the T8 and T9 vertebrae. Therefore, the T9 spinal cord segment is located well above the displaced posterior fracture fragment of the L1 vertebral body and the medullary cone, and it would not be damaged in this patient. **Choice C** (T11) is incorrect. The eleventh thoracic (T11) spinal cord segment lies posterior to the bodies of the T10 and T11 vertebrae. Therefore, the T11 spinal cord segment is located well above the displaced posterior fracture fragment of the L1 vertebral body and the medullary cone, and it would not be damaged in this patient. **Choice D** (L2) is incorrect. The second lumbar (L2) spinal cord segment lies posterior to the vertebral body of T12. Therefore, the L2 spinal cord segment is located well above the displaced posterior fracture fragment of the L1 vertebral body and the medullary cone, and it would not be damaged in this patient. The spinal nerve roots of L2 may be damaged by the displaced posterior fracture fragment; however, this question asks specifically for the spinal cord segment that would be damaged.

Chapter 7

Lower Limb

QUESTIONS

Select the single best answer.

1 A physician tests the patellar tendon reflex as shown. A normal response of the involuntary contraction of the quadriceps femoris muscle is noted. This reflex confirms the integrity of what nerve?

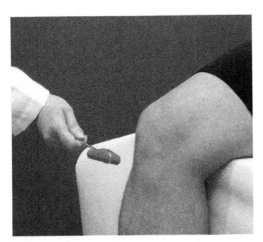

(A) Tibial nerve
(B) Deep fibular nerve
(C) Superficial fibular nerve
(D) Obturator nerve
(E) Femoral nerve

2 On the given radiograph, a fractured tarsal bone is identified by the black arrow with accompanying impaction of the tarso-metatarsal joint. What bone, articulating with the fourth and fifth metatarsal bones, is fractured?

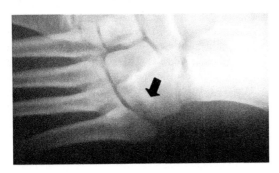

(A) Navicular
(B) Cuboid
(C) Talus
(D) Calcaneus
(E) Lateral cuneiform

3 Despite slamming on her brakes, a 23-year-old female driver crashes into the back of a car that stopped suddenly. During impact, her foot is severely dorsiflexed resulting in severe pain. At the ER, she explains to the attending physician that she thinks she has broken her foot. A lateral plain film of the foot reveals the fracture indicated by the white arrow. Which of the following bones is fractured in this patient?

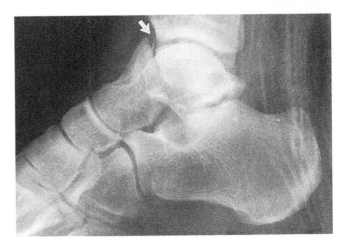

(A) Navicular
(B) Sustentaculum tali
(C) Talus
(D) Calcaneus
(E) Cuboid

4 A 70-year-old man reports an inability to climb stairs and stand up from a sitting position. Further examination also shows weakness when laterally rotating the thigh against resistance. What nerve is most likely compromised in this patient?
(A) Femoral nerve
(B) Obturator nerve
(C) Sciatic nerve
(D) Superior gluteal nerve
(E) Inferior gluteal nerve

5 A physician tests the calcaneal tendon (ankle jerk) reflex as shown. A normal response of plantar flexion of the ankle joint is noted. This myotatic (deep tendon) reflex confirms the integrity of what nerve?

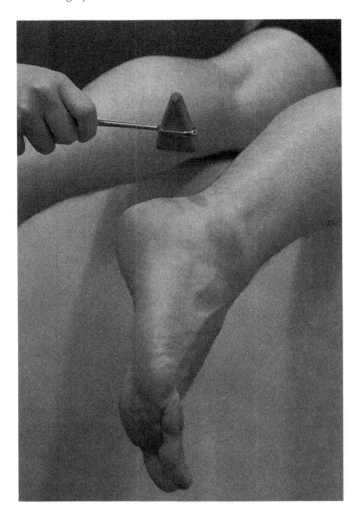

(A) Tibial nerve
(B) Deep fibular nerve
(C) Superficial fibular nerve
(D) Medial plantar nerve
(E) Lateral plantar nerve

6 A 21-year-old female basketball player lands on her opponent's foot after jumping to rebound the basketball. Her foot is forcefully inverted, and when leaving the court, she tells her trainer that she twisted or sprained her ankle. After getting her ankle taped for support, she reenters the game. What ligament was most likely damaged?
(A) Calcaneofibular ligament
(B) Anterior talofibular ligament
(C) Posterior talofibular ligament
(D) Plantar calcaneonavicular ligament
(E) Medial (deltoid) ligament

7 A 76-year-old man recently had coronary bypass surgery in which the small saphenous vein was harvested to establish coronary blood flow. Following the procedure, he complained of numbness and paresthesia in the limb from which the vein was removed. The given photo highlights the cutaneous area affected in the patient. No motor loss was noted. What nerve was most likely damaged during harvesting of the vein for transplantation?

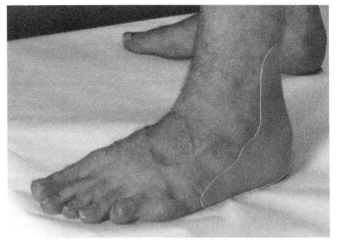

(A) Sural nerve
(B) Saphenous nerve
(C) Superficial fibular nerve
(D) Deep fibular nerve
(E) Lateral plantar nerve

8 A 36-year-old man arrives at the ER unconscious and with a suspected spinal cord injury after being involved in a motor vehicle accident. If the physician wants to localize the spinal cord lesion, what reflex would test the integrity of the L1-2 spinal cord segment?
(A) Anocutaneous reflex
(B) Patellar reflex
(C) Plantar reflex
(D) Calcaneal reflex
(E) Cremasteric reflex

9 Human feet are everted so that their soles lie fully on the ground during ambulation. What muscle is developmentally unique to humans, inserts into the base of the fifth metatarsal, and assists in eversion (or pronation)?
(A) Extensor digitorum longus
(B) Extensor digitorum brevis
(C) Fibularis longus
(D) Fibularis tertius
(E) Flexor digiti minimi brevis

10 A 15-year-old girl, unaware that she is pregnant, borrows her friend's Accutane (retinoic acid; vitamin A) to combat an acne problem. She uses the Accutane for about 2 months, which corresponds to weeks 7 to 15 of the embryonic development of her fetus. Which of the following skeletal elements is most likely to be absent in the newborn infant?
(A) Ilium
(B) Femur
(C) Patella
(D) Tibia
(E) Phalanges

11 A 25-year-old woman is brought to the emergency room in severe pain due to an ankle injury. She tells the attending physician she was wearing high-heel shoes, stepped off the curb into the street, lost her balance and landed awkwardly, causing her foot to turn extremely outward (eversion). Which of the following ligaments is most likely damaged?
(A) Plantar calcaneonavicular (spring) ligament
(B) Calcaneofibular ligament
(C) Deltoid ligament
(D) Anterior talofibular ligament
(E) Plantar calcaneocuboid (long plantar) ligament

12 A 75-year-old female patient fell in a hospital and landed on her hip. The given AP X-ray reveals fragmentation of her proximal femur. Which of the following muscles is most likely detached in association with the fracture fragment?

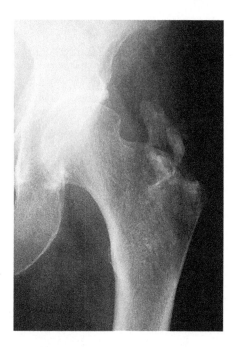

(A) Gluteus maximus
(B) Gluteus medius
(C) Iliopsoas
(D) Biceps femoris
(E) Sartorius

13 Two 11-year-old boys sneak up on their friend from behind. In surprising their friend, they shove him suddenly, which forcefully pushes his hips forward while he is standing relaxed talking to other friends. Which of the following ligaments best resists anterior dislocation of the head of the femur?
(A) Iliofemoral ligament
(B) Pubofemoral ligament
(C) Ischiofemoral ligament
(D) Lacunar ligament
(E) Ligament of the head of the femur

14 A 15-year-old girl is struck by a car while crossing the street. She suffers numerous pelvic injuries, including tearing of the sacrotuberous ligament. The damage to this ligament will most likely cause direct trauma to which of the following muscles?

(A) Gluteus maximus
(B) Gluteus medius
(C) Gluteus minimus
(D) Gemelli
(E) Obturator externus

15 A 16-year-old boy making a powerful move out of the starting blocks to begin a 100-m sprint feels intense pain below his right knee and collapses to the ground, unable to straighten his leg. The given plain film of the lateral knee reveals an avulsion fracture at the area indicated by the white arrowhead, with the fracture fragment identified by the white arrow. Which of the following muscles is most likely detached?

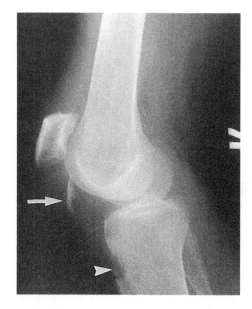

(A) Gastrocnemius
(B) Tibialis anterior
(C) Adductor magnus
(D) Rectus femoris
(E) Semitendinosus

16 When standing upright, the femur moves into the locked position by slightly hyperextending, gliding posteriorly, and medially rotating on the tibial plateaus. Which of the following muscles acts to initiate the unlocking of the knee?
(A) Biceps femoris
(B) Gastrocnemius
(C) Popliteus
(D) Sartorius
(E) Plantaris

17 A roofing installer falls off a high ladder and lands with the sole of his right foot hitting the ground first. He suffers a fracture and inferior displacement of the sustentaculum tali of the calcaneus. Which of the following structures is most likely torn?
(A) Tendon of the tibialis posterior muscle
(B) Tendon of the flexor hallucis longus (FHL) muscle
(C) Tendons of the flexor digitorum brevis muscle
(D) Small saphenous vein
(E) Plantar arterial arch

18 A soccer player injures his left knee when he twists the flexed knee while trying to avoid another player. While performing a knee examination, his physician pulls the flexed knee toward her (the physician's) body, as shown in the illustration. This clinical test is a check for the integrity of which of the following ligaments?

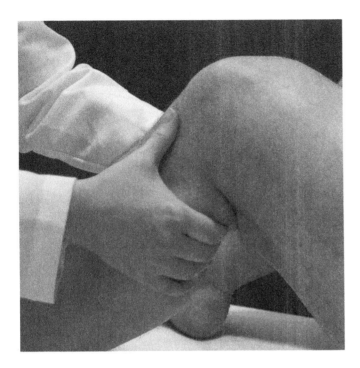

(A) Tibial (medial) collateral ligament (TCL)
(B) Fibular (lateral) collateral ligament (FCL)
(C) Anterior cruciate ligament (ACL)
(D) Posterior cruciate ligament (PCL)
(E) Patellar ligament

19 A veteran infantry soldier develops painful flat feet after several years of service including hundreds of miles of marches. The pain is particularly acute on the medial aspect of his sole. Which of the following structures is most likely strained in this condition?

(A) Calcaneal (Achilles) tendon
(B) Plantar calcaneocuboid (long plantar) ligament
(C) Extensor retinaculum
(D) Tendon of the fibularis (peroneus) longus muscle
(E) Plantar calcaneonavicular (spring) ligament

20 A 62-year-old man recently had coronary bypass surgery in which the great saphenous vein was harvested for reestablishing coronary blood flow. Following the procedure, he complained of loss of sensation in the cutaneous area noted in the given photo in the limb from which the vein was harvested. Which of the following nerves was most likely damaged during the surgery?

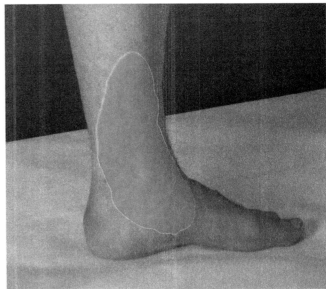

(A) Sural nerve
(B) Obturator nerve
(C) Saphenous nerve
(D) Deep fibular (peroneal) nerve
(E) Superficial fibular (peroneal) nerve

21 A young man suffers a dislocation of the right hip in a car accident. During recovery, he finds he has an abnormal gait in which his left hip sinks when he lifts that foot to take a step, as shown in the right frame (C) of the given diagram. The problem may be the result of damage to which of the following structures?

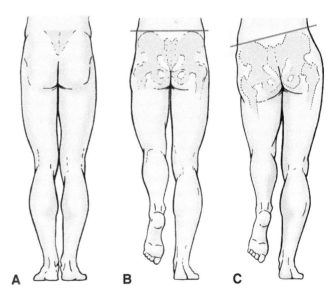

(A) Right gluteus maximus and inferior gluteal nerve
(B) Left gluteus maximus and superior gluteal nerve
(C) Left gluteus medius and inferior gluteal nerve
(D) Right gluteus medius and superior gluteal nerve
(E) Right gluteus minimus and inferior gluteal nerve

22 A 72-year-old woman slips and falls on a wet floor, fracturing the neck of her right femur. Subsequent physical examination in the ER shows her right foot is laterally rotated, and the right lower extremity appears slightly shorter than the left. Which of the following muscles is mainly responsible for the rotated posture of the right limb?

(A) Semitendinosus

(B) Adductor longus

(C) Gluteus maximus

(D) Rectus femoris

(E) Gracilis

23 A 36-year-old woman injured in an automobile accident tells the paramedics at the scene that her upper thigh hurts badly and she can barely flex her hip. A plain film of the hip joint reveals an avulsion fracture of the proximal femur, indicated by the open white arrow, and a fracture fragment identified by the solid white arrow. Which of the following muscles is most likely detached?

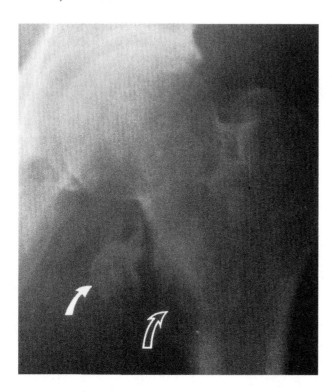

(A) Adductor magnus

(B) Iliopsoas

(C) Rectus femoris

(D) Biceps femoris

(E) Sartorius

24 A rugby player injures his left extended knee when hit from the lateral side by a defender trying to tackle him. While performing a knee examination, his physician applies pressure to his lateral thigh and medial leg (as shown in the illustration). This clinical test is a check for the integrity of which of the following ligaments?

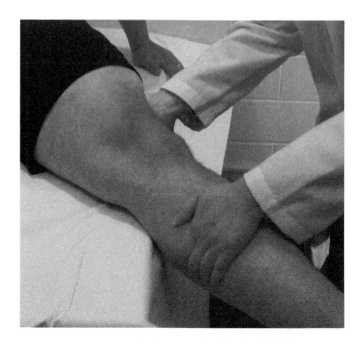

(A) Tibial (medial) collateral ligament (TCL)

(B) Fibular (lateral) collateral ligament (FCL)

(C) Anterior cruciate ligament (ACL)

(D) Posterior cruciate ligament (PCL)

(E) Patellar ligament

25 A 55-year-old woman recently had pelvic surgery during which cancerous lymph nodes were removed from the lateral wall of her pelvis. During a postoperative examination, she says she has been having painful muscle spasms in her thigh. Which of the following muscles is most likely involved?

(A) Sartorius

(B) Biceps femoris

(C) Tensor muscle of fascia lata

(D) Vastus medialis

(E) Gracilis

26 A 6-year-old boy playing barefooted in his backyard steps on a piece of broken glass and suffers a large transverse cut on his sole, at the level of the midfoot. In the emergency room, the examining physician determines the cut is to the depth of the first layer of the plantar muscles. Which of the following structures is most likely damaged in this injury?

(A) Plantar arterial arch

(B) Tendons of the flexor digitorum longus muscle

(C) Tendon of the fibularis (peroneus) longus muscle

(D) Abductor hallucis muscle

(E) Superficial fibular (peroneal) nerve

27 A man working in a junkyard trips and falls into a pile of scrap metal, suffering a deep cut immediately posterior to the lateral malleolus. Which of the following is most likely to be injured?

(A) Saphenous nerve

(B) Tendon of the fibularis (peroneus) tertius

(C) Tendon of the fibularis (peroneus) longus

(D) Posterior tibial artery

(E) Great saphenous vein

28 A physician performs some simple muscle tests on a 35-year-old male patient when he complains of weakness in his lower limbs. In the physical test illustrated below, the patient is asked to touch his buttocks with his heel while working against resistance. What muscle group is being tested?

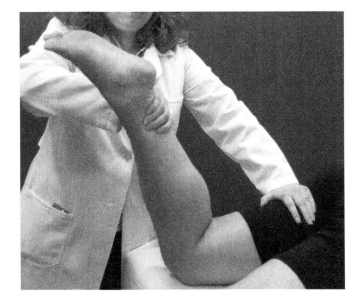

(A) Quadriceps femoris
(B) Hamstrings
(C) Adductors
(D) Triceps surae
(E) Plantar flexors

29 A patient presents with extreme pain due to arterial insufficiency in the posterior femoral compartment. This compartment of the thigh receives its blood supply mainly from the perforating arteries. An arteriogram confirms partial occlusion of the artery that gives rise to these perforating arteries. What artery is occluded in the arteriogram?

(A) Femoral artery
(B) Profunda femoris artery
(C) Obturator artery
(D) Popliteal artery
(E) Medial femoral circumflex artery

30 A 25-year-old man suffers a gunshot wound to the calf that severs the posterior tibial artery at its origin. Which of the following vessels will not receive blood flow immediately following the injury?

(A) Anterior tibial artery
(B) Inferior medial genicular artery
(C) Dorsalis pedis artery
(D) Popliteal artery
(E) Fibular (peroneal) artery

31 A 65-year-old man with a history of heavy smoking visits his physician complaining of intermittent pain in his feet, accompanied by pallor and coldness of his feet. The physician suspects vascular insufficiency and takes a pulse of the dorsalis pedis artery. That pulse is best palpated at which of the following locations?

(A) Immediately anterior to the medial malleolus
(B) Immediately anterior to the lateral malleolus
(C) Between the tendons of the extensor hallucis longus and extensor digitorum longus muscles
(D) Between the tendons of the extensor digitorum longus and fibularis (peroneus) tertius muscles
(E) Immediately lateral to the tendon of the fibularis (peroneus) tertius muscle

32 An elderly man falls on an icy sidewalk outside his home and cannot get up. He tells the attending paramedics that he has a lot of pain in his right hip. Following inconclusive analysis of an AP X-ray, the given coronal MRI reveals a nondisplaced fracture of the right femoral neck, as noted by the black arrow. Branches of which of the following arteries are most likely to be damaged in this injury?

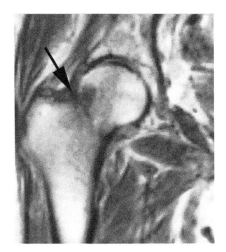

(A) Femoral artery
(B) Obturator artery
(C) Lateral circumflex femoral artery
(D) Medial circumflex femoral artery
(E) Inferior gluteal artery

33 The relative positions of blood vessels can sometimes be explained in terms of rotation of the limbs during development. For example, upon entering the femoral triangle the femoral artery resides ____ to the femoral vein, whereas in the popliteal fossa the popliteal artery lies ____ to the popliteal vein.

(A) medial…posterior
(B) lateral…deep
(C) lateral…posterior
(D) medial…superficial
(E) anterior…lateral

34 Due to torsioning of the lower limb and merging of separate premuscle masses during development, certain adult lower limb muscles are supplied by two separate nerves. These interneural fusions are termed "hybrid muscles". Which of the following is a hybrid muscle?

(A) Adductor magnus
(B) Gastrocnemius
(C) Rectus femoris
(D) Semimembranosus
(E) Tibialis anterior

35 A 23-year-old female medical student notices she was gaining weight due to a sedimentary lifestyle and compulsive studying. Therefore, she decides to run in a marathon and starts her training by running 6 miles each morning before class. After 2 weeks, she presents with right lateral knee pain and inflammation, specifically in the area of the lateral femoral epicondyle. This pain intensifies throughout her morning jogs, especially when her right foot strikes the ground or when she is running downhill. What is most likely diagnosis in this patient?

(A) Sprained fibular (lateral) collateral ligament (FCL)
(B) Patellofemoral pain syndrome
(C) Iliotibial band syndrome (ITBS)
(D) Torn lateral meniscus
(E) Pes anserinus bursitis

36 A 47-year-old woman walks with difficulty into the ER and presents with pain, inflammation, and tenderness on the outside of her right foot. She reports she sprained her ankle, an inversion injury, while stepping off a sidewalk wearing 3-in. high heels. The given X-ray reveals an avulsion fracture on her lateral foot. The white arrow identifies the fracture fragment. What muscle is most likely injured, given the site of the fracture?

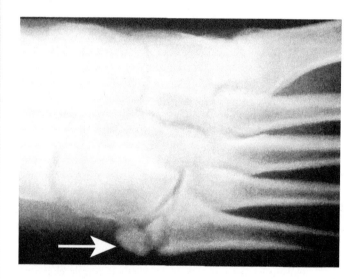

(A) Extensor digitorum longus
(B) Fibularis brevis
(C) Fibularis longus
(D) Fibularis tertius
(E) Flexor digiti minimi brevis

37 A 32-year-old male farmer cuts the medial aspect of his midthigh when climbing over a barbwire fence. Though he bandages the wound, he reports to the ER 5 days later with an infected wound, high fever (102.7°), and lymphadenitis (swollen lymph nodes). Given the location of the injury, which groups of nodes would be the first to receive drainage from the infected wound?

(A) Popliteal
(B) External iliac
(C) Deep inguinal
(D) Horizontal group of superficial inguinal
(E) Vertical group of superficial inguinal

38 As part of a physical examination to evaluate lower limb function, a physician places her hands on the dorsum of the patient's foot and asks the patient to dorsiflex the ankle joint against resistance, as shown. What nerve is the doctor testing?

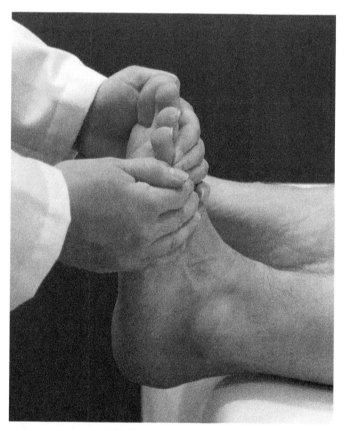

(A) Tibial nerve
(B) Deep fibular nerve
(C) Superficial fibular nerve
(D) Medial plantar nerve
(E) Lateral plantar nerve

39 A 35-year-old male prisoner received a right gluteal intramuscular (IM) injection during a visit to the infirmary. Following the injection, the man experienced a painful, swollen right leg. Within a month, he complained that his right leg started to shrink. Examination revealed muscle wasting with fasciculations in the L4-S1 distribution and marked weakness in dorsiflexion, inversion, and eversion at the ankle joint. He also exhibited a typical high-steppage gait indicating right foot drop. What nerve was most likely damaged during the gluteal IM injection?

(A) Superior gluteal nerve
(B) Common fibular nerve
(C) Tibial nerve
(D) Inferior gluteal nerve
(E) Sciatic nerve

40 A 22-year-old soldier is injured from shrapnel from an improvised explosive device in the right upper thigh, below the midpoint of the inguinal ligament. Though he received field dressings from a medic, he arrives at the military hospital having lost copious amounts of blood. What sign and/or symptom would accompany this patient's presentation?

(A) Increased pulse in the right dorsalis pedis artery

(B) Tachycardia

(C) Warm right foot

(D) Increased hematocrit

(E) Hypertension

41 A rising second-year medical student spends his summer hiking the Appalachian Trial with a 100-lb backpack in tow. After a month of hiking 30-mi/day (48-km/day), he notices numbness, tingling, and burning sensations in the lateral aspect of his right upper thigh. His symptoms are exacerbated by his backpack pressing on the area surrounding his right anterior superior iliac spine. What nerve is most likely affected?

(A) Femoral branch of genitofemoral nerve

(B) Saphenous nerve

(C) Anterior cutaneous branches of femoral nerve

(D) Lateral femoral cutaneous nerve

(E) Iliohypogastric nerve

42 After spending 2 days moving heavy furniture out of her house, a 56-year-old woman goes to an emergency room in acute pain. The patient reports nausea, vomiting, and severe abdominal pain. On examination, the doctor discovers a painful, globular mass located inferior and lateral to the pubic tubercle. Given her presentation and history, what is the most likely diagnosis?

(A) Indirect inguinal hernia

(B) Direct inguinal hernia

(C) Femoral hernia

(D) Lymphadenitis of superficial inguinal nodes

(E) Fractured hip

43 A 16-year-old boy was fishing barefoot in a muddy river when the plantar surface of his foot was cut by unseen debris. He suffers a large transverse cut, penetrating the first two layers of his plantar musculature, in the area of the first cuneiform bone. In the emergency room, his physician notes a complete inability to flex and abduct the big toe and numbness on the plantar aspect of the three medial toes. Which of the following nerves is most likely damaged?

(A) Medial plantar nerve

(B) Lateral plantar nerve

(C) Sural nerve

(D) Deep fibular nerve

(E) Superficial fibular nerve

44 A tall 17-year-old man is crammed into the front passenger seat of an automobile when the speeding car slides off a wet road and slams its front bumper into a road guardrail. The passenger's left shin slams against the dashboard with an impact just below the knee. He reports to the emergency room with considerable knee pain, tenderness, and a pronounced limp during walking. With the patient lying supine, his hips flexed at 45 degrees, knees flexed at 90 degrees, and feet flat on the table, the physician notes a widened space, or sag, in the sulcus between the tibia and the femur. When the physician pushes the left tibia posteriorly, as noted in the photo, a pronounced laxity is noted in the left knee when compared to the right. What structure is most likely damaged?

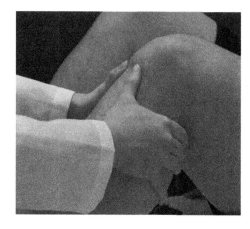

(A) Anterior cruciate ligament (ACL)

(B) Posterior cruciate ligament (PCL)

(C) Tibial (medial) collateral ligament (TCL)

(D) Fibular (lateral) collateral ligament (FCL)

(E) Patellar ligament

45 An overweight woman participates in her first rugby match without proper training and conditioning. Upon catching the opening kickoff, she awkwardly twists her right knee, screams in pain, and falls to the ground. The team manager notes her patella is dislocated, residing on the lateral side of her knee. After straightening the woman's knee, the patellar dislocation is reduced (goes back into place). To prevent future dislocation of the patella, what specific muscle should be targeted during rehabilitation?

(A) Vastus intermedius

(B) Vastus lateralis

(C) Vastus medialis

(D) Rectus femoris

(E) Tibialis anterior

46 A 32-year-old mixed martial arts fighter could not continue his fight after receiving a side leg kick to the neck of his left fibula. The fighter reported paresthesia and numbness on the entire dorsum of his left foot. During his physical examination, the patient often stumbled with his left toes dragging on the floor during the swing phase of his gait. Asymmetry in his normal foot position was also noted by the physician (see photo) as well as weakness in eversion of the foot at the ankle joint. What nerve was damaged?

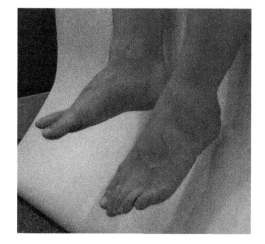

(A) Tibial nerve
(B) Deep fibular nerve
(C) Superficial fibular nerve
(D) Common fibular nerve
(E) Sciatic nerve

47   A 35-year-old male recreational basketball player heard a loud pop in his left knee while pivoting in a squatted position. He finished playing several more games, but 3 days later he went to an orthopedic surgeon reporting persistent pain, inflammation, and stiffness in his knee, and he admitted it felt like his knee was "going to give out" when he descended stairs. During a knee examination, the physician noted tenderness along the joint line and a clicking sound while placing a valgus stress on the lateral side of the flexed left knee. During a deep knee bend, the patient experienced pain in the bottom of the motion as shown in the figure. An MRI would confirm damage to what knee structure?

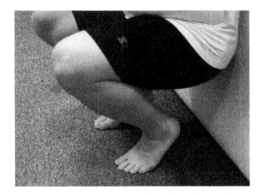

(A) Tibial (medial) collateral ligament (TCL)
(B) Fibular (lateral) collateral ligament (FCL)
(C) Anterior cruciate ligament (ACL)
(D) Meniscus
(E) Patella

48   As part of a physical examination to evaluate lower limb function, a physician asks a patient to abduct her second through fifth toes. What specific nerve is the doctor testing?
(A) Sural nerve
(B) Deep fibular nerve
(C) Superficial fibular nerve
(D) Medial plantar nerve
(E) Lateral plantar nerve

49   Following surgery to repair a broken right tibia, a 22-year-old patient is placed in a short leg cast. Several hours later, she complains of extreme pain, numbness with a "pins and needles sensation," inflammation, and abnormal pressure on the anterior and lateral aspects of the affected lower leg. The cast is removed, and the physician notes weakness in dorsiflexion of the foot and toes, a weak dorsalis pedis arterial pulse, and sensory loss between the first and second toes. What nerve is most likely damaged?
(A) Tibial nerve
(B) Deep fibular nerve
(C) Superficial fibular nerve
(D) Medial plantar nerve
(E) Lateral plantar nerve

50   As part of a physical examination to evaluate lower limb function, a physician asks her patient to stand on his tiptoes, as shown. What nerve is the doctor testing?

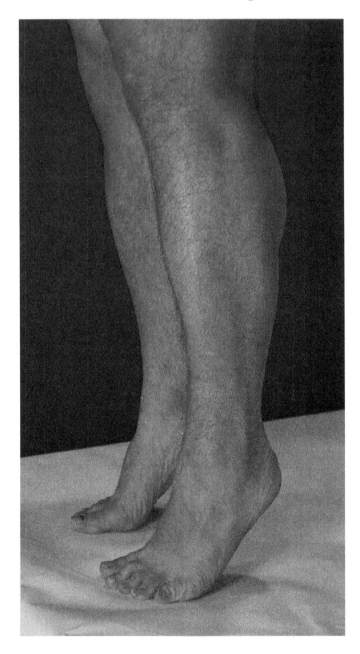

(A) Tibial nerve
(B) Deep fibular nerve
(C) Superficial fibular nerve
(D) Sural nerve
(E) Saphenous nerve

ANSWERS AND DISCUSSION

1 **The answer is E: Femoral nerve.** A positive response to the patellar reflex confirms the integrity of the femoral nerve and the L2-4 spinal segments, from which this nerve arises. The femoral nerve supplies the motor innervation to the anterior compartment of the thigh, including the iliacus, sartorius, articularis genu, the lateral aspect of the pectineus muscle, and the four muscles of the quadriceps femoris tested in this patient: vastus medialis, vastus lateralis, vastus intermedius, and rectus femoris. Loss of the femoral nerve supplying the quadriceps femoris would lead to weakness in extending the knee and flexing the thigh (via the rectus femoris muscle which crosses the hip joint). The saphenous nerve, a sensory branch of the femoral nerve, supplies the skin and subcutaneous tissue on the anterior and medial aspects of the knee, leg, and foot. Therefore, a patellar myotatic (deep tendon) reflex tests the integrity of the femoral nerve. **Choice A** (Tibial nerve) is incorrect. The tibial nerve is a terminal branch of the sciatic nerve that supplies the posterior compartment of the leg. It does not supply innervation to the quadriceps femoris muscle and is not involved with the patellar myotatic reflex. **Choice B** (Deep fibular nerve) is incorrect. The deep fibular nerve is a terminal branch of the common fibular nerve that supplies innervation to the anterior compartment of the leg. It does not supply innervation to the quadriceps femoris muscle, which resides in the anterior compartment of the thigh, so it is not involved with the patellar myotatic reflex. **Choice C** (Superficial fibular nerve) is incorrect. The superficial fibular nerve is a terminal branch of the common fibular nerve that supplies innervation to the lateral compartment of the leg. It is not involved with the patellar myotatic reflex. **Choice D** (Obturator nerve) is incorrect. The obturator nerve supplies motor innervation to the muscles of the medial compartment of the thigh, including the medial half of the **P**ectineus muscle, **O**bturator externus, **G**racilis, and the **A**dductor muscles: adductor brevis, adductor longus, and the medial (adductor) half of the adductor magnus. The mnemonic for muscles innervated by the obturator nerve is "POGA." Because it does not innervate the quadriceps femoris muscles, it is not involved with the patellar myotatic reflex.

2 **The answer is B: Cuboid.** The given radiograph reveals a fractured cuboid bone, which is identified by the black arrow. The cuboid is a tarsal bone named for its cube-like shape. It is the most lateral bone in the distal row of tarsal bones, where it articulates proximally with the calcaneus and distally with the fourth and fifth metatarsal bones. It is the only bone involved with both the transverse tarsal and tarsometatarsal joints. The tarsus, or proximal foot, consists of seven bones: **T**alus, **C**alcaneus, **N**avicular, **M**edial cuneiform, **I**ntermediate cuneiform, **L**ateral cuneiform, and **C**uboid. A mnemonic for the tarsal bones is "Tiger Cubs Need MILC," which lists the superior tarsal bones first and then names each distal tarsal bone in the right foot in a clockwise pattern. **Choice A** (Navicular) is incorrect. The navicular (**L**: little ship) is a flattened, boat-shaped bone located between the talus proximally and the three cuneiform bones distally. **Choice C** (Talus) is incorrect. The talus (**L**: ankle bone) is located between the malleoli of the fibula and tibia and is the only tarsal bone without tendinous or muscular attachments. It articulates with the navicular bone anteriorly and the calcaneus bone inferiorly. **Choice D**

(Calcaneus) is incorrect. The calcaneus (**L**: heel bone) is the largest and strongest tarsal bone. With its superior surface articulating with the talus, this bone transmits the majority of the forces generated by the weight of the bone from the talus to the ground during standing. Its anterior surface articulates with the cuboid. **Choice E** (Lateral cuneiform) is incorrect. The lateral cuneiform (**L**: wedge-shaped) articulates with the navicular located posterior, the third metatarsal located anterior, the cuboid positioned lateral, and the intermediate cuneiform bone located medial.

3 **The answer is C: Talus.** The radiograph reveals a displaced (Hawkins Type II) fracture of the neck of the talus. The talus (**L**: ankle bone) is located between the malleoli of the fibula and tibia and is the only tarsal bone without tendinous or muscular attachments. It articulates with the navicular bone anteriorly and the calcaneus bone inferiorly. A fracture of the neck of the talus is often seen when a patient is involved in a high impact accident with the foot placed in an exaggerated dorsiflexed position at the ankle joint. These types of fractures were first reported in pilots who were forcefully applying pressure to their rudder with their foot during airplane crashes in World War I, but they are now more commonly seen in motor vehicle accidents due to forcefully slamming on the brakes during impact. Displaced fractures of the neck of the talus can increase in severity and receive a higher Hawkins classification (II, III, or IV). As severity of the displacement increases, so does the risk of avascular necrosis due to interruption of the complex blood supply of the talus. **Choice A** (Navicular) is incorrect. The navicular is a flattened, boat-shaped bone located between the talus proximally and the three cuneiform bones distally. It is the bone located distally to the fractured talus in this radiograph. **Choice B** (Sustentaculum tali) is incorrect. The sustentaculum tali, a bony ledge of the calcaneus that projects off the medial side of this bone, supports the head of the talus. This osteological feature is located inferior to the fractured talus in this radiograph. **Choice D** (Calcaneus) is incorrect. The calcaneus, or heel bone, is the largest and strongest tarsal bone. With its superior surface articulating with the talus, this bone transmits the majority of the forces generated by the weight of the bone from the talus to the ground during standing. This bone is located inferior and posterior to the fractured talus in this radiograph. **Choice E** (Cuboid) is incorrect. The cuboid bone, named for its cube-like shape, is the most lateral bone in the distal row of tarsal bones, where it articulates proximally with the calcaneus and distally with the fourth and fifth metatarsals. It is the only bone involved with both the transverse tarsal and tarsometatarsal joints. This bone can be identified anterior to the calcaneus in this radiograph.

4 **The answer is E: Inferior gluteal nerve.** The inferior gluteal nerve innervates the gluteus maximus. This muscle produces lateral rotation and extension of the thigh at the hip joint, especially when the thigh is in a flexed position (rising from a sitting position or climbing stairs). The gluteus maximus can be tested by placing the patient in a prone position and asking them to perform a straight leg lift. During this functional test, the examiner should observe and palpate the contraction of this muscle. **Choice A** (Femoral nerve) is incorrect. The femoral nerve supplies the motor innervation to the anterior compartment of the thigh. In general, loss of the femoral nerve would lead to weakness in extending the knee and flexing the thigh. The patient was having difficulty extending the thigh at the hip joint, so the femoral nerve can be eliminated. **Choice B** (Obturator nerve) is incorrect. The obturator nerve supplies motor innervation to the muscles of the medial compartment of the thigh. These muscles collectively adduct the thigh. However, the individual components also participate in additional actions: lateral (external) rotation of the thigh (obturator externus), flexion of the hip (adductor brevis; adductor magnus), and flexion and medial rotation of the leg (gracilis). However, this patient was having trouble with extension of the thigh at the hip joint, which is not a function of the obturator nerve. **Choice C** (Sciatic nerve) is incorrect. The sciatic nerve supplies the **B**iceps femoris, posterior half of the **A**dductor magnus, **S**emitendinosus, and **S**emimembranosus. The mnemonic for the muscles innervated by the sciatic nerve is "BASS." Three of these muscles, the long head of the biceps femoris, semitendinosus, and semimembranosus, comprise the hamstrings, which (along with the short head of the biceps femoris) form the posterior compartment of the thigh. Collectively, these muscles extend the thigh at the hip joint and flex the leg at the knee joint. Though this patient is having trouble extending the thigh at the hip joint, loss of the sciatic nerve would not explain the observed weakness in external rotation of the thigh. Also, the gluteus maximus, and not the hamstrings, is the strongest muscle in extension of the thigh, and it acts primarily when force is needed, as in climbing stairs. **Choice D** (Superior gluteal nerve) is incorrect. The superior gluteal nerve supplies motor innervation to the gluteus medius, gluteus minimus, and tensor fasciae latae muscles. Loss of this innervation would lead to weakness in abducting and medially rotating the thigh at the hip joint. These muscles are also responsible for keeping the pelvis level during the swing phase of gait.

5   **The answer is A: Tibial nerve.** A positive response to the calcaneal (Achilles) tendon reflex causes plantar flexion of the ankle joint via the contractions of the gastrocnemius and soleus muscles, which insert distally into the calcaneal tendon. These muscles are innervated by the tibial nerve, and the plantar flexion of the ankle joint confirms the integrity of this nerve and the S1-2 spinal segments, from which this nerve is primarily derived. The tibial nerve is a terminal branch of the sciatic nerve that supplies the posterior compartment of the leg, including the superficial compartment where the gastrocnemius and soleus muscles reside. **Choice B** (Deep fibular nerve) is incorrect. The deep fibular nerve is a terminal branch of the common fibular nerve that innervates the anterior compartment of the leg. It does not supply the muscles inserting into the calcaneal tendon, which reside in the posterior compartment of the leg, so it is not involved with the calcaneal myotatic reflex. **Choice C** (Superficial fibular nerve) is incorrect. The superficial fibular nerve is a terminal branch of the common fibular nerve that innervates the lateral compartment of the leg. It is not involved with the calcaneal myotatic reflex. **Choice D** (Medial plantar nerve) is incorrect. The tibial nerve divides into the medial and lateral plantar nerves, which innervate the muscles in the sole of the foot. The medial plantar nerve, which is homologous to the median nerve in the hand, innervates the following intrinsic foot muscles: first **L**umbrical, **A**bductor hallucis,

Flexor digitorum brevis, and **F**lexor hallucis brevis. The mnemonic for muscles supplied by the medial plantar nerve is the "LAFF" muscles. Because this nerve does not supply muscles that cross the ankle joint, it cannot be responsible for the plantar flexion seen in this calcaneal myotatic reflex test. **Choice E** (Lateral plantar nerve) is incorrect. The tibial nerve divides into the medial and lateral plantar nerves to innervate the muscles of the sole of the foot. The lateral plantar nerve, which is homologous to the ulnar nerve in the hand, innervates all of the intrinsic foot muscles, with the exception of the four "LAFF" muscles supplied by the medial plantar nerve. Because this nerve does not supply muscles that cross the ankle joint, it cannot be responsible for the plantar flexion seen in this calcaneal myotatic reflex test.

6   **The answer is B: Anterior talofibular ligament.** The ankle is the most frequently injured major joint in the body. Torn ligaments (ankle sprains) are commonly seen following inversion injuries, where the joint is twisted on a weight-bearing plantar flexed foot (as described in this patient). The most commonly sprained ankle ligament is the anterior talofibular ligament on the lateral side of the ankle, and this injury results in instability of the joint. If this ankle injury were more severe, additional ligaments of the lateral side of the ankle would also be involved, specifically the calcaneofibular and posterior talofibular ligaments. **Choice A** (Calcaneofibular ligament) is incorrect. The calcaneofibular ligament is often injured in severe ankle sprains following forced inversion of the foot but only after the anterior talofibular ligament would have incurred damage. However, in this athlete, the ankle sprain was not severe and she was able to continue playing. Therefore, the calcaneofibular ligament was most likely not involved. **Choice C** (Posterior talofibular ligament) is incorrect. The posterior talofibular ligament would only be damaged in the most severe cases of forced inversion of the ankle joint following injury to the anterior talofibular and calcaneofibular ligaments. Given the nature of this injury, the anterior talofibular ligament was the only ligament involved. **Choice D** (Plantar calcaneonavicular ligament) is incorrect. The plantar calcaneonavicular (spring) ligament connects the sustentaculum tali of the calcaneus with the plantar surface of the navicular bone. It supports the head of the talus and helps maintain the medial longitudinal arch of the foot. This ligament would not be involved with a sprained (or twisted) ankle. **Choice E** (Medial [deltoid] ligament) is incorrect. The medial (deltoid) ligament of the ankle reinforces the medial aspect of the ankle joint and would be injured during forced eversion injuries. This ligament is much stronger than the lateral ligaments of the ankle (calcaneofibular, anterior talofibular, posterior talofibular ligaments) and would not be involved in this inversion injury.

7   **The answer is A: Sural nerve.** The sural nerve is formed in the distal posterior aspect of the leg by the convergence of the medial sural cutaneous nerve (off the tibial nerve) and the lateral sural cutaneous nerve (off the common fibular nerve). This nerve parallels the small saphenous vein coursing in between the calcaneal tuberosity and lateral malleolus of the fibula, and it is at this location that this vein is often harvested for transplantation. Damage to the sural nerve would lead to numbness and paresthesia in the posterior leg, particularly to the dorsal aspect of the fifth toe and lateral malleolus of the fibula, as seen in this patient. **Choice B** (Saphenous nerve) is incorrect. The saphenous nerve is a terminal sensory branch of the femoral nerve, which traverses medially through the adductor canal in the thigh. It supplies cutaneous (sensory) innervation from the medial side of the leg and foot, including the medial malleolus of the tibia. Due to the lateral location of the sensory deficits, this nerve would not be involved in this patient. **Choice C** (Superficial fibular nerve) is incorrect. The superficial fibular nerve is a terminal branch of the common fibular nerve that supplies motor innervation to the lateral compartment of the leg and sensory innervation from the anterior aspect of the distal leg and dorsum of the foot. Its sensory distribution does not correspond to this patient's deficits. **Choice D** (Deep fibular nerve) is incorrect. The deep fibular nerve is a terminal branch of the common fibular nerve that supplies motor innervation to the anterior compartment of the leg and sensory innervation from the web space between the great toe and the second toe. This sensory deficit is not seen in this patient. **Choice E** (Lateral plantar nerve) is incorrect. The tibial nerve divides into the medial and lateral plantar nerves to innervate the muscles in the sole of the foot. The lateral plantar nerve, which is homologous to the ulnar nerve in the hand, innervates the majority of the intrinsic foot muscles. The sensory innervation of the lateral plantar nerve is limited to the plantar aspect of the foot, specifically the lateral sole of the foot and the lateral 1.5 toes.

8   **The answer is E: Cremasteric reflex.** The cremasteric reflex is a cutaneous reflex that tests the integrity of the L1-2 spinal cord segments. Lightly stroking the superior and medial parts of the thigh stimulates the sensory fibers of the ilioinguinal nerve (the afferent limb of this reflex), which, in turn, stimulates the contraction of the cremaster muscle to pull up the testis on the ipsilateral side. This efferent limb of the reflex is activated by the motor fibers of the genital (cremasteric) branch of the genitofemoral nerve. The genitofemoral nerve is formed by the ventral rami of L1-2. **Choice A** (Anocutaneous reflex) is incorrect. The anocutaneous reflex (or anal wink test) is a cutaneous reflex that tests the integrity of the S2-4 spinal cord segments due to the innervation of this aspect of the perineum by the pudendal nerve. **Choice B** (Patellar reflex) is incorrect. The patellar reflex is a deep tendon reflex that confirms the integrity of the L2-4 spinal segments. Striking the patellar tendon elicits contraction of the quadriceps muscles, which are innervated by the femoral nerve, comprised of the ventral rami of L2-4. **Choice C** (Plantar reflex) is incorrect. The plantar (Babinski) reflex is a cutaneous reflex that confirms the integrity of the corticospinal tract within the central nervous system. Rubbing the lateral side of the sole of the foot from the heel to the toes with a blunt instrument should cause a normal adult response, which is flexion of the toes and eversion of the foot. **Choice D** (Calcaneal reflex) is incorrect. The calcaneal (Achilles or ankle jerk) reflex is a deep tendon reflex that confirms the integrity of the tibial nerve and the S1-2 spinal segments, from which this nerve is primarily derived. The tibial nerve is a terminal branch of the sciatic nerve that supplies the posterior compartment of the leg, including the superficial compartment containing the gastrocnemius and soleus muscles, which contract in a normal response to this reflex.

9   **The answer is D: Fibularis tertius.** The fibularis (peroneus) tertius muscle arises off the distal portion of the extensor digitorum longus muscle and attaches to the dorsal surface of the base of the fifth metatarsal. This muscle is rarely found in other primates and is functionally linked to efficient terrestrial bipedalism. Though this muscle may be highly variable in human specimens, it is important in eversion of the foot during ambulation and may have a proprioceptive role to guard against excessive inversion of the foot at the ankle joint. **Choice A** (Extensor digitorum longus) is incorrect. The extensor digitorum longus arises off the superiolateral aspect of the tibia and interosseous membrane and inserts into the middle and distal phalanges of the lateral four digits. This muscle extends the lateral four digits and dorsiflexes the ankle. It does not insert into the base of the fifth metatarsal or assist in eversion. It does give rise to the fibularis tertius muscle distally. **Choice B** (Extensor digitorum brevis) is incorrect. The extensor digitorum brevis is an intrinsic foot muscle that inserts into the middle phalanges of the lateral four digits to extend these toes. It does not insert into the base of the fifth metatarsal or assist in eversion. **Choice C** (Fibularis longus) is incorrect. The fibularis longus muscle arises off the proximal aspect of the fibula and inserts into the base of the first metatarsal and medial cuneiform bone. This muscle is important in eversion of the foot; however, it can be eliminated due to its medial insertion in the foot. **Choice E** (Flexor digiti minimi brevis) is incorrect. The flexor digiti minimi brevis arises from the base of the fifth metatarsal and inserts into the base of the proximal phalanx of the fifth digit. It does not participate in eversion of the foot, so this answer can be easily eliminated.

10   **The answer is E: Phalanges.** Accutane (retinoic acid; vitamin A) is a useful therapeutic drug in relieving skin disorders such as acne. However, it also is a recognized teratogenic agent that should not be utilized during pregnancy. Both upper and lower limbs follow the same pattern of development, except that corresponding events occur slightly later (by ~2 days) in the lower limb. One aspect of this pattern is that development proceeds along the proximo-distal axis of the limb, with the more proximal skeletal elements differentiating first, followed by the more distal structures. Overall, the major formative events take place from late week 4 to week 8. In this case, the Accutane was used during the later stages of limb development. The structures most likely affected are the most distal elements, the phalanges. **Choice A** (Ilium) is incorrect. Because of the timing of the mother's use of Accutane, the more distal skeletal components, which are the last to differentiate, are most likely affected. The ilium, a bony component of the coxal or hip bone, would not be affected. **Choice B** (Femur) is incorrect. Because of the timing of the mother's use of Accutane, the more distal skeletal components, which are the last to differentiate, are most likely affected. The femur would not be affected. **Choice C** (Patella) is incorrect. Because of the timing of the mother's use of Accutane, the more distal skeletal components, which are the last to differentiate, are most likely affected. The patella, a sesamoid bone in the quadriceps tendon, would not be affected. **Choice D** (Tibia) is incorrect. Because of the timing of the mother's use of Accutane, the more distal skeletal components, which are the last to differentiate, are most likely affected. The tibia, a long bone in the leg, would not be affected.

11 **The answer is C: Deltoid ligament.** The injury in this patient is one of excessive eversion of the foot. Therefore, the ligament damaged is on the medial aspect of the ankle, where it is positioned to resist eversion. The deltoid ligament is a four-part structure that in total resembles the triangular Greek letter Delta. It covers the medial side of the ankle, extending from its apex on the medial malleolus of the tibia down to its base on the navicular, calcaneus, and talus. It functions to resist excessive eversion of the foot. Due to its intrinsic strength, the deltoid ligament may not rupture but instead cause an avulsion fracture of the medial malleolus. **Choice A** (Plantar calcaneonavicular [spring] ligament) is incorrect. The plantar calcaneonavicular ligament is located in the plantar aspect of the foot, where it connects the sustentaculum tali of the calcaneus to the navicular bone. It helps support the head of the talus and the medial longitudinal arch of the foot. It is termed the spring ligament because it contains a high density of elastic fibers that provide spring to the foot during plantar flexion. **Choice B** (Calcaneofibular ligament) is incorrect. The calcaneofibular ligament, one of the three ligaments on the lateral aspect of the ankle, runs from the calcaneus to the lateral malleolus of the fibula, as its name indicates. It resists excessive inversion of the foot at the ankle joint, rather than eversion. **Choice D** (Anterior talofibular ligament) is incorrect. This ligament, like the calcaneofibular ligament, resists excessive inversion of the foot at the ankle joint, rather than eversion. It connects the head and neck of the talus with the lateral malleolus of the fibula. The third component of the lateral ligament is the posterior talofibular ligament. **Choice E** (Plantar calcaneocuboid [long plantar] ligament) is incorrect. The plantar calcaneocuboid ligament is located in the plantar aspect of the foot. It is a relatively long structure that runs from the plantar side of the calcaneus to the cuboid and bases of the lateral metatarsal bones. It forms a deep canal for the tendon of the fibularis (peroneus) longus muscle and helps to support the lateral longitudinal arch of the foot.

12 **The answer is B: Gluteus medius.** The given AP X-ray reveals fragmentation of the greater trochanter, a large superolateral projection of the proximal end of the femur. The greater trochanter serves as the insertion site for the gluteus medius and minimus muscles, which are involved with abduction and medial rotation of the hip joint. These two muscles also keep the pelvis level when the ipsilateral hip is bearing weight during gait. Fragmentation of the greater trochanter would most likely include detachment of the gluteus medius and minimus muscles. Moreover, additional muscles insert into the greater trochanter to produce lateral rotation of the hip, such as the piriformis, obturator externus, obturator internus, and superior and inferior gemelli (which attach onto the tendon of the obturator internus and by default onto the greater trochanter). In this discussion, the trochanteric fossa is considered part of the greater trochanter, which explains the inclusion of muscles involved with lateral rotation. **Choice A** (Gluteus maximus) is incorrect. The gluteus maximus arises from the ilium of the hip (or coxal) bone, sacrum and coccyx, and sacrotuberous ligament. It inserts partly into the gluteal tuberosity of the femur, but mostly into the iliotibial tract, which attaches into the lateral condyle of the tibia. Due to its course, the gluteus maximus is a powerful extensor and lateral rotator of the thigh, with a notable influence on the leg. However, the given X-ray reveals fragmentation of the greater

trochanter, so the gluteus maximus muscle is not involved in this fracture. **Choice C** (Iliopsoas) is incorrect. The given plain film of the hip joint identifies a fragmentation fracture of the greater trochanter of the femur. However, the lesser trochanter is the insertion site for the iliopsoas muscle, so this muscle is not involved. **Choice D** (Biceps femoris) is incorrect. The two heads of the biceps femoris originate from the ischial tuberosity and the linea aspera and supracondylar line of the femur, respectively. This muscle inserts into the lateral side of the head of the fibula. Because this muscle is not associated with the greater trochanter of the femur, the biceps femoris muscle is not involved in this fracture. **Choice E** (Sartorius) is incorrect. The sartorius muscle originates from the anterior superior iliac spine and inserts into the medial surface of the tibia. Because this muscle is not associated with the greater trochanter of the femur, the sartorius muscle is not involved in this fracture.

13 **The answer is A: Iliofemoral ligament.** In this situation, the hip is pushed into hyperextension with forces directed to produce anterior dislocation of the head of the femur. Thus, the ligament best positioned to resist this force crosses the anterior aspect of the hip joint. The iliofemoral ligament is a large, Y-shaped structure that crosses the front of the hip from the anterior inferior iliac spine and acetabular rim down to the intertrochanteric line of the femur. It is the largest ligament that reinforces the front of the hip joint, and resists hyperextension by tightening the head of the femur into the acetabulum. **Choice B** (Pubofemoral ligament) is incorrect. This ligament reinforces the hip joint capsule inferiorly and anteriorly as it runs from the pubic part of the acetabular rim to the neck of the femur. Its primary function is to resist hyperabduction of the hip. **Choice C** (Ischiofemoral ligament) is incorrect. The ischiofemoral ligament is a relatively weak structure that reinforces the posterior aspect of the hip joint. It attaches from the ischial portion of the acetabular rim to the neck of the femur medial to the base of the greater trochanter. Thus, its primary role is to resist medial rotation of the thigh plus aiding in resisting extension. **Choice D** (Lacunar ligament) is incorrect. The lacunar ligament is a reflection of fibers from the inguinal ligament down to the pubic tubercle. It forms part of the floor of the inguinal canal and the medial wall of the femoral ring (canal). While it is a notable structure in differentiating femoral from inguinal herniae, it is not part of the hip joint. **Choice E** (Ligament of the head of the femur) is incorrect. This ligament (also called the round ligament of the head of the femur or ligamentum teres capitis femoris) is a relatively weak structure that runs from the floor of the acetabular fossa to the small fovea in the head of the femur. It has little importance in strengthening the hip joint. However, this ligament is notable because in early life it usually carries the small nutrient artery supplying the epiphysis of the head of the femur.

14 **The answer is A: Gluteus maximus.** The sacrotuberous ligament runs from the lower lateral sacrum and the coccyx to the ischial tuberosity. It is important in stabilizing the sacroiliac joint and, together with the sacrospinous ligament, defines the lesser sciatic foramen. Furthermore, it provides the gluteus maximus muscle additional firm surface area for origin of its fibers. It is important to notice that skeletal muscle fibers do not always attach only to bone. They may utilize any available structure to increase the surface area for attachment of fibers. Since muscle force production is directly proportional to the physiological cross-sectional area of a muscle, increasing the space available for packing in muscle fibers is an important mechanical aspect of muscle anatomy. **Choice B** (Gluteus medius) is incorrect. This muscle attaches only to bone, the superior aspect of the greater trochanter. This muscle is not located close to the sacrotuberous ligament. **Choice C** (Gluteus minimus) is incorrect. The gluteus minimus, like the gluteus medius, attaches to the superior aspect of the greater trochanter. This muscle is not located in proximity to the sacrotuberous ligament. **Choice D** (Gemelli) is incorrect. The small gemellus superior and inferior muscles originate from bony locales (ischial spine and ischial tuberosity, respectively) and attach onto the tendon of the obturator internus muscle in order to exert their actions against the greater trochanter of the femur. They pass deep to the sacrotuberous ligament, but do not attach onto it. **Choice E** (Obturator externus) is incorrect. Both the obturator externus and internus muscles take most of their origins from the surfaces of the obturator membrane. Thus, both muscles are additional examples of muscles that use ligaments to increase the surface area available for muscle fiber attachment.

15   **The answer is D: Rectus femoris.**   This plain film of the lateral knee indicates an avulsion fracture of the tibial tuberosity (white arrowhead), which is the insertion site for the quadriceps femoris muscles (rectus femoris and the vastus muscles [lateralis, medialis, and intermedius]) via the patellar ligament. Sudden, powerful muscle actions may cause avulsion fractures of the attachments of muscles. In this case, the push out of the starting blocks involves sudden, powerful extension of the right knee, which is the main action of the quadriceps. Because of the insertion onto the tibial tuberosity (via the patella), the force of the contraction of the quadriceps muscles may avulse the tibial tuberosity off the anterior surface of the tibia, resulting in the fragmented tibial tuberosity (white arrow), being pulled superiorly above the knee joint into the anterior thigh. The inability to straighten the leg reflects the loss of extension of the knee from detachment of the quadriceps. **Choice A** (Gastrocnemius) is incorrect. The gastrocnemius is included in the posterior superficial compartment of the leg. It lies across the posterior aspect of the knee and contributes to flexion of that joint. Because it inserts into the calcaneal tendon (tendo calcaneus; Achilles tendon), contraction of the gastrocnemius may cause an avulsion fracture of the calcaneal tuberosity. However, an avulsion fracture of the tibial tuberosity was shown on the given radiograph. **Choice B** (Tibialis anterior) is incorrect. The tibialis anterior is a member of the anterior compartment of the leg. It has an extensive origin from the lateral condyle and upper half of the lateral surface of the tibia and the interosseous membrane of the leg, and it crosses the anterior aspect of the ankle to insert onto the dorsum of the foot, thus producing dorsiflexion and inversion of the foot. It is commonly involved in the painful condition of shin splints. **Choice C** (Adductor magnus) is incorrect. This muscle is contained in the medial (adductor) compartment of the thigh. It runs from the ischial tuberosity to an extensive insertion along the linea aspera, medial supracondylar line, and adductor tubercle of the femur. It acts to adduct and flex the hip. **Choice E** (Semitendinosus) is incorrect. This hamstring muscle is part of the posterior compartment of the

thigh. It originates from the ischial tuberosity and inserts via its long cord-like tendon onto the medial side of the proximal tibia, acting to extend the hip and flex the knee.

16   **The answer is C: Popliteus.**   As described in the question, holding the upright posture during standing includes locking the knee in a stable position. Locking is a complex event in which the femur slightly hyperextends, glides posterior, and rotates medially on the tibial condyles. Therefore, unlocking the knee (necessary in shifting from standing to locomoting) must call for the reverse movements. The popliteus lies deep and obliquely across the posterior aspect of the knee, from the lateral condyle of the femur to the posterior aspect of the proximal tibia. It unlocks the knee by initiating flexion and laterally rotating the femur on the tibia. **Choice A** (Biceps femoris) is incorrect. The biceps femoris descends from the ischium and femur, crosses the lateral posterior aspect of the knee, and attaches onto the head of the fibula. It extends the hip, flexes the knee after unlocking, and laterally rotates the leg when the knee is flexed. **Choice B** (Gastrocnemius) is incorrect. The gastrocnemius attaches to the femoral condyles, crosses the posterior side of the knee, and inserts onto the posterior calcaneus via the calcaneal tendon (tendo calcaneus; Achilles tendon). It flexes the knee after unlocking and plantar flexes the foot. **Choice D** (Sartorius) is incorrect. This long strap-like muscle crosses the anterior thigh from lateral (anterior superior iliac spine) to medial (proximal medial tibia). Because of its oblique course, it contributes to flexion, lateral rotation, and abduction of the hip and flexion of the knee. While it does participate in flexion of the knee, it does not unlock the knee, but acts after the popliteus has unlocked the knee joint. **Choice E** (Plantaris) is incorrect. This very small muscle originates just above the popliteus, from the lower lateral supracondylar line of the femur. However, rather than following the line of the popliteus, it descends through the leg to attach onto the posterior calcaneus. While the plantaris is generously described as participating in flexion of the knee and plantar flexion of the foot, in reality it contributes virtually no forces to those movements and may be primarily proprioceptive in function.

17   **The answer is B: Tendon of the flexor hallucis longus (FHL) muscle.**   The sustentaculum tali is a bony ledge projecting off the medial side of the calcaneus, as seen in the given drawing. It supports the head of the talus and serves as a pulley-like device for the tendon of the FHL. This tendon emerges from the posterior deep compartment of the leg and turns through a groove on the inferior side of the sustentaculum tali to align itself with the hallux. Thus, the FHL uses the sustentaculum tali to change its direction and improve its mechanical efficiency. Likewise, the obturator internus tendon uses the lesser sciatic notch as a pulley to change its line of action. Because of their intimate relationship, a fracture of the sustentaculum tali immediately endangers the FHL tendon. **Choice A** (Tendon of the tibialis posterior muscle) is incorrect. This tendon accompanies the tendon of the FHL out of the posterior deep compartment of the leg. However, the tibialis posterior tendon crosses the medial side of the ankle by hugging the posterior side of the medial malleolus to reach the medial aspect of the foot. Thus, the tibialis posterior also utilizes a bony prominence as a pulley to alter its line of action. **Choice C** (Tendons of the flexor digitorum brevis muscle) is incorrect. The flexor digitorum brevis muscle is located in the first muscle layer in the plantar side of the foot and is not related to the sustentaculum tali. However, the flexor digitorum longus is the third member of the posterior deep compartment of the leg. Its tendon does cross the medial side of the ankle in close company with the FHL and tibialis posterior. **Choice D** (Small saphenous vein) is incorrect. This important cutaneous vein arises from the lateral end of the dorsal venous arch of the foot. It ascends into the leg by crossing the ankle posterior to the lateral malleolus. It is at this location that the small saphenous vein is often harvested for vein grafting procedures. **Choice E** (Plantar arterial arch) is incorrect. The plantar arterial arch is located deep in the plantar aspect of the foot, crossing the metatarsals. It is formed from the lateral plantar artery and the deep plantar artery (a branch of the dorsalis pedis artery).

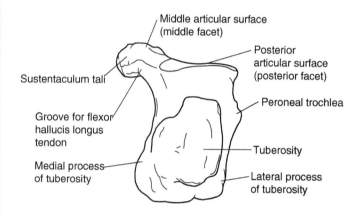

18 **The answer is C: Anterior cruciate ligament (ACL).** The illustration shows testing for the anterior drawer sign, an indicator of the integrity of the ACL. The cruciate ligaments cross each other in essentially the sagittal (anterior to posterior) plane within the knee joint capsule. They are named according to their tibial attachments: the ACL attaches anteriorly on the intercondylar eminence of the tibia and the PCL attaches more posteriorly. Functionally, the ACL (the weaker of the two cruciates) resists anterior sliding of the tibia on the femur when the foot is free (or posterior sliding of the femur on the tibia when the foot is fixed) and hyperextension of the knee. It is commonly injured (along with the TCL and the medial meniscus) in athletes who receive a blow to the lateral side of the leg, which forcefully twists their flexed knee when the foot is planted on the ground. Rupture of the ACL allows the free tibia to be unduly displaced anteriorly relative to the femur. Thus, in the indicated test the femur is fixed and the physician pulls the free tibia forward, as in opening a drawer, to check the range of movement. A positive drawer test (sign) is one in which the tibia can be displaced abnormally forward, indicating damage to the ACL. **Choice A** (Tibial [medial] collateral ligament [TCL]) is incorrect. The TCL supports the medial side of the knee, attaching to the medial femoral epicondyle and the medial tibial condyle. It is tightly stretched in knee extension, resisting medial displacement of these bones. Therefore, the appropriate clinical test for integrity of the TCL is the valgus test, abducting the leg at the knee. Very importantly, the TCL is firmly attached to the medial meniscus. Tearing of the TCL (e.g., due to a blow to the lateral side of the knee) may tear and/or detach the medial meniscus. The

ACL, TCL, and medial meniscus are often damaged together in sports injuries resulting from a lateral impact to the knee when the foot is planted and the knee flexed. This combination injury is termed the "unhappy triad" of the knee joint. **Choice B** (Fibular [lateral] collateral ligament [FCL]) is incorrect. The FCL supports the lateral side of the knee, attaching to the lateral femoral epicondyle and the head of the fibula. As with the TCL, it is taut in knee extension, resisting that and lateral displacement of the leg. Thus, the appropriate clinical test for integrity of the FCL is the varus test, adducting the leg at the knee. Notably, the FCL does not attach to the lateral meniscus, eliminating damage to that structure in cases of tearing of the FCL. **Choice D** (Posterior cruciate ligament [PCL]) is incorrect. The PCL resists posterior sliding of the tibia on the femur when the foot is free (or anterior sliding of the femur on the tibia when the foot is fixed) and hyperflexion of the knee. Because it is shorter, straighter, and stronger than the ACL, the PCL is injured less frequently. It may tear when the anterior knee hits the ground when flexed. Rupture of the PCL allows the free tibia to be unduly displaced posterior under the fixed femur. Thus, in clinical testing, the femur is fixed and the physician pushes the free tibia backward, as in closing a drawer, to check the range of movement. In this case, a positive drawer test (sign) is one in which the tibia can be displaced abnormally backward, indicating damage to the PCL. **Choice E** (Patellar ligament) is incorrect. The patellar ligament is, in actuality, the terminal end of the quadriceps tendon, attaching those four muscles to the tibial tuberosity. Damage to the patellar ligament is indicated by displacement of the patella into the anterior thigh and/or a deficit in knee extension. Interestingly and conveniently, a segment of the patellar ligament may be used for surgical repair of the closely neighboring ACL.

19 **The answer is E: Plantar calcaneonavicular (spring) ligament.** The condition of "flat-foot" (pes planus; talipes planus; "fallen arch") is that in which the medial longitudinal arch of the foot significantly lowers or collapses altogether. This collapse may cause pain due to stretching of the plantar muscles and ligaments, and eversion and abduction of the forefoot leading to excessive wear on the medial side of the soles of shoes. The medial longitudinal arch of the foot is higher and more mechanically significant than the lateral longitudinal arch. It runs through the talus, calcaneus, navicular, cuneiforms, and the three medial metatarsal bones. It is supported largely by the plantar calcaneonavicular (spring) ligament and the tendon of the flexor hallucis longus muscle. Thus, collapse of this arch is likely to put significant strain on the spring ligament. **Choice A** (Calcaneal [Achilles] tendon) is incorrect. The calcaneal tendon (tendo calcaneus; Achilles tendon) is the tendon of insertion for the gastrocnemius and soleus muscles onto the tuberosity of the calcaneus (posterior aspect of the heel). It does not enter the sole of the foot and does not provide support to the arches of the foot. **Choice B** (Plantar calcaneocuboid [long plantar] ligament) is incorrect. The plantar calcaneocuboid ligament is located in the sole of the foot, running from the plantar side of the calcaneus forward to the cuboid and lateral metatarsals. That is, it underlies and supports the lateral longitudinal arch of the foot. The plantar calcaneocuboid (long plantar) ligament may be strained somewhat in fully pronounced flat foot. However, that would normally be secondary to strain of the plantar calcaneonavicular (spring) ligament. **Choice C** (Extensor retinaculum) is incorrect. The extensor retinaculum is a two-part (superior and inferior) band of deep fascia across the anteroinferior leg and dorsum of the foot. It is important in binding and stabilizing the extensor tendons that emerge from the anterior compartment of the leg to pass into the dorsum of the foot. **Choice D** (Tendon of the fibularis [peroneus] longus muscle) is incorrect. This very long tendon enters the deep lateral plantar aspect of the foot and runs across the foot to attach onto the base of the first metatarsal and medial cuneiform. Due to its course, the tendon supports the lateral longitudinal arch of the foot and enables the muscle to participate in eversion and plantar flexion of the foot at the ankle joint.

20   **The answer is C: Saphenous nerve.**   The cutaneous area indicated in the illustration is that of the saphenous nerve, the longest branch of the femoral nerve. The saphenous nerve becomes cutaneous at the medial aspect of the knee, and descends through the leg into the foot in company with the great saphenous vein. It innervates the skin on the medial side of the leg and foot. Because of its close relationship to the great saphenous vein, this nerve is vulnerable to injury in surgery involving the vein (e.g., harvesting of the vein for coronary bypass or repair of varicosities). **Choice A** (Sural nerve) is incorrect. The sural nerve is derived from both the tibial and common fibular (peroneal) nerves in the proximal posterior leg. It supplies the skin on the posterior leg and lateral side of the ankle, heel, and foot. It travels in company with the small saphenous vein and is vulnerable in surgery involving that vessel. **Choice B** (Obturator nerve) is incorrect. The obturator nerve supplies most of the muscles in the medial (adductor) compartment of the thigh and also has a small cutaneous territory in the medial thigh. The cutaneous branches may be damaged in surgery of the upper segment of the great saphenous vein. **Choice D** (Deep fibular [peroneal] nerve) is incorrect. This nerve is one of the terminal branches of the common fibular (peroneal) nerve. It supplies the muscles in the anterior compartment of the leg and dorsum of the foot and has a small cutaneous area in the contiguous skin between the first and second toes. **Choice E** (Superficial fibular [peroneal] nerve) is incorrect. This nerve represents the other terminal branch of the common fibular (peroneal) nerve. It supplies the two muscles in the lateral compartment of the leg and has a large cutaneous territory in the lateral side of the lower leg and most of the dorsum of the foot.

21   **The answer is D: Right gluteus medius and superior gluteal nerve.**   In normal gait, when one foot is lifted off the ground in taking a step, that side of the pelvis becomes unsupported and is subject to falling or sagging due to gravity. Normally, the gluteus medius and minimus muscles on the opposite (contralateral; supported) side act to abduct their side of the pelvis against the lower limb, thus preventing sinking of the unsupported side. The gluteus medius and minimus are innervated by the superior gluteal nerve. Abnormal gait, in which the unsupported side of the pelvis sinks, indicates damage to the contralateral (supported) side of the superior gluteal nerve and/or the gluteus medius and/or minimus muscles. Clinically, this presentation is referred to as a positive Trendelenburg sign. **Choice A** (Right gluteus maximus and inferior gluteal nerve) is incorrect. The gluteus maximus is innervated by the inferior gluteal nerve. However, this muscle does not play a role in

prevention of the sagging of the pelvis (positive Trendelenburg sign) to the contralateral side because its primary action is strong extension of the hip joint. **Choice B** (Left gluteus maximus and superior gluteal nerve) is incorrect. Though the superior gluteal nerve does supply the gluteus medius and minimus involved in this presentation, the gluteus maximus muscle does not play a role in prevention of the sagging of the pelvis (positive Trendelenburg sign) to the contralateral side. Moreover, the muscle was listed on the left side, which is also incorrect. **Choice C** (Left gluteus medius and inferior gluteal nerve) is incorrect. Muscles on the unsupported side are not responsible for the sinking of the pelvis (positive Trendelenburg sign). Also, the inferior gluteal nerve supplies the gluteus maximus, not the gluteus medius and minimus muscles that are involved in this presentation. **Choice E** (Right gluteus minimus and inferior gluteal nerve) is incorrect. The right gluteus minimus is a correct component in the presentation of a positive Trendelenburg sign. However, this muscle is innervated by the superior gluteal nerve rather than the inferior gluteal nerve.

22   **The answer is C: Gluteus maximus.**   Several muscles cross the femoral neck and would react to the fracture by contracting, thus pulling the distal segment of the limb upward over the fracture and shortening the limb. The gluteus maximus inserts partly into the gluteal tuberosity of the femur, but mostly into the iliotibial tract, which attaches into the lateral condyle of the tibia. Thus, the gluteus maximus is a powerful extensor and lateral rotator of the thigh, with a notable influence on the leg. In this case, the strong gluteus maximus is responsible for the distinctive lateral rotation of the limb. **Choice A** (Semitendinosus) is incorrect. The semitendinosus muscle primarily flexes the knee and extends the hip as well as contributing to medial rotation of the leg rather than lateral rotation. **Choice B** (Adductor longus) is incorrect. The adductor longus muscle primarily adducts the thigh. It does not contribute to either medial or lateral rotation of the leg. **Choice D** (Rectus femoris) is incorrect. The rectus femoris muscle extends the leg at the knee joint and contributes to flexion at the hip joint, but it does not contribute to either medial or lateral rotation of the leg. **Choice E** (Gracilis) is incorrect. The gracilis muscle contributes to medial rotation of the leg rather than lateral rotation.

23   **The answer is B: Iliopsoas.**   The given plain film of the hip joint identifies an avulsion fracture of the lesser trochanter of the femur. This osteological feature is the insertion site for the iliopsoas muscle, the major flexor of the hip. Thus, fracture of the lesser trochanter detaches the iliopsoas from the femur, resulting in pain in the upper thigh and a severe deficit in ability to flex the hip. **Choice A** (Adductor magnus) is incorrect. The adductor magnus inserts into the posterior and medial femur far inferior to the lesser trochanter. Its main action is to adduct the thigh. In addition, its adductor part contributes to flexion of the hip, contrasting its hamstring component, which extends the thigh. **Choice C** (Rectus femoris) is incorrect. The rectus femoris is part of the quadriceps femoris group of muscles. These muscles insert through the patellar ligament into the tibial tuberosity and act to extend the knee. Additionally, the rectus femoris is the only muscle in the quadriceps that crosses the hip joint, thus contributing to flexion of the hip. **Choice D** (Biceps femoris) is incorrect. This hamstring muscle inserts into the head of the fibula. It extends the hip and flexes the knee. **Choice E** (Sartorius) is incorrect. The long, strap-like sartorius runs obliquely across the thigh to its insertion into the upper medial tibia. It acts in flexion and lateral rotation of the hip and flexion and medial rotation of the knee.

24 **The answer is A: Tibial (medial) collateral ligament (TCL).**   The TCL supports the medial side of the knee, attaching to the medial femoral epicondyle and the medial tibial condyle. It is tightly stretched in knee extension, resisting medial displacement of these bones. Therefore, the appropriate clinical test for integrity of the TCL, the valgus test, is to abduct the leg at the knee (as shown in the figure). Very importantly, the TCL is firmly attached to the medial meniscus. Tearing of the TCL (e.g., due to a blow to the lateral side of the knee) may tear and/or detach the medial meniscus. The ACL, TCL, and medial meniscus are often damaged together in sports injuries resulting from a lateral impact to the knee when the foot is planted and the knee flexed. This combination injury is termed the "unhappy triad" of the knee joint. **Choice B** (Fibular [lateral] collateral ligament [FCL]) is incorrect. The FCL supports the lateral side of the knee, attaching to the lateral femoral epicondyle and the head of the fibula. As with the TCL, it is taut in knee extension, resisting that and lateral displacement of the leg. Thus, the appropriate clinical test for integrity of the FCL, the varus test, is to adduct the leg at the knee. Notably, the FCL does not attach to the lateral meniscus, eliminating damage to that structure in cases of tearing of the FCL. **Choice C** (Anterior cruciate ligament [ACL]) is incorrect. The ACL resists anterior sliding of the tibia on the femur when the foot is free (or posterior sliding of the femur on the tibia when the foot is fixed) and hyperextension of the knee. It is commonly injured (along with the tibial collateral ligament and the medial meniscus) in athletes who receive a blow to the lateral side of the leg, which forcefully twists their flexed knee when the foot is planted on the ground. Rupture of the ACL allows the free tibia to be unduly displaced anteriorly under the fixed femur. The integrity of the ACL is tested by looking for an anterior drawer sign, in which the femur is fixed and the physician pulls the free tibia forward, as in opening a drawer, to check the range of movement. A positive drawer test (sign) is one in which the tibia can be displaced abnormally forward, indicating damage to the ACL. **Choice D** (Posterior cruciate ligament [PCL]) is incorrect. The PCL resists posterior sliding of the tibia on the femur when the foot is free (or anterior sliding of the femur on the tibia when the foot is fixed) and hyperflexion of the knee. Because it is shorter, straighter, and stronger than the ACL, the PCL is injured less frequently. It may tear when the anterior knee hits the ground when flexed. Rupture of the PCL allows the free tibia to be unduly displaced posteriorly under the fixed femur. Thus, in clinical testing, the femur is fixed and the physician pushes the free tibia backward, as in closing a drawer, to check the range of movement. In this case, a positive drawer test (sign) is one in which the tibia can be displaced abnormally backward, indicating damage to the PCL. **Choice E** (Patellar ligament) is incorrect. The patellar ligament is, in actuality, the terminal end of the quadriceps tendon, attaching those four muscles to the tibial tuberosity. Damage to the patellar ligament is indicated by displacement of the patella into the anterior thigh and/or a deficit in knee extension.

25 **The answer is E: Gracilis.**   All the nerves supplying the lower limb originate within the abdominal and/or pelvic cavities, from the lumbar and/or sacral plexuses. Therefore, all these nerves must have positional relationships to and must penetrate through the abdominal or pelvic walls in order to reach the lower limb. The obturator nerve crosses the lateral wall of the pelvis on its way to the obturator canal and into the lower limb, and may be damaged in surgery or trauma to the lateral pelvic wall. Ultimately, it supplies the muscles in the medial compartment of the thigh, including the gracilis. Trauma to the efferent fibers within the obturator nerve may produce spasms or dysfunction in any of these muscles. **Choice A** (Sartorius) is incorrect. The sartorius is a member of the anterior compartment of the thigh, controlled by the femoral nerve. The femoral nerve does not cross the lateral pelvic wall in its path to the lower limb. Instead, it runs lateral and parallel to the psoas major muscle, outside the true pelvic cavity. **Choice B** (Biceps femoris) is incorrect. The biceps femoris is located in the posterior compartment of the thigh. It is supplied by both the tibial and common fibular (peroneal) nerves. These nerves exit the pelvis through the greater sciatic foramen as components of the sciatic nerve. Neither nerve is related to the lateral pelvic wall. **Choice C** (Tensor muscle of fascia lata) is incorrect. The tensor muscle of fascia lata (tensor fasciae latae) is innervated by the superior gluteal nerve. This nerve also exits the pelvis through the greater sciatic foramen and is well removed from the lateral pelvic wall. **Choice D** (Vastus medialis) is incorrect. The vastus medialis is part of the quadriceps femoris muscles in the anterior compartment of the thigh. It is supplied by the femoral nerve, which does not cross the lateral pelvic wall in its path to the lower limb. Instead, it runs lateral and parallel to the psoas major muscle, outside the true pelvic cavity.

26 **The answer is D: Abductor hallucis muscle.**   The muscles and associated structures in the plantar aspect of the foot are organized into four layers from superficial (layer 1) to deep (layer 4). The first layer includes the abductor hallucis muscle as well as the abductor digiti minimi and the flexor digitorum brevis. **Choice A** (Plantar arterial arch) is incorrect. The plantar arterial arch (deep plantar arch) is an anastomotic vessel formed by the lateral plantar artery and the deep plantar branch of the dorsalis pedis artery. The lateral plantar artery portion (providing the main flow into the plantar arch) is initially located in the plane between the first and second layers of plantar muscles and then courses deeper, between the third and fourth layers. The contribution of the dorsalis pedis artery pierces between the first and second metatarsals into the deepest plantar layer. **Choice B** (Tendons of the flexor digitorum longus muscle) is incorrect. These tendons are located in the second layer of plantar muscles, with the quadratus plantae and the tendon of the flexor hallucis longus. The four lumbrical muscles are also found here, attached to the tendons of the flexor digitorum longus. **Choice C** (Tendon of the fibularis [peroneus] longus muscle) is incorrect. This long tendon crosses the foot deep to the fourth layer of plantar muscles. Some authors include this tendon as a member of the fourth layer. **Choice E** (Superficial fibular [peroneal] nerve) is incorrect. The superficial fibular nerve emerges from the lateral compartment of the leg and distributes its terminal cutaneous branches across the dorsum of the foot.

27 **The answer is C: Tendon of the fibularis (peroneus) longus.** Several structures that enter or exit the foot do so via close positional relationships to the medial and lateral malleoli. As a result, these bony prominences serve as important landmarks for locating structures at the ankle. Also, because a horizontal axis through the malleoli forms the axis of rotation about which flexion and extension of the foot occur, the positions of muscle tendons relative to the malleoli determine plantar flexion versus dorsiflexion. The tendons of the fibularis (peroneus) longus and brevis muscles pass tightly against the posterior side of the lateral malleolus as they leave the lateral compartment of the leg and cross the ankle. Therefore, both muscles act to produce plantar flexion of the foot and may be injured in trauma posterior to the lateral malleolus. **Choice A** (Saphenous nerve) is incorrect. The saphenous nerve enters the medial aspect of the foot by crossing the ankle anterior to the medial malleolus, in close company with the great saphenous vein. **Choice B** (Tendon of the fibularis [peroneus] tertius) is incorrect. The fibularis tertius is a member of the anterior compartment of the leg. Its tendon crosses the anterior aspect of the ankle, bound by the extensor retinaculum. It is the most lateral tendon from the anterior compartment but does not have a particularly close relation to the lateral malleolus. Because it does pass anterior to the malleoli, the tendon of the fibularis tertius muscle participates in dorsiflexion of the foot at the ankle joint and eversion of the foot at the subtalar and transverse tarsal joints. **Choice D** (Posterior tibial artery) is incorrect. This vessel descends through the tibial side of the posterior compartment of the leg and crosses the ankle posterior to the medial malleolus before it terminates by dividing into the medial and lateral plantar arteries. **Choice E** (Great saphenous vein) is incorrect. The great saphenous vein originates from the medial end of the dorsal venous arch in the foot. It ascends into the leg by crossing the ankle anterior to the medial malleolus, in close company with the saphenous nerve.

28 **The answer is B: Hamstrings.** Muscle function is best tested by working individual or groups of muscles against resistance while in their optimal mechanical alignment. This patient is being asked to flex his leg against resistance to test the hamstring muscles in the posterior compartment of the thigh. While some other muscles (e.g., gracilis, gastrocnemius) do contribute to flexion of the leg, the hamstrings are by far the major flexors at the knee. **Choice A** (Quadriceps femoris) is incorrect. The four quadriceps femoris muscles are parts of the anterior compartment of the thigh. Their major action is extension of the knee. Thus, testing of this group is best accomplished by asking the patient to extend the knee against resistance from the flexed position. **Choice C** (Adductors) is incorrect. The adductors are the muscles of the medial compartment of the thigh. Their major action is adduction of the thigh. The basic test for integrity here is adduction of the thigh against resistance, as in working with a Thighmaster. **Choice D** (Triceps surae) is incorrect. The triceps surae ("three heads of the calf") group is composed of the gastrocnemius (with two heads) and soleus (with one head) muscles in the posterior superficial compartment of the leg. The primary action of this group is plantar flexion of the foot. Testing can be accomplished by plantar flexion against resistance from the prone position, or, by asking the patient to stand on their tiptoes. **Choice E** (Plantar flexors) is incorrect. The terms "plantar flexion" and "dorsiflexion" refer specifically to flexion and extension, respectively, of the foot and digits. These terms are not used to describe flexion and extension at other joints. "Plantar flexors" refers to multiple muscle groups. Plantar flexion of the foot is produced mainly by the triceps surae muscles, with notable assistance from the muscles in the lateral and posterior deep compartments of the leg. Plantar flexion of the digits is the product of certain muscles in the posterior deep compartment of the leg and the plantar muscles in the foot.

29 **The answer is B: Profunda femoris artery.** The profunda femoris artery (deep femoral artery; deep artery of the thigh) gives off the perforating arteries that supply blood to the posterior femoral compartment. Arising from the femoral artery, the profunda femoris artery gives off the medial and lateral circumflex femoral arteries before it descends to give off a series of (usually four in number) perforating arteries. These arteries are so named because they pierce (perforate) through the adductor magnus muscle to reach the posterior compartment of the thigh. The perforating arteries supply the adductor magnus and hamstring muscles of the posterior compartment of the thigh. **Choice A** (Femoral artery) is incorrect. The femoral artery gives rise to the profunda femoris artery, which in turn gives off the perforating branches. **Choice C** (Obturator artery) is incorrect. The obturator artery is a branch of the internal iliac artery within the pelvic cavity. It enters the thigh through the obturator canal and divides into anterior and posterior branches, which envelope the adductor brevis muscle. The obturator artery supplies the adductor muscles in the medial compartment of the thigh. **Choice D** (Popliteal artery) is incorrect. The popliteal artery is the direct continuation of the femoral artery in the popliteal fossa. It gives rise to five genicular arteries that form an extensive anastomotic network around the knee. **Choice E** (Medial femoral circumflex artery) is incorrect. This vessel arises from the femoral or profunda femoris artery high within the femoral triangle. It supplies the muscles in the upper medial thigh and the hip joint. This important vessel is one component of the cruciate anastomosis around the hip and also provides the main supply to the head and neck of the femur.

30 **The answer is E: Fibular (peroneal) artery.** The posterior tibial artery supplies the posterior compartments of the leg and the plantar aspect of the foot. A major branch is the fibular (peroneal) artery, which supplies the fibular side of the posterior compartment of the leg. **Choice A** (Anterior tibial artery) is incorrect. The popliteal artery terminates by dividing into the anterior and posterior tibial arteries. In this case, blood will initially continue to flow into the anterior tibial artery and into the anterior compartment of the leg despite disruption of the posterior tibial artery. **Choice B** (Inferior medial genicular artery) is incorrect. Both the inferior medial and inferior lateral genicular arteries are branches of the popliteal artery within the popliteal fossa, proximal to the terminal branching of the popliteal artery. Thus, blood flow into these vessels is spared in this injury. **Choice C** (Dorsalis pedis artery) is incorrect. The dorsalis pedis artery is the direct continuation of the anterior tibial artery into the dorsum of the foot. **Choice D** (Popliteal artery) is incorrect. The popliteal artery runs through the popliteal fossa and ends by dividing into the anterior and posterior tibial arteries at approximately the lower border of the popliteus muscle.

31 **The answer is C: Between the tendons of the extensor hallucis longus and extensor digitorum longus muscles.** The dorsalis pedis pulse is an important indicator of peripheral vascular integrity. The dorsalis pedis artery is the direct continuation of the anterior tibial artery into the dorsum of the foot. Its pulse is normally easy to palpate, as the vessel is subcutaneous and lies against the navicular and cuneiform bones, just lateral to the tendon of the extensor hallucis longus. Because of the prominence of the extensor hallucis longus and extensor digitorum longus tendons, the vessel can be located between them by asking the patient to slightly dorsiflex the digits. **Choice A** (Immediately anterior to the medial malleolus) is incorrect. The dorsalis pedis artery begins midway between the malleoli on the dorsum of the ankle. It is not immediately related to either malleolus. **Choice B** (Immediately anterior to the lateral malleolus) is incorrect. The dorsalis pedis artery begins midway between the malleoli on the dorsum of the ankle. It is not immediately related to either malleolus. **Choice D** (Between the tendons of the extensor digitorum longus and fibularis [peroneus] tertius muscles) is incorrect. This location is too far lateral from the normal position of the dorsalis pedis artery. **Choice E** (Immediately lateral to the tendon of the fibularis [peroneus] tertius muscle) is incorrect. This location is too far lateral from the normal position of the dorsalis pedis artery.

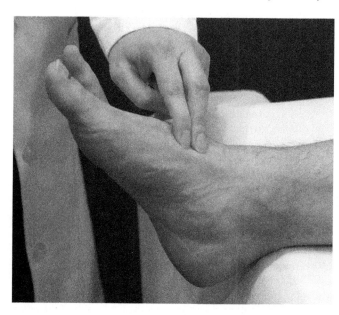

32 **The answer is D: Medial circumflex femoral artery.** The given coronal MRI reveals a nondisplaced femoral neck fracture of the right hip. The medial circumflex femoral artery is important because it supplies most of the blood to the neck and head of the femur. Fracture of the femoral neck may damage this major supply route, creating the possibility of avascular (ischemic) necrosis of the head of the femur. **Choice A** (Femoral artery) is incorrect. The femoral artery gives rise to the profunda femoris artery, which usually gives rise to the medial circumflex femoral artery. However, the medial circumflex femoral may sometimes arise from the femoral artery. **Choice B** (Obturator artery) is incorrect. The obturator artery supplies the medial compartment of the thigh. In addition, it sends a small acetabular branch into the hip joint. This vessel gives rise to the artery to the head of the femur, which follows the ligament of the head of the femur to reach the

femoral head. This artery is usually pronounced in children but may or may not be present or sufficient in adults. When sufficient, it is an important collateral route for blood to reach the femoral head. If the neck of the femur is fractured and the main blood supply to the head is compromised by disruption of the branches of the medial circumflex femoral artery, the flow through the artery to the head of the femur may save the head from avascular necrosis. **Choice C** (Lateral circumflex femoral artery) is incorrect. This vessel usually branches off the profunda femoris artery but may arise from the femoral artery. It supplies the lateral aspect of the thigh, gives branches that anastomose with the medial circumflex femoral artery around the femoral neck and greater trochanter, and enters into the formation of the cruciate anastomosis around the hip. **Choice E** (Inferior gluteal artery) is incorrect. This artery is a branch of the internal iliac artery within the pelvis. It enters the gluteal region, supplies the gluteus maximus, and contributes to the formation of the cruciate anastomosis.

33 **The answer is B: lateral...deep.** The upper and lower limbs rotate in opposite directions during the 7th week of development. The upper limb rotates 90 degrees laterally, resulting in digit no. 1 (the thumb; pollux) lying on the lateral side of the hand. The lower limb rotates 90 degrees medially, resulting in digit no. 1 (the big toe; hallux) lying on the medial side of the foot. At the base of the femoral triangle, where the large vessels enter the lower limb proper from the pelvis, the femoral artery resides lateral to the femoral vein. As the vessels descend through the thigh, they rotate positions relative to each other in the same way the entire limb rotated during development (i.e., 90 degrees medially). Thus, when they reach the popliteal fossa the vessels are essentially stacked on top of one another, with the popliteal artery lying anterior (deep) to the popliteal vein. In mentally reconstructing anatomical directions here, it is important to remember that the vessels are located on the anterior aspect of the thigh in the femoral triangle, but on the posterior aspect of the limb in the popliteal fossa. **Choice A** (medial...posterior) is incorrect. The femoral artery resides lateral to the femoral vein and the popliteal artery lies anterior (=deep) to the popliteal vein. In this question, remember that recognizing either position as incorrect immediately renders the entire choice incorrect. **Choice C** (lateral...posterior) is incorrect. While the femoral artery does reside lateral to the femoral vein, the popliteal artery lies anterior (deep) to the popliteal vein. Remember the direction of rotation of the lower limb. **Choice D** (medial... superficial) is incorrect. Both positions are incorrect here. The femoral artery is lateral to the femoral vein and the popliteal artery is deep to the popliteal vein. **Choice E** (anterior...lateral) is incorrect. In this choice, the correct positions of the femoral and popliteal arteries are reversed. The femoral artery is lateral to the femoral vein, whereas the popliteal artery is anterior (deep) to the popliteal vein.

34 **The answer is A: Adductor magnus.** Hybrid muscles have two distinct parts, each supplied by a different peripheral nerve, reflecting the complex development of the muscle. The two hybrid muscles in the lower limb are the adductor magnus and the biceps femoris, both located in the thigh. The adductor magnus is composed of an adductor portion (supplied by the obturator nerve that controls the adductor muscles in the medial femoral compartment) and a hamstring portion (innervated by the tibial nerve that supplies most of the hamstring muscles in the posterior femoral compartment). The biceps femoris is composed of a larger hamstring (long head) portion (supplied by the tibial nerve) and a smaller gluteal (short head) portion (supplied by the common fibular [peroneal] nerve). The pectineus may or may not be considered a hybrid muscle. It is normally entirely supplied by the femoral nerve. However, it may be innervated by the obturator nerve, and sometimes may be supplied by both the femoral and obturator nerves. **Choice B** (Gastrocnemius) is incorrect. Despite having two heads arising from the femur, the muscle is part of the posterior superficial compartment of the leg and is supplied entirely by the tibial nerve. **Choice C** (Rectus femoris) is incorrect. This muscle is a member of the anterior femoral compartment and is supplied entirely by the femoral nerve. **Choice D** (Semimembranosus) is incorrect. This hamstring muscle is a component of the posterior femoral compartment, along with the biceps femoris and semitendinosus. It is controlled by the tibial nerve. Remember that the sciatic nerve is actually a bundling of the tibial and common fibular (peroneal) nerves. Do not be confused by more generalized references that ascribe the innervation of the hamstrings to the sciatic nerve versus more specific references (such as here) that differentiate the tibial and common fibular components of the sciatic nerve. **Choice E** (Tibialis anterior) is incorrect. This muscle is located in the anterior compartment of the leg. It is supplied entirely by the deep fibular (deep peroneal) nerve.

35   **The answer is C: Iliotibial band syndrome (ITBS).** ITBS is one of the leading causes of lateral knee pain in runners, and it is often seen in runners who increase the intensity of their workouts too rapidly. The iliotibial band (tract) is a lateral thickening of the fascia lata that extends inferiorly to the anterolateral aspect of the lateral condyle of the tibia and stabilizes the knee during running. When the knee is flexed at approximately 45 degrees, the iliotibial tract passes posterior to the lateral femoral epicondyle. In distance runners and cyclists, repeated flexion and extension of the knee cause friction on the lateral femoral epicondyle due to the iliotibial band rubbing against the bone. ITBS, and its associated pain and inflammation of the lateral knee, is exacerbated by downhill running and chronic repetitive foot strikes during long runs. **Choice A** (Sprained fibular [lateral] collateral ligament [FCL]) is incorrect. Lateral knee pain can generally be traced to three anatomical sites: ITBS (seen in this patient), a torn lateral meniscus, and a sprained FCL. The latter two scenarios usually follow trauma to the knee joint, which was not reported in this patient and can be ruled out as a diagnosis. FCL sprains are usually due to a blow to the medial side of the knee, which sprains or tears the FCL; however, this type of trauma was not reported in this patient. **Choice B** (Patellofemoral pain syndrome) is incorrect. Patellofemoral pain syndrome is often seen in runners who increase the intensity of their workouts too rapidly. This syndrome results from imbalances in the forces controlling patellar tracking during knee flexion and extension, and patients present with anterior knee pain that is described as being around, underneath, or behind the patella. While this syndrome is similar in presentation to ITBS, it can be distinguished from ITBS due to the presence of anterior knee pain versus the lateral knee pain seen in this patient. **Choice D** (Torn lateral meniscus) is incorrect. Though a patient with a torn lateral meniscus would report lateral knee pain, this presentation is usually due to trauma, particularly when the flexed knee is twisted. Patients with torn menisci present with pain, inflammation, tenderness, popping or clicking of the joint, and knee joint instability. Though this patient had lateral knee pain with some of these signs and symptoms, there was no trauma reported, which would make a meniscus tear unlikely. **Choice E** (Pes anserinus bursitis) is incorrect. The pes anserinus (**L**: foot of a goose) is the combined tendon insertions of the **S**artorius, **G**racilis, and semi**T**endinosus muscles (mnemonics: 1. SGT, an abbreviation for sergeant, and 2. "Say Grace Before Tea," which takes into account the presence of the anserine **B**ursa) at the medial border of the tuberosity of the tibia. Pes anserinus bursitis is often seen in athletic overuse; however, it would be responsible for medial knee pain, not the lateral knee pain seen in this patient.

36   **The answer is B: Fibularis brevis.** The fibularis (peroneus) brevis muscle attaches to the dorsal surface of the tuberosity on the lateral side of the base of the fifth metatarsal, which is where the avulsion fracture is seen in this X-ray. During extreme inversion injuries, force from this muscle can avulse the tuberosity at the base of the fifth metatarsal. When diagnosing fractures of the fifth metatarsal, a physician must distinguish among an avulsion fracture (as seen on this X-ray), a stress fracture normally located at the midshaft, and a Jones fracture, which is a fracture through the proximal fifth metatarsal that enters the intermetatarsal joint. With the fifth metatarsal, blood supply is less than adequate as it progresses distally along this bone, so treatments for each type of fracture will vary. **Choice A** (Extensor digitorum longus) is incorrect. The extensor digitorum longus inserts into the middle and distal phalanges of the lateral four digits. This muscle extends the lateral four digits and dorsiflexes the ankle. It does not insert into the tuberosity located at the base of the fifth metatarsal, so it would not be involved in the avulsion fracture seen in this patient. **Choice C** (Fibularis longus) is incorrect. The fibularis (peroneus) longus muscle inserts into the base of the first metatarsal and medial cuneiform bone. This muscle is important in eversion of the foot; however, it can be eliminated due to its medial insertion in the foot. **Choice D** (Fibularis tertius) is incorrect. The fibularis (peroneus) tertius muscle attaches to the dorsal surface at the base of the fifth metatarsal. Due to its dorsal attachment, an avulsion fracture involving this muscle would not involve the tuberosity located at the base of the fifth metatarsal, which is shown avulsed in this patient. Remember, the fibularis tertius muscle is located in the anterior leg compartment and is important in eversion of the foot during ambulation. **Choice E** (Flexor digiti minimi brevis) is incorrect. The flexor digiti minimi brevis inserts into the base of the proximal phalanx of the fifth digit. It does not participate in eversion of the foot, so it would not be injured in this inversion ankle injury.

37   **The answer is E: Vertical group of superficial inguinal.** The vertical group of superficial inguinal lymph nodes receives superficial lymph vessels from the territory drained by the great saphenous vein (including the medial aspect of the thigh) and lies along its termination near the saphenous hiatus. Efferent lymphatic vessels from this group of superficial inguinal nodes drain into deep inguinal nodes. Given the location of the injury and the patient's presentation, this group of lymph nodes is most likely to receive the initial drainage from the infected wound. **Choice A** (Popliteal) is incorrect. The popliteal nodes are located in the popliteal fossa and receive lymphatic drainage from the lateral side of the leg and foot, which corresponds to the area drained by the small saphenous vein, and from deep lymph vessels accompanying the anterior and posterior tibial arteries. The efferent lymphatic vessels leaving the popliteal nodes drain into deep lymph vessels of the lower limb that parallel the major vessels before reaching the deep inguinal nodes. **Choice B** (External iliac) is incorrect. The external iliac lymph nodes lie along the external iliac vessels above the superior pelvic aperture and receive lymphatic drainage from the inguinal lymph nodes, abdominal wall below the level of the umbilicus, and the pelvic viscera. Efferent vessels from the external iliac nodes drain into common iliac nodes. These nodes are not the first nodes affected in this patient due to the site of the injury (medial thigh). **Choice C** (Deep inguinal) is incorrect. The deep inguinal nodes receive lymph from deep lymphatic vessels in the lower limb that travel with the arteries, from the superficial inguinal nodes (horizontal and vertical groups), from the popliteal nodes, and from the glans and body of the clitoris or penis. Efferent vessels from the deep inguinal nodes drain into external iliac nodes. Though the deep inguinal nodes could be involved with this infection, they would not be the first nodes affected in this patient due to the site of the injury (medial thigh). **Choice D** (Horizontal group of superficial inguinal) is incorrect. The horizontal group of superficial inguinal lymph nodes is located approximately 2 cm below the inguinal ligament and receives lymphatic drainage from the lateral buttocks, lower anterior abdomen wall, and the perineum. An infected cut on the medial thigh would not send lymph to this group of nodes.

38 **The answer is B: Deep fibular nerve.** The deep fibular (peroneal) nerve is a terminal branch of the common fibular nerve that supplies motor innervation to the four muscles of the anterior compartment of the leg: (1) tibialis anterior, (2) extensor digitorum longus, (3) extensor hallucis longus, and (4) fibularis (peroneus) tertius. These four muscles are responsible for dorsiflexion of the ankle. The deep fibular nerve also innervates the extensor digitorum brevis and extensor hallucis brevis, which are intrinsic muscles of the foot, sends articular branches to joints it crosses, and supplies cutaneous innervation to the first interdigital cleft. The deep fibular nerve is responsible for dorsiflexion of the foot at the ankle joint, and the segmental innervation of this movement is L4 and L5. **Choice A** (Tibial nerve) is incorrect. The tibial nerve is a terminal branch of the sciatic nerve that supplies the posterior muscles of the knee joint and leg, including the superficial compartment where the gastrocnemius and soleus muscles reside. The tibial nerve is responsible for plantar flexion of the foot at the ankle joint, and the segmental innervation of this movement is S1 and S2. **Choice C** (Superficial fibular nerve) is incorrect. The superficial fibular nerve is a terminal branch of the common fibular nerve that supplies motor innervation to the two muscles (fibularis longus and brevis) of the lateral compartment of the leg and cutaneous (sensory) innervation to the distal third of the anterior surface of the leg and dorsum of the foot. These muscles are primarily responsible for eversion of the foot at the ankle joint, and the segmental innervation of

this movement is L5 and S1. **Choice D** (Medial plantar nerve) is incorrect. The tibial nerve divides into the medial and lateral plantar nerves to innervate muscles of the sole of the foot. The medial plantar nerve, which is homologous to the median nerve in the hand, innervates the following intrinsic foot muscles: first **L**umbrical, **A**bductor hallucis, **F**lexor digitorum brevis, and **F**lexor hallucis brevis. The mnemonic for muscles supplied by the medial plantar nerve is the "LAFF" muscles. Because this nerve does not supply muscles that cross the ankle joint, it cannot be responsible for the dorsiflexion being tested here. **Choice E** (Lateral plantar nerve) is incorrect. The tibial nerve divides into the medial and lateral plantar nerves to innervate muscles of the sole of the foot. The lateral plantar nerve, which is homologous to the ulnar nerve in the hand, innervates all of the intrinsic foot muscles, with the exception of the four "LAFF" muscles supplied by the medial plantar nerve. Because this nerve does not supply muscles that cross the ankle joint, it cannot be responsible for the dorsiflexion being tested in this patient.

39 **The answer is E: Sciatic nerve.** The sciatic nerve is formed by the anterior rami of L4-S3 and is located in the inferior medial quadrant of the buttock. This nerve supplies the muscles in the posterior compartment of the thigh and bifurcates into the tibial nerve and common fibular nerves in the popliteal fossa. The patient exhibits damage to the L4-S1 distribution of this nerve, which would severely limit inversion (L4, L5), eversion (L5, S1), and dorsiflexion (L4, L5) of the foot at the ankle joint. The inability to dorsiflex the foot also has led to foot drop. This prisoner received an improperly placed gluteal IM injection, which either directly damaged his sciatic nerve or the damage to the nerve was caused secondarily due to infection (possibly from an improperly sanitized needle). Properly administered gluteal IM injections are placed posterior to the anterior superior iliac spine and anterior to the tubercle of the iliac crest along the superior border of the gluteus maximus muscle (see diagram on next page). These injections penetrate skin, fascia, and muscles, which allows absorption of the injected substance into the IM veins located in the area of the tensor fasciae latae muscle. **Choice A** (Superior gluteal nerve) is incorrect. The superior gluteal nerve supplies motor innervation to the gluteus medius, gluteus minimus, and tensor fasciae latae muscles. Loss of this innervation would lead to weakness in abducting and medially rotating the thigh at the hip joint. These muscles are also responsible for keeping the pelvis level during the swing phase of gait. Though the superior gluteal nerve is formed by the anterior rami of L4-S1, damage to this nerve would not cause the paresis (weakness) seen in this patient at the ankle joint. **Choice B** (Common fibular nerve) is incorrect. The common fibular (peroneal) nerve is a terminal branch of the sciatic nerve that usually does not arise until the sciatic nerve bifurcates in the apex of the popliteal fossa. This nerve further divides into the deep and superficial fibular nerves, which supply the motor innervation to the anterior and lateral compartments of the leg, respectively. Damage to the common fibular nerve would lead to the symptoms seen in this patient (i.e., weakness in inversion, eversion, and dorsiflexion of the foot at the ankle joint as well as foot drop). However, a gluteal IM injection would not affect this nerve directly due to its origin, which is usually in the apex of the popliteal fossa. **Choice C** (Tibial nerve) is incorrect. The tibial nerve is a terminal branch of the sciatic nerve that usually does not arise until the sciatic nerve bifurcates in the apex of the popliteal fossa. This nerve supplies the posterior compartment of the leg and is important in plantar flexion of the foot at the ankle joint. Weakness in plantar flexion was not noted in this patient, and more importantly, a gluteal IM injection would not affect this nerve directly due to its origin, which is usually in the popliteal fossa. **Choice D** (Inferior gluteal nerve) is incorrect. The inferior gluteal nerve innervates the gluteus maximus and is formed by the anterior rami of L5-S2. This muscle is involved with lateral rotation and extension of the thigh at the hip joint, especially when the thigh is in a flexed position (rising from a sitting position or climbing stairs). Damage to the inferior gluteal nerve would not produce weakness in movements of the ankle joint.

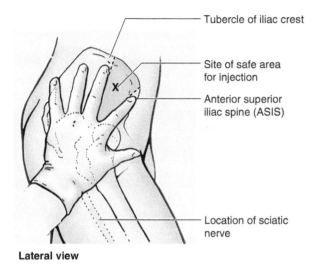

Tubercle of iliac crest

Site of safe area for injection

Anterior superior iliac spine (ASIS)

Location of sciatic nerve

Lateral view

40 **The answer is B: Tachycardia.** Tachycardia (rapid beatings of the heart) would be seen in this patient. Acute blood loss induces the following hemodynamic changes: tachycardia, hypotension (subnormal arterial blood pressure), generalized arteriolar vasoconstriction, and generalized venoconstriction. **Choice A** (Increased pulse in right dorsalis pedis artery) is incorrect. Due to the hemodynamic changes associated with acute blood loss, the pulse in the right dorsalis artery would be diminished due to generalized arteriolar vasoconstriction, which greatly reduces peripheral blood flow to ensure that vital organs in the thorax are receiving blood. **Choice C** (Warm right foot) is incorrect. Due to the hemodynamic changes associated with acute blood loss, the right foot would feel cold due to generalized arteriolar vasoconstriction. **Choice D** (Increased hematocrit) is incorrect. Due to the hemodynamic changes associated with acute blood loss, the hematocrit (the proportion of blood volume that is occupied by red blood cells) would be decreased from the normal 46% value seen in men due to the loss of blood. Lowered hematocrit levels imply significant hemorrhage. **Choice E** (Hypertension) is incorrect. Due to the hemodynamic changes associated with acute blood loss, hypertension (high arterial blood pressure) would not be seen in this patient due to the severe blood loss. Due to his blood loss, the patient would be hypotensive.

41 **The answer is D: Lateral femoral cutaneous nerve.** This case is the classic presentation of meralgia paresthetica, an entrapment of the lateral femoral cutaneous nerve as it passes under the inguinal ligament in proximity to the anterior superior iliac spine. Impingement of the lateral femoral cutaneous nerve causes abnormal sensations of burning, pain, and numbness in the distribution of this nerve, which is the lateral portion of the upper thigh. Meralgia paresthetica may be called "bikini brief syndrome" because it is seen in individuals who have gained considerable weight in a short period (e.g., in pregnancy), and the entrapment of the nerve can be caused by tight undergarments. In this case, the student's backpack rested near the anterior superior iliac spine, which led to his presentation. **Choice A** (Femoral branch of genitofemoral nerve) is incorrect. The femoral branch of the genitofemoral nerve is formed by the ventral rami of L1-2. This nerve supplies the upper medial aspects of the thigh. Due to the lateral location of the symptoms in this patient, this nerve is not involved. **Choice B** (Saphenous nerve) is incorrect. The saphenous nerve is a terminal sensory branch of the femoral nerve, which traverses medially through the adductor canal in the thigh to supply the medial side of the leg and foot, including the medial malleolus of the tibia. Due to the location of the sensory deficits in the upper lateral thigh, this nerve is not involved in this patient's presentation. **Choice C** (Anterior cutaneous branches of femoral nerve) is incorrect. The anterior cutaneous branches of the femoral nerve supply the upper medial aspect of the thigh. These nerves are derived from L2-4 and are too far medial to elicit the symptoms in this medical student. **Choice E** (Iliohypogastric nerve) is incorrect. The iliohypogastric nerve arises primarily from the ventral ramus of L1, with possible contributions from T12. This nerve runs above the anterior superior iliac spine within the anterolateral muscular wall of the abdomen. The iliohypogastric nerve supplies the suprapubic region of the abdomen rather than the lateral thigh.

42 **The answer is C: Femoral hernia.** The femoral ring is a weakened aspect in the anterior abdominal wall through which a femoral hernia enters the femoral canal. This type of hernia often contains abdominal viscera and is more common in females due to their wider pelves. Femoral herniae are also more susceptible to strangulation, in which case the blood supply can be interrupted due to the sharp boundaries of the femoral ring, particularly the lacunar ligament. Strangulation can lead to ischemia, sharp pain, and necrosis of the impinged tissue. Because this patient is female and the sudden onset of her symptoms following strenuous lifting, strangulation of a femoral hernia is the most likely diagnosis. Her nausea and vomiting may be due to a small bowel obstruction or may be a result of the severe pain due to the ischemia associated with the hernia. The location of the globular mass may be difficult to distinguish from indirect or direct inguinal herniae. However, several studies suggest CT imaging can differentiate between these hernia types. Direct inguinal herniae rarely occur in females. Males are three to four times more likely to have an indirect inguinal hernia, due to the embryological descent of the testes. **Choice A** (Indirect inguinal hernia) is incorrect. An indirect inguinal hernia is usually a congenital hernia that results when abdominal cavity contents herniate through a patent processus vaginalis, or in an adult, the inguinal canal. The hernia passes through the deep and superficial inguinal rings and descends into the scrotum in males. Indirect inguinal herniae are three to four times more common in men and do not usually evoke the high incidence of strangulation seen in femoral herniae. **Choice B** (Direct inguinal hernia) is incorrect. A direct inguinal hernia is an acquired hernia that results when abdominal cavity contents herniate through a weakness in the anterior abdominal wall in the inguinal (Hesselbach) triangle. The hernia exits through the superficial inguinal ring but does not usually descend into the scrotum. Direct inguinal herniae are rare in women. In fact, some references cite groin herniae as 25 times more likely to occur in men. **Choice D** (Lymphadenitis of superficial inguinal nodes) is incorrect. Lymphadenitis (swollen lymph nodes) of the superficial inguinal nodes could be responsible for the globular mass detected in this patient. However, the history of this patient does not include a recent bacterial or viral infection, which would cause these lymph nodes to be tender and swollen. Lymph nodes affected by cancer could also appear as a globular mass. However, when affected by cancer, these nodes are enlarged but usually not painful. Most importantly, the pain in this patient is acute, which would rule out lymph node involvement, especially due to the patient's history of onset after heavy lifting. **Choice E** (Fractured hip) is incorrect. No trauma was reported by the patient, so a fractured hip can be easily eliminated as a choice, especially due to the location of the globular mass inferolateral to the pubic tubercle.

43 **The answer is A: Medial plantar nerve.** The medial plantar nerve, which is homologous to the median nerve in the hand, innervates four intrinsic foot muscles: first Lumbrical, Abductor hallucis, Flexor digitorum brevis, and Flexor hallucis brevis (mnemonic = "LAFF" muscles). This nerve supplies cutaneous innervation to the medial three and a half toes on the plantar surface of the foot. The given photo shows the sensory distribution of the medial plantar nerve, but please remember that the other cutaneous nerves of the plantar aspect of the foot (lateral plantar nerve on the lateral aspect, tibial nerve proximally, and saphenous nerve medially) will have some overlap with this distribution pattern. Due to the depth of the cut, the medial plantar nerve, which travels between the first and second layers of the plantar foot musculature, was most likely severed, resulting in loss of cutaneous sensation to the plantar surface of the medial three toes and loss of motor innervation to the abductor hallucis and flexor hallucis brevis. The tendon of the flexor hallucis longus muscle, which resides in the second layer of plantar foot musculature, would have also been severed by this cut. Despite being innervated by the tibial nerve, the tendon of this muscle would have been severed due to the depth of the cut, resulting in the complete inability to flex the big toe, seen in this patient. **Choice B** (Lateral plantar nerve) is incorrect. The lateral plantar nerve, which is homologous to the ulnar nerve in the hand, innervates all of the intrinsic foot muscles, with the exception of the four muscles supplied by the medial plantar nerve. This nerve also provides cutaneous (sensory) innervation to the lateral one and a half toes. Due to the location of the laceration near the first (or medial) cuneiform bone and the symptoms of this patient, this nerve was not severed in this injury. **Choice C** (Sural nerve) is incorrect. The sural nerve is a cutaneous nerve, so the motor deficits seen in this patient (weakness in flexing and abducting the big toe) would not be possible. The course of this nerve parallels the small saphenous vein, and damage to the sural nerve would lead to numbness and paresthesia in the dorsal aspect of the lateral fifth toe and lateral malleolus of the fibula. **Choice D** (Deep fibular nerve) is incorrect. The deep fibular (peroneal) nerve supplies motor innervation to the four muscles of the anterior compartment of the leg and two intrinsic muscles of the foot: extensor digitorum brevis and extensor hallucis brevis. Its cutaneous territory lies between the first and the second toes on the dorsal surface of the foot. So, the deep fibular nerve is not involved in this patient. **Choice E** (Superficial fibular nerve) is incorrect. The superficial fibular nerve supplies motor innervation to the two muscles (fibularis longus and brevis) of the lateral compartment of the leg and cutaneous (sensory) innervation to the distal third of the anterior surface of the leg and dorsum of the foot. Because the patient did not present with weakness during eversion of the foot at the ankle joint or numbness on the dorsum of the foot, this nerve was not damaged in this patient.

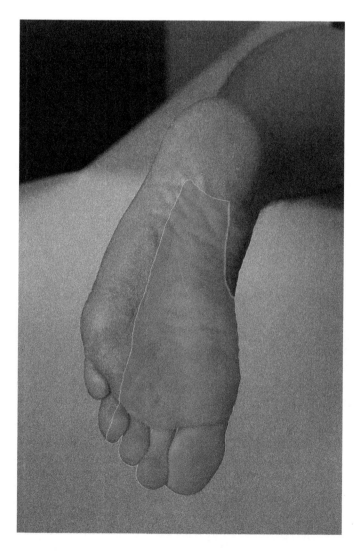

44 **The answer is B: Posterior cruciate ligament (PCL).** The PCL resists posterior sliding of the tibia on the femur when the foot is free (or anterior sliding of the femur on the tibia when the foot is fixed) and hyperflexion of the knee. Because it is shorter, straighter, and stronger than the ACL, the PCL is injured less frequently; however, PCL damage can occur in dashboard injuries (as seen in this patient) or contact sports when the anterior shin hits the ground when the knee is flexed. Rupture of the PCL allows the free tibia to be unduly displaced posterior under the fixed femur. Thus, in clinical testing as shown in the given figure, the femur is fixed and the physician pushes the free tibia backward, as in closing a drawer, to check the range of movement. In this case, a positive posterior drawer test (sign) is one in which the tibia can be displaced abnormally backward, indicating damage to the PCL. This sign was seen in this patient. **Choice A** (Anterior cruciate ligament [ACL]) is incorrect. The ACL resists anterior sliding of the tibia on the femur when the foot is free (or posterior sliding of the femur on the tibia when the foot is fixed) and hyperextension of the knee. It is commonly injured (along with the tibial collateral ligament and the medial meniscus) in athletes who receive a blow to the lateral side of the leg, which forcefully twists their flexed knee when the foot is planted on the ground. Rupture of the ACL allows the free tibia to be unduly displaced anteriorly under the fixed femur. Thus, in the drawer test the femur is fixed and the physician pulls the free tibia forward, as in opening a drawer, to check the range of movement. A positive anterior drawer test (sign) is one in which the tibia can be displaced abnormally forward, indicating damage to the ACL. **Choice C** (Tibial [medial] collateral ligament [TCL]) is incorrect. The TCL supports the medial side of the knee, attaching to the medial femoral epicondyle and the medial tibial condyle. It is tightly stretched in knee extension, resisting medial displacement of these bones. Therefore, the appropriate clinical test for integrity of the TCL is the valgus test, to abduct the leg at the knee, and abnormal results for this test were not reported in this patient. Very importantly, the TCL is firmly attached to the medial meniscus. Tearing of the TCL (e.g., due to a blow to the lateral side of the knee) may tear and/ or detach the medial meniscus. The ACL, TCL, and medial meniscus are often damaged together in sports injuries resulting from a lateral impact to the knee when the foot is planted and the knee flexed. This combination injury is termed the "unhappy triad" of the knee joint. **Choice D** (Fibular [lateral] collateral ligament [FCL]) is incorrect. The FCL supports the lateral side of the knee, attaching to the lateral femoral epicondyle and the head of the fibula. As with the tibial collateral ligament, it is taut in knee extension, resisting that and lateral displacement of the leg. Therefore, this ligament may have also been damaged in this accident; however, the appropriate clinical test for integrity of the FCL is the varus test, to adduct the leg at the knee, which was not mentioned in this clinical vignette. Notably, the FCL does not attach to the lateral meniscus, eliminating damage to that structure in cases of tearing of the FCL. **Choice E** (Patellar ligament) is incorrect. The patellar ligament conducts force from the terminal end of the quadriceps tendon, attaching those four muscles to the tibial tuberosity. Damage to the patellar ligament is indicated by displacement of the patella into the anterior thigh and/ or a deficit in knee extension, which was not noted in this patient.

45   **The answer is C: Vastus medialis.** The vastus medialis muscle, a component of the quadriceps femoris, inserts into the patella and the tibial tuberosity through the common quadriceps tendon and patellar ligament. This muscle helps extend the leg at the knee joint, but it also maintains a medial pull on the patella, reducing the lateral, dislocating force. The patella is stabilized by the vastus medialis muscle and the prominent femoral condyles, which usually prevent lateral dislocation during flex-

ing of the leg at the knee joint. Moreover, the vastus medialis muscle helps stabilize the patella within the patellar groove to control the tracking of the patella when the knee is bent and straightened. Females are at a greater risk of dislocating the patella due to the width of their hips, which tends to cause genu valgum ("knocked-knee" appearance). In this patient, her conditioning was suspect, so strengthening the quadriceps femoris muscle, especially the vastus medialis, should stabilize the patella, hold it within the patellar groove, and decrease the incidence of future patellar dislocations. **Choice A** (Vastus intermedius) is incorrect. The vastus intermedius muscle, the central deep component of the quadriceps femoris, inserts into the patella and the tibial tuberosity through the common quadriceps tendon and patellar ligament. This muscle helps extend the leg at the knee joint. Due to its insertion into the superior aspect of the patella, this muscle does not provide a medial pull on the patella, so targeting this muscle specifically in rehabilitation would not prevent lateral dislocation of the patella. However, strengthening the entire quadriceps femoris muscle would help keep the patella in the patellar groove. **Choice B** (Vastus lateralis) is incorrect. The vastus lateralis muscle (lateral head of the quadriceps femoris) inserts into the patella and the tibial tuberosity through the common quadriceps tendon and patellar ligament. This muscle helps extend the leg at the knee joint. Due to its insertion into the lateral aspect of the patella, the orientation of its muscle fibers will not prevent lateral dislocation of the patella. **Choice D** (Rectus femoris) is incorrect. The rectus femoris muscle (anterior [superficial] head of the quadriceps femoris) inserts into the patella and the tibial tuberosity through the common quadriceps tendon and patellar ligament. This muscle helps extend the leg at the knee joint and also flexes the thigh at the hip joint because it is the only component of the quadriceps femoris to cross the hip joint. Due to its insertion into the superior aspect of the patella, this muscle does not provide a medial pull on the patella, so targeting this muscle specifically in rehabilitation would not prevent lateral dislocation of the patella. However, strengthening the entire quadriceps femoris muscle would help keep the patella in the patellar groove. **Choice E** (Tibialis anterior) is incorrect. The tibialis anterior muscle does not insert into the patella, so targeting this muscle during physical therapy and rehabilitation would not prevent future dislocations of the patella.

46   **The answer is D: Common fibular nerve.** The common fibular (peroneal) nerve, a terminal branch of the sciatic nerve, courses around the neck of the fibula. It is at this site that this nerve is particularly prone to injury via trauma, such as a kick to the side of the leg. Distal to this location, the common fibular nerve divides into the deep and superficial fibular nerves, which supply the motor innervation to the anterior and lateral compartments of the leg, respectively. Damage to the common fibular nerve would lead to all of the symptoms seen in this patient, such as weakness in eversion and dorsiflexion of the foot at the ankle joint, foot drop, and loss of sensation to the dorsum of the foot. **Choice A** (Tibial nerve) is incorrect. The tibial nerve is a terminal branch of the sciatic nerve that supplies the posterior muscles of the knee joint and leg. Damage to this nerve would cause an inability to stand on one's tiptoes, not the foot drop and other signs and symptoms present in this patient. **Choice B** (Deep fibular nerve) is incorrect. The deep fibular (peroneal) nerve is a terminal branch of the common fibular nerve that supplies motor innervation to the muscles of the anterior compartment of the leg. These muscles are responsible for dorsiflexion of the ankle, and damage to the deep fibular nerve would result in foot drop, seen in the image. However, the cutaneous innervation of the deep fibular nerve supplies only a small area between the first and second toes, not the entire dorsum of the foot, which is primarily supplied by the superficial fibular nerve. This involvement of the superficial fibular nerve suggests the lesion is more proximal. **Choice C** (Superficial fibular nerve) is incorrect. The superficial fibular nerve is a terminal branch of the common fibular nerve that supplies motor innervation to the muscles of the lateral compartment of the leg, responsible for eversion of the foot at the ankle joint. It also supplies cutaneous (sensory) innervation to the distal third of the anterior surface of the leg and dorsum of foot. Both motor (weakness in eversion) and sensory (paresthesia on dorsum of foot) symptoms are present in this patient; however, a lesion to the superficial fibular nerve would not explain the foot drop of the patient. This involvement of the anterior leg compartment indicates that the lesion is more proximal. **Choice E** (Sciatic nerve) is incorrect. The sciatic nerve is formed by the anterior rami of L4-S3 and supplies the muscles in the posterior compartment of the thigh. The sciatic nerve bifurcates into the tibial and common fibular nerves in the popliteal fossa. Because this nerve usually gives off its terminal branches in the popliteal fossa, it is unlikely to be damaged by impact to the fibular neck.

47   **The answer is D: Meniscus.**   The menisci are crescent-shaped intraarticular fibrocartilages found in the knees. These cartilaginous structures serve to dissipate force between the femur and the tibia by acting as shock absorbers, to increase knee joint congruence by forming shallow fossae that receive the femoral condyles, and to help distribute the synovial fluid of the knee joint. A meniscus usually tears during abnormal twisting of the flexed knee, usually eliciting a loud pop, as noted by this patient. Patients present with the listed symptoms and also may experience limited range of motion in the knee joint. If a meniscal tear is suspected, a McMurray test can be implemented by the physician by placing a valgus stress on the flexed knee of the patient. A clicking sound or pain along the joint line represents a "positive McMurray test." An MRI is taken to verify the suspected meniscal tear. Although X-rays do not show meniscal tears, it is standard practice to X-ray the affected knee joint to look for other causes of knee pain, such as osteoarthritis. **Choice A** (Tibial [medial] collateral ligament [TCL]) is incorrect. The TCL supports the medial side of the knee, attaching to the medial femoral epicondyle and the medial tibial condyle. It is tightly stretched in knee extension, resisting medial displacement of these bones. Therefore, the appropriate clinical test for integrity of the TCL is to abduct the leg while placing a valgus stress on the knee joint. Very importantly, the TCL is firmly attached to the medial meniscus. Tearing of the TCL (e.g., due to a blow to the lateral side of the knee) may tear and/or detach the medial meniscus. The ACL, TCL, and medial meniscus are often damaged together in sports injuries resulting from a lateral impact to the knee when the foot is planted and the knee flexed. This combination injury is termed the "unhappy triad" of the knee joint. Due to the absence of considerable impact to the medial aspect of the knee, TCL damage is unlikely. Moreover, a TCL tear would most likely lead to considerable

pain, which would have made it unlikely for him to continue playing. **Choice B** (Fibular [lateral] collateral ligament [FCL]) is incorrect. The FCL supports the lateral side of the knee, attaching to the lateral femoral epicondyle and the head of the fibula. As with the TCL, it is taut in knee extension, resisting that and lateral displacement of the leg. Thus, the appropriate clinical test for integrity of the FCL is to adduct the leg while placing a varus stress on the knee joint. Notably, the FCL does not attach to the lateral meniscus, eliminating damage to that structure in cases of tearing of the FCL. Due the absence of considerable impact to the lateral aspect of the knee, FCL damage is unlikely. Moreover, a FCL tear would most likely lead to considerable pain, which would have made it unlikely for him to continue playing. **Choice C** (Anterior cruciate ligament [ACL]) is incorrect. An ACL rupture may also elicit a loud pop and lead to instability in the knee joint during descent of stairs. However, the patient would most likely not be able to continue playing and would have sought medical attention immediately. The integrity of the ACL is tested via an anterior drawer test. When the tibia can be displaced abnormally forward away from the femur, damage to the ACL is verified. It is important to note that the ACL is commonly injured (along with the tibial collateral ligament and the medial meniscus) in athletes who receive a blow to the lateral side of the leg, which forcefully twists their flexed knee when the foot is planted on the ground. In this patient, joint line pain and clicking of the knee during the McMurray test indicate damage to the meniscus. **Choice E** (Patella) is incorrect. The patella (kneecap) is a sesamoid bone within the quadriceps tendon that increases the leverage of the knee joint. This bone can be damaged via a direct blow or fall onto the anterior aspect of the knee. The deep knee bend can differentiate between damage to the patella and the menisci. Patients with patellar issues would experience pain while rising from the deep knee bend position. In this patient, pain was elicited at the bottom of the deep knee bend, which indicates damage to the meniscus.

48   **The answer is E: Lateral plantar nerve.**   The lateral plantar nerve, which is homologous to the ulnar nerve in the hand, innervates all of the intrinsic foot muscles, with the exception of the four muscles supplied by the medial plantar nerve. The lateral plantar nerve innervates the dorsal interossei of the foot and the abductor digiti minimi muscles, which are responsible for abduction of the lateral four toes. **Choice A** (Sural nerve) is incorrect. The sural nerve is a cutaneous nerve, so it would not be responsible for abduction of the lateral four toes. The course of this nerve parallels the small saphenous vein, and damage to the sural nerve would lead to numbness and paresthesia in the dorsal aspect of the lateral fifth toe and lateral malleolus of the fibula. No motor deficits would be seen. **Choice B** (Deep fibular nerve) is incorrect. The deep fibular (peroneal) nerve supplies motor innervation to the four muscles of the anterior compartment of the leg and two intrinsic muscles of the foot: extensor digitorum brevis and extensor hallucis brevis. Neither of these two foot muscles is involved with abduction of the toes. **Choice C** (Superficial fibular nerve) is incorrect. The superficial fibular nerve supplies motor innervation to the two muscles (fibularis longus and brevis) of the lateral compartment of the leg and cutaneous (sensory) innervation to the distal third of the anterior surface of the leg and dorsum of the foot. These muscles are primarily responsible for eversion of the foot at the ankle joint and are not responsible for any toe movements. **Choice D** (Medial plantar nerve) is incorrect. The medial plantar nerve, which is homologous to the median nerve in the hand, innervates four intrinsic foot muscles: first Lumbrical, Abductor hallucis, Flexor digitorum brevis, and Flexor hallucis brevis. The mnemonic for muscles supplied by the medial plantar nerve is the "LAFF" muscles. Though it would be responsible for abduction of the first toe, the medial plantar nerve is not responsible for abduction of the lateral four toes, which are being tested in this patient.

49   **The answer is B: Deep fibular nerve.**   The deep fibular nerve supplies motor innervation to the anterior compartment of the leg and sensory innervation to the space between the first and second toes. The muscles within this compartment are responsible for dorsiflexion of the ankle. This patient is suffering from anterior leg compartment syndrome. The signs and symptoms of anterior leg compartment syndrome can be remembered by the following mnemonic: the five "P's," which are Pain, Pallor (white appearance due to lack of blood supply), Paresthesia (abnormal sensations), Paralysis, and Pulselessness. Anterior compartment syndrome of the leg is caused by increased intracompartmental pressure due to bleeding from the trauma or the improper casting of the lower leg. If this intracompartmental pressure is not relieved, the venous outflow will be obstructed, which will exacerbate the symptoms. The resulting ischemia leads to previously mentioned symptoms and necrosis of the muscles and the deep fibular nerve, which supplies the anterior compartment of the leg. Severe anterior compartment syndrome is corrected surgically by incising the strong, nonyielding crural fascia to relieve the pressure. **Choice A** (Tibial nerve) is incorrect. The tibial nerve supplies the posterior muscles of the knee joint and leg, so it would be responsible for plantar flexion of the foot at the ankle joint, not dorsiflexion, which is affected in this patient. **Choice C** (Superficial fibular nerve) is incorrect. The superficial fibular nerve is a terminal branch of the common fibular nerve that supplies motor innervation to the two muscles (fibularis longus and brevis) of the lateral compartment of the leg and cutaneous (sensory) innervation to the distal third of the anterior surface of the leg and dorsum of foot. These muscles are primarily responsible for eversion of the foot at the ankle joint; however, dorsiflexion of the foot is affected in this patient. **Choice D** (Medial plantar nerve) is incorrect. The tibial nerve divides into the medial and lateral plantar nerves to innervate muscles of the sole of the foot. The medial plantar nerve, which is homologous to the median nerve in the hand, innervates only intrinsic foot muscles. Because this nerve does not supply muscles that cross the ankle joint, it cannot be responsible for weakness in dorsiflexion at the ankle joint. **Choice E** (Lateral plantar nerve) is incorrect. The tibial nerve divides into the medial and lateral plantar nerves to innervate muscles of the sole of the foot. The lateral plantar nerve,

which is homologous to the ulnar nerve in the hand, innervates most of the intrinsic foot muscles. Because this nerve does not supply muscles that cross the ankle joint, it cannot be responsible for weakness in dorsiflexion at the ankle joint.

50   **The answer is A: Tibial nerve.**   The tibial nerve is a terminal branch of the sciatic nerve that supplies the posterior muscles of the knee joint and leg, including the three muscles of the superficial compartment (gastrocnemius, soleus, and plantaris) and four muscles of the deep compartment (popliteus, flexor hallucis longus, flexor digitorum longus, tibialis posterior). The tibial nerve is responsible for plantar flexion of the foot at the ankle joint, which is being tested in this patient, and the segmental innervation of this movement is S1 and S2. Distally, the tibial nerve divides into the medial and lateral plantar nerves. **Choice B** (Deep fibular nerve) is incorrect. The deep fibular (peroneal) nerve is a terminal branch of the common fibular nerve that supplies motor innervation to the four muscles of the anterior compartment of the leg: (1) tibialis anterior, (2) extensor digitorum longus, (3) extensor hallucis longus, and (4) fibularis (peroneus) tertius. These four muscles are responsible for dorsiflexion of the ankle. The deep fibular nerve also innervates the extensor digitorum brevis and extensor hallucis brevis, which are intrinsic muscles of the foot, sends articular branches to joints it crosses, and supplies cutaneous innervation to the first interdigital cleft. The deep fibular nerve is responsible for dorsiflexion of the foot at the ankle joint, and the segmental innervation of this movement is L4 and L5. **Choice C** (Superficial fibular nerve) is incorrect. The superficial fibular nerve is a terminal branch of the common fibular nerve that supplies motor innervation to the two muscles (fibularis longus and brevis) of the lateral compartment of the leg and cutaneous (sensory) innervation to the distal third of the anterior surface of the leg and dorsum of foot. These muscles are primarily responsible for eversion of the foot at the ankle joint, and the segmental innervation of this movement is L5 and S1. **Choice D** (Sural nerve) is incorrect. The sural nerve supplies cutaneous innervation to the dorsal aspect of the lateral fifth toe and lateral malleolus of the fibula. This sensory nerve, which approximates the course of the small saphenous vein, is formed in the inferoposterior aspect of the leg by the convergence of the medial sural cutaneous nerve (off the tibial nerve) and the lateral sural cutaneous nerve (off the common fibular nerve). Damage to the sural nerve would only produce sensory deficits, so it is not responsible for plantar flexion of the foot at the ankle joint. **Choice E** (Saphenous nerve) is incorrect. The saphenous nerve is a terminal sensory branch of the femoral nerve, which traverses medially through the adductor canal in the thigh to supply the medial side of the leg and foot, including the medial malleolus of the tibia. Damage to the saphenous nerve would only produce sensory deficits, so it is not responsible for plantar flexion of the foot at the ankle joint.

Chapter 8

Upper Limb and Mammary Gland

QUESTIONS

Select the single best answer.

1 Physical examination of a 40-year-old man injured in an automobile accident indicates that he has suffered nerve damage affecting his left upper limb. The patient exhibits significant weakness when pronating his left forearm and flexing his left wrist. What nerve is most likely damaged?

(A) Median nerve
(B) Ulnar nerve
(C) Superficial branch of the radial nerve
(D) Deep branch of the radial nerve
(E) Musculocutaneous nerve

2 A 50-year old man falls off a ladder while cleaning his windows, landing on the ground as seen in the given drawing. He does not seek medical aid, believing his general soreness will go away with time. However, after several months, he develops a postural deformity of his left upper limb that includes an adducted, medially rotated, and extended shoulder, extended elbow, and pronated forearm. The injury and subsequent condition reflect damage to what structure?

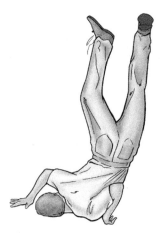

(A) Upper trunk of the brachial plexus
(B) Lower roots of the brachial plexus
(C) Posterior divisions of the brachial plexus
(D) Medial cord of the brachial plexus
(E) Lateral root of the median nerve

3 A 21-year-old man goes to his college campus health clinic complaining of soreness in his left wrist after falling on an outstretched hand during a basketball game the previous day. He is supporting his left wrist and indicates that the pain worsens with movement and is minimized with inactivity. There is no loss of feeling in his hand, nor does he have trouble grasping or holding objects. The physician exacerbates the wrist pain by applying pressure to the base of the thumb in the anatomical snuffbox (see photo). Radiographic imaging will confirm a break of which carpal bone?

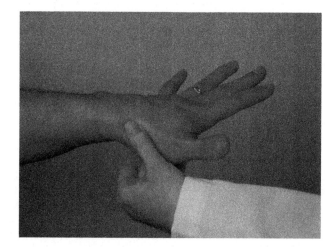

(A) Capitate
(B) Scaphoid
(C) Hamate
(D) Trapezium
(E) Pisiform

4 As a result of chronic stress associated with an intense high school weight-lifting program, a 15-year-old boy suffers an avulsion fracture of the greater tubercle of the humerus. In the ER, he displays difficulty initiating abduction of the upper limb. Which of the following muscles was involved in this fracture?

(A) Supraspinatus
(B) Long head of biceps brachii
(C) Long head of triceps
(D) Subscapularis
(E) Infraspinatus

5 During an attempted suicide, a depressed young woman slashes her wrist with a straight razor. She cuts just proximal to the pisiform bone to the depth of the superficial aspect of the flexor retinaculum before passing out at the sight of her own blood. As a result of this wound, she may suffer a neuromuscular deficit that results in which of the following?

(A) Weakness in pronation
(B) Inability to abduct the thumb
(C) Weakness in flexion of the thumb
(D) Weakness in opposition of the thumb
(E) Inability to adduct the thumb

6 As part of a physical examination to evaluate muscle function in the hand, a physician holds the proximal interphalangeal joint of his patient's index finger in the extended position and instructs him to try to flex the distal interphalangeal joint, as shown below. Which of the following muscles is the doctor testing?

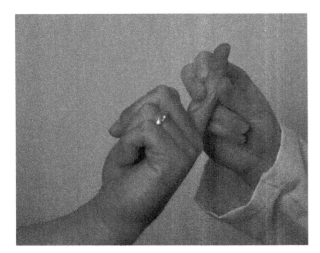

(A) Flexor digitorum profundus (FDP)
(B) Extensor indicis
(C) First lumbrical
(D) First dorsal interosseous
(E) Flexor digitorum superficialis (FDS)

7 A 17-year-old boy comes to the emergency room after a hard fall onto the lateral aspect of his left shoulder during a high school basketball game. He complains of generalized pain during shoulder motion. On physical examination, the distal end of the clavicle is prominent and distinctly palpable. Radiological findings confirm the diagnosis of a severe (grade 3) shoulder separation. Which of the following features is a component of this condition?

(A) Dislocated head of the humerus
(B) Torn coracoclavicular ligament
(C) Fractured clavicle
(D) Dislocated sternal end of the clavicle
(E) Torn anterior glenohumeral (GH) ligament

8 An 18-year-old boy is cut severely on the lateral wall of his right chest during a knife fight. Following healing, his scapula moves away from the thoracic wall when he leans on his right hand, giving the appearance indicated in the given photo. Which of the following nerves is likely damaged?

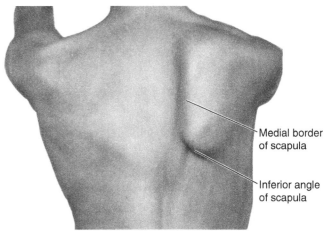

Medial border of scapula

Inferior angle of scapula

(A) Axillary nerve
(B) Thoracodorsal nerve
(C) Long thoracic nerve
(D) Dorsal scapular nerve
(E) Suprascapular nerve

9 On his downswing, an amateur golfer strikes the hard earth with his club and feels pain in his right wrist. During a subsequent physical examination, he complains of wrist pain that is exacerbated by gripping, displays point tenderness in his medial wrist, and complains of numbness and weakness in his pinky finger (fifth digit). What carpal bone, identified by the white arrow on the given X-ray, is most likely fractured in this patient?

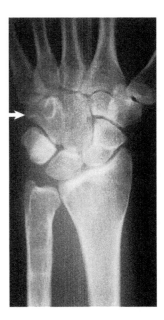

(A) Capitate
(B) Hamate
(C) Lunate
(D) Pisiform
(E) Scaphoid

10 The given anteroposterior (AP) X-ray depicts a humeral shaft fracture in a 22-year-old man. Given the location of the fracture, which of the following structures is most likely damaged?

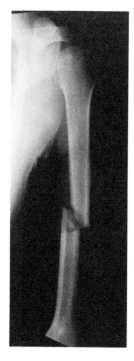

(A) Posterior circumflex humeral artery
(B) Ulnar nerve
(C) Axillary nerve
(D) Profunda brachii artery
(E) Median nerve

11 A 23-year-old man was injured in a motor vehicle accident and X-rays confirmed a displaced distal radius fracture in his left forearm. Upon examination, the patient exhibits weakened pronation, weakened flexion of the index and middle fingers at the distal interphalangeal joints, and weakened flexion of the interphalangeal joint of the thumb. When asked to make the "okay" sign (make a circle with the thumb and index finger), the patient is unable to make a round circle, producing a "collapsed circle" on the affected hand (see photo). No areas of sensory loss are detected. Which nerve is most likely damaged?

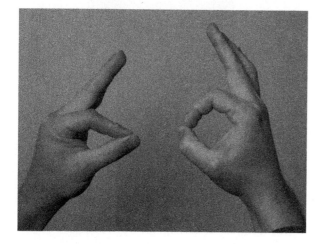

(A) Deep branch of the radial nerve
(B) Superficial branch of the radial nerve
(C) Anterior interosseous nerve
(D) Median nerve, proximal to the carpal tunnel
(E) Recurrent branch of the median nerve

12 A 23-year-old medical student complains of loss of sensation in the skin on the medial edge of her left hand, including the entire fifth digit. The associated motor deficit probably involves weakness in which of the following?
(A) Pronation
(B) Abduction of the wrist
(C) Extension of the wrist
(D) Abduction of the index finger
(E) Flexion of the interphalangeal joints of the index finger

13 A dermatologist performed a biopsy on a suspicious mole on the right side of the posterior neck of a 57-year-old male construction worker. Pathology confirmed a malignant melanoma, so the physician excised a substantial amount of tissue surrounding the mole. After the procedure, the patient experienced difficulty elevating his right shoulder and lifting his right arm over his head. No sensory deficits were seen. What nerve was most likely damaged in this patient?
(A) Accessory nerve
(B) Axillary nerve
(C) Dorsal scapular nerve
(D) Long thoracic nerve
(E) Thoracodorsal nerve

14 A 19-year-old man arrives at his campus health clinic complaining of soreness in his right wrist. He explains he landed on an outstretched hand when he was tackled in a rugby match. He indicates that the pain worsens with movement and is minimized by stabilization of the wrist. There are no sensory deficits in his hand nor does he have trouble grasping or holding objects. Pressure applied to the anatomic snuffbox between the extensor pollicis brevis and extensor pollicis longus tendons produces no pain. Radiographic studies show no fractures but reveal an anterior dislocation of a bone in the proximal row of carpal bones. What carpal bone is most likely dislocated in this patient?
(A) Scaphoid
(B) Lunate
(C) Capitate
(D) Triquetrum
(E) Trapezium

15 A 36-year-old man broke a window with his fist to rescue his child from a house fire. The man sustained a laceration to the lateral aspect of his right forearm, but he only showed a sensory deficit (numbness and paresthesia) to the dorsolateral aspect of his hand (as denoted by the shaded area within the given photo). What nerve was most likely damaged?

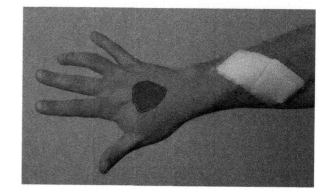

(A) Dorsal cutaneous branch of the ulnar nerve
(B) Lateral cutaneous nerve of the forearm
(C) Posterior cutaneous nerve of the forearm
(D) Deep branch of the radial nerve
(E) Superficial branch of the radial nerve

16 An anesthesiologist administers an anesthetic solution into the axillary sheath of a 19-year-old college baseball player in preparation for repair of the ulnar collateral ligament of the elbow. After 5 minutes, the patient experiences numbness and paresthesia distal to the middle aspect of the arm; however, the medial aspect of the arm and elbow remain sensitive to pain. What nerve provides sensory innervation to the sensitive area and was not blocked by the anesthetic solution?

(A) Long thoracic nerve
(B) Median nerve
(C) Medial cutaneous nerve of the arm
(D) Intercostobrachial nerve
(E) Ulnar nerve

17 A 17-year-old male football player suffers a shoulder injury and arrives at the ER 2 hours after the injury. The physician diagnoses a shoulder dislocation, and after administration of a local anesthetic solution, the doctor repositions the head of the humerus into the glenoid cavity of the scapula (reduction). No fractures are seen on X-rays. However, the patient displays weakness in abduction and external rotation at the shoulder. A loss of sensation is also noted at the superior and lateral aspects of the arm. What nerve was most likely damaged in this injury?

(A) Axillary nerve
(B) Median nerve
(C) Ulnar nerve
(D) Radial nerve
(E) Musculocutaneous nerve

18 A physician tests the myotatic biceps reflex as shown. A normal response of involuntary contraction of the biceps brachii muscle is noted. This reflex confirms the integrity of what nerve?

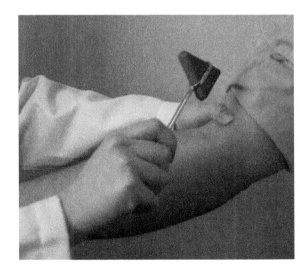

(A) Axillary nerve
(B) Median nerve
(C) Ulnar nerve
(D) Radial nerve
(E) Musculocutaneous nerve

19 A 21-year-old male college student reports to the student health clinic on Monday morning, the day after the Super Bowl. He explains that he was intoxicated and lost consciousness with his upper limbs draped over the back of a couch. He complains of numbness and paresthesia over the dorsum of his hand on the radial side and is unable to support the weight of his left hand when the hand is placed in a pronated position (see photo). What nerve was most likely damaged in this individual?

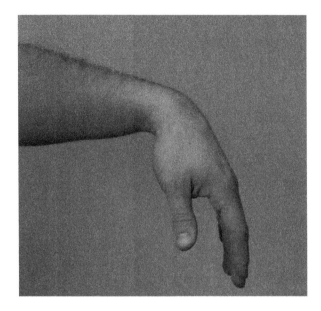

(A) Axillary nerve
(B) Median nerve
(C) Ulnar nerve
(D) Radial nerve
(E) Musculocutaneous nerve

20 A 50-year female equestrian is thrown from a startled horse and dragged by the reins, which were wrapped around her left wrist, for some distance. At the ER, she is experiencing pain and paresthesia in the axilla and medial aspect of her upper limb. Despite being left-handed, she has marked weakness in the movements of her dominant hand, especially abduction and adduction of the fingers. What structure was most likely damaged in this woman?

(A) Upper trunk of the brachial plexus
(B) Lower trunk of the brachial plexus
(C) Posterior cord of the brachial plexus
(D) Lateral cord of the brachial plexus
(E) Long thoracic nerve

21 A child is born to a young woman who had utilized thalidomide to help relieve her morning sickness early in her pregnancy. The infant suffers the congenital defects shown here. She is missing the proximal segments of both upper and lower limbs. The hands and feet that are present are attached to the trunk of the body and resemble small seal's flippers. Which of the following is the correct term for this malformation?

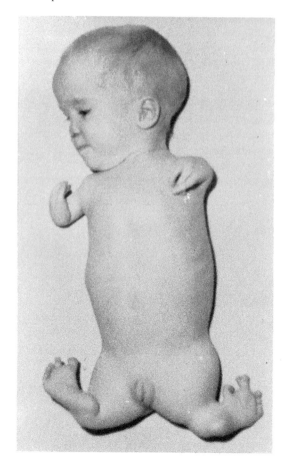

(A) Supinator
(B) Brachialis
(C) Pronator teres
(D) Biceps brachii
(E) Brachioradialis

23 A 65-year-old man is brought to the emergency room after being attacked in his office by a disgruntled co-worker. The attacker reportedly used a long, narrow-bladed letter-opener to inflict multiple stab wounds to the man's back. Physical examination shows a puncture wound in the posterior axillary fold. The patient presents with weakness in extension, adduction, and medial rotation of his arm. Which of the following muscles is most likely cut in this injury?

(A) Pectoralis minor
(B) Latissimus dorsi
(C) Levator scapulae
(D) Serratus anterior
(E) Teres minor

24 Physical examination of a 45-year-old man who had been stabbed in the back of the shoulder shows a deep wound penetrating into the quadrangular space of the shoulder, causing bleeding from the severed blood vessels there. Which of the following neural structures is most likely damaged as well?

(A) Musculocutaneous nerve
(B) Lateral cord of the brachial plexus
(C) Radial nerve
(D) Axillary nerve
(E) Medial cutaneous nerve of the arm

(A) A dysplasia
(B) A duplication defect
(C) Micromelia
(D) Meromelia
(E) Amelia

22 A 23-year-old competitive weight lifter goes to his physician complaining of pain in his proximal forearm. During his examination, the pain is exacerbated by flexion of the elbow and supination of the forearm against resistance. A lateral radiograph shows chronic microtrauma to the proximal radius, marked by the black arrows. Which of the following muscles attaches to, and most likely damaged, this osteological process?

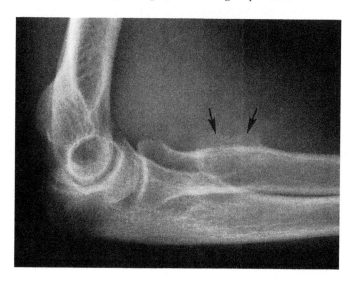

25 The pectoralis minor muscle is an important landmark in identifying and describing neighboring structures in the chest and axillary regions. Which of the following relationships of the pectoralis minor is correct?

(A) The lateral cord of the brachial plexus lies lateral to the muscle
(B) The clavipectoral triangle lies lateral to the muscle
(C) The anterior axillary lymph nodes lie along the medial border of the muscle
(D) The lateral wall of the axillary fossa includes the muscle
(E) The second part of the axillary artery lies deep to the muscle

26 Lateral rotation of the arm is an important mechanical component of "bringing the arm back" when preparing to throw an object. What muscle acts to produce lateral rotation of the arm?

(A) Supraspinatus
(B) Teres major
(C) Latissimus dorsi
(D) Subscapularis
(E) Teres minor

27 The lateral cord of the brachial plexus is named because it lies immediately lateral to which of the following structures?

(A) Long head of the biceps brachii muscle
(B) Axillary artery
(C) Subclavian vein
(D) Surgical neck of the humerus
(E) Pectoralis minor muscle

28 "Pronator teres syndrome" is a condition in which one of the following nerves is excessively compressed where it passes between the two heads of the pronator teres muscle. Which of the following nerves is entrapped?
(A) Deep branch of radial nerve
(B) Median Nerve
(C) Deep branch of ulnar nerve
(D) Superficial branch of ulnar nerve
(E) Musculocutaneous nerve

29 The pulse of the radial artery is readily palpable where the vessel passes which of the following structures?
(A) Across the anterior aspect of the lateral epicondyle of the humerus
(B) Between the tendons of the palmaris longus and flexor carpi ulnaris
(C) Lateral to the tendon of the flexor carpi radialis
(D) Superficial to the tendons of the extensor pollicis brevis and abductor pollicis longus
(E) Superficial to the carpal tunnel

30 A 74-year-old man complains of pain in his right hand and fingers when he works with his hands for a while. Thorough testing reveals insufficient blood flow into the deep palmar arch. Occlusion of which of the following arteries is the most likely cause of this condition?
(A) Posterior interosseous artery
(B) Ulnar artery
(C) Anterior interosseous artery
(D) Radial artery
(E) Inferior ulnar collateral artery

31 In both the upper and lower limbs, the superficial veins begin in a dorsal cutaneous arch that drains into medial and lateral cutaneous veins aligned mainly along the first and fifth digit sides of the limb. Which of the following veins in the upper limb is the equivalent of the great saphenous vein in the lower limb?
(A) Radial vein
(B) Ulnar vein
(C) Brachial vein
(D) Basilic vein
(E) Cephalic vein

32 The given X-ray reveals a fracture of the proximal humerus, indicated by the black arrow. Given the location of the fracture, what artery is most likely damaged in this patient?

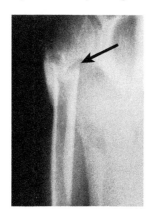

(A) Posterior circumflex humeral artery
(B) Brachial artery
(C) Deep brachial (profunda brachii) artery
(D) Subscapular artery
(E) Superior ulnar collateral artery

33 During an attempted suicide, a depressed young woman slashes the front of her wrist with a razor blade. However, she cuts only to the depth of the superficial aspect of the flexor retinaculum before passing out at the sight of her own blood. Which of the following muscle tendons may be severed?
(A) Flexor digitorum superficialis
(B) Brachioradialis
(C) Flexor pollicis longus
(D) Abductor pollicis longus
(E) Flexor carpi radialis

34 A 17-year-old man has pain and moderate swelling over the dorsomedial aspect and in the hypothenar area of his right hand after punching a locker over a dispute with his girlfriend. What is the most likely finding on an X-ray of his hand?
(A) Dislocation of the fifth metacarpophalangeal joint
(B) Fracture of the triquetral bone
(C) Fracture of the proximal phalanx of the ring finger
(D) Fracture of the proximal phalanx of the little finger
(E) Fracture of the fifth metacarpal bone

35 A right-handed 21-year-old college student visits his physician because of pain in his right shoulder that developed after starting a summer job on a construction crew 2 weeks ago. He explains that on his job site he regularly lifts heavy construction materials over his head. During physical examination, the patient experiences sharp pain in the range of 80 to 150 degrees of abduction at the glenohumeral joint. What is the most likely diagnosis?
(A) Infraspinatus tendonitis
(B) Supraspinatus tendonitis
(C) Acromioclavicular (AC) joint arthritis
(D) Degenerative arthritis of the shoulder
(E) Broken clavicle

36 A 56-year-old woman was stopped at a light when her car was rear-ended by another car. She had her right arm on the steering wheel, and the impact caused forced flexion at her elbow. Several months later, she comes to her physician complaining of numbness and a "pins and needles" sensation in her right little finger when she talks on the phone, rests her head on her right hand at work, or spends most of her day typing at work. She also notices the quality of her typing and her ability to play the violin have diminished. Which nerve is compressed at what location?
(A) Ulnar nerve in the elbow
(B) Ulnar nerve in the wrist
(C) Median nerve in the wrist
(D) Median nerve in the elbow
(E) Median nerve in the axilla

37 As part of a physical examination to evaluate intrinsic hand muscle function, a physician holds three fingers in the extended position, and instructs the patient to flex the proximal interphalangeal joint of the free finger, as shown. Which of the following muscles is the doctor specifically testing?

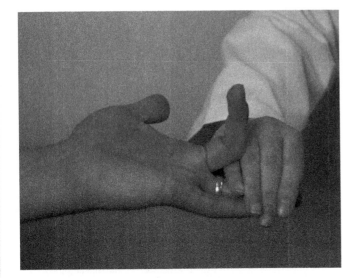

(A) Flexor digitorum profundus (FDP)
(B) Extensor digitorum
(C) Second lumbrical
(D) Dorsal interosseous
(E) Flexor digitorum superficialis (FDS)

38 Because of repeated bad needle sticks, a heroin addict develops an infected abscess in the floor of the cubital fossa. Which of the following structures is the abscess most likely to invade first?
(A) Brachioradialis muscle
(B) Pronator teres muscle
(C) Brachialis muscle
(D) Head of the radius
(E) Olecranon fossa of the humerus

39 The traditional radical mastectomy includes removal of the pectoralis major muscle. Which of the following movements is most affected postoperatively by this surgical procedure?
(A) Adduction of the arm
(B) Abduction of the arm
(C) Extension of the arm
(D) Lateral rotation of the arm
(E) Depression of the arm

40 The lateral thoracic artery provides the main blood supply to the lateral side of the chest wall, including much of the breast. To deter excessive blood loss during a surgical procedure involving the breast, a surgeon can clamp the lateral thoracic artery near its origin. Which of the following arteries gives rise to this artery?

(A) First part of the axillary artery
(B) Second part of the axillary artery
(C) Third part of the axillary artery
(D) Third part of the subclavian artery
(E) First part of the brachial artery

41 Following a radical mastectomy procedure, a surgeon plans to conduct a breast reconstruction utilizing a latissimus dorsi muscle flap. What nerve will the surgeon need to keep intact during the surgical dissection of the chest wall to prevent atrophy of the muscle flap?
(A) Long thoracic nerve
(B) Intercostobrachial nerve
(C) Medial pectoral nerve
(D) Thoracodorsal nerve
(E) Axillary nerve

42 An 80-year-old woman comes to the physician because of a lump in her right breast. Physical examination shows a 2-cm mass in the right breast with dimpling of the overlying skin and peau d'orange (edema of the breast with the skin assuming the appearance of an orange peel). Examination of a biopsy specimen confirms a diagnosis of carcinoma. Involvement of what structure is the most likely cause of this patient's skin dimpling?
(A) Clavipectoral fascia
(B) Suspensory ligaments
(C) Lactiferous ducts
(D) Retromammary space
(E) Pectoralis major

43 As part of a physical examination to evaluate intrinsic hand muscle function, a physician asks the patient to assume the Z-position (seen in photo) with his hand, which involves flexion of the metacarpophalangeal joints and extension of the interphalangeal joints of the fingers. Which of the following nerves is being tested in assuming this position?

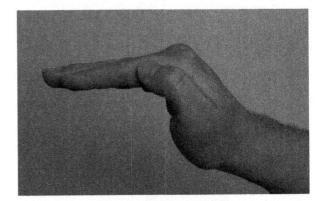

(A) Deep branch of radial nerve
(B) Superficial branch of radial nerve
(C) Recurrent branch of median nerve
(D) Deep branch of ulnar nerve
(E) Superficial branch of ulnar nerve

44 A 10-year-old boy was running across a parking lot when he tripped and received lacerations on the base of his thumb from a broken glass bottle. On examination, his thumb was unable to oppose to his fingers, and the thumb also showed weakness when abducting and flexing. No sensory deficits were reported. What nerve was most likely severed?

(A) Deep branch of radial nerve
(B) Superficial branch of radial nerve
(C) Recurrent branch of median nerve
(D) Deep branch of ulnar nerve
(E) Superficial branch of ulnar nerve

45 A 48-year-old woman is diagnosed with a malignant tumor in the superolateral quadrant of the right breast, including the axillary tail. If it metastasizes, this cancer will most likely spread first to which of the following locations?

(A) Lateral axillary lymph nodes
(B) Anterior axillary lymph nodes
(C) Deep cervical lymph nodes
(D) Parasternal lymph nodes
(E) Contralateral breast lymph nodes

46 A 48-year-old woman falls on an icy sidewalk and lands on her right elbow. She suffers a midshaft humeral fracture, as seen on the given X-ray. The attending physician wants to assess whether the nerve residing in the spiral groove of the humerus is damaged. What sign or symptom would confirm damage to this nerve?

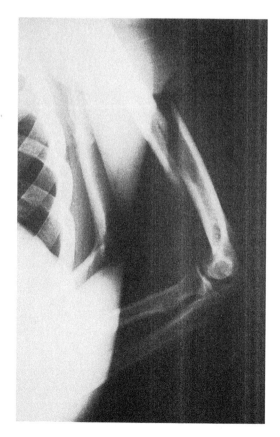

(A) Numbness on the lateral (radial) aspect of the forearm
(B) Numbness of the medial aspect of the upper arm
(C) Numbness over the superolateral aspect of the upper arm
(D) Weakness extending the wrist and fingers
(E) Weakness in grip strength

47 Organization of the axillary lymph nodes into Levels I, II, and III for breast cancer treatment is based on the location of the nodes relative to which of the following muscles?

(A) Pectoralis minor
(B) Pectoralis major
(C) Latissimus dorsi
(D) Serratus anterior
(E) Subscapularis

48 A 37-year-old factory worker fractures multiple bones distal to the elbow when his hand and forearm are crushed by equipment dropped by a faulty hydraulic lift. Which of the following bones, if fractured, would most likely develop avascular necrosis?

(A) Distal radius
(B) Midshaft ulna
(C) Fifth metacarpal
(D) Lunate
(E) Scaphoid

49 As part of a physical examination to evaluate muscle function in the hand, a physician holds the four fingers (digits 2 through 5) and asks the patient to spread their fingers, as shown below. What muscle(s) is/are the doctor testing?

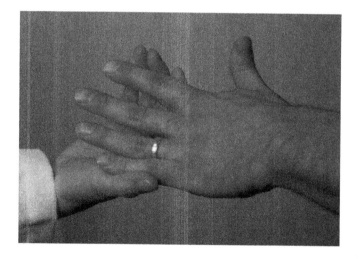

(A) Lumbrical muscles
(B) Palmar interosseous muscles
(C) Dorsal interosseous muscles
(D) Flexor digitorum superficialis
(E) Flexor digitorum profundus

50 A 52-year-old retired professional cyclist, who still rides his bike 400 miles per week, comes to his physician complaining of hand problems. The physician notes hyperextension of the ring and little fingers at the metacarpophalangeal joints and flexion at the interphalangeal joints within the same fingers (see photo). During examination, the patient has no weakness in flexion or adduction of the wrist. What nerve is compressed at what location?

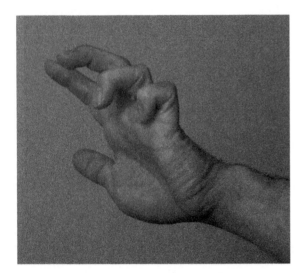

(A) Ulnar nerve in the elbow
(B) Ulnar nerve in the wrist
(C) Median nerve in the wrist
(D) Median nerve in the elbow
(E) Median nerve in the axilla

51 A 3-year-old girl is brought to the emergency room holding her right arm with the elbow flexed and the forearm pronated. She refuses to move her arm and complains her elbow "hurts a lot." Her mother reports they were holding hands and running in the park when the child tripped. The mother pulled on the child's hand to prevent her from hitting the ground. Given the nature of this injury and the age of the patient, what structure is most likely damaged?

(A) Interosseous membrane of forearm
(B) Quadrate ligament
(C) Radial collateral ligament of elbow
(D) Ulnar collateral ligament of elbow
(E) Anular ligament of radius

ANSWERS AND DISCUSSION

1 **The answer is A: Median nerve.** The median nerve controls pronation through the actions of the pronator teres and pronator quadratus muscles in the anterior compartment of the forearm. It also controls much of flexion of the wrist and lateral digits via the actions of most of the other muscles in that compartment. **Choice B** (Ulnar nerve) is incorrect. The ulnar nerve controls 1½ muscles in the anterior compartment of the forearm (flexor carpi ulnaris and the ulnar half of the flexor digitorum profundus) and most of the intrinsic muscles of the hand. However, neither of these 1½ forearm muscles produces pronation. **Choice C** (Superficial branch of the radial nerve) is incorrect. The superficial branch of the radial nerve is entirely cutaneous, carrying sensation from the dorsolateral part of the hand. So, cutting this nerve would not result in weakness in pronation of the forearm or flexion of the wrist. **Choice D** (Deep branch of the radial nerve) is incorrect. The deep branch of the radial nerve supplies the posterior compartment of the forearm. It influences supination via motor control of the supinator muscle, but not pronation. **Choice E** (Musculocutaneous nerve) is incorrect. The musculocutaneous nerve supplies the anterior compartment of the arm, and then continues distally via its termination as the lateral cutaneous nerve of the forearm. It contributes significantly to control of supination by its innervation of the biceps brachii muscle, but has no effect on wrist flexion.

2 **The answer is A: Upper trunk of the brachial plexus.** The illustration shows an injury in which the cervicobrachial angle (the angle between the neck and shoulder) is stretched widely. This abnormal impact eventually results in the postural presentation of a "waiter's tip" deformity (Erb-Duchenne palsy). This combination of injury and postural deformity is related to damage to both the C5 and C6 roots or upper trunk of the brachial plexus. The C5 and C6 roots converge to form the upper trunk of the brachial plexus and contribute heavily to the suprascapular, axillary, and musculocutaneous nerves. The suprascapular nerve supplies the supraspinatus and infraspinatus muscles. The axillary nerve controls the deltoid and teres minor muscles. The musculocutaneous nerve supplies the anterior compartment of the arm (coracobrachialis, biceps brachii, brachialis muscles). Therefore, a significant weakness in abduction and lateral rotation of the shoulder, flexion of the shoulder and elbow, and supination of the forearm would result from this brachial plexus injury. The ultimate postural deformity is a contracture effect in which the intact muscles act unopposed to draw the limb into a position that is the opposite of the actions of the affected muscles. **Choice B** (Lower roots of the brachial plexus) is incorrect. The lower roots (C8, T1) have a strong projection into the ulnar nerve. Trauma here would result in an ultimate postural deformity of "claw hand" due to the loss of flexion of the medial digits. That injury does not match this patient's clinical presentation. **Choice C** (Posterior divisions of the brachial plexus) is incorrect. The posterior divisions supply the radial, axillary, upper and lower subscapular, and thoracodorsal nerves. The primary postural effect resulting from trauma here would be a case of "wrist drop" expressed due to loss of the extensor muscles innervated by the radial nerve. **Choice D** (Medial cord of the brachial plexus) is incorrect. The medial cord projects into the ulnar and median nerves. Damage to the ulnar nerve will result in "claw hand."

The classic median nerve deformity of "ape hand" probably would not be realized because the median nerve also receives a strong input from the lateral cord. **Choice E** (Lateral root of the median nerve) is incorrect. The median nerve is formed by lateral and medial roots derived from the lateral and medial cords, respectively. Trauma to either root would weaken the territory of the median nerve but likely not result in the classic median nerve postural defect of "ape hand." The lateral root does not contribute to the suprascapular and axillary nerves, which have been affected in this patient.

3 **The answer is B: Scaphoid.** The most commonly fractured carpal bone is the scaphoid that forms the floor of the anatomical snuffbox. This area is a fossa located between the three long tendons of the thumb (tendons of abductor pollicis longus and extensor pollicis brevis laterally and tendon of the extensor pollicis longus medially). The scaphoid bone is frequently broken when an individual falls with an outstretched hand and lands on the palm with the hand abducted. A broken scaphoid bone is commonly seen in individuals under the age of 30. The scaphoid is broken due to its unfortunate position between the downward force transmitted by the weight of the upper limb and the upward force due to the impact of hitting the floor. The proximal aspect of a broken scaphoid bone can suffer from avascular necrosis due to its blood supply entering the bone distally. **Choice A** (Capitate) is incorrect. The capitate is located centrally in the distal row of carpal bones and articulates with most of the carpal bones (the triquetrum, pisiform, and trapezium being the exceptions). This bone is not located in the floor of the anatomical snuffbox, so it was not the most likely bone injured in this patient. **Choice C** (Hamate) is incorrect. The hamate is located in the distal row of carpal bones on the ulnar side. It is not related to the anatomical snuffbox, so it would not produce pain in the base of the thumb when broken. **Choice D** (Trapezium) is incorrect. The trapezium is located at the base of the thumb, but it is not commonly fractured when a person falls with an outstretched hand. A mnemonic for the position of the trapezium is "trapezium articulated with the thumb." **Choice E** (Pisiform) is incorrect. The pisiform is located in the proximal carpal row and is a sesamoid bone located within the tendon of the flexor carpi ulnaris muscle. Its position on the ulnar side of the wrist would not cause pain in the anatomical snuffbox.

4 **The answer is A: Supraspinatus.** The greater tubercle of the humerus is the insertion site of three (of the four) rotator cuff muscles: supraspinatus, infraspinatus, and teres minor. Avulsion of this structure could result in detachment of any of these rotator cuff muscles, depending upon the size and scope of the fracture. However, the wrestler is unable to initiate abduction of the upper limb, which implies damage to the supraspinatus muscle. **Choice B** (Long head of biceps brachii) is incorrect. This muscle originates from the supraglenoid tubercle of the scapula and passes between the greater and lesser tubercles of the humerus, in the intertubercular (bicipital) groove. Detachment of the tendon of this muscle causes the biceps brachii to bulge in the anterior arm. Avulsion of the biceps brachii muscle is not related to the greater tubercle of the humerus. **Choice C** (Long head of triceps) is incorrect. The long head of the triceps brachii muscle originates from the infraglenoid tubercle of the scapula and inserts on the olecranon process of the ulna. It would not be involved in avulsion of the greater tubercle of the humerus. **Choice D** (Subscapularis) is incorrect. The fourth rotator cuff muscle, subscapularis, inserts onto the lesser tubercle of the humerus, so it would not be directly involved with this avulsion injury. **Choice E** (Infraspinatus) is incorrect. The infraspinatus muscle does insert onto the middle aspect of the greater tubercle of the humerus; however, damage to this muscle would result in weakness in external rotation at the shoulder joint, not the problems with abduction seen in this patient.

5   **The answer is E: Inability to adduct the thumb.**   The location of the cut, superficial to the flexor retinaculum, indicates injury to the ulnar nerve. This nerve controls most of the intrinsic muscles of the hand, including the adductor pollicis. Because this muscle is the sole adductor of the thumb, the result will be inability to adduct that digit. **Choice A** (Weakness in pronation) is incorrect. Pronation is controlled by branches of the median nerve to the pronator teres and pronator quadratus muscles. These are located proximal to the site of the injury. **Choice B** (Inability to abduct the thumb) is incorrect. Abduction of the thumb is governed by the radial nerve (to abductor pollicis longus) and the recurrent branch of the median nerve (to abductor pollicis brevis) at sites removed from the injury. **Choice C** (Weakness in flexion of the thumb) is incorrect. Flexion of the thumb is controlled by branches of the median nerve at locations proximal (to flexor pollicis longus) and distal (to flexor pollicis brevis) to the cut flexor retinaculum (transverse carpal ligament). However, the reported laceration was superficial to this ligament and proximal to the pisiform bone, so the median nerve would not have been damaged. **Choice D** (Weakness in opposition of the thumb) is incorrect. Opposition of the thumb is controlled by the recurrent branch of the median nerve (to opponens pollicis), distal to the injury site.

6   **The answer is A: Flexor digitorum profundus (FDP).**   Flexion of the distal interphalangeal joint in digits 2 to 5 is produced by the FDP. The actions of this muscle are being tested in this illustration. **Choice B** (Extensor indicis) is incorrect. The extensor indicis extends the index finger (digit 2), which enables this finger to extend independent of the other fingers. Because the muscle arises from the distal third of the ulna and the interosseous membrane, it also acts to extend the hand at the wrist. The extensor indicis muscle is not involved in flexion of the distal interphalangeal joint, which is being tested in this patient. **Choice C** (First lumbrical) is incorrect. The first lumbrical muscle extends the interphalangeal joints of the index (second) finger and flexes the metacarpophalangeal joint of the same finger. The first lumbrical is an intrinsic hand muscle that arises off the tendon of the flexor digitorum profundus and inserts into the extensor expansion of the index finger. This muscle is not involved with flexion of the distal interphalangeal joint. **Choice D** (First dorsal interosseous) is incorrect. The primary movement of the first dorsal interosseous is abduction of the index finger. However, because it inserts into the extensor expansion, it also extends the interphalangeal joints of the index (second) finger and flexes the metacarpophalangeal joint of the same finger. This muscle is not involved with flexion of the distal interphalangeal joint. **Choice E** (Flexor digitorum superficialis [FDS]) is incorrect. The FDS acts at the proximal interphalangeal joint in digits 2 to 5 and influences the distal interphalangeal joint by binding the tendons of the FDP. However, when the proximal interphalangeal joint is held in extension, the influence of the FDS is eliminated, allowing testing of only the FDP.

7   **The answer is B: Torn coracoclavicular ligament.**   "Shoulder separation" describes a dislocation of the acromioclavicular joint. In its most severe form (grade 3), the condition includes a tearing of both the intrinsic acromioclavicular ligament and the extrinsic coracoclavicular ligament. As a result, the scapula separates from the clavicle and falls away due to the weight of the upper limb. Thus, the distal end of the clavicle is prominent. **Choice A** (Dislocated head of the humerus) is incorrect. Dislocations of the GH joint easily occur inferiorly due to its lack of muscular and ligamentous support. Thus, damage to the axillary nerve often occurs following inferior displacment of the head of humerus from the GH joint. However, the acromioclavicular joint, which is more proximal, was injured in this patient. Dislocations of the glenohumeral joint in other directions are more difficult (but not impossible) because of the support of the rotator cuff muscles (anteriorly and posteriorly) and the coracoacromial arch (superiorly). **Choice C** (Fractured clavicle) is incorrect. Radiological imaging would have detected a fractured clavicle, but these tests confirmed a shoulder separation and not a fractured clavicle. **Choice D** (Dislocated sternal end of the clavicle) is incorrect. Due to its intrinsic strength, dislocation of the sternoclavicular (SC) joint is rare. Most dislocations of the SC joint occur in persons less than 25 years of age following a fracture of the epiphysial plate of the clavicle. The epiphysis at the proximal end of the clavicle does not close until approximately age 25. Though this patient was under the age of 25, his injury was localized to the acromioclavicular joint. **Choice E** (Torn anterior glenohumeral [GH] ligament) is incorrect. Three GH ligaments reinforce the anterior part of the joint capsule; however, the GH joint was not involved in this patient.

8   **The answer is C: Long thoracic nerve.**   The photo demonstrates a case of "winged scapula," indicative of a lesion of the long thoracic nerve and subsequent paralysis of the serratus anterior muscle. The nerve runs down the lateral thoracic wall, on the superficial aspect of the serratus anterior, where it is unusually exposed (for a motor nerve) and vulnerable to injury, especially when the limb is elevated. Lesion of the nerve denervates the serratus anterior. This results in the medial border and inferior angle of the scapula pulling away from the posterior chest wall, giving the scapula a wing-like appearance when the affected limb is protracted. Additionally, the affected arm cannot be abducted above the horizontal plane because the serratus anterior is not available to superiorly rotate the glenoid cavity of the scapula to allow full abduction. **Choice A** (Axillary nerve) is incorrect. This nerve passes deeply through the axilla, around the surgical neck of the humerus, to supply the teres minor and deltoid muscles. Lesion here would result in significant weakness in abduction of the arm and wasting of the rounded contour of the shoulder. **Choice B** (Thoracodorsal nerve) is incorrect. This nerve runs inferior through the axilla to supply the latissimus dorsi muscle. Loss of the nerve would result in weakness in extension and medial rotation of the arm, plus wasting of the posterior axillary fold. **Choice D** (Dorsal scapular nerve) is incorrect. This nerve courses into the upper, medial part of the back and the lower neck to supply the levator scapulae and rhomboid muscles. Paralysis of these muscles would result in weakness in elevation and retraction of the scapula and perhaps wasting of the contour of the back under the trapezius muscle. **Choice E** (Suprascapular nerve) is incorrect. The suprascapular nerve runs through the suprascapular notch and into the supraspinous and infraspinous fossae to supply the supraspinatus and infraspinatus muscles. Lesion of this nerve would result in weakness in the rotator cuff affecting the initiation of abduction (supraspinatus) and external rotation (infraspinatus) of the shoulder and wasting of the muscular contour of the posterior aspect of the scapula.

9 **The answer is B: Hamate.** The hamate bone is identified by the white arrow in the given X-ray. This bone resides in the medial (ulnar) aspect of the distal row of carpal (wrist) bones. Stress fractures can occur to this bone, particularly within its hook, which appears as a radiodense oval on this radiograph. This type of fracture is frequently seen in golfers due to the positioning of the proximal aspect of the golf club within their grip. A fracture of the hamate results in pain, which is exacerbated by gripping and point tenderness in the skin overlying the bone. The numbness and weakness in the medial aspect of the hand, seen in this patient, are due to impingement of the ulnar nerve. Remember, the eight carpal (wrist) bones form two rows that contain four bones each. The proximal row (from lateral to medial) is composed of the scaphoid, lunate, triquetrum, and pisiform. The distal row (from lateral to medial) is composed of the trapezium, trapezoid, capitate, and hamate. To remember the carpal bones as listed, some students use the mnemonic: "Some Lovers Try Positions That They Can't Handle". In a standard posteroanterior plane film, the medial aspect of the wrist can be deceiving to the untrained eye. Here, the pisiform overlies the triquetrum, and the seemingly single radiopacity might not be distinguished as two separate bones. Instead, the distinctive hook of the hamate bone may be mistaken for the pisiform. **Choice A** (Capitate) is incorrect. The capitate (L: head) is a head-shaped bone that is the largest of the carpal bones. Its position is noted by its articulation with the third metacarpal distally. **Choice C** (Lunate) is incorrect. The lunate (L: moon) is a moon-shaped bone between the scaphoid and triquetral bones. It articulates with the radius proximally, and its position makes it the most commonly dislocated carpal bone. **Choice D** (Pisiform) is incorrect. The pisiform (L: pea) is a pea-shaped sesamoid bone that lies on the palmar aspect of the triquetrum bone. **Choice E** (Scaphoid) is incorrect. The scaphoid (G: boat) is a boat-shaped bone that is the largest of the carpal bones located in the proximal row. Its articulation with the radius proximally makes it the most commonly fractured carpal bone, especially when a person falls and impacts an abducted, outstretched hand.

10 **The answer is D: Profunda brachii artery.** It is important to recognize where neurovascular structures have close positional relations to each other and to underlying bony structures in order to predict the likely second order functional consequences of damage to the bones. In the given AP X-ray, the midshaft of the humerus is fractured slightly distal to the radial groove. At this point, the profunda brachii vessels (deep vessels of the arm) and the radial nerve emerge from the radial groove in a bundle tightly wrapped against the body of the humerus. A fracture here may readily damage any of these neurovascular structures. Lesion of the vessels may produce swelling in the posterior compartment of the arm and loss of supply to the muscles therein. Lesion of the nerve will result in major motor and sensory deficits in the posterior aspect of the forearm and hand. **Choice A** (Posterior circumflex humeral artery) is incorrect. This vessel travels in companionship with the axillary nerve around the surgical neck of the humerus. Fractures here are the most common injuries to the proximal end of the humerus, especially in the elderly. **Choice B** (Ulnar nerve) is incorrect. In the arm, the ulnar nerve travels with the superior ulnar collateral artery. Both lie in contact with the posterior side of the large, projecting medial epicondyle of the humerus as they cross the elbow. **Choice C** (Axillary nerve) is incorrect. The axillary nerve travels in companionship with the posterior circumflex humeral artery around the surgical neck of the humerus. Fractures here are the most common injuries to the proximal end of the humerus, especially in the elderly. **Choice E** (Median nerve) is incorrect. This large nerve travels with the brachial vessels down the anterior midline of the arm. The nerve lies close to the distal end of the humerus, where it may be damaged due to fractures of the condyle.

11 **The answer is C: Anterior interosseous nerve.** The anterior interosseous nerve is a branch of the median nerve in the distal part of the cubital fossa, and it courses distally on the interosseous membrane. It supplies the deep forearm flexors, including the flexor digitorum profundus of digits 2 and 3, the flexor pollicis longus, and the pronator quadratus. Loss of this nerve would cause weakness in pronation due to denervation of the pronator quadratus. This injury would also result in inability to flex the distal interphalangeal joints of the index and middle fingers and the interphalangeal joint of the thumb due to denervation of the flexor digitorum profundus and flexor pollicis longus, respectively. This deficit would lead to the collapsed "O.K. sign" indicated in the photo. Because compromising the anterior interosseous nerve would not result in any cutaneous sensory deficits, it is this nerve that was most likely damaged by the displaced end of the left radius. **Choice A** (Deep branch of the radial nerve) is incorrect. The deep branch of the radial nerve arises from the radial nerve in the cubital fossa, dives deep to pierce the supinator muscle, and supplies all the muscles in the posterior compartment of the forearm. Damage to this nerve would lead to "wrist drop" in the patient due to the flexors of the forearm being unopposed and an inability to extend at the wrist. **Choice B** (Superficial branch of the radial nerve) is incorrect. The superficial branch of the radial nerve arises from the radial nerve in the cubital fossa. This nerve is entirely a sensory nerve, supplying the dorsum of the hand and fingers. Because the patient has motor deficits, this nerve was not damaged by the displaced radius. **Choice D** (Median nerve proximal to the carpal tunnel) is incorrect. The median nerve proximal to the carpal tunnel would not be injured because damaging this nerve would lead to a significant sensory loss over the thumb and the adjacent two and a half fingers in addition to motor loss to the thenar eminence (opponens pollicis, abductor pollicis brevis, and flexor pollicis brevis muscles) and the first two lumbrical muscles. So, the median nerve was not injured proximal to the carpal tunnel. **Choice E** (Recurrent [thenar] branch of median nerve) is incorrect. The recurrent (thenar) branch of the median nerve innervates most of the thenar muscles, including the abductor pollicis brevis, opponens pollicis, and superficial head of the flexor pollicis brevis. Cutting this nerve would lead to atrophy of the thenar muscular complex, a condition known as "ape hand." In this condition, the patient would not be able to oppose the thumb and second finger. Though this nerve has no sensory distribution, it is unlikely that it was involved due to the weakness when pronating the forearm.

12 **The answer is D: Abduction of the index finger.** The sensory deficit occurs in the cutaneous territory of the ulnar nerve. This nerve controls most of the intrinsic muscles of the hand, including the first dorsal interosseous muscle, which controls abduction of the index finger. The four dorsal interosseous muscles of the hand are innervated by the deep branch of the ulnar nerve and function to abduct digits 2 to 4. Remember that two fingers (the thumb and little finger) have their own muscles dedicated to abduction. Also, remember the mnemonic "DAB," which stands for **D**orsal interossei **AB**duct the fingers. Thus, the associated motor deficit for the ulnar nerve on this list would be loss of abduction of the index finger. **Choice A** (Pronation) is incorrect. Pronation is governed by the median nerve, which supplies the pronator teres and pronator quadratus muscles. **Choice B** (Abduction of the wrist) is incorrect. Abduction of the wrist is controlled by the median nerve (supplying the flexor carpi radialis) and the radial nerve (supplying the extensor carpi radialis longus and brevis). **Choice C** (Extension of the wrist) is incorrect. Extension of the wrist is produced by the radial nerve acting mainly on the extensor carpi radialis longus and brevis and the extensor carpi ulnaris muscles. **Choice E** (Flexion of the interphalangeal joints of the index finger) is incorrect. Flexion of the interphalangeal joints of the index finger is controlled by branches of the median nerve, which supply the flexor digitorum superficialis muscle (to flex the proximal interphalangeal joint of the second finger) and the flexor digitorum profundus muscle (to flex the distal interphalangeal joint of the index finger).

13 **The answer is A: Accessory nerve.** The accessory nerve (CN XI) traverses the posterior triangle of the neck to reach the deep surface of the trapezius muscle after it innervates the sternocleidomastoid muscle. Its position within the triangle is superficial, and it is at this location that this nerve is vulnerable to injury. Damage to the distal accessory nerve would inhibit elevation of the scapula and lateral rotation of the scapula during abduction greater than 90 degrees. Both of these actions were affected in this patient. **Choice B** (Axillary nerve) is incorrect. The axillary nerve travels through the quadrangular space to reach the deltoid and teres minor muscles. While a lesion of this nerve would affect abduction of the arm, the axillary nerve is not found in the neck, instead arising distally from the posterior cord of the brachial plexus. Moreover, damage to the axillary nerve would cause a sensory deficit in the upper lateral arm, which was not reported. **Choice C** (Dorsal scapular nerve) is incorrect. This nerve courses into the upper, medial part of the back and the lower neck to supply the levator scapulae and rhomboid muscles. Paralysis of these muscles would result in weakness in elevation and retraction of the scapula and perhaps wasting of the contour of the back under the trapezius muscle. **Choice D** (Long thoracic nerve) is incorrect. The long thoracic nerve is a branch of the upper three roots (C5-C7) of the brachial plexus. It descends along the medial wall of the axilla and travels superficial to the serratus anterior muscle, which it innervates. This nerve is coalescing

in the deep, most inferior region of the neck, so it would not be injured in the location of the incision. Damage to the long thoracic nerve would lead to "winging of the scapula," when the patient is asked to protract the affected shoulder. **Choice E** (Thoracodorsal nerve) is incorrect. This nerve runs inferiorly through the axilla to supply the latissimus dorsi muscle. Loss of the nerve would result in weakness in extension and medial rotation of the arm, plus wasting of the posterior axillary fold.

14 **The answer is B: Lunate.** The lunate is shaped like a moon, thus its name. It is situated in the center of the proximal row of carpal bones where it articulates with the radius. This bone is the most commonly dislocated carpal bone, which leads to severe carpal instabilities. This dislocation often occurs in association with a trans-scaphoid fracture. It is important to note that scaphoid fractures are often difficult to see in radiographic imaging; however, these fractures can be detected frequently by applying direct pressure to the anatomical snuffbox. **Choice A** (Scaphoid) is incorrect. The scaphoid bone is located in the proximal row and is the most frequently fractured carpal bone. As the weight of the body is transmitted through the upper limb onto the outstretched hand and the impact of the fall exerts pressure back upon the limb, the scaphoid bone is crushed by these opposing forces and is subsequently fractured, usually along its narrowest part. The scaphoid bone is clinically relevant due to the frequency of fractures in younger patients and the poor vascularization of its proximal part. Avascular necrosis is often a postfracture complication that slows the healing of this bone. **Choice C** (Capitate) is incorrect. The capitate is located in the distal row of carpal bones, so this selection can be easily eliminated. **Choice D** (Triquetrum) is incorrect. The triquetrum is located in the proximal row of carpal bones and may be involved in a severe dislocation of the wrist. Specifically, the triquetrum can be displaced in Stage III wrist dislocations when the triquetrolunate interosseous ligament is damaged. However, tearing this interosseous intercarpal ligament would only occur following dislocation of the lunate bone, which is the most commonly dislocated carpal bone. **Choice E** (Trapezium) is incorrect. The trapezium bone helps form the distal floor of the anatomic snuffbox and forces would be exerted on this bone during the fall. However, it is not located in the proximal row of carpal bones. Moreover, this four-sided bone is rarely fractured or dislocated due to its shape and construction.

15 **The answer is E: Superficial branch of the radial nerve.** The superficial branch of the radial nerve is entirely cutaneous, carrying sensation from the dorsolateral part of the hand from the anatomical snuffbox to the midline of the fourth finger. This nerve is vulnerable as it runs posteriorly between the brachioradialis and extensor carpi radialis longus tendons toward the dorsum of the hand. This nerve was damaged at this location, but the area of sensory loss is less than expected due to the overlap from cutaneous branches of the ulnar and median nerves. **Choice A** (Dorsal cutaneous branch of the ulnar nerve) is incorrect. The dorsal cutaneous branch of the ulnar nerve passes posterior between the ulna and flexor carpi ulnaris to supply the subcutaneous tissue of the dorsal aspect of the posteromedial aspect of the hand, medial to the midline of the fourth finger. Its medial location and its sensory distribution make it an unlikely choice to be involved with this patient.

Choice B (Lateral cutaneous nerve of the forearm) is incorrect. The lateral cutaneous nerve of the forearm is the continuation of the musculocutaneous nerve, which exits the arm between the biceps brachii and brachialis muscles. It supplies the skin on the lateral aspects of the forearm and wrist but would not be responsible for the numbness and paresthesia seen in this patient because the sensory deficit is distal to this nerve's normal distribution. **Choice C** (Posterior cutaneous nerve of the forearm) is incorrect. The posterior cutaneous nerve of the forearm arises from the radial nerve and passes in close proximity to the lateral intermuscular septum of the arm near the origin of the brachioradialis. As its name implies, it supplies the posterior aspect of the forearm, but it does not extend past the wrist. Therefore, it would not be the nerve damaged in this patient. **Choice D** (Deep branch of the radial nerve) is incorrect. The deep branch of the radial nerve is entirely motor in its distribution to the posterior muscles of the forearm. Its lack of cutaneous innervation makes this choice easy to eliminate.

16   **The answer is D: Intercostobrachial nerve.**   The intercostobrachial nerve is the lateral cutaneous branch of the second intercostal nerve. As its name implies, it leaves the thorax by exiting between the second and third ribs (between the ribs = intercosto-) to supply cutaneous innervation to the axilla and medial aspect of the arm (brachium). In some instances, it may also supply skin distal to the elbow. The anesthetic solution would block all of the distal branches of the brachial plexus residing within the axillary sheath, thus sparing the intercostobrachial nerve. **Choice A** (Long thoracic nerve) is incorrect. The long thoracic nerve does not have a cutaneous distribution and provides only motor innervation to the serratus anterior. Because the long thoracic nerve arises from the ventral rami of C5-C7, it would not be affected by the anesthetic solution, especially if an occlusive tourniquet was utilized to retain the solution. Such a procedure is used to prevent spread of the anesthetic into the neck where it could affect the phrenic nerve and negatively affect respiration. **Choice B** (Median nerve) is incorrect. The median nerve does not branch proximal to the elbow, and its sensory distribution is limited to distal to the wrist. Furthermore, this nerve would be blocked by effective administration of the anesthetic reagent. **Choice C** (Medial cutaneous nerve of the arm) is incorrect. The medial cutaneous nerve of the arm arises from the medial cord of the brachial plexus, and it would be blocked by effective administration of the anesthetic solution into the axillary sheath. This nerve would also provide sensation to the area (medial aspect of the arm) that remains sensitive to pain, but it should be blocked by the drug. **Choice E** (Ulnar nerve) is incorrect. The ulnar nerve does not branch proximal to the elbow, and its sensory distribution is limited to distal to the wrist. Furthermore, this nerve would be blocked by effective administration of the anesthetic solution.

17   **The answer is A: Axillary nerve.**   The axillary nerve may be damaged in approximately one of seven shoulder dislocations. This nerve innervates the deltoid and teres minor muscles as well as supplying innervation to the skin overlying the deltoid in the superolateral aspect of the arm. Loss of innervation to the deltoid muscle would explain the weakness in abduction of the upper limb. The teres minor assists the infraspinatus muscle in external rotation of the shoulder. **Choice B** (Median nerve) is incorrect. The median nerve does not branch proximal to the elbow, and its sensory distribution is limited to the hand. The median nerve could not be responsible for the patient's motor and sensory deficits. **Choice C** (Ulnar nerve) is incorrect. The ulnar nerve can be damaged during shoulder dislocations; however, its sensory distribution is limited to distal to the wrist, and the first muscle it innervates is in the forearm (flexor carpi ulnaris). Therefore, the ulnar nerve could not be responsible for this patient's motor and sensory deficits. **Choice D** (Radial nerve) is incorrect. The radial nerve supplies motor innervation to the posterior compartments of the arm and forearm. Damage to this nerve would cause weakness in extending at the elbow and wrist joints. The radial nerve gives rise to the posterior cutaneous nerves of the arm and forearm as well as the inferior lateral cutaneous nerve of the arm. However, it would not affect the superior lateral cutaneous nerve of the arm, arising from the axillary nerve, which was damaged in this patient. The radial nerve would also not affect abduction and external rotation of the shoulder. **Choice E** (Musculocutaneous nerve) is incorrect. The musculocutaneous nerve can be damaged during shoulder dislocations; however, this nerve supplies the motor innervation to the anterior compartment of the arm. Trauma to this nerve would lead to weakness in flexing the elbow and supinating the forearm. Its sensory distribution is limited to the lateral aspect of the forearm, so it was not the nerve damaged in this patient.

18   **The answer is E: Muculocutaneous nerve.**   A positive response to the myotatic biceps reflex confirms the integrity of the musculocutaneous nerve and the C5 and C6 spinal segments, from which this nerve arises. The musculocutaneous nerve supplies motor innervation and proprioception to the muscles in the anterior compartment of the arm, including the coracobrachialis, biceps brachii (tested here), and brachialis. Lesioning the musculocutaneous nerve would lead to loss of proprioception and weakness in flexing the elbow (via the biceps brachii and brachialis muscles) and supinating the forearm (via the biceps brachii), resulting in a negative myotatic biceps reflex. **Choice A** (Axillary nerve) is incorrect. The axillary nerve innervates the deltoid and teres minor muscles as well as the skin overlying the deltoid in the superolateral aspect of the arm. Loss of innervation to the deltoid muscle would cause weakness in abduction of the upper limb. The teres minor and posterior head of the deltoid are responsible for external rotation of the shoulder. **Choice B** (Median nerve) is incorrect. The median nerve innervates 6.5 of the 8 anterior forearm muscles. This nerve would help with flexion of the forearm at the elbow; however, the myotatic biceps reflex test specifically tests the innervation of the biceps brachii muscle, which is innervated by the musculocutaneous nerve. **Choice C** (Ulnar nerve) is incorrect. The ulnar nerve innervates only 1.5 muscles of the forearm, specifically the flexor carpi ulnaris and the ulnar side of the flexor digitorum profundus. This nerve also innervates most of the intrinsic muscles of the hand. It is not involved with the myotatic biceps reflex test. **Choice D** (Radial nerve) is incorrect. The radial nerve supplies motor innervation to the posterior compartments of the arm and forearm. Damage to this nerve would cause weakness in extension at the elbow and wrist joints. The radial nerve is responsible for the posterior cutaneous nerves of the arm and forearm as well as the inferior lateral cutaneous nerve of the arm. However, it is responsible for extension at the elbow, not the flexion of the elbow tested with the myotatic biceps reflex test.

19 **The answer is D: Radial nerve.** This case represents a classic presentation of "Saturday Night Palsy," where the radial nerve is compressed against the humerus in the arm. Remember, the radial nerve supplies motor innervation to the posterior compartments of the arm and forearm, so damage to this nerve would cause weakness in extending the elbow and wrist. This patient is unable to extend the wrist when the hand is placed in a pronated position ("wrist drop"), implying damage to the radial nerve. Moreover, the superficial branch of the radial nerve is responsible for cutaneous innervation over much of the dorsum of the hand, which explains the numbness and paresthesia in his hand. **Choice A** (Axillary nerve) is incorrect. The axillary nerve innervates the deltoid and teres minor muscles as well as the skin overlying the deltoid in the superolateral aspect of the arm. Compressing the axillary nerve would not affect wrist function or cause paresthesia distal to the wrist, which was seen in this student. **Choice B** (Median nerve) is incorrect. The median nerve is responsible for flexion at the wrist; however, this patient is having trouble with wrist extension. The sensory distribution for the median nerve is primarily on the palmar side of the hand rather than the dorsum of the hand, which is seen in this patient. **Choice C** (Ulnar nerve) is incorrect. The ulnar nerve is responsible for sensory innervation on the dorsum of the hand that is limited to the ulnar side (medial to the midline of the fourth finger). Damage to the ulnar nerve would not result in "wrist drop," which is an indication of a radial nerve injury. The ulnar nerve does supply motor innervation to most of the intrinsic muscles of the hand. **Choice E** (Musculocutaneous nerve) is incorrect. The musculocutaneous nerve supplies motor innervation to the anterior compartment of the arm and cutaneous innervation to the lateral aspect of the forearm. Therefore, damage to this nerve would not affect wrist function.

20 **The answer is B: Lower trunk of the brachial plexus.** This woman has experienced a lower brachial plexus injury due to forced abduction of the upper limb during the accident. This injury presents with numbness and paresthesia in the C8 and T1 dermatomes, which supply the axilla and medial aspect of her upper limb. These nerve roots primarily supply the medial cord of the brachial plexus, which creates the ulnar nerve. Due to damage to the ulnar nerve, she is experiencing weakness in the movement of her left hand. The abduction and adduction of the fingers are controlled by the deep branch of the ulnar nerve by supplying the dorsal interosseous and palmar interosseous muscles, respectively. **Choice A** (Upper trunk of the brachial plexus) is incorrect. Damage to the upper trunk of the brachial plexus results in Erb-Duchenne palsy ("waiter's tip malformation"). In this injury, the patient presents with significant weakness in abduction and lateral rotation of the shoulder, flexion of the shoulder and elbow, and supination of the forearm. **Choice C** (Posterior cord of the brachial plexus) is incorrect. The posterior cord of the brachial plexus gives rise to the axillary and radial nerves. Damage to the axillary nerve causes weakness in abduction of the shoulder due to loss of the deltoid muscle. Damage

to the radial nerve results in inability to extend at the elbow or wrist (leading to "wrist drop"). However, this patient had significant weakness in the movements of the hand, which implies damage to the contributions of the ulnar nerve. **Choice D** (Lateral cord of the brachial plexus) is incorrect. Damage to the lateral cord of the brachial plexus results in signs and symptoms similar to those seen in Erb-Duchenne palsy, or the "waiter's tip malformation." In this injury, the patient presents with significant weakness in abduction and lateral rotation of the shoulder, flexion of the shoulder and elbow, and supination of the forearm. **Choice E** (Long thoracic nerve) is incorrect. A lesion of the long thoracic nerve leads to a "winged scapula" due to the subsequent paralysis of the serratus anterior muscle. Additionally, the affected arm cannot be abducted above the horizontal plane because the serratus anterior is not available to superiorly rotate the glenoid cavity of the scapula to allow full abduction. This deficit was not seen in this patient.

21 **The answer is D: Meromelia.** Thalidomide was once used widely to help combat morning sickness during pregnancy. Following a wave of children born with limb malformations, the medication was discovered to be a significant teratogen and was taken off the market. Currently, thalidomide is being used to treat AIDS and cancer patients, raising concerns of a new rash of children born with limb defects. The specific malformation in this case is termed meromelia, a partial absence of limb segments. Meromelia is a type of reduction defect, in which whole or partial limb components are absent. Because of the resemblance of the limbs to a seal's flippers, this defect is also termed phocomelia ("seal limb"). **Choice A** (A dysplasia) is incorrect. Dysplasias are malformations in which elements are malformed. In this case, limb components are missing rather than malformed. **Choice B** (A duplication defect) is incorrect. Duplication defects are characterized by the presence of supernumerary (extra) elements. An example is polydactyly, in which extra digits are present. **Choice C** (Micromelia) is incorrect. Micromelia ("small limb") is a type of dysplasia. In this, the limb segments are present but are abnormally short. **Choice E** (Amelia) is incorrect. Amelia ("without limb") is a type of reduction defect in which an entire extremity is absent.

22 **The answer is D: Biceps brachii.** The lateral X-ray reveals chronic microtrauma to the radial tuberosity, which is the insertion site for the biceps brachii muscle. In this weightlifter, the damage to the radial tuberosity is most likely due to overuse of the biceps brachii and the concomitant stress placed upon the radial tuberosity by lifting significant weight loads. The biceps brachii muscle produces flexion of the elbow (and shoulder) and is the powerful supinator of the forearm, explaining why these actions exacerbated the pain in this patient. **Choice A** (Supinator) is incorrect. The supinator muscle attaches onto the proximal shaft of the radius rather than the radial tuberosity, so it would not cause damage to the radial tuberosity. Moreover, the supinator muscle acts to produce lower resistance supination and does not flex the elbow. **Choice B** (Brachialis) is incorrect. The brachialis muscle is a powerful flexor of the elbow. However, it is not related to the radial tuberosity as it attaches onto the coronoid process and tuberosity of the ulna. Furthermore, the brachialis muscle does not act in supination. **Choice C** (Pronator teres) is incorrect.

The pronator teres muscle contributes somewhat to flexion of the elbow. However, it inserts onto the midshaft portion of the radius, and its main action is pronation. In this patient, pain was exacerbated by supination against resistance. **Choice E** (Brachioradialis) is incorrect. The brachioradials muscle is a notable flexor of the elbow. However, it attaches to the styloid process at the distal end of the radius and is not related to the radial tuberosity. Also, the brachioradialis muscle does not act in supination.

23 **The answer is B: Latissimus dorsi.** The axilla is a large, pyramidal space between the side of the chest and the upper part of the brachium. Its major importance is as a passageway from the root of the neck to the upper limb. The axilla is demarcated by four walls: anterior, posterior, medial, lateral. The posterior wall is composed of the latissimus dorsi, teres major, and subscapularis muscles. The posterior axillary fold forms the palpable lower margin of the wall and is composed of the latissimus dorsi and teres major. The subscapularis is not part of the posterior axillary fold. Damage to the latissimus dorsi would severely hinder adduction, extension, and medial rotation of the arm. **Choice A** (Pectoralis minor) is incorrect. The pectoralis minor contributes to the formation of the anterior wall of the axilla. The pectoralis major forms the bulk of the anterior wall and creates the noticeable anterior axillary fold. **Choice C** (Levator scapulae) is incorrect. The levator scapulae muscle passes out of the neck to attach onto the superior angle of the scapula. It is far removed from any of the walls of the axilla and does not contribute to rotation and adduction of the arm. **Choice D** (Serratus anterior) is incorrect. The serratus anterior lies against the thoracic wall and forms much of the medial wall of the axilla along with the thoracic wall. It fixes the scapula to the thoracic wall and has no affect on rotation of the arm. **Choice E** (Teres minor) is incorrect. The teres minor is located immediately above the teres major. However, it is not a component of the posterior wall of the axilla and normally contributes to lateral rotation of the arm.

24 **The answer is D: Axillary nerve.** The quadrangular space of the shoulder is an important passageway allowing the posterior humeral circumflex vessels and their companion axillary nerve to pass from the axilla to the posterior aspect of the shoulder. The neurovascular bundle runs across the surgical neck of the humerus to enter the quadrangular space. The space itself (sometimes termed the lateral axillary hiatus) is formed by four structures: teres major, teres minor, long head of the triceps, surgical neck of the humerus. The vessels contribute to the collateral network around the shoulder. The axillary nerve supplies the teres minor and deltoid muscles and a cutaneous area on the superolateral aspect of the arm (i.e., the skin overlying the lower aspect of the deltoid muscle). **Choice A** (Musculocutaneous nerve) is incorrect. The musculocutaneous nerve is a terminal branch of the lateral cord of the brachial plexus within the axilla. It supplies the anterior compartment of the arm and is not related to the quadrangular space. **Choice B** (Lateral cord of the brachial plexus) is incorrect. The lateral cord occupies a relatively lateral position in the axilla but is not related to the quadrangular space. The axillary nerve originates from the posterior cord of the brachial plexus. **Choice C** (Radial nerve) is incorrect. The radial and axillary

nerves are the terminal branches of the posterior cord of the brachial plexus. The radial nerve runs through the radial (spiral) groove in the midshaft of the humerus to emerge through the lower triangular space, just below the quadrangular space, and enter the posterior compartment of the arm. **Choice E** (Medial cutaneous nerve of the arm) is incorrect. The medial cutaneous nerve of the arm is a branch of the medial cord of the brachial plexus. It is far removed from the quadrangular space.

25 **The answer is E: The second part of the axillary artery lies deep to the muscle.** The pectoralis minor muscle overlies the axillary artery in such a way as to divide it into three parts: first (prepectoral; medial), second (subpectoral; deep), third (postpectoral; lateral). The first part is medial to the pectoralis minor, running from the lateral border of the first rib to the medial border of the pectoralis minor. The second part is deep to the muscle. The third part is lateral to the pectoralis minor, running from the lateral border of the muscle to the inferior border of the teres major muscle. **Choice A** (The lateral cord of the brachial plexus lies lateral to the muscle) is incorrect. The cords of the brachial plexus are so named by their positions relative to the second part of the axillary artery. **Choice B** (The clavipectoral triangle lies lateral to the muscle) is incorrect. The clavipectoral triangle lies medial to the pectoralis minor, between the muscle and the clavicle. This fascia-roofed space is noteworthy because it is pierced by the lateral pectoral nerve (on its way to the clavicular head of the pectoralis major), branches of the thoracoacromial artery, and the cephalic vein (on its way to empty into the axillary vein). **Choice C** (The anterior axillary lymph nodes lie along the medial border of the muscle) is incorrect. The anterior (pectoral; level 1) group of axillary lymph nodes lie along the lateral border of the pectoralis minor. **Choice D** (The lateral wall of the axillary fossa includes the muscle) is incorrect. The pectoralis minor forms the anterior wall of the axillary fossa, along with the pectoralis major.

26 **The answer is E: Teres minor.** Throwing motions are complex mechanical events that involve multiple muscles interacting in moment-to-moment changing ways, with rotation of the humerus being one important outcome. The four rotator cuff muscles (supraspinatus, infrapsinatus, teres minor, subscapularis), plus several other muscles that cross the glenohumeral joint, contribute significant forces to rotation of the arm. The teres minor and infraspinatus (i.e., half the rotator cuff group) lie completely across the posterior aspect of the glenohumeral joint and are primary lateral (external) rotators. These muscles are aided by the posterior fibers of the deltoid muscle. **Choice A** (Supraspinatus) is incorrect. The supraspinatus is one of the rotator cuff muscles. However, it does not produce rotation. It lies across the superior aspect of the glenohumeral joint and initiates abduction of the arm from the rest position. **Choice B** (Teres major) is incorrect. The teres major arises posteriorly from the inferior angle of the scapula and crosses the glenohumeral joint to its anteriorly located insertion into the medial lip of the intertubercular groove of the humerus. Thus, the teres major muscle acts to adduct and medially (internally) rotate the arm rather than laterally rotate. It is not a member of the rotator cuff muscles. **Choice C** (Latissimus dorsi) is incorrect. The latissimus dorsi muscle arises posteriorly from the spinous processes of the inferior six thoracic vertebrae and the thoracolumbar fascia and crosses the glenohumeral joint anteriorly to insert into the floor of the intertubercular sulcus of the humerus. Thus, the latissimus dorsi muscle acts to extend, adduct, and medially rotate the humerus rather than laterally rotate. It is not a member of the rotator cuff muscles. **Choice D** (Subscapularis) is incorrect. The subscapularis muscle is part of the rotator cuff. In common with the teres major and latissimus dorsi muscles, it crosses the glenohumeral joint from posterior to anterior, thus producing medial rotation and adduction of the arm. It is not responsible for external (lateral) rotation of the arm.

27 **The answer is B: Axillary artery.** The brachial plexus is divided into five geographic parts: **R**oots (or ventral rami of C5-T1), **T**runks, **D**ivisions, **C**ords, terminal **B**ranches (or Nerves). These sections of the brachial plexus can be remembered with the mnemonics, "**R**eal **T**ruckers **D**rink **C**old **B**eer" or "**R**emember **T**hose **D**arn **C**ervical **N**erves". The cords are named according to their important positional relationship to the second part of the axillary artery, deep to the pectoralis minor muscle. Here, the nerves form a cradle-like bed for this segment of the vessel as it passes through the axilla. Thus, the lateral cord is located lateral, the medial cord is medial, and the posterior cord is posterior to the axillary artery. **Choice A** (Long head of the biceps brachii muscle) is incorrect. The long head of the biceps brachii muscle lies lateral to all three cords of the brachial plexus. **Choice C** (Subclavian vein) is incorrect. This vessel is located well proximal to the cords of the brachial plexus, medial to the first rib. **Choice D** (Surgical neck of the humerus) is incorrect. This part of the humerus is located distal and lateral to all three cords of the brachial plexus. **Choice E** (Pectoralis minor muscle) is incorrect. The pectoralis minor lies superficial (anterior) to the cords of the brachial plexus. This muscle divides the axillary artery into its three parts. Thus, it defines the second part of the artery and creates the situation for naming the cords of the plexus.

28 **The answer is B: Median nerve.** Each of the five terminal branches of the brachial plexus (musculocutaneous, median, ulnar, radial, and axillary nerves) passes through a muscular or osseofascial tunnel at some point in its distribution, where it may be subject to entrapment in a tunnel syndrome. The pronator teres muscle arises via two heads, one from the medial epicondyle of the humerus and the other from the coronoid process of the ulna, with a tendinous arch connecting them. The median nerve exits the cubital fossa and enters the forearm by passing between these heads, where it may be unduly compressed in a pronator teres syndrome. This condition would influence much of the median nerve territory in the forearm plus the entire median nerve territory in the hand. **Choice A** (Deep branch of the radial nerve) is incorrect. The radial nerve descends from the arm into the cubital fossa, where it divides into superficial and deep branches. The deep branch of the radial nerve pierces the supinator muscle, winds around the proximal end of the radius within the substance of that muscle, and passes into the deep posterior compartment of the forearm as the posterior interosseous nerve. The nerve may be entrapped within the supinator, resulting in a supinator syndrome. Such

a condition would affect the deeper, more distal extensor muscles arising in the forearm and some sensory areas in the wrist joints. **Choice C** (Deep branch of the ulnar nerve) is incorrect. The ulnar nerve enters the hand superficial to the flexor retinaculum, runs through a groove between the pisiform and hook of the hamate (Guyon canal), and divides into superficial and deep branches at the base of the hypothenar eminence. The deep branch curls deeply there and enters the deep lying adductor/interosseous compartment in the palmar aspect of the hand. Compression of the ulnar nerve in Guyon canal may cause a Guyon tunnel syndrome, which affects the hypothenar muscles, medial two lumbricals, all interossei, adductor pollicis, and a large sensory area on both palmar and dorsal sides of the hand. **Choice D** (Superficial branch of the ulnar nerve) is incorrect. The superficial branch of the ulnar nerve does not enter a tunnel and is not subject to a tunnel syndrome. This nerve supplies the palmaris brevis muscle but is mostly cutaneous across the palmar and dorsal aspects of the medial third of the hand. **Choice E** (Musculocutaneous nerve) is incorrect. This nerve penetrates the coracobrachialis muscle, supplies the three flexor muscles in the anterior compartment of the arm, and continues into the forearm as the lateral cutaneous nerve of the forearm. Entrapment of the nerve within the coracobrachialis is rare.

29 **The answer is C: Lateral to the tendon of the flexor carpi radialis.** The most common location for measuring pulse rate is on the radial artery at the wrist. Here, the vessel lies on the anterior side of the distal end of the radius, lateral to the tendon of the flexor carpi radialis. It is covered only by skin and a thin superficial fascia and can be palpated easily against the radius. Note the placement of the index and middle fingers of the physician in the given photo. **Choice A** (Across the anterior aspect of the lateral epicondyle of the humerus) is incorrect. The radial artery originates in the cubital fossa as one of the two terminal branches of the brachial artery (the ulnar artery is the other). The radial recurrent artery branches off the radial artery just below its origin and ascends across the anterior aspect of the lateral epicondyle of the humerus. However, the radial recurrent artery lies on muscle and is not normally palpable. **Choice B** (Between the tendons of the palmaris longus and flexor carpi ulnaris) is incorrect. The ulnar artery enters the hand superficial to the flexor retinaculum, lateral to the pisiform and medial to the hook of the hamate. The ulnar pulse may be palpable slightly lateral to the insertion of the flexor carpi ulnaris onto the pisiform, between it and the tendon of the palmaris longus. **Choice D** (Superficial to the tendons of the extensor pollicis brevis and abductor pollicis longus) is incorrect. The radial pulse is also available in the anatomical snuffbox, where the radial artery crosses the floor of that space between the tendons of the extensor pollicis longus and brevis muscles. In entering the snuffbox, the artery passes deep (not superficial) to the tendons of the abductor pollicis longus and extensor pollicis brevis muscles. **Choice E** (Superficial to the carpal tunnel) is incorrect. As noted above, the ulnar artery enters the hand superficial to the flexor retinaculum, thus, superficial to the carpal tunnel. The superficial palmar branch of the radial artery usually runs through the thenar muscles and is not palpable.

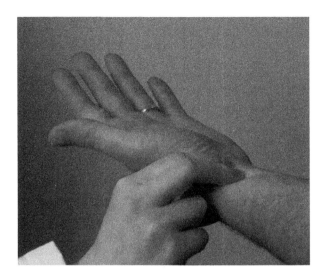

the hand. The alignment of the great saphenous and cephalic veins with the first digits in the limbs denotes them as developmental equivalents. **Choice A** (Radial vein) is incorrect. The radial vein is a deep vena comitans, a vein that accompanies another structure; in this case, it travels with the radial artery. Like most deep veins of the limbs, this vein actually exists as two veins that travel as companions to the radial artery and are called venae commitantes. Being a deep vein, the radial vein is not an equivalent structure to the subcutaneous great saphenous vein. **Choice B** (Ulnar vein) is incorrect. The ulnar vein is a deep vena comitans, a vein that accompanies the ulnar artery. The ulnar vein also exists as two venae commitantes that travel collaterally to the ulnar artery within the same connective tissue sheath. The ulnar vein is not an equivalent structure to the great saphenous vein. **Choice C** (Brachial vein) is incorrect. The brachial vein is a deep, paired venae commitantes that accompanies the brachial artery. This vein is not an equivalent structure to the great saphenous vein due to its deep course within the arm. **Choice D** (Basilic vein) is incorrect. The basilic vein is a cutaneous vessel that ascends the medial aspect of the arm, in alignment with the fifth digit in the hand. Thus, it is actually on the opposite side of the limb for equivalence with the great saphenous vein. Instead, the basilic vein is the counterpart of the small saphenous vein.

30 **The answer is D: Radial artery.** The radial and ulnar arteries anastomose to form the superficial and deep palmar arches. However, the superficial palmar arch is formed mainly by the ulnar artery, whereas the deep palmar arch is formed primarily by the radial artery. Thus, the insufficiency in this case is most likely due to reduced flow in the radial artery. **Choice A** (Posterior interosseous artery) is incorrect. The posterior interosseous artery branches off the common interosseous artery, which is derived from the ulnar artery in the proximal forearm. The posterior interosseous artery supplies the posterior compartment of the forearm. This artery does not reach the wrist and does not contribute blood to the palmar arterial arches. **Choice B** (Ulnar artery) is incorrect. The ulnar artery provides the primary supply into the superficial palmar arterial arch. The deep palmar arch is formed primarily by the radial artery, and it is the reduced flow of the radial artery most likely present in this patient. **Choice C** (Anterior interosseous artery) is incorrect. The anterior interosseous artery branches off the common interosseous artery, which is derived from the ulnar artery in the proximal forearm. The anterior interosseous artery supplies the anterior compartment of the forearm as well as the distal posterior forearm via its posterior terminal branch. This artery does reach the wrist, but it does not contribute blood to the palmar arterial arches. **Choice E** (Inferior ulnar collateral artery) is incorrect. This artery branches off the brachial artery just above the elbow. It passes distally across the anterior side of the medial epicondyle of the humerus to form a collateral connection with the anterior ulnar recurrent branch of the ulnar artery. This vessel is far removed from the hand.

31 **The answer is E: Cephalic vein.** The great saphenous vein is a large cutaneous vessel that ascends the medial aspect of the lower limb to ultimately drain into the femoral vein at the top of the limb. The cephalic vein is a distinctive cutaneous vessel that ascends the lateral aspect of the arm to ultimately drain into the axillary vein. At first glance, these two veins might seem to be traveling opposite venous routes. However, notice that each vein is aligned along the first digit side (great toe and thumb) of its respective limb. Remember that the upper and lower limbs rotate in opposite directions during their development, resulting in the great toe placed on the medial side of the foot and the thumb on the lateral side of

32 **The answer is A: Posterior circumflex humeral artery.** The radiograph shows a fracture of the surgical neck of the humerus. The posterior humeral circumflex artery, accompanied by the axillary nerve, lies against the posterior aspect of the surgical neck as it passes into the quadrangular space of the shoulder. This fracture places both of these structures in immediate danger. **Choice B** (Brachial artery) is incorrect. The brachial artery travels down the midline of the arm, close to the median nerve. It is not immediately endangered by the fracture of the surgical neck. **Choice C** (Deep brachial, or profunda brachii, artery) is incorrect. The deep brachial artery wraps tightly around the midshaft of the humerus, in the radial (spiral) groove. It, along with the radial nerve with which it travels, would be endangered by a fracture through the radial groove of the humerus. **Choice D** (Subscapular artery) is incorrect. The subscapular artery is the largest branch of the axillary artery. It descends along the axillary border of the scapula and is not in contact with the humerus. **Choice E** (Superior ulnar collateral artery) is incorrect. This artery is a branch of the brachial artery. It descends through the arm, moves into company with the ulnar nerve, and takes a close relation to the posterior aspect of the medial epicondyle of the humerus. This vessel would be endangered by a fracture of the medial epicondyle rather than a surgical neck fracture.

33 **The answer is E: Flexor carpi radialis.** The flexor retinaculum (transverse carpal ligament) is a thickening of investing deep fascia on the anterior (ventral) aspect of the wrist that forms the roof of the carpal tunnel. All issues related to the carpal tunnel revolve around an understanding of what structures are contained within the carpal tunnel versus the positions of structures outside the tunnel. The tendons of the flexor carpi radialis and palmaris longus muscles, plus the ulnar nerve and ulnar artery, lie against the superficial aspect of the flexor retinaculum. Any of these structures may be lesioned by a superficial cut across the front (anterior side) of the wrist. **Choice A** (Flexor digitorum superficialis) is incorrect.

The tendons of this muscle are contained within the carpal tunnel, deep to the flexor retinaculum. **Choice B** (Brachioradialis) is incorrect. This muscle inserts onto the base of the styloid process of the radius. Thus, its tendon is proximal and lateral to the flexor retinaculum, and therefore unrelated to the carpal tunnel. **Choice C** (Flexor pollicis longus) is incorrect. The tendons of this muscle are contained within the carpal tunnel, deep to the flexor retinaculum. **Choice D** (Abductor pollicis longus) is incorrect. This muscle is a member of the posterior compartment of the forearm. Its tendon loops out of that compartment to attach onto the lateral side of the base of the first metacarpal (the lateral base of the thumb). Thus, it is well removed from the flexor retinaculum and the carpal tunnel.

34   **The answer is E: Fracture of the fifth metacarpal bone.**   Fracture of the fifth metacarpal bone is called a "boxer's fracture" because this injury is often seen after an individual improperly punches a solid object with a clenched fist. The impact on the head of the fifth metacarpal causes the distal shaft of this bone to fracture. Skilled pugilists are trained to direct the impact of the clenched fist on the heads of the first and second metacarpals to avoid this type of injury. **Choice A** (Dislocation of the fifth metacarpophalangeal joint) is incorrect. This type of injury is rare, and a dislocation of the fifth metacarpophalangeal joint would have been detected by the physician on examination. **Choice B** (Fracture of the triquetral bone) is incorrect. This carpal bone is rarely fractured in this type of impact. **Choice C** (Fracture of the proximal phalanx of the ring finger) is incorrect. The impact of the clenched fist would have been localized to the head of the fifth metacarpal. Damage to the proximal phalanx of the ring finger would have occurred only if the fist was not clenched during impact. **Choice D** (Fracture of the proximal phalanx of the little finger) is incorrect. The impact of the clenched fist would have been localized to the head of the fifth metacarpal. Damage to the proximal phalanx of the little finger would have occurred only if the fist was not clenched during impact.

35   **The answer is B: Supraspinatus tendonitis.**   This patient is experiencing shoulder impingement syndrome, in which impingement of the supraspinatus tendon leads to supraspinatus tendonitis. Supraspinatus tendonitis is a result of stressful repetitive overhead motions, such as lifting heavy objects, which this patient noted in his summer job. This type of tendonitis presents with a painful arc of motion (between 80 and 150 degrees in this patient) during abduction of the upper limb. **Choice A** (Infraspinatus tendonitis) is incorrect. Infraspinatus tendonitis would lead to pain during external rotation at the glenohumeral joint against resistance, which is not noted in this patient. **Choice C** (Acromioclavicular (AC) joint arthritis) is incorrect. AC joint arthritis would result following repeated movements that wear away the cartilage surfaces in the AC joint. It can also be seen after repeated shoulder separations. However, due to the age of this patient and the fact that he was only participating in construction during the summer, this diagnosis is unlikely. **Choice D** (Degenerative arthritis of the shoulder) is incorrect. Given the young age of this patient, degenerative arthritis of the shoulder is extremely unlikely. **Choice E** (Broken clavicle) is incorrect. The patient is reporting pain only during abduction of the upper limb. A broken clavicle presents with constant pain and results from trauma; however, trauma was not reported in this patient.

36   **The answer is A: Ulnar nerve in the elbow.**   Situations in which peripheral nerves are compressed or otherwise entrapped where they pass through narrow spaces ("tunnels") in muscles and/or osseo-fascial units are generally referred to as "tunnel syndromes." Such conditions may result in periodic or constant motor and/or sensory deficits. The ulnar nerve crosses the elbow in a narrow space between the olecranon process and the medial epicondyle of the humerus, on the posteromedial (ulnar) side of the joint. The ulnar nerve can be compressed between these bony landmarks or between the humeral and ulnar heads of the attachment of the flexor carpi ulnaris. Compression of the ulnar nerve within these areas leads to "cubital tunnel syndrome." The symptoms are exacerbated during events where flexion of the elbow narrows these passageways and compresses the ulnar nerve at the elbow joint. The patient's cubital tunnel syndrome would explain the paresthesia and numbness on the medial aspect of the hand and the diminished fine motor control of the intrinsic hand muscles. Her condition originated due to the forced flexion of the elbow in the motor vehicle accident, which compressed the ulnar nerve in the cubital tunnel. **Choice B** (Ulnar nerve in the wrist) is incorrect. The ulnar nerve can be compressed between the pisiform and hook of the hamate at the wrist in a condition termed "ulnar canal syndrome" or "Guyon tunnel syndrome." This entrapment syndrome presents with similar signs and symptoms as seen in this patient. However, the ability to flex the wrist would not be affected. In this patient, trauma to the wrist was not reported. **Choice C** (Median nerve in the wrist) is incorrect. The median nerve is often compressed at the wrist in "carpal tunnel syndrome" because this nerve travels deep to the transverse carpal ligament (flexor retinaculum of the wrist) within the carpal tunnel. This entrapment syndrome presents with paresthesia of the lateral fingers as well as an inability to oppose the thumb and a wasting of the thenar eminence. These symptoms were not reported in this patient. **Choice D** (Median nerve in the elbow) is incorrect. The median nerve is not usually compressed by forced flexion of the elbow because it lies loosely on the flexor surface of the joint deep to the bicipital aponeurosis. The median nerve can be compressed in the proximal forearm as it passes between the two heads of the pronator teres. However, the symptoms in this patient were due to forced flexion of the elbow and involve the ulnar nerve. **Choice E** (Median nerve in the axilla) is incorrect. The median nerve would not be damaged in the axilla without significant trauma. Damage to the median nerve in the axilla would lead to weakness in flexing the wrist, loss of pronation of the forearm, and wasting of the thenar muscles. However, these signs and symptoms were not reported.

37   **The answer is E: Flexor digitorum superficialis (FDS).**   The FDS muscle flexes the proximal interphalangeal joints in digits 2 to 5. In this patient, this muscle is being tested in the third (middle) finger. By holding the other fingers in extension, the physician is eliminating the influences of the FDP muscles, which flex the distal interphalangeal joints in digits 2 to 5. **Choice A** (Flexor digitorum profundus [FDP]) is incorrect. Flexion of the distal interphalangeal joint in digits 2 to 5 is produced by the FDP; however, the physician is testing flexion of the proximal interphalangeal joint in the middle finger, which is controlled by the FDS muscle. **Choice B** (Extensor digitorum) is incorrect. The extensor digitorum extends fingers #2 to #5. This muscle can easily be eliminated because the physician is testing a muscle on the flexor side of the hand. **Choice C** (Second lumbrical) is incorrect. The second lumbrical muscle extends the interphalangeal joints of the middle (third) finger and flexes the metacarpophalangeal joint of the same finger. The third lumbrical is an intrinsic hand muscle that arises off the tendon of the FDP and inserts into the extensor expansion of the middle finger. This muscle does not control flexion of the proximal interphalangeal joint. **Choice D** (Dorsal interosseous) is incorrect. The primary action of the dorsal interosseous muscles is to abduct the fingers. However, because these muscles insert into the extensor expansion, they also extend the interphalangeal joints of the middle (third) finger and flex the metacarpophalangeal joint of the same finger. Although the dorsal interossei are not involved with flexion of the distal interphalangeal joint, it is important to remember the middle (third) finger forms the axis of movement of the hand. Therefore, this finger has two dorsal interossei attached to it to enable abduction away from the midline in either direction.

38 **The answer is C: Brachialis muscle.**   The cubital fossa is a triangular intermuscular space located anterior to the elbow, comparable to the popliteal fossa in the lower limb. It is an important transition zone between the arm and the forearm, containing major blood vessels and nerves. The roof of the cubital fossa is subcutaneous tissue carrying superficial veins, such as the median cubital vein, which is the most common site for venipuncture in the upper limb. The floor of the fossa is formed by two muscles: brachialis and supinator. Either of these muscles could house the deep abscess caused by repeated needle injections in the cubital fossa. **Choice A** (Brachioradialis muscle) is incorrect. The brachioradialis muscle forms the lateral wall of the cubital fossa. **Choice B** (Pronator teres muscle) is incorrect. The pronator teres muscle forms the medial wall of the cubital fossa. **Choice D** (Head of the radius) is incorrect. The head of the radius lies deep to the muscular floor of the cubital fossa, within the elbow joint complex. **Choice E** (Olecranon fossa of the humerus) is incorrect. The olecranon fossa is located on the posterior distal aspect of the humerus, well removed from the cubital fossa.

39 **The answer is A: Adduction of the arm.**   In a traditional (Halsted) radical mastectomy, both the pectoralis major and minor muscles are removed with the breast and associated axillary tissue. The primary actions of the pectoralis major are adduction, flexion, and medial rotation of the arm. These actions are weakened but not lost postoperatively. Other neighboring muscles (e.g., subscapularis, latissimus dorsi, biceps brachii, anterior deltoid) also perform these actions and can compensate somewhat for loss of the pectoralis major. **Choice B** (Abduction of the arm) is incorrect. Abduction of the arm is performed by the supraspinatus, deltoid, and serratus anterior muscles. Removing the pectoralis major would not affect abduction of the arm. In fact, abduction, extension, and lateral rotation of the arm are the antagonistic actions to the pectoralis major. **Choice C** (Extension of the arm) is incorrect. The pectoralis major helps with flexion of the arm, not extension (the antagonistic action). The latissimus dorsi and posterior part of the deltoid help with extension of the arm. **Choice D** (Lateral rotation of the arm) is incorrect. The pectoralis major helps with medial rotation of the arm, not lateral rotation of

the arm (the antagonistic action). The infraspinatus, teres minor, and posterior part of the deltoid help with lateral rotation of the arm. **Choice E** (Depression of the arm) is incorrect. The pectoralis major muscle acts to adduct, flex, and medial rotate the arm. Therefore, a radical mastectomy would affect these actions.

40 **The answer is B: Second part of the axillary artery.**   The lateral thoracic wall receives significant arterial supply from the branches of the axillary artery. The axillary artery is divided into three parts by the overlying pectoralis minor muscle. The lateral thoracic artery, along with the thoracoacromial trunk, typically branches from the second part of the axillary artery, deep to the pectoralis minor. It descends along the lateral border of the pectoralis minor to supply the lateral aspect of the chest wall, including much of the breast and the serratus anterior muscle. However, this vessel is variable and may originate from other source points. Remember, arteries are often named for the regions they supply, not necessarily for their branching patterns. **Choice A** (First part of the axillary artery) is incorrect. This segment typically gives rise to one branch: the superior (or supreme) thoracic artery, which has a small distribution to the superolateral chest wall. **Choice C** (Third part of the axillary artery) is incorrect. This part typically gives rise to three branches: the subscapular artery and the anterior and posterior circumflex humeral arteries. The lateral thoracic and subscapular arteries may originate as a common trunk. **Choice D** (Third part of the subclavian artery) is incorrect. The subclavian artery is divided into three parts by the anterior scalene muscle. Usually, the third part of the subclavian artery has no branches; however, the dorsal scapular artery may occasionally arise from this location. More importantly, none of the branches of the subclavian artery supply the lateral chest wall. **Choice E** (First part of the brachial artery) is incorrect. The distribution of the brachial artery is limited to the upper limb; it does not supply the lateral chest wall.

41 **The answer is D: Thoracodorsal nerve.**   Successful transposition of muscle flaps in reconstructive surgery hinges largely on maintaining the neurovascular pedicles that supply the muscle. The latissimus dorsi muscle is innervated by the thoracodorsal (middle subscapular) nerve, a branch of the posterior cord of the brachial plexus. Lesion of this nerve during dissection of the chest wall will cause loss of the muscle flap. **Choice A** (Long thoracic nerve) is incorrect. The long thoracic nerve supplies the serratus anterior muscle. Damage to this nerve would cause a "winged scapula." **Choice B** (Intercostobrachial nerve) is incorrect. The intercostobrachial nerve is actually the lateral cutaneous branch of the second thoracic nerve and is entirely sensory in innervation. This nerve arises from the chest wall underneath the second rib and travels distally to give sensory innervation to the skin of the medial arm. **Choice C** (Medial pectoral nerve) is incorrect. The medial pectoral nerve innervates the pectoralis minor and major muscles. It would have been cut during the removal of these muscles during the radical mastectomy. **Choice E** (Axillary nerve) is incorrect. The axillary nerve traverses the quadrangular space (accompanying the posterior circumflex humeral artery) to supply the teres minor and deltoid muscles as well as give cutaneous innervation to the upper lateral aspect of the arm.

42 **The answer is B: Suspensory Ligaments.** Fibrous lobar septa are connective tissue partitions that separate the glandular lobes of the breast and compartmentalize breast tissue. These septa run through the depth of the breast from the dermis of the skin to the underlying pectoral fascia and are most pronounced in the superior aspect of the breast, where they are termed suspensory (Cooper's) ligaments of the breast. Edema and/or tumor growth within the breast can apply traction on the suspensory ligaments, and this tension causes dimpling of the skin that resembles an orange peel. **Choice A** (Clavipectoral fascia) is incorrect. This sleeve of connective tissue extends from the clavicle to the deep fascia of the axilla and envelopes the subclavius and pectoralis minor muscles. It does not enter the breast. **Choice C** (Lactiferous ducts) is incorrect. Each of the 15 to 20 glandular lobes of the breast is drained by a lactiferous duct that opens in the lactiferous sinus and then onto the nipple. Edema and/or tumor growth within the breast may apply traction to these ducts. However, the result of such traction is typically inversion of the nipple rather than dimpling of the skin. **Choice D** (Retromammary space) is incorrect. The retromammary space (or bursa) is a loose connective tissue plane between the breast and pectoral fascia, which contains a small amount of fat and allows the breast some degree of mobility on the pectoral fascia. It does not send connective tissue extensions into the substance of the breast and would not lead to dimpling of the skin due to the presence of an abnormal growth within the breast. **Choice E** (Pectoralis major muscle) is incorrect. The pectoralis major underlies the breast but does not send fibers into the breast. It does not influence the appearance of the skin of the breast.

43 **The answer is D: Deep branch of ulnar nerve.** The deep branch of the ulnar nerve innervates most of the intrinsic muscles of the hand, including the hypothenar muscles, medial two lumbrical muscles, the palmar and dorsal interossei, adductor pollicis, and the deep head of the flexor pollicis brevis. Specifically, the palmar interossei, dorsal interossei, and lumbrical muscles insert into the extensor digital expansion to provide, collectively, flexion of the metacarpophalangeal joints and extension of the interphalangeal joints of the fingers. All of these muscles, with the exception of the first and second lumbrical muscles, are innervated by the deep branch of the ulnar nerve, so this nerve is being tested by placing the hand in the Z-position. If the deep branch of the ulnar nerve were severed, the hand would assume the opposite of the Z-position, which is called "claw hand." **Choice A** (Deep branch of radial nerve) is incorrect. The radial nerve descends from the arm into the cubital fossa, where it divides into superficial and deep branches. The deep branch of the radial nerve pierces the supinator muscle, winds around the proximal end of the radius within the substance of that muscle, and passes into the deep posterior compartment of the forearm as the posterior interosseous nerve. The nerve may be entrapped within the supinator, resulting in supinator syndrome. Such a condition would affect the deeper, more distal extensor muscles arising in the forearm and some sensory areas in the wrist joints. It is not responsible for the Z position of the hand. **Choice B** (Superficial branch of radial nerve) is incorrect. The superficial branch of the radial nerve arises from the radial nerve in the cubital fossa. This nerve is purely a sensory nerve, supplying the dorsum of the hand and fingers. Because it does not have a motor component, this nerve would not be responsible for assuming the Z position of the hand. **Choice C** (Recurrent branch of median nerve) is incorrect. The recurrent (thenar) branch of the median nerve innervates most of the thenar muscles, including the abductor pollicis brevis, opponens pollicis, and superficial head of the flexor pollicis brevis. Cutting this nerve would lead to atrophy of the thenar muscular complex, a condition known as "ape hand." The recurrent branch of the median nerve does not supply muscles outside of the thumb, so it would not be responsible for assuming the hand's Z position. **Choice E** (Superficial branch of ulnar nerve) is incorrect. The superficial branch of the ulnar nerve arises from the ulnar nerve distal to the flexor retinaculum. This nerve supplies cutaneous branches to the anterior surface of the medial one and a half fingers. The palmaris brevis is the only muscle supplied by this nerve, and this muscle tightens the skin of the medial surface of the palm. Therefore, this nerve would not be responsible for the Z position of the hand.

44 **The answer is C: Recurrent branch of median nerve.** The recurrent (thenar) branch of the median nerve lies subcutaneously in the thenar eminence and can be damaged by lacerations in this area. This nerve innervates most of the thenar muscles, including the **O**pponens pollicis, **A**bductor pollicis brevis, and superficial head of the **F**lexor pollicis brevis (mnemonic = "OAF"). Opposition of the thumb would be lost by cutting the recurrent branch of the median nerve. Though the abductor pollicis brevis is denervated, the abductor pollicis longus, innervated by the deep branch of the radial nerve, is still intact. Also, the flexor pollicis longus, innervated by the anterior interosseous nerve, would still allow flexion at the interphalangeal joint of the thumb. Cutting the recurrent branch of the median nerve would lead to atrophy of the thenar muscular complex, a condition known as "ape hand." **Choice A** (Deep branch of the radial nerve) is incorrect. The deep branch of the radial nerve is also called the posterior interosseous nerve as it exits from the supinator muscle. It innervates the abductor pollicis longus and extensor pollicis longus and brevis muscles, which form the boundaries of the anatomical snuffbox. Cutting this nerve would cause loss of extension of the thumb and weakness in abduction. However, the puncture was on the thenar eminence, and the radial nerve does not travel there. **Choice B** (Superficial branch of the radial nerve) is incorrect. The superficial branch of the radial nerve arises from the radial nerve in the cubital fossa. This nerve is purely cutaneous, supplying sensation to the dorsum of the hand and fingers. Because it does not have a motor component, this nerve would not be responsible for the deficit in thumb function. **Choice D** (Deep branch of ulnar nerve) is incorrect. The deep branch of the ulnar nerve innervates most of the intrinsic muscles of the hand, including the hypothenar muscles, medial two lumbrical muscles, the palmar and dorsal interossei, adductor pollicis, and the deep head of the flexor pollicis brevis. With a small motor supply to the thenar compartment (specifically the deep head of the flexor pollicis brevis), this nerve could not cause a substantial loss of function in the thenar eminence. **Choice E** (Superficial branch of the ulnar nerve) is incorrect. The superficial branch of the ulnar nerve arises from the ulnar nerve distal to the flexor retinaculum. This nerve supplies cutaneous branches to the anterior surface of the medial one and a half fingers. The palmaris brevis is the only muscle supplied by this nerve, and this muscle tightens the skin of the medial surface of the palm. Therefore, this nerve would not be responsible for substantial loss of motor function in the thumb.

45 **The answer is B: Anterior axillary lymph nodes.** The primary lymphatic drainage route for the lateral half of the breast (including the axillary tail) plus part of the medial half of the breast is first into the anterior (pectoral; Level 1) axillary lymph nodes. These lymph nodes are located along the lateral border of the pectoralis minor muscle. Further metastasis would spread progressively to the central axillary (Level 2) nodes, then the apical axillary (Level 3) nodes. **Choice A** (Lateral axillary lymph nodes) is incorrect. These nodes, located along the distal segment of the axillary vein, collect the lymphatic drainage from most of the upper limb. They drain to the central axillary (Level 2) nodes. **Choice C** (Deep cervical lymph nodes) is incorrect. These nodes are located in the neck, along the internal jugular vein, and collect lymph from the head and neck. **Choice D** (Parasternal lymph nodes) is incorrect. The parasternal (internal thoracic) nodes lie along the internal thoracic vessels within the chest. Most of the medial half of the breast sends its lymphatic drainage primarily to these nodes. **Choice E** (Contralateral breast lymph nodes) is incorrect. Small areas of the medial aspect of the breast may send an accessory lymphatic drainage across the midline to the contralateral nodes of the opposite breast. Due to the site of the tumor, this lymphatic drainage pattern is unlikely.

46 **The answer is D: Weakness extending the wrist and fingers.** The radial nerve is particularly vulnerable during midshaft humeral fractures because it is located directly against the bone in this region. The radial nerve innervates the extensor muscles of the arm and forearm and also carries sensory innervation from the posterior aspect of the arm, forearm, and hand and the lateral aspect of the arm (but not the forearm). Depending upon the exact placement of the fracture, the nerve fibers that innervate the triceps brachii may have already left the radial nerve. However, the fibers innervating the extensors of the wrist and fingers would still be bundled in the radial nerve and would be vulnerable to damage during a fracture of this type. **Choice A** (Numbness on the lateral [radial] aspect of the forearm) is incorrect. The radial nerve innervates the skin on the posterior aspect of the arm and forearm and the lateral aspect of the lower arm. The lateral (radial) aspect of the forearm is innervated primarily by the lateral cutaneous nerve of the forearm, the terminal branch of the musculocutaneous nerve. **Choice B** (Numbness of the medial aspect of the upper arm) is incorrect. The skin over the medial aspect of the upper arm is innervated by the medial cutaneous nerve of the arm (medial brachial cutaneous nerve) that originates from the medial cord of the brachial plexus. This nerve would be protected from the humeral fracture due to its location. **Choice C** (Numbness over the superolateral aspect of the upper arm) is incorrect. The cutaneous innervation of the superolateral aspect of the upper arm is derived from the axillary nerve that shares a common origin with the radial nerve from the posterior cord of the brachial plexus. Though both nerves arise from the posterior cord, the axillary and radial nerves separate proximal to the site of the fracture, thus leaving the axillary nerve undamaged by the fracture. **Choice E** (Weakness in grip strength) is incorrect. While the pain associated with the fracture would affect the integrity of all muscle activity in the limb, all of the muscles used for gripping (flexing the wrist and digits) are innervated by the median and ulnar nerves, which do not have close relations to the fracture site.

47 **The answer is A: Pectoralis minor.** The pectoralis minor muscle forms a portion of the anterior axillary wall and is used as a marker to organize the contained groups of axillary lymph nodes. In a clinical context, the axillary nodes are organized into three major groups (Level 1, 2, and 3) that denote the progressive lymph drainage of the breast. Level 1 (anterior; pectoral) nodes are located along the lateral border of the pectoralis minor. Level 2 (central; deep) nodes are situated in the center of the axilla, deep (posterior) to the pectoralis minor. Level 3 (apical; medial) nodes are positioned in the apex of the axilla, superior to the upper medial border of the pectoralis minor. Detection of cancer cells in each increasing number level of nodes indicates progressively greater metastasis of the disease out of the breast. **Choice B** (Pectoralis major) is incorrect. The pectoralis major and minor form the anterior axillary wall. However, the pectoralis major muscle is not used to classify the positions of the axillary lymph nodes or levels of metastasis. **Choice C** (Latissimus dorsi) is incorrect. The latissimus dorsi muscle helps to form the posterior wall of the axilla along with the subscapularis and teres major muscles. Due to its posterior location, it is not an important landmark for classification of axillary lymph nodes in breast cancer. **Choice D** (Serratus anterior) is incorrect. This muscle contributes to the formation of the medial wall of the axilla, along with the thoracic cage. This muscle is not an important landmark for classification of axillary lymph nodes in breast cancer. **Choice E** (Subscapularis) is incorrect. The subscapularis muscle helps to form the posterior wall of the axilla along with the latissimus dorsi and teres major muscles. Due to its posterior location, this muscle is not an important landmark for classification of axillary lymph nodes in breast cancer.

48 **The answer is E: Scaphoid.** The proximal segment of the scaphoid bone has a poor supply of blood because the palmar carpal branch of the radial artery enters the distal part of the scaphoid and then supplies blood proximally. This small artery is often severed during fractures of the scaphoid bone leading to avascular necrosis, or death of the bone due to poor blood supply. Remember, the scaphoid is the most commonly fractured carpal bone, but a fracture within this bone is often not seen on initial radiographs. Radiographs taken several weeks later will show the fracture due to bone resorption at the fracture site. **Choice A** (Distal radius) is incorrect. The distal radius is often fractured in older individuals who fall on their outstretched hand. This fracture of the distal radius is called a Colles fracture ("dinner fork deformity") due to its appearance on a lateral radiograph. However, the distal radius has an adequate blood supply and is not prone to avascular necrosis. **Choice B** (Midshaft ulna) is incorrect. A fracture of the midshaft ulna is not prone to avascular necrosis due to its adequate blood supply. **Choice C** (Fifth metacarpal) is incorrect. The fifth metacarpal is often fractured when an individual improperly punches a solid object with a clenched fist, as in a "boxer's fracture." This bone is not prone to avascular necrosis due to its adequate blood supply. **Choice D** (Lunate) is incorrect. The lunate is the most commonly dislocated carpal bone, which leads to severe carpal instabilities. This dislocation often occurs in association with a trans-scaphoid fracture. If this bone were fractured in this work-related accident, it would not be prone to avascular necrosis due to its adequate blood supply.

49 **The answer is C: Dorsal interosseous muscles.** The primary action of the dorsal interossei is to abduct the fingers, which is being tested in this photo. It is also important to remember the dorsal interossei insert into the extensor digital expansion, so these muscles work with the palmar interossei and the lumbrical muscles to extend the interphalangeal joints and flex the metacarpophalangeal joints. The nerve being tested in this patient, via abduction of the fingers, is the deep branch of the ulnar nerve. A mnemonic is "DAB", which stands for **D**orsal interossei **AB**duct the fingers. **Choice A** (Lumbrical Muscles) is incorrect. The lumbrical muscles arise off the flexor digitorum profundus tendons and insert into the lateral (radial) aspect of the extensor digital expansion. Due to their course and insertion, the lumbrical muscles extend the interphalangeal joints and flex the metacarpophalangeal joints. These intrinsic hand muscles are not being tested when a patient abducts the fingers against resistance. **Choice B** (Palmar interosseous muscles) is incorrect. The primary action of the three palmar interossei is to adduct the index finger, ring finger, and little finger toward the axis of the hand, which is the middle finger. The deep branch of the ulnar nerve supplies the palmar interossei. A mnemonic is "PAD", which stands for **P**almar interossei **AD**duct the fingers. It is also important to remember the palmar interossei insert into the extensor digital expansion, so these muscles work in concert with the dorsal interossei and the lumbrical muscles to extend the interphalangeal joints and flex the metacarpophalangeal joints of the fingers. **Choice D** (Flexor digitorum superficialis) is incorrect. The flexor digitorum superficialis muscle flexes the proximal interphalangeal joint in digits 2 to 5, and influences the distal interphalangeal joint by binding the tendons of the flexor digitorum profundus muscle. Flexion of the proximal interphalangeal joints of the fingers is not being tested in this patient. **Choice E** (Flexor digitorum profundus) is incorrect. The flexor digitorum profundus muscle is responsible for flexion of the distal interphalangeal joint in digits 2 to 5; however, this action is not being tested in this photo.

50 **The answer is B: Ulnar nerve in the wrist.** The ulnar nerve can become compressed between the pisiform and hook of the hamate at the wrist in a condition termed "ulnar canal syndrome" or "Guyon tunnel syndrome." This entrapment syndrome is especially seen in professional cyclists who spend countless hours placing pressure on the hook of the hamate bone as they grasp their handlebars. This "handlebar neuropathy" presents with hyperextension of the metacarpophalangeal joints and flexion at the interphalangeal joints of the fourth and fifth fingers. The "clawing" of these two fingers is accompanied by sensory loss in the medial side of the hand. **Choice A** (Ulnar nerve in the elbow) is incorrect. The ulnar nerve crosses the elbow in a narrow space between the olecranon process and the medial epicondyle of the humerus, on the posteromedial (ulnar) side of the joint. Compression of the ulnar nerve at this location leads to "cubital tunnel syndrome" and presents with hand deficits similar to those seen in this patient. However, this patient does not exhibit weakness in flexion or adduction of the wrist. Sparing of these actions indicates that damage to the ulnar nerve must be distal to the elbow. **Choice C** (Median nerve in the wrist) is incorrect. The median nerve is often compressed at the wrist in "carpal tunnel syndrome" because it travels deep to the transverse carpal ligament (flexor retinaculum of the wrist) within the carpal tunnel. This entrapment syndrome presents with paresthesia of the lateral fingers as well as an inability to oppose the thumb and a wasting of the thenar eminence. Damage to the median nerve would not lead to the postural deformity seen in the medial two fingers in this patient. **Choice D** (Median nerve in the elbow) is incorrect. The median nerve is not usually compressed by forced flexion of the elbow because it lies loosely on the flexor surface of the joint deep to the bicipital aponeurosis. The median nerve can be compressed in the proximal forearm as it passes between the two heads of the pronator teres. However, damage to the median nerve would not lead to this patient's postural deformity in the medial two fingers. **Choice E** (Median nerve in the axilla) is incorrect. The median nerve would not be damaged in the axilla without significant trauma. Damage to the median nerve in the axilla would lead to weakness in flexing the wrist, loss of pronation of the forearm, and wasting of the thenar muscles. However, these signs and symptoms were not reported.

51 **The answer is E: Anular ligament of radius.** The anular ligament of the radius encircles and holds the head of the radius in the radial notch of the ulna (see diagram on next page). This ligament enables pronation and supination of the forearm. However, the head of the radius can be pulled distally out of this anular ligament resulting in a subluxation or dislocation of the radial head, which is frequently called "nursemaid's elbow." This injury is often seen in children, particularly girls, between the ages of 1 to 3 years old. It occurs when an extended arm is pulled, commonly during a fall, and the individual holding the hand does not let go, as reported in this case. Subluxation and dislocation of the radial head are also seen when the child is swinging while being held by the hands. **Choice A** (Interosseous membrane of the forearm) is incorrect. The interosseous membrane of the forearm connects the interosseous borders of the radius and ulna. This membrane would not be injured in this type of the injury, especially because the patient complains of pain in the elbow region. **Choice B** (Quadrate ligament) is incorrect. The quadrate ligament passes from the distal margin of the radial notch of the ulna to the neck of the radius. Damage to this ligament is rare in this type of injury when the extended arm is pulled. **Choice C** (Radial collateral ligament of elbow) is incorrect. The radial collateral ligament of the elbow extends from the lateral epicondyle of the humerus to the anular ligament of the radius. This ligament would be injured in forced adduction of the elbow joint, which was not seen in this patient. **Choice D** (Ulnar collateral ligament of elbow) is incorrect. The ulnar collateral ligament of the elbow extends from the medial epicondyle of the humerus to the coronoid process and olecranon of the ulna. This ligament would be injured in forced abduction of the elbow joint, which was not seen in this patient. This ligament is also frequently injured in athletes who use an overhead throwing motion. When the athlete releases the ball during their throwing motion, the ulna is pulled from the humerus, which can damage this ligament. American baseball pitchers often need surgery to repair the ulnar collateral ligament of the elbow, which is commonly termed "Tommy John surgery."

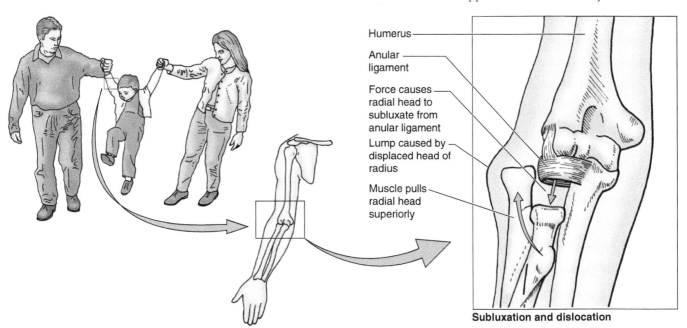

Humerus

Anular ligament

Force causes radial head to subluxate from anular ligament

Lump caused by displaced head of radius

Muscle pulls radial head superiorly

Subluxation and dislocation

Chapter 9

Head and Neck

QUESTIONS

Select the single best answer.

1. A 59-year-old man with a herpes zoster infection within the mandibular division of the trigeminal nerve (CN V₃) complains of weakness when opening his mouth. A comprehensive evaluation reveals that his problems are due to difficulty protruding the mandible, and when protrusion is accomplished the mandible deviates to the left side, as seen in the figure. What muscle is most likely weakened?

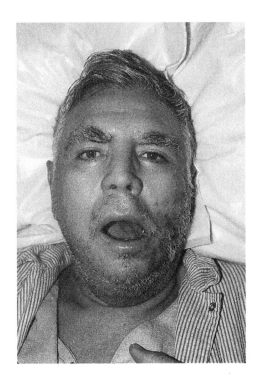

(A) Anterior belly of digastric
(B) Lateral pterygoid
(C) Masseter
(D) Medial pterygoid
(E) Temporalis

2. A 64-year-old male professional angler is diagnosed with a skin melanoma above his right eyebrow after years of excessive sun exposure. His dermatologist removes this cancerous lesion, but the doctor needs to rule out possible metastasis. What group of lymph nodes would his physician first check for possible spread of the cancer?

(A) Deep cervical
(B) Retroauricular
(C) Parotid
(D) Submental
(E) Submandibular

3. A 68-year-old man arrived at the ER with sudden onset of the worst headache of his life, lethargy, and nuchal rigidity. He quickly loses consciousness and dies. Autopsy reveals no traumatic injury; however, the man's subarachnoid space is filled with blood, as seen in the photo. Damage to what blood vessel most likely led to the death of this patient?

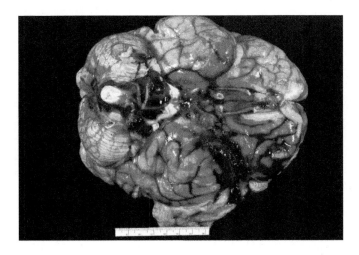

(A) Common carotid artery
(B) Middle meningeal artery
(C) Facial artery
(D) Superior cerebral veins
(E) Cerebral arterial circle

4. A 15-year-old young man developed cavernous sinus thrombophlebitis after a 1-week history of a single acne-like lesion at the anterior tip of his nose. He presented with a headache, periorbital edema, diplopia, and a fever (103°F or 39.4°C). What vein is the most likely route for the spread of this infection to the cavernous sinus?

(A) Ophthalmic
(B) Superior cerebral
(C) Great cerebral (of Galen)
(D) Maxillary
(E) Supraorbital

5 A 27-year-old man comes to his doctor complaining that the floor of his mouth is painful and swollen. Bimanual palpation and later computed tomography show an 8-mm stone (sialolith) in the right submandibular salivary duct, as indicated by the arrow in the figure. If the submandibular duct is partially obstructed, where would the physician observe salivation in the oral cavity after applying pressure to the right submandibular gland?

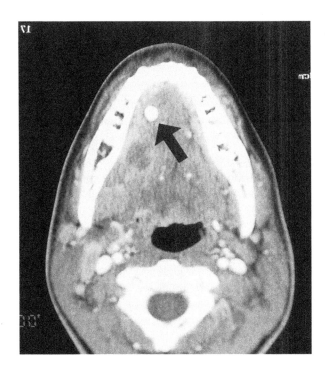

(A) Second maxillary molar tooth
(B) Oral vestibule
(C) Palatine mucosa
(D) Sublingual fold
(E) Lingual frenulum

6 A 65-year-old man complains of a persistent nosebleed. His physician uses a cotton swab to apply pressure at the source, the inferior and posterior aspects of the lateral nasal wall. Which artery is the most likely source of the bleeding?
(A) Greater palatine
(B) Infraorbital
(C) Facial
(D) Anterior ethmoidal
(E) Sphenopalatine

7 A 16-year-old girl experiences mild ptosis and miosis (pupillary constriction) in her right eye following resection of a lymphangioma from the apex of her right lung, as seen in the photo. Vision in each eye is normal. These findings are most likely due to a lesion involving which structure on the right?

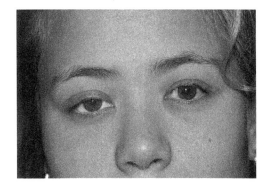

(A) Cervical posterior roots
(B) Thoracic posterior roots
(C) Thoracic anterior roots
(D) Thoracic posterior primary rami
(E) Thoracic gray rami communicantes

8 A 75-year-old man tells his physician he has been having progressively more trouble opening his left eye because his upper eyelid tends to droop. Which of the following muscles is most likely weakened?
(A) Orbicularis oculi
(B) Frontalis
(C) Levator palpebrae superioris
(D) Superior rectus
(E) Orbital muscle

9 Mandibulofacial dysostosis (Treacher-Collins syndrome) is a developmental disorder characterized by craniofacial deformities, including malformed or absent ears, zygomatic and mandibular hypoplasia, and downward slanting eyes exhibiting ptosis of the lateral eyelids, as shown in the photo. This condition is the result of lack of migration of neural crest cells into what pharyngeal arch?

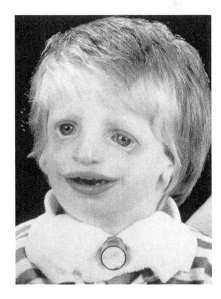

(A) First pharyngeal arch
(B) Second pharyngeal arch
(C) Third pharyngeal arch
(D) Fourth pharyngeal arch
(E) Fifth pharyngeal arch

10 A 68-year-old man was choking on a piece of steak at a family restaurant. Despite attempts to dislodge the food via abdominal thrusts (or the Heimlich maneuver), his upper airway remained blocked. An emergency medical technician (EMT), eating at the scene, performed an emergency tracheotomy to enable the man to breathe. Which subcutaneous structure was most likely cut during this procedure?

(A) Cricoid cartilage
(B) Thyrohyoid membrane
(C) Cricothyroid membrane
(D) Tracheal rings
(E) Isthmus of thyroid gland

11 A 7-year-old boy was kicked in the right side of his head during a sledding accident. He arrived at the ER with no loss of consciousness but complained of a severe headache and vomiting. A computed tomography (CT) scan revealed a biconvex hyperdense extraaxial collection of blood, indicated by the arrows in the figure. What blood vessel is the most likely source of the bleed?

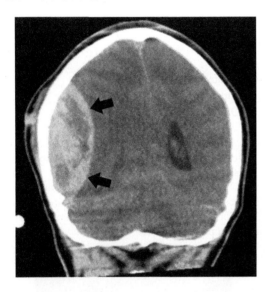

(A) Superficial temporal artery
(B) Middle meningeal artery
(C) Superior cerebral veins
(D) Cerebral arterial circle (of Willis)
(E) Middle cerebral artery (MCA)

12 A newborn infant exhibits labored, gasping breathes and unusual vocal tones when crying. Thorough examination reveals the child has malformed vocal folds due to displaced attachments of the vocal ligaments. Which of the following structures is most likely defective in this condition?

(A) Arytenoid cartilages
(B) Cricoid cartilage
(C) Epiglottic cartilage
(D) Corniculate cartilages
(E) Cuneiform cartilages

13 A baby girl presents with a disproportionately wide skull with a short occipitofrontal diameter, as depicted in the given surface shaded CT reconstruction. What cranial suture most likely closed prematurely to result in this cranial deformity?

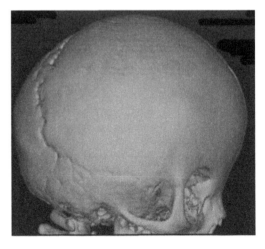

(A) Sphenosquamous
(B) Sphenoparietal
(C) Lambdoid
(D) Coronal
(E) Sagittal

14 A 22-year-old man receives a stab wound in the left anterior cervical region, at the C2 vertebral level. The wound was 3 cm deep and located anterior to the sternocleidomastoid muscle (SCM) and superior to the greater horn of the hyoid bone. During a postoperative examination, the patient displays dysarthria, or difficulty speaking. Which of the following structures is most likely damaged?

(A) Hypoglossal nerve
(B) Accessory nerve
(C) Mandibular division of trigeminal nerve
(D) Lingual branch of glossopharyngeal nerve
(E) Roots of the brachial plexus

15 A 60-year-old female yodeler with a 43-year history of smoking complains of pain during swallowing and hoarseness in her voice. A fiberoptic endoscopy reveals a laryngeal squamous cell carcinoma at the location identified by the arrow within the given figure. What structure is most likely affected by this laryngeal cancer?

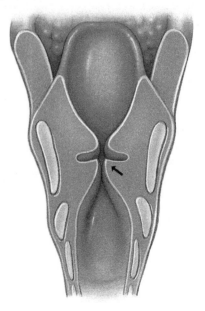

(A) Infraglottic cavity
(B) Vocal folds
(C) Vestibular folds
(D) Laryngeal vestibule
(E) Epiglottis

16 A 9-year-old girl with a history of strep throat has her palatine tonsils surgically removed. She returns to the hospital 3 days later with a high fever and chest pain. A physician orders a CT scan, which revealed spread of infection into the superior mediastinum. What is the most likely route for this infection to descend through the neck to reach the superior mediastinum?

(A) Parapharyngeal space
(B) Retropharyngeal space
(C) Buccal space
(D) Carotid sheath
(E) Suprasternal space

17 A 23-year-old man was punched in the left eye in a bar fight, which resulted in periorbital edema and ecchymosis. In the ER, the man refuses to open his eye, and when his eyelids are pried opened he exhibits vertical diplopia, specifically when asked to look up. A coronal CT reformat image reveals asymmetry in the left orbit and the superior antrum of the maxillary sinus, apparent in the given image. What is the most likely cause of the patient's diplopia?

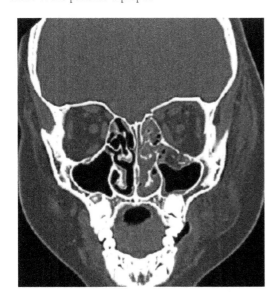

(A) Paralysis of lateral rectus muscle
(B) Entrapment of inferior rectus muscle
(C) Detached retina
(D) Paralysis of superior oblique muscle
(E) Damage to infraorbital nerve

18 A 23-year-old female professional student wakes up with a facial nerve (CN VII or Bell) palsy. What muscle will continue to function despite this affliction?

(A) Zygomaticus major
(B) Levator labii superioris
(C) Buccinator
(D) Masseter
(E) Platysma

19 A newborn baby girl is unable to move her head to the right, even when her pediatrician tries to assist the movement, as seen in the photo. Her range of motion in the neck is limited in rotation and lateral bending, and her head posture is abnormally tilted toward the right and her chin is elevated and turned toward the left side. What muscle is most likely responsible for the baby's abnormal range of movement and head posture?

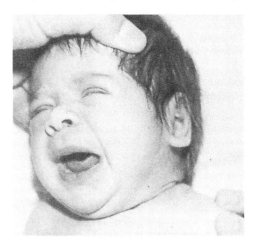

(A) Platysma
(B) Trapezius
(C) Sternocleidomastoid
(D) Masseter
(E) Digastric

20 A professional student finds out she has a perfect score on the anatomy portion of her board examination and her muscles of facial expression produce a long anticipated smile. What muscle is assisting her in elevating her labial commissure bilaterally to smile?

(A) Zygomaticus major
(B) Zygomaticus minor
(C) Levator labii superioris
(D) Buccinator
(E) Orbicularis oris

21 A physician noticed a keyhole appearance of the right pupil in a 21-year-old woman characteristic of a defect of the iris known as coloboma, as seen in the photo. When asked about her affected eye, the patient responds that she was born with the condition. What is the most likely cause of this coloboma of the iris?

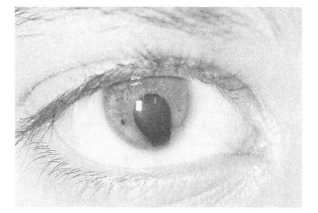

(A)   Traumatic damage to the sphincter muscle of the pupil
(B)   Interruption of neural crest cell migration
(C)   Persistent pupillary membrane
(D)   Failure of fusion of the retinal fissure
(E)   Lack of fusion of inner and outer layers of the optic cup

22   A 62-year-old male factory worker went to his doctor complaining of a progressive hearing loss. Audiometric tests reveal an inability to detect high-frequency sound waves, but the rest of his hearing scores within the normal range. What is the most likely location of injury for this sensorineural hearing loss?

(A)   Tympanic membrane
(B)   External acoustic meatus
(C)   Hair cells in the apex of the cochlea
(D)   Hair cells located in the middle of the cochlea
(E)   Hair cells in the base of the cochlea

23   A 4-year-old girl presents with nausea, vomiting, papilledema, and a headache, which is more severe when she wakes up in the morning. A sagittal T1-weighted MRI reveals a medulloblastoma, outlined in the image, in the posterior cranial fossa. Its location has compressed the 4th ventricle, impeding the flow of cerebrospinal fluid (CSF) from the 3rd ventricle via the cerebral aqueduct, indicated by the black arrow. The MRI shows massive dilation of the lateral and 3rd ventricles, shallow cortex, and effaced sulci within the cerebral hemispheres. Which of the following selections describes this condition?

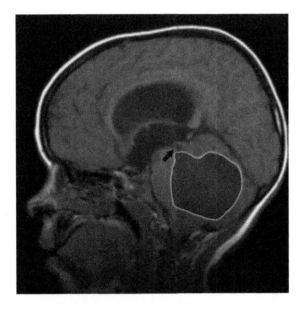

(A)   Dandy-Walker syndrome
(B)   Chiari malformation
(C)   Noncommunicating hydrocephalus
(D)   Congenital communicating hydrocephalus
(E)   Acquired communicating hydrocephalus

24   A 36-year-old woman comes to her physician complaining of heart palpitations, weight loss, anxiety, insomnia, fatigue, and amenorrhea. The physician palpates a 1.5-cm mass on her neck, which elevates when she swallows, located inferior to the cricoid cartilage yet off the midline. What is the most likely structure involved with her presentation?

(A)   Enlarged deep cervical lymph node
(B)   Thyroid nodule
(C)   Benign parathyroid adenoma
(D)   Thyroglossal duct cyst
(E)   Branchial cyst

25   During preparation to extract the right maxillary (upper) canine tooth, a dentist has difficulty anesthetizing this tooth and its associated gingivae. Therefore, the dentist administers a regional nerve block, depicted in the given photo, in which the anesthetic syringe needle penetrates the oral mucosa at the apex of the maxillary vestibule and is pushed beyond the roots of the teeth. Due to this injection, the patient experiences numbness and paresthesia within the upper canine and neighboring teeth, as well as the skin of the right inferior eyelid, cheek, lateral nose, and upper lip. What nerve was blocked and produced the described numbness?

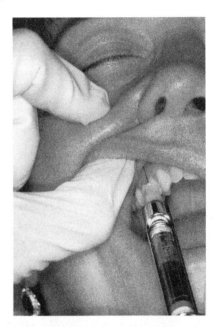

(A)   Anterior superior alveolar
(B)   External nasal
(C)   Infratrochlear
(D)   Infraorbital
(E)   Nasopalatine

26   A 36-year-old man flips over the handlebars of his motorcycle and falls on the asphalt pavement, striking his head. He was not wearing a helmet. Although alert after the fall, he has a clear nasal discharge that tests positive for glucose. The patient most likely has a fracture of which of the following bones?

(A)   Ethmoid
(B)   Vomer
(C)   Sphenoid
(D)   Maxilla
(E)   Frontal

27   A 42-year-old man has a lymph node biopsy in the left side of his lateral cervical region or posterior triangle of his neck. After closure of the wound, the physician asks the patient to rotate his head to the right against resistance, as shown in the photo. What nerve is the doctor assessing with this test?

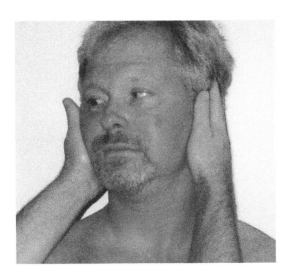

(A) Hypoglossal

(B) Accessory

(C) Mandibular division of trigeminal

(D) Great auricular

(E) Upper trunk of the brachial plexus

28 A 10-year-old boy was admitted to the hospital with a sore throat, earache, and high fever. On examination, he had severely swollen palatine tonsils (tonsillitis). What nerve carries the sensory input for most of the patient's symptoms?

(A) Greater palatine

(B) Lesser palatine

(C) Vagus

(D) Posterior superior alveolar

(E) Glossopharyngeal

29 A 10-year-old girl presents with a smooth, round neck mass the size of a golf ball at the upper third of the anterior border of her right sternocleidomastoid muscle, as seen in the photo. Her mother says this once small, peanut-sized mass grew without pain or inflammation after it became noticeable 2 months previously. The mass does not affect the girl's daily activities. What is the most likely diagnosis for the pictured mass?

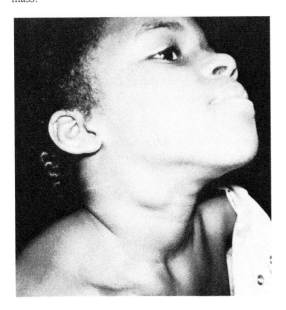

(A) Thyroglossal cyst

(B) Branchial cyst

(C) Undescended thymus

(D) Preauricular cyst

(E) Ectopic palatine tonsil

30 A 31-year-old woman with an ongoing, long-term history of alcoholism becomes pregnant. The embryo she is carrying suffers a neural crest insufficiency during the critical period of development. Which of the following structures is most likely to be malformed as a result of this condition?

(A) Laryngeal cartilages

(B) Parietal bones

(C) Maxillary bones

(D) Common carotid arteries

(E) Thyroid gland

31 A 17-year-old girl uses Accutane, an acne drug implicated in interfering with normal development of the facial primordia, early in her unexpected pregnancy. Examination of the newborn reveals the craniofacial defect seen in the photo. In this case, the defect is related to failure of fusion of what craniofacial processes?

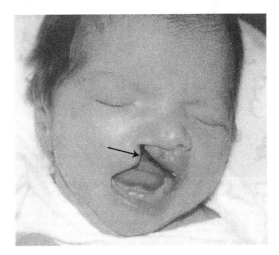

(A) Maxillary and medial nasal processes

(B) Opposite maxillary processes

(C) Medial and lateral nasal processes

(D) Maxillary and lateral nasal processes

(E) Opposite medial nasal processes

32 A young child suffers a debilitating condition that includes progressive degeneration of the motor axons that innervate the masseter muscle. Which of the following muscles is most likely to exhibit the same fate?

(A) Genioglossus

(B) Tensor tympani

(C) Orbicularis oris

(D) Levator veli palatini

(E) Stylopharyngeus

33 A 25-year-old woman notes the pictured asymmetry in her neck when she tenses the skin of her inferior face and neck. This asymmetry may be due to a limited mesodermal migration in which of the following embryonic structures?

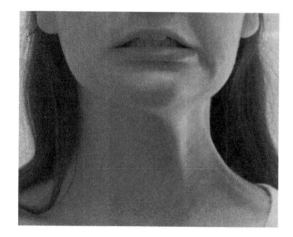

(A) First pharyngeal arch
(B) Second pharyngeal arch
(C) Third pharyngeal arch
(D) Fourth pharyngeal arch
(E) Fifth pharyngeal arch

34 A 78-year-old man presents with signs of reduced blood flow into the right side of his face. His physician wishes to take a pulse of the facial artery on both sides to help evaluate the situation. The pulse of the facial artery can be readily palpated at which of the following locations?
(A) Lateral side of the body of the hyoid bone
(B) Inferior edge of the zygomatic arch
(C) Apex of the zygomatic bone
(D) Lateral surface of the nasal bone
(E) Inferior margin of the body of the mandible

35 Holoprosencephaly is a complex of developmental abnormalities characterized by the loss of midline structures to greater or lesser degrees. The pictured infant suffers multiple aspects of this disorder, including the midline cleft indicated. This specific developmental malformation is termed "premaxillary agenesis," developmental failure of formation of the intermaxillary segment of the face. Which of the following structures is most likely to be affected in this condition?

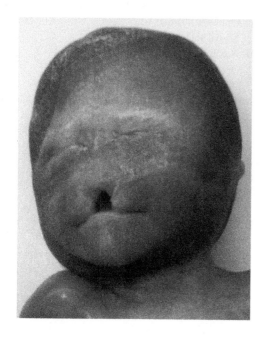

(A) Nasal bones
(B) Soft palate
(C) Inferior nasal conchae
(D) Philtrum
(E) Mandibular incisors

36 Startled by a loud noise while shaving his head with a straight razor, a young man accidentally cuts his scalp, severing branches of the supraorbital and superficial temporal vessels. The scalp wound appears modest but bleeds profusely. In what layer of the scalp do the severed vessels reside?
(A) Skin
(B) Dense connective tissue
(C) Epicranial aponeurosis
(D) Loose connective tissue
(E) Pericranium

37 A 9-year-old girl suffers from the mumps, causing unilateral inflammation of her right parotid gland, as seen in the photo. The girl is experiencing great pain due to the stretched capsule of the parotid gland. Her physician is also concerned about the condition of the structures contained within the gland. Which of the following structures may be directly compressed in this situation?

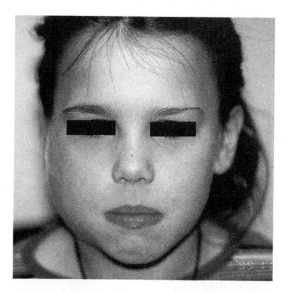

(A) Buccal nerve of CN V_3
(B) Auriculotemporal nerve
(C) Posterior belly of the digastric muscle
(D) External jugular vein
(E) Facial artery

38 As a result of facial injuries suffered in an automobile accident, a 17-year-old girl is unable to close her lips together tightly. Which of the following muscles is paralyzed?
(A) Zygomaticus major
(B) Buccinator
(C) Levator labii superioris
(D) Orbicularis oris
(E) Mentalis

39 A 50-year-old man presents with recurring dizziness, ataxia, vertigo, aphasia, and weakness in his right upper limb. A magnetic resonance angiogram (MRA) revealed a stenosis of the right subclavian artery (marked by the arrow) and poststenotic dilatation, which led to the diagnosis of subclavian steal syndrome. In this condition, blood is shunted from the left side arterial tree via collateral flow into the right side circulation. Through which of the following ipsilateral vessels is blood entering the right subclavian artery distal to the stenosis?

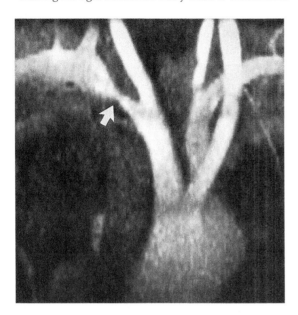

(A) Internal thoracic artery
(B) Common carotid artery
(C) Vertebral artery
(D) Superior thyroid artery
(E) Suprascapular artery

40 A newborn infant has difficulty in breastfeeding due to unilateral atrophy in the area of the face occupied by the levator labii superioris, levator anguli oris, and lateral upper part of the orbicularis oris muscles. This region of the face is derived from which of the following embryonic sources?

(A) Maxillary process
(B) Mandibular process
(C) Frontal process
(D) Lateral nasal process
(E) Medial nasal process

41 A tumor growing at the base of the skull impinges upon the opening indicated by the arrow, severely compressing its contents. Which of the following conditions is the most likely result?

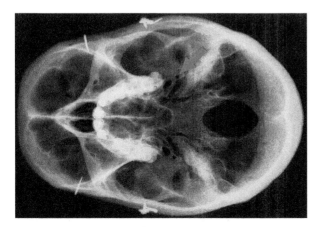

(A) Venous drainage from the base of the brain is obstructed
(B) Mucus secretion in the oral floor is reduced
(C) Sensation from the mandibular teeth is lost
(D) Motor control of the upper pharynx is lost
(E) Arterial supply to the dura mater is reduced

42 A 43-year-old man presents with loss of control of facial expression across the entire right side. The corner of his mouth droops on the right side, but he can clench his jaw and chew on demand. During examination, his physician also notes loss of hearing on the right side, and the patient has difficulty maintaining balance while standing on one foot. The patient's corneal (blink) reflex is absent in the right eye, but cutaneous sensation is normal on the entire face. The physician orders radiographic imaging in anticipation of finding a tumor. What is the most likely location of the tumor?

(A) Internal acoustic meatus
(B) Foramen ovale
(C) Foramen rotundum
(D) Geniculum of the facial canal
(E) Stylomastoid foramen

43 An 8-year-old boy suffers a fracture at the base of the skull from the impact of a terrorist bomb explosion. The skull trauma includes a lesion of the vagus nerve. Damage at which of the indicated openings would injure the vagus nerve?

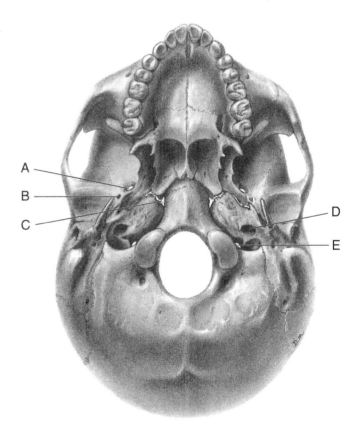

44 During a difficult childbirth, a physician uses obstetric forceps to grip the infant's head as an aid to extracting her from the birth canal. However, the forceps are misapplied at the right stylomastoid foramen and crush its contents at the opening of the foramen. Which of the following ipsilateral deficits is the baby most likely to suffer?

(A) Reduced blood flow to the inner ear
(B) No sensation in the external acoustic meatus
(C) Inability to close the eyelids
(D) Lack of taste on the body of the tongue
(E) Inability to tense the eardrum

45 Which of the following labeled areas indicates the petrous portion of the temporal bone?

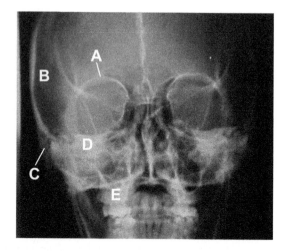

46 If normal evagination of the endodermal lining of the embryonic pharynx does not take place between the pharyngeal (branchial) arches, the pharyngeal (branchial) pouches will not form. Maldevelopment of the first pharyngeal pouch during embryonic weeks 4 to 5 is most likely to result in a congenital disorder of which of the following structures?
(A) Thyroid gland
(B) Thymus gland
(C) Parathyroid glands
(D) Facial muscles
(E) Tympanic cavity

47 A 35-year-old man complains to his physician that he feels congested, has trouble with nasal breathing, and is experiencing a yellowish nasal mucus discharge. He also mentions that his right side upper molar teeth ache terribly. A thorough physical examination reveals maxillary sinusitis. The discharge from this sinus initially drains into the nasal cavity at which of the labeled points within this drawing of the lateral nasal wall?

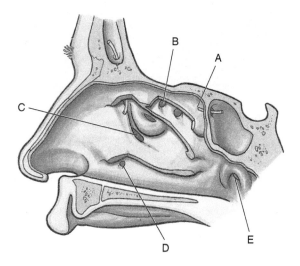

48 A 45-year-old man is in surgery. While seated at the head of the operating table, the anesthesiologist periodically checks the patient's pulse by palpating the artery located anterior to the tragus of the external ear. Which of the following arteries is being utilized to monitor the patient's pulse?
(A) Maxillary
(B) Posterior auricular
(C) Superficial temporal
(D) Facial
(E) Internal carotid

49 A 32-year-old woman undergoes LASIK refractive surgery to improve her visual acuity and rid herself of eyeglasses. To combat dry eyes, a common complication of this surgery, her ophthalmologist inserts a silicone plug, marked by an arrow in the given photo, to block drainage of tears from the patient's left eye. Obstruction of what structure prevents tears from entering the lacrimal apparatus?

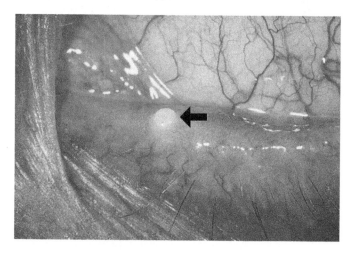

(A) Lacrimal punctum
(B) Lacrimal canaliculus
(C) Lacrimal sac
(D) Nasolacrimal duct
(E) Inferior nasal meatus

50 In the process of removing cervical lymph nodes during a radical neck dissection, a surgeon mistakenly lesions the ansa cervicalis. Which of the following deficits may occur?
(A) Decreased blood flow to the larynx
(B) Lymphedema in the carotid triangle of the neck
(C) Reduced sensation in the skin over the posterior triangle of the neck
(D) Paralysis of several infrahyoid (strap) muscles
(E) Paralysis of the intrinsic laryngeal muscles

51 Identify the structure indicated with the letter "X" in this X-ray of the lateral neck.

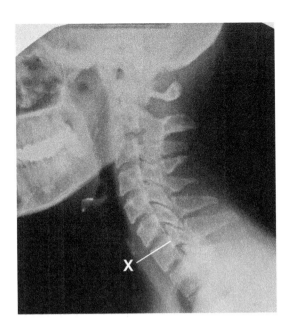

(A) Vertebral body
(B) Pedicle
(C) Intervertebral disc space
(D) Superior articular process
(E) Inferior articular process

52 A paralyzed right true vocal fold is most likely associated with which of the following situations?
(A) Repair of a patent ductus arteriosus
(B) Repair of an aortic aneurysm
(C) A gunshot wound below the second rib
(D) Surgical removal of the thyroid gland
(E) Obstruction of the thoracic duct

53 Lesion of the trunks of the brachial plexus is most likely to occur from a penetrating wound into which of the following labeled areas in the given drawing of the neck regions?

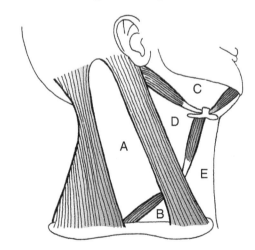

54 A 47-year-old man has trouble with double vision (diplopia) after striking his head on the steering wheel in a car accident. During a subsequent eye examination, his ophthalmologist asks him to first look inward (toward his nose) and then upward (toward the ceiling). The integrity of which of the following extraocular muscles is being tested?

(A) Superior oblique
(B) Inferior oblique
(C) Lateral rectus
(D) Inferior rectus
(E) Superior rectus

55 Which of the labeled structures is derived from the body of the first cervical vertebra in this labeled X-ray showing a transoral view of the upper cervical vertebrae?

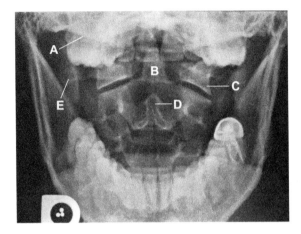

56 During extraction of her impacted wisdom teeth, a 22-year-old woman suffers damage to her right inferior alveolar nerve. Which of the following conditions is most likely to result?
(A) Inability to compress the cheek
(B) Paresthesia of the lower lip
(C) Weakness in closing the jaw
(D) Decreased salivary flow
(E) Reduced taste in the body of the tongue

57 The following computed tomography (CT) scan shows a left crescent-shaped extraaxial hematoma, indicated by the arrows, compressing the brain of a 17-year-old woman, who impacted the front of her head on the steering wheel during a head-on motor vehicular accident. Given the radiologic imaging results and the history of the accident, what blood vessel(s) is/are the most likely source for this cerebral hemorrhage?

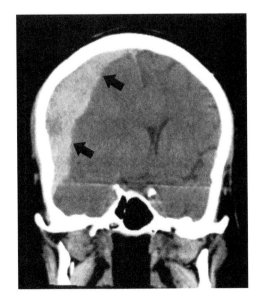

(A) Middle meningeal artery
(B) Superficial temporal artery
(C) Cerebral arterial circle
(D) Superior cerebral veins
(E) Occipital artery

58 A 35-year-old woman comes to her dentist complaining of tenderness and pain in her cheek near the parotid gland, as well as bad breath and a foul-tasting mouth at meal times. A radiopaque fluid is injected into the parotid duct system through cannulation, and this sialography of the parotid duct confirms blockage by a calculus (sialolith). What muscle, through which the parotid duct passes, is most likely causing the stenosis where the sialolith now resides, blocking the drainage of the parotid duct?

(A) Buccinator
(B) Mentalis
(C) Temporalis
(D) Orbicularis oris
(E) Masseter

59 A 33-year-old woman presents with rapid weight gain, particularly in the trunk and face with sparing of the limbs, excess sweating, thinning of the skin, and hirsutism (facial male-pattern hair growth). A full examination also reveals bitemporal hemianopsia (or tunnel vision). What of the following labeled areas on the given X-ray of the lateral skull will be of most interest to the physician?

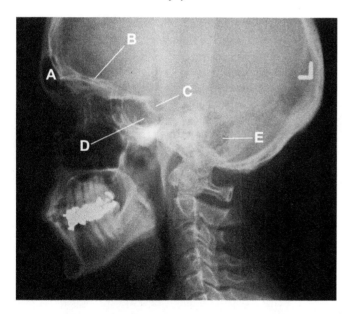

60 A tumor is discovered embedded in the posterior wall of the tympanic cavity in a 45-year-old man. If the tumor erodes through this wall, which of the following structures will it first encounter?

(A) Internal jugular vein
(B) Tympanic membrane
(C) Internal carotid artery
(D) Brain
(E) Facial nerve

61 An 8-year-old boy comes to his physician with a painless and smooth mass located in the midline of his neck at the level of the hyoid bone, as noted by the arrow in the given photo. This palpable, midline neck mass was asymptomatic, but due to recent expansion, it has caused difficulty and pain when swallowing. When he swallows or protrudes his tongue, the mass moves superiorly. What is the most likely diagnosis?

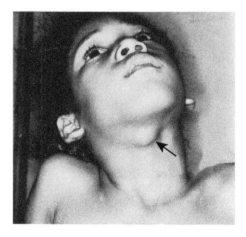

(A) Enlarged deep cervical lymph node
(B) Thyroid nodule
(C) Benign parathyroid adenoma
(D) Thyroglossal duct cyst
(E) Branchial cyst

62 During a fight between two construction workers, one man strikes the other with a hammer at the pterion of the skull. Which of the following bones may be fractured?

(A) Zygomatic process of the temporal bone
(B) Greater wing of the sphenoid bone
(C) Mastoid process of the temporal bone
(D) Lateral pterygoid plate of the sphenoid bone
(E) Coronoid process of the mandible

63 The given photo shows a superior view of the head of a baby boy with scaphocephaly. Which of the following sutures closed prematurely in this infant?

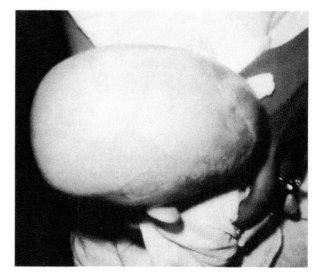

(A) Coronal

(B) Sagittal

(C) Lambdoid

(D) Metopic

(E) Squamous

64 A bony overgrowth narrows the pterygomaxillary fissure, compressing the third part of the maxillary artery. As a result, blood flow will be reduced in which of the following arteries?

(A) Superficial temporal

(B) Sphenopalatine

(C) Inferior alveolar

(D) Middle meningeal

(E) Ophthalmic

65 A 17-year-old woman presents with an anterior dislocation of her temporomandibular joint (TMJ), as shown in the diagram. With her mandible stuck in the protruded (protracted) position, her dentist pulls the mandible inferiorly to enable the tone of a muscle to retrude (retract) the mandible to its normal position. Which muscle returns the mandibular condyle back into its normal position after it clears the articular eminence?

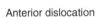

Anterior dislocation

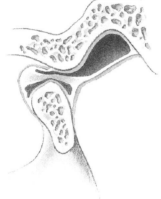

(A) Lateral pterygoid

(B) Masseter

(C) Medial pterygoid

(D) Stylohyoid

(E) Temporalis

66 During a mixed martial arts (MMA) fight, one fighter punched his opponent in the anterior neck, resulting in a fracture of the hyoid bone. Which of the following muscles would be most directly affected by this injury?

(A) Palatopharyngeus

(B) Stylopharyngeus

(C) Superior pharyngeal constrictor

(D) Middle pharyngeal constrictor

(E) Inferior pharyngeal constrictor

67 A 40-year-old woman suffers from headaches, nausea, vomiting, and multiple lower cranial nerve involvement. Her physician orders a CT soft tissue neck study, and the given coronal CT shows a mass lesion (tumor) centered at the jugular foramen and identified by arrows. This tumor has destroyed the jugular foramen and hypoglossal canal on the right side and damaged the cranial nerves traversing these foramina. In this patient, which of the following functions will remain intact?

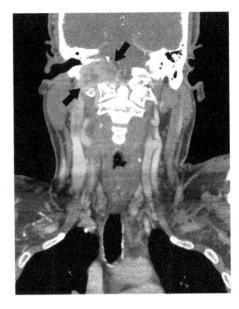

(A) Control of the true vocal fold

(B) Taste in the anterior two thirds of the tongue

(C) Symmetric protrusion of the tongue

(D) Sensation in the tympanic cavity

(E) Elevation of the shoulder

68 The external laryngeal nerve of a 23-year-old man becomes ensnared and tightly compressed by a tortuous superior thyroid artery, which parallels the course of this nerve. Which of the following functions is most likely to be affected?

(A) Sensation above the true vocal fold

(B) Sensation below the true vocal fold

(C) Abduction of the vocal cord

(D) Tension of the vocal cord

(E) Depression of the hyoid bone

69 An 82-year-old woman develops a dural meningioma (tumor) that compresses the confluence of the dural venous sinuses. On the given contrast venogram from an angiographic series, drainage from which of the following labeled vessels would be impeded by the tumor?

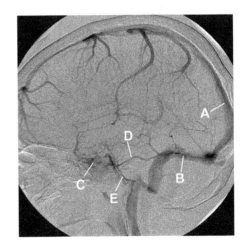

(A) Superior sagittal sinus

(B) Transverse sinus

(C) Cavernous sinus

(D) Superior petrosal sinus

(E) Inferior petrosal sinus

70 A 9-year-old girl with a history of middle ear infections presents with pain, tenderness, and inflammation located posterior to her right auricle. What is the most likely diagnosis, given her current symptoms?

(A) Otitis externa

(B) Blockage of pharyngotympanic tube

(C) Mastoiditis

(D) Perforated tympanic membrane

(E) Ménière syndrome

71 A 21-year-old professional boxer receives a series of powerful punches to the side of his face, which fractures the left mandible slightly superior to the mandibular angle as indicated by the arrow on the given CT scan. Resultant muscle spasticity causes his jaw to close, making it difficult to remove his mouthpiece. Which of the following muscles is acting to close the jaw?

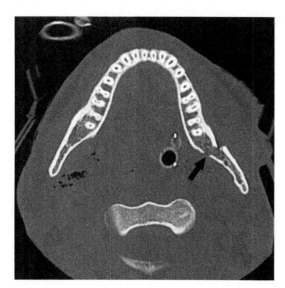

(A) Temporalis

(B) Lateral pterygoid

(C) Zygomaticus major

(D) Masseter

(E) Posterior digastric

72 As part of an initial oral examination of a new patient, a dental hygienist inspects the vestibule of the mouth. Which of the following structures is encountered in this area?

(A) Lingual frenulum

(B) Opening of the parotid duct

(C) Opening of the submandibular duct

(D) Uvula

(E) Palatine tonsil

73 Genetic testing of a baby boy with facial and cardiovascular anomalies reveals a small deletion in chromosome 22, specifically 22q11.2. This 22q11.2 deletion (DiGeorge) syndrome often results in migration defects of neural crest cells within the pharyngeal pouches. In this DiGeorge syndrome patient, the thymus and inferior parathyroid glands are absent. Which of the following pharyngeal pouches is most likely affected?

(A) First

(B) Second

(C) Third

(D) Fourth

(E) Fifth

74 While participating in a bar fight, the orbit of a 25-year-old man is pierced by a broken pool cue stick, which extends back to the superior orbital fissure. Which of the following nerves is most likely damaged?

(A) Optic nerve

(B) Facial nerve

(C) Mandibular division of trigeminal

(D) Maxillary division of trigeminal

(E) Ophthalmic division of trigeminal

75 A physician examines a 53-year-old woman and notes deviation of the uvula to the right and asymmetry in the elevation of the soft palate, with the palatal arch of the left side sagging when compared to the right. The muscles involved in these abnormal findings are most likely derived from the mesoderm of what pharyngeal arch?

(A) First

(B) Second

(C) Third

(D) Fourth

(E) Sixth

ANSWERS AND DISCUSSION

1 **The answer is B: Lateral pterygoid.** The lateral pterygoid muscle acts on the temporomandibular joint (TMJ) to cause protrusion (or protraction) of the mandible. During the contraction of the lateral pterygoid muscle, the mandibular condyle slides anterior (translation) to be located inferior to the articular eminence of the temporal bone, which enables the mouth to open passively due to gravity. Acting unilaterally, the lateral pterygoid muscle produces side-to-side movements. So, the patient has all of the signs of a paralyzed lateral pterygoid muscle on the left side, including weakness protruding the mandible, weakness opening the oral fissure (or mouth), and the lateral deviation of the mandible during protrusion. In this patient, herpes zoster, or shingles, is a painful skin rash affecting the mandibular division (or motor root) of the trigeminal nerve (CN V₃). Shingles is seen in patients who have had previous exposure to the varicella zoster virus, which causes chickenpox in children or young adults. After the initial exposure to chickenpox, this virus can reside latent in ganglia of an individual for years. If this individual becomes immunocompromised, the skin (or dermatomes supplied by the infected ganglia) can develop shingles, a painful skin rash, which blisters, breaks open, crusts over, and then disappears. In this patient, the herpetic lesions were found in the sensory distribution of the left CN V₃, which means the virus resides in the trigeminal (or semilunar) ganglion. This herpes zoster infection also affected the motor root of CN V₃, which is why the lateral pterygoid muscle displayed weakness in this patient. **Choice A** (Anterior belly of digastric) is incorrect. The anterior belly of the digastric muscle is a suprahyoid muscle that assists in the elevation of the hyoid bone during swallowing. It has no role in the deviation of the mandible during protrusion. **Choice C** (Masseter) is incorrect. The masseter primarily works to close the jaw. Though its superficial fibers may play a limited role in protrusion of the mandible, it is the deviation of the mandible to the left that signals involvement of the left lateral pterygoid muscle. **Choice D** (Medial pterygoid) is incorrect. The medial pterygoid functions to elevate the mandible. Though it may play a limited role in protrusion of the mandible, it is the deviation of the mandible to the left that signals involvement of the left lateral pterygoid muscle. **Choice E** (Temporalis) is incorrect. The temporalis muscle is also involved with elevation of the mandible leading to closure of the jaw; however, its middle and oblique fibers are the primary retractors of the mandible. These actions did not display weakness in this patient.

2 **The answer is C: Parotid.** The parotid lymph nodes receive lymphatic drainage from the lateral part of the anterior scalp, anterior part of the auricle, and the lateral part of the face, including the upper and lower eyelids. Due to the site of the skin melanoma above the right eyebrow, the physician must first check the parotid lymph nodes for spread of cancer. This task can be accomplished by sentinel lymph node mapping, which is a technique for locating the lymph node that is most likely to receive primary drainage from the melanoma. The sentinel node, identified by this procedure, is the most likely lymph node to contain cancer and can be surgically removed if lymphogenous spread of cancer is suspected. **Choice A** (Deep cervical) is incorrect. The deep cervical lymph nodes run along the internal jugular vein to return lymph to the systemic venous return at the junction of the internal jugular and subclavian veins (or the venous angle). This set of lymph nodes receives lymphatic drainage from deep structures within the neck, including the larynx and pharynx. These lymph nodes would receive secondary drainage of the tumor site if the cancer is more advanced in staging; however, the deep cervical lymph nodes would not be the first nodes to be checked by the physician. **Choice B** (Retroauricular) is incorrect. The retroauricular lymph nodes receive lymphatic drainage from the posterior part of the auricle and lateral aspects of the middle scalp. However, these areas do not include the anterior scalp above the forehead where the melanoma was located in this patient. **Choice D** (Submental) is incorrect. The submental lymph nodes receive lymphatic drainage from the middle part of the lower lip, chin, frenulum and tip of the tongue, and the anterior floor of the mouth. These submental lymph nodes can be adversely affected by prolonged smokeless tobacco (or cigar) use, in which the tobacco is placed posterior to the lower lip and anterior to the lower incisor teeth. Knowledge of the lymphatic drainage of the oral cavity is important clinically because oral and pharyngeal cancer is the sixth most common malignancy reported worldwide. Early detection is crucial because the 5-year survival rate for oral cancer is only 50%. However, this patient's melanoma, located above the right eyebrow, would not drain to the submental lymph nodes. **Choice E** (Submandibular) is incorrect. The submandibular lymph nodes receive lymphatic drainage from the lateral parts of the anterior two thirds of the tongue, upper lips, lateral aspects of the lower lip, cheek, and nose. Concerning the oral cavity, the submandibular lymph nodes receive everything that is not directly drained by the submental nodes, which also eventually drain into the submandibular nodes. Prolonged use of chewing tobacco can pathologically alter the labial mucosa in the lateral aspects of the mouth. However, this patient's melanoma, located above the right eyebrow, would not drain to the submandibular lymph nodes.

3 **The answer is E: Cerebral arterial circle.** The cerebral arterial circle (of Willis) is an anastomoses of arteries located on the inferior surface of the brain in the area of the interpeduncular fossa, optic chiasm, and hypothalamus. These vessels are prone to saccular (berry) aneurysm, particularly where the arteries join together. Upon rupturing, blood spills into the subarachnoid space, causing the subarachnoid hemorrhage seen in autopsy. Remember that all major vessels of the brain travel within the subarachnoid space, and subarachnoid hemorrhages are one of the few cerebral hemorrhages that can occur in the absence of trauma, often seen following rupture of a saccular aneurysm within the cerebral arterial circle. The three cardinal signs and symptoms of a subarachnoid hemorrhage are (1) loss of consciousness (lethargy), (2) nuchal rigidity (stiff neck), and (3) a sudden onset of the "worst headache of your life," which were all present in this patient. **Choice A** (Common carotid artery) is incorrect. The common carotid artery, which gives rise to the internal and external carotid arteries at the level of the fourth cervical vertebra, is a major artery of the neck that lies outside of the skull. If this artery were lacerated, it would not cause the sudden onset of the severe headache seen in this patient due to its extracranial location. **Choice B** (Middle meningeal artery) is incorrect. This artery, which supplies blood to the dura mater, is often torn following impact to the side of the head, fracturing the skull in the area of the pterion. The anterior division of the middle meningeal artery is at risk if the pterion, an osteological feature on the side of the head that marks the junction of the parietal, frontal, squamous temporal, and sphenoid bones, is fractured because this artery runs in close proximity to the pterion. A traumatic blow to the side of the head, and subsequent fracture of the pterion, leads to an epidural hemorrhage as the blood pools between the endosteal layer of the dura mater and the calvaria. Because no trauma was reported and blood was not found in the epidural space, this option can be eliminated. **Choice C** (Facial artery) is incorrect. The facial artery lies outside of the skull. If this artery were lacerated, it would not cause the signs and symptoms, sudden onset of the worst headache of his life, lethargy, and nuchal rigidity, seen in this patient. **Choice D** (Superior cerebral veins) is incorrect. Traumatic impact to the front of the head can tear the superior cerebral veins. The impact shears the superior cerebral veins as they empty into the superior sagittal sinus, leading to a subdural hematoma. Because no trauma was reported in this patient, this option can be eliminated.

4   The answer is A: Ophthalmic.   Both the superior and inferior ophthalmic veins provide a pathway for the spread of infection from the anterior tip of the nose to the cavernous sinus as these veins connect the facial vein to the cavernous sinus. Because the facial vein does not contain valves, infection would spread in the direction of least physical resistance. An infection arising on the tip of the nose may spread to the cavernous sinus causing thrombophlebitis. The "danger triangle of the face" stretches from the labial commissures bilaterally to the bridge of the nose. Any lacerations within this triangle, such as the acne pustules frequently seen in maturing adolescents, can cause an infection in the facial vein, which may spread to the cavernous sinus. Remember that veins of the face and the scalp do NOT contain valves, which is clinically relevant due to the potential spread of infection. The symptoms seen in this patient, headache, fever, and periorbital edema were due to the spread of the infection through the ophthalmic veins to the cavernous sinus. Once the infection resided in the cavernous sinus, it could affect the cranial nerves, oculomotor nerve (CN III), trochlear nerve (CN IV), and abducent nerve (CN VI), which control the extraocular muscles, leading to the diplopia, or double vision, seen in this patient. **Choice B** (Superior cerebral) is incorrect. The superior cerebral vein drains blood from the superolateral aspects of the cerebrum into the superior sagittal sinus. Though these veins are clinically significant because they are often disrupted from a traumatic blow to the front of head resulting in a subdural cerebral hemorrhage, they do not communicate with the cavernous sinus and would not be involved with spread of infection from the tip of the nose. **Choice C** (Great cerebral [of Galen]) is incorrect. The great cerebral vein (of Galen) merges with the inferior sagittal dural venous sinus to form the straight dural venous sinus. It is a single, midline vein that drains deep structures of the brain. The great cerebral vein does not communicate with the cavernous sinus and would not drain blood from the tip of the nose. **Choice D** (Maxillary) is incorrect. The maxillary vein is formed by the drainage of the pterygoid plexus of veins, located between the temporalis and lateral pterygoid muscles in the infratemporal region, and drains into the retromandibular vein. The maxillary vein does not directly communicate with the cavernous sinus; however,

it can communicate with the ophthalmic veins through the pterygoid plexus via the inferior orbital fissure. However, the maxillary vein is located some distance away from the "danger triangle of the face" and is unlikely to be involved. **Choice E** (Supraorbital) is incorrect. The supraorbital vein drains the anterosuperior aspects of the scalp, but it is not involved with venous drainage of the tip of the nose, where the infection originated in this patient. Though this vein does drain into the ophthalmic veins, it is not the correct answer due to the location of the lesion on the tip of the nose.

5   The answer is E: Lingual frenulum.   The openings of the submandibular ducts reside on either side of the lingual frenulum, and the saliva produced by the submandibular glands drains through the sublingual caruncles (or papillae), openings at the base of the lingual frenulum. By applying pressure to the right submandibular gland, the physician would look at the lingual frenulum for the salivary secretions of the submandibular glands. If no salivation is observed, then the right submandibular salivary duct is completely obstructed. **Choice A** (Second maxillary molar tooth) is incorrect. The duct of the parotid gland drains saliva into the oral vestibule via a small opening opposite the second maxillary molar teeth on either side of the oral cavity. In this case, the physician needs to look for the drainage of the submandibular duct, which is at the sublingual caruncle located within the base of the lingual frenulum. **Choice B** (Oral vestibule) is incorrect. The duct of the parotid gland drains saliva into the oral vestibule via a small opening opposite the second maxillary molar teeth on either side of the oral cavity. In this case, the physician needs to look for the drainage of the submandibular duct, which is at the sublingual caruncle located within the base of the lingual frenulum. **Choice C** (Palatine mucosa) is incorrect. The ducts of the palatine glands reside deep to the mucosa of the hard palate, and they drain their mucous secretions into the superior aspect of the oral cavity. In this case, the physician needs to look for the drainage of the submandibular duct, which is at the sublingual caruncle located within the base of the lingual frenulum. **Choice D** (Sublingual folds) is incorrect. The sublingual folds lie in the floor of the mouth and represent the location of the drainage of the sublingual glands. The small sublingual ducts conduct saliva into the oral cavity through numerous openings within the sublingual folds.

6   The answer is E: Sphenopalatine.   The sphenopalatine artery supplies most of the blood to the nasal cavity, particularly the inferior and posterior aspects of the nasal cavity. Therefore, it is highly probable that the sphenopalatine artery, a terminal branch of the maxillary artery, was the source of the epistaxis (nosebleed) in this patient, as seen in the given illustration located on the next page. **Choice A** (Greater palatine) is incorrect. The greater palatine artery supplies blood primarily to the hard palate; however, it may supply a small amount of blood to the anterior and inferior aspects of nasal cavity via its communication with the sphenopalatine artery through the incisive canal. However, due to the location of the injury in this patient, the greater palatine artery would not be involved with this persistent nosebleed. **Choice B** (Infraorbital) is incorrect. The infraorbital artery courses in the roof of the maxillary sinus to give blood to this area as well as the superior canine and incisor teeth, inferior aspect of the orbit, and superior aspect of the lip. The infraorbital artery would not be responsible for

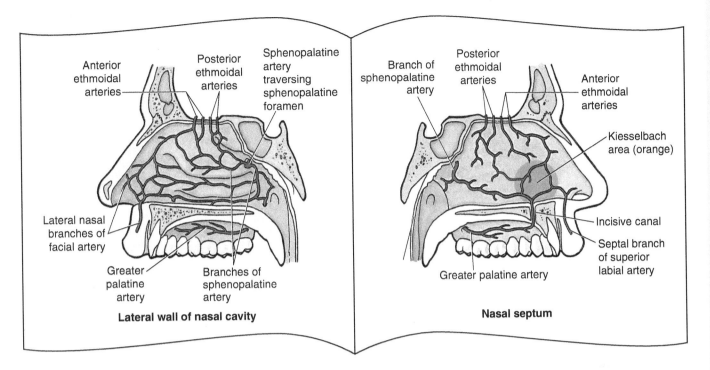

Anterior ethmoidal arteries

Posterior ethmoidal arteries

Sphenopalatine artery traversing sphenopalatine foramen

Lateral nasal branches of facial artery

Greater palatine artery

Branches of sphenopalatine artery

Lateral wall of nasal cavity

Branch of sphenopalatine artery

Posterior ethmoidal arteries

Anterior ethmoidal arteries

Kiesselbach area (orange)

Incisive canal

Septal branch of superior labial artery

Greater palatine artery

Nasal septum

the nosebleed seen in this patient. **Choice C** (Facial) is incorrect. The lateral nasal branch of the facial artery would supply the anterior and inferior aspects of the nasal cavity in the region of the vestibule; however, bleeding of this artery would be easily stopped by applying pressure to the alae of the nose. **Choice D** (Anterior ethmoidal) is incorrect. The anterior ethmoidal artery supplies the anterior, superior aspect of the nasal cavity after entering the nasal cavity through the cribiform plate of the ethmoid bone. This artery does not supply blood to posterior and inferior aspect of the lateral nasal wall, which is the location of the bleed in this patient.

7   **The answer is C: Thoracic anterior roots.** This patient is exhibiting miosis (constriction of the pupil) and ptosis (drooping of the eyelid), which are cardinal signs/symptoms of a loss of sympathetic fibers to the head (Horner syndrome). The only structure in this list that carries sympathetic fibers to the head is the anterior roots of the thoracic spinal nerves (T1-3). These anterior roots convey presynaptic sympathetic neurons to the T1-3 mixed spinal nerves, enter the sympathetic chain ganglia via the white rami communicantes, and ascend to synapse in the superior cervical ganglion. The postsynaptic sympathetic neurons are distributed to the head by following blood vessels within the associated periarterial plexi. Remember that the sympathetic chain ended at the first cervical level, so sympathetic fibers must follow blood vessels to reach their endpoint. In this patient, ptosis (drooping of the upper eyelid) and miosis (pupillary constriction) were noted, and these signs indicate the interruption of the sympathetic innervation to the head. The thoracic anterior roots are the only component of the sympathetic nervous system listed in these choices, and these anterior roots of T1-3 were interrupted during the resection of the lymphangioma in this patient. Knowledge of the sympathetic distribution to the head is vital to understanding the innervation of the head.

Choice A (Cervical posterior roots) is incorrect. The patient is exhibiting a loss of sympathetic innervation to the head, due to the ptosis and miosis noted in the patient. The sympathetic nervous system is a thoracolumbar system, consisting of presynaptic cell bodies that reside in the intermediolateral cell column (IML), which exists from the vertebral levels of T1 through L2 (or L3). The cervical posterior (dorsal) roots are an incorrect answer because posterior roots only contain afferent (or sensory) information, and the autonomic nervous system is an entirely efferent (or motor) system. Moreover, presynaptic sympathetic fibers would ONLY reside in the anterior (ventral) roots of T1-L2 (or L3). Because the IML is somatotopically organized, the sympathetic fibers going to the head would exist in the IML from T1-3, and they would ONLY exist in the anterior (ventral) roots of these specific spinal nerves. **Choice B** (Thoracic posterior roots) is incorrect. The posterior (dorsal) roots contain only afferent (sensory) information. The autonomic nervous system is an entirely efferent (motor) system, which eliminates this option. **Choice D** (Thoracic posterior primary rami) is incorrect. Postsynaptic sympathetic fibers would exist in thoracic posterior (dorsal) primary rami in order to vasoconstrict or vasodilate the blood vessels going to the area supplied by these nerves, specifically the epaxial back muscles and the skin overlying these muscles. However, the patient is exhibiting a loss of sympathetic innervation to the head. Sympathetic fibers in the thoracic posterior (dorsal) primary rami have already synapsed in the sympathetic chain and would not be distributed to the head. **Choice E** (Thoracic gray rami communicantes) is incorrect. Sympathetic fibers in a thoracic gray rami communicantes have already synapsed in the sympathetic chain and would be distributed to the vertebral level at which they synapsed. Therefore, these sympathetic fibers in the thoracic region would not reach the head and would not be involved in the clinical signs/symptoms of this patient.

8 **The answer is C: Levator palpebrae superioris.** The levator palpebrae superioris muscle attaches into the tarsal plate and skin of the upper eyelid and is the primary elevator of the eyelid. Weakness in this muscle results in ptosis (drooping) of the upper eyelid and may reflect a problem with the oculomotor nerve (CN III). The oculomotor nerve provides the motor control for the levator palpebrae superioris and most (4 of 6) of the extraocular muscles. The levator palpebrae superioris is assisted by the superior tarsal muscle, a thin smooth muscle sheet in the upper eyelid innervated by sympathetic fibers. **Choice A** (Orbicularis oculi) is incorrect. The orbicularis oculi is a muscle of facial expression that acts to close the eye, forming a sphincter-like arrangement around the orbit and extending into the eyelids. Functional deficits of the orbicularis oculi muscle result in loss of the ability to blink, which endangers the health of the eye by hampering proper spread of tears across the eyeball. **Choice B** (Frontalis) is incorrect. The frontalis muscle is the anterior component of the epicranius muscle in the scalp. It elevates the eyebrows and produces the horizontal wrinkles across the forehead, occurring when a person looks up (superior). **Choice D** (Superior rectus) is incorrect. The superior rectus muscle is one of the extraocular muscles. It attaches onto the sclera on the superior aspect of the eye and acts as the primary elevator of the eyeball. **Choice E** (Orbital muscle) is incorrect. The orbital muscle is a rudimentary smooth (nonstriated) muscle sling across the orbit that helps to support and position the eyeball within the orbit.

9 **The answer is A: First pharyngeal arch.** Mandibulofacial dysostosis (Treacher-Collins syndrome) affects derivatives of the first pharyngeal arch, specifically the migration of the neural crest cells into the arch. The cranial neural crests of the first pharyngeal arch are responsible for formation of the mandible, malleus, incus, squamous portion of the temporal bone, temporal bone, palatine bone, and vomer. As the figure shows, this patient exhibits micrognathia (small lower jaw), malar (zygomatic) hypoplasia, and malformed external ears, and this craniofacial deformities clearly indicate problems with the neural crest migration of the first pharyngeal arch. Mandibulofacial dysostosis is seen in 1 in 10,000 births. **Choice B** (Second pharyngeal arch) is incorrect. Neural crest cells of the second pharyngeal arch are responsible for formation of the stapes, styloid processes, and the upper body and lesser horns of the hyoid bone. Malformation of these structures derived from the second pharyngeal arch would not lead to the characteristic craniofacial deformities seen in a patient with mandibulofacial dysostosis (Treacher-Collins syndrome). **Choice C** (Third pharyngeal arch) is incorrect. Neural crest cells of the third pharyngeal arch are responsible for formation of the lower body and greater horns of the hyoid bone. Malformation of these third pharyngeal arch structures would not lead to the characteristic craniofacial deformities seen in a patient with mandibulofacial dysostosis. **Choice D** (Fourth pharyngeal arch) is incorrect. Neural crest cells of the fourth pharyngeal arch are not responsible for any skeletal elements. Therefore, failure of the neural crest cell migration of the fourth pharyngeal arch structures would not lead to any craniofacial deformities, and this option can be easily eliminated. **Choice E** (Fifth pharyngeal arch) is incorrect. The fifth pharyngeal arch only exists transiently in human embryologic growth and development. No structures are derived from the fifth pharyngeal arch in adults, so this option can be easily eliminated.

10 **The answer is C: Cricothyroid membrane.** In an emergency tracheotomy, the cricothyroid membrane is incised in order to establish a direct airway for the patient. This procedure is also called a cricothyrotomy or cricothyroidotomy, and it is used as a last resort to circumvent upper airway obstructions. The cricothyroid membrane is an important component of the conus elasticus, which is composed of the vocal ligaments, median cricothyroid membrane, and lateral cricothyroid membranes. The cricothyroid membrane is the perfect location to perform an emergency tracheotomy because of several nearby palpable landmarks, and it is located below the (true) vocal folds, which serve as the main inspiratory sphincter of the larynx. Do not confuse the emergency tracheotomy with a tracheostomy, which is a procedure performed in a hospital setting and involves surgically creating a hole in the cartilaginous rings of the trachea. **Choice A** (Cricoid cartilage) is incorrect. Due to the thickness of the cricoid cartilage, incising through this cartilage would be difficult outside the hospital setting. Moreover, an incised cricoid cartilage would need surgical intervention to heal due to its lack of blood supply. Moreover, damaging the cricoid cartilage would be detrimental to the integrity of the larynx and the laryngeal skeleton. **Choice B** (Thyrohyoid membrane) is incorrect. Though it is easily palpated due to its position above the laryngeal prominence (or the "Adam's apple"), the thyrohyoid membrane is located between vertebral levels C3 and C4 and may not establish a direct airway. To combat against an upper airway obstruction, the cricothyroid membrane (between vertebral levels C5 and C6) would be a better option. Damage to the thyrohyoid membrane could also compromise the superior laryngeal artery and the internal branch of the superior laryngeal nerve, which pierce this membrane to enter the larynx. **Choice D** (Tracheal rings) is incorrect. In a tracheostomy, a hole is created surgically in the cartilaginous rings of the trachea. However, this procedure is usually performed in a hospital setting under sterile conditions. Damage to the thyroid gland and infrahyoid muscles can easily occur if a tracheostomy is not performed correctly. Incising the cricothyroid membrane would be a much easier means of establishing an airway, especially considering the emergency conditions surrounding this patient's choking incident. **Choice E** (Isthmus of the thyroid gland) is incorrect. Cutting through the isthmus of the thyroid gland would not establish an airway for this patient, so this option can be easily eliminated. Due to its location at the seventh cervical vertebra, this glandular tissue is often transected or resected during a tracheostomy, when the tracheal rings are incised. However, a tracheostomy is performed in a hospital setting under sterile conditions.

11 **The answer is B: Middle meningeal artery.** The middle meningeal artery is often torn following impact to the side of the head, fracturing the skull in the area of the pterion. The pterion, an osteological feature on the side of the head that marks the junction of the parietal, frontal, squamous temporal, and sphenoid bones, is prone to fracture following traumatic impact to the side of the head, which this boy experienced during his sledding accident. The middle meningeal artery, specifically its anterior division, runs in close proximity to the pterion, so a fracture of this weakened area of the lateral skull may lacerate the middle meningeal artery, which frequently leads to an epidural hemorrhage as the blood pools between the endosteal layer of the dura mater and the calvaria. This epidural hemorrhage was confirmed by the CT scan showing a biconvex hyperdense extraaxial collection of blood pooling beneath the pterion in the epidural space, which is characteristic of an epidural hematoma. Also, note the edema at the place of impact located extracranially in this patient's scalp. Remember that a CT scan reveals "blood and bone," and due to it being inexpensive relative to an MRI, it is the perfect diagnostic tool in trauma. The symptoms displayed in this patient, including a severe headache and vomiting, are signs of increased intracranial pressure (ICP) due to the extravasation of blood from the middle meningeal artery compressing brain tissue within the skull. **Choice A** (Superficial temporal artery) is incorrect. The superficial temporal artery, the terminal branch of the external carotid artery, lies outside of the skull. If this artery were lacerated, bleeding of the scalp would be profuse. Due to its extracranial location, damage to the superficial temporal artery would not cause the vomiting seen in this patient, which is indicative of increased ICP. **Choice C** (Superior cerebral veins) is incorrect. Traumatic impact to the front of the head can tear the superior cerebral veins. The impact shears the superior cerebral veins as they empty into the superior sagittal sinus, leading to a subdural hemorrhage (or dural border hematoma). Due to the location of the trauma and the pooling blood revealed on the CT scan, these veins were not damaged. **Choice D** (Cerebral arterial circle) is incorrect. The cerebral arterial circle (of Willis) is an anastomoses of arteries located on the ventral surface of the brain in the area of the interpeduncular fossa, optic chiasm, and hypothalamus. These vessels are prone to saccular (berry) aneurysm, particularly where the arteries join together. Upon rupturing, blood spills into the subarachnoid space because all major vessels of the brain travel within the subarachnoid space. Subarachnoid hemorrhages are often seen in the absence of trauma, and the three cardinal signs and symptoms of a subarachnoid hemorrhage are (1) loss of consciousness (lethargy), (2) nuchal rigidity (stiff neck), and (3) a sudden onset of the "worst headache of your life", which were not present in this patient. **Choice E** (Middle cerebral artery [MCA]) is incorrect. The MCA travels deep within the brain in between the frontal and temporal lobes, so it should not be involved in fracture in the area of the pterion. If the MCA was compromised, it would lead to a subarachnoid hemorrhage, which was not evident on the provided CT scan.

12   **The answer is A: Arytenoid cartilages.**   The paired vocal ligaments (true vocal cords) are contained within the free, upper, thickened edges of the conus elasticus. Each of these ligaments stretches from its anterior attachment near the midline on the deep side or posterior surface of the thyroid cartilage to its posterior attachment on the vocal process of the arytenoid cartilage. Rotation and translation of the arytenoid cartilages and tilting of the thyroid cartilage determine the tension and position of the vocal ligaments. These conditions control the size and shape of the rima glottidis and the tension and vibration of the vocal folds. Thus, malformed vocal ligaments affect both respiration and phonation. **Choice B** (Cricoid cartilage) is incorrect. The single (unpaired) cricoid cartilage is the only completely circular cartilage in the respiratory tract. It articulates with the thyroid and arytenoid cartilages via synovial joints that permit regulation of the vocal folds. **Choice C** (Epiglottic cartilage) is incorrect. The epiglottic cartilage is a single (unpaired), roughly spoon-shaped structure that attaches to the posterior surface of the thyroid cartilage. Elevation of the larynx against the backward movement of the tongue during swallowing allows the epiglottis to act like a trap door in closing the laryngeal inlet.

Choice D (Corniculate cartilages) is incorrect. The corniculate cartilages are small, paired structures contained within the free margins of the aryepiglottic folds. They may aid in supporting these folds. **Choice E** (Cuneiform cartilages) is incorrect. The cuneiform cartilages are small, paired structures contained within the free margins of the aryepiglottic folds. They may aid in supporting these folds.

13   **The answer is D: Coronal.**   Premature closure of the coronal suture leads to brachycephaly (G: short head), which leads to a disproportionately wide skull with a short occipitofrontal diameter. The surface shaded CT reconstruction shows the complete closure of the coronal suture and depicts the characteristic square-shaped skull with a short occipitofrontal diameter seen following premature closure of the coronal suture. Brachycephaly is more common in females, and surgical intervention can be implemented to remove bone from both coronal sutures. Interestingly, some infants wear molding caps to treat cranial deformities, if surgical intervention is not required. If only one side of the coronal suture closes prematurely, the infant would present with an asymmetric cranium, a condition known as plagiocephaly. Craniosynostosis is the term that refers generally to the premature fusion of the cranial sutures. **Choice A** (Sphenosquamous) is incorrect. The sphenosquamous suture is a dense, fibrous connective tissue joint located on the side of the skull between the greater wing of the sphenoid bone and the squamous portion of the temporal bone. This suture later closes to help form the pterion, which is clinically relevant due to the fractures located at this structurally weak area on the side of the head, which may cause epidural hemorrhage via damage to the middle meningeal artery. The premature closure of this suture, as well as the sagittal, parietotemporal, and sphenoparietal sutures, can be involved with scaphocephaly (G: boat-shaped skull). **Choice B** (Sphenoparietal) is incorrect. The sphenoparietal suture is a dense, fibrous connective tissue joint located on the side of the skull between the greater wing of the sphenoid bone and the parietal bone. This suture later closes to help form the pterion, which is clinically relevant due to the fractures located at this structurally weak area on the side of the head, which may cause epidural hemorrhage via damage to the middle meningeal artery. The premature closure of this suture, as well as the sagittal, parietotemporal, and sphenosquamous sutures, can be involved with scaphocephaly (G: boat-shaped skull). **Choice C** (Lambdoid) is incorrect. The lambdoid suture is a dense, fibrous connective tissue joint located on the back of the skull that connects the occipital bone with the posterior aspect of the parietal bone and petrous portion of the temporal bone. If only one side of the lambdoid suture closes prematurely, the infant would present with a twisted and asymmetric cranium, a condition known as plagiocephaly. **Choice E** (Sagittal) is incorrect. The sagittal suture is a dense, fibrous connective tissue joint located between the two parietal bones in the midline of the skull. The premature closure of this suture, as well as the parietotemporal, sphenosquamous, and sphenoparietal sutures, can be involved with scaphocephaly (G: boat-shaped skull), which presents as a long and narrow cranium.

14   **The answer is A: Hypoglossal nerve.**   The left hypoglossal nerve (CN XII) is located in the anterior cervical region at the location of the stab wound. CN XII innervates all of the intrinsic muscles of the tongue and most of its extrinsic muscles with the lone exception being the palatoglossus muscle, innervated by the vagus nerve (CN X). Therefore, damage to the right CN XII would produce dysarthria, or difficult speaking, which was seen in this patient due to the loss of innervation to the tongue musculature. Though not noted in this patient, damage to the hypoglossal nerve also causes ipsilateral deviation of the tongue due to the unopposed muscular contractions of the contralateral genioglossus muscle. The mnemonic "The tongue licks the wound" will help you remember that the tongue deviates to the ipsilateral side in a lower motor neuron lesion of CN XII. **Choice B** (Accessory nerve) is incorrect. The accessory nerve (CN XI) passes deep to the SCM and to the investing layer of deep cervical fascia and courses posterolaterally into the lateral cervical region (posterior triangle of neck). Cutting this nerve would not produce the dysarthria displayed in this patient because CN XI innervates only the SCM and the trapezius muscle, which are primarily involved in head and shoulder movements. Also, the accessory nerve is not located in the anterior cervical region in the location of the stab wound. **Choice C** (Mandibular division of trigeminal nerve) is incorrect. The mandibular (third) division of the trigeminal nerve (CN V$_3$) is the only division of the trigeminal nerve (CN V) that supplies motor innervation. It supplies the muscles derived from the mesoderm of the first pharyngeal arch, including the four muscles of mastication (temporalis, masseter, lateral pterygoid, and medial pterygoid) and four additional muscles: **M**ylohoid, **A**nterior belly of the Digastric, **T**ensor Tympani, and **T**ensor Veli Palatini (mnemonic = "MATT"). These muscles play no role in the dysarthria noted in this patient, and CN V$_3$ is not located in close proximity to the stab wound. **Choice D** (Lingual branch of glossopharyngeal nerve) is incorrect. The lingual branch of the glossopharyngeal nerve (CN IX) enters the posterior one third of the tongue to provide general sensation and taste to the region. It does not provide any motor innervation, so this nerve would not be involved with the dysarthria noted in this patient. Moreover, due to the location of the knife wound, this nerve would not be affected. **Choice E** (Roots of the brachial plexus) is incorrect. The roots of the brachial plexus represent the anterior (ventral) rami of C5-8 and T1, and these nerves emerge between the anterior and middle scalene muscles in the lateral cervical region (posterior triangle of neck). The roots of the brachial plexus are located too inferior to be damaged by the knife.

15 **The answer is B: Vocal folds.**   The squamous cell carcinoma is identified on the mucosal surface at the inferiomedial border of the laryngeal ventricle, which would be the location of the vocal cords. The most common presenting symptom in laryngeal cancer, particularly in glottic tumors such as this one, is hoarseness of the voice while some people experience odynophagia (painful swallowing). **Choice A** (Infraglottic cavity) is incorrect. The infraglottic cavity is the inferior part of the laryngeal cavity, so it lies inferior to the vocal folds and is continuous with the lumen of the trachea. Its inferior boundary would be the inferior border of the cricoid cartilage. **Choice C** (Vestibular folds) is incorrect. The laryngeal ventricle (laryngeal sinus) is a recess extending laterally within the middle portion of the laryngeal cavity. This recess lies between the superior vestibular folds and the inferior vocal folds. **Choice D** (Laryngeal vestibule) is incorrect. The laryngeal vestibule is located between the laryngeal inlet and the vestibular folds, and it represents

the superior part of the laryngeal cavity. **Choice E** (Epiglottic cartilage) is incorrect. The epiglottic cartilage would form the anterior wall of the laryngeal vestibule, so it resides in the superior part of the laryngeal cavity above the vestibular folds.

16 **The answer is B: Retropharyngeal space.**   The retropharyngeal space is the most frequent route for infection to spread through the neck into the superior mediastinum. This potential space exists between the prevertebral fascia and the anterior lamina of the prevertebral fascia, and it extends from the base of the skull to the superior mediastinum to the level of the third thoracic vertebra. The retropharyngeal space allows movement of the esophagus, pharynx, larynx, and trachea relative to the vertebral column, but it is clinically important due to its potential to provide a conduit for the spread of infection into the mediastinum. **Choice A** (Parapharyngeal space) is incorrect. The parapharyngeal space is located between the lateral wall of the upper pharynx, the medial pterygoid muscle, and the cervical vertebrae. An infection residing in this potential space is unable to reach the superior mediastinum, unless it communicates directly with the retropharyngeal space. **Choice C** (Buccal space) is incorrect. The buccal space exists between the deep surface of the parotid gland and the mucosa of the cheek. An infection residing in this potential space is unable to reach the superior mediastinum. **Choice D** (Carotid sheath) is incorrect. The carotid sheath is a fascial investment that extends from the base of the skull to the root of the neck, and it does communicate with the mediastinum of the thorax. So, this fascial space does offer a potential pathway for the spread of infection into the mediastinum; however, based upon the source of the infection in the tonsillar fossa, the retropharyngeal space is the best answer to this question. **Choice E** (Suprasternal space) is incorrect. The suprasternal space is located above the manubrium of the sternum, and it is a narrow interval located between a split in the investing layer of the deep cervical fascia. This space would allow a communication between the anterior jugular veins to pass, but it would not allow an infection to spread through the neck and into the mediastinum.

17 **The answer is B: Entrapment of the inferior rectus muscle.**   The coronal CT (computed tomography) reformat image reveals a fractured orbital floor and the downward herniation of orbital contents into the superior antrum of the left maxillary sinus, leading to the entrapment of the inferior rectus muscle. In this CT, there is no visibility of the inferior rectus muscle within the left orbit because this extraocular muscle and orbital fat have herniated through the acquired defect in the floor of the orbit. The displacement, and subsequent impingement, of the inferior rectus muscle within the fractured floor of the orbit causes the vertical diplopia (double vision) in this patient. In this patient, this orbital ("blowout") fracture was caused by the traumatic blow to the left eye. **Choice A** (Paralysis of the lateral rectus muscle) is incorrect. The lateral rectus muscle of the orbit is innervated by the abducent nerve (CN VI), and it is the only muscle innervated by CN VI. Paralysis of this muscle would lead to horizontal diplopia as the left pupil would be resting in the adducted position due to the unopposed action of the other extraocular muscles. However, due to blowout fracture site in the floor of the orbital rim and the patient exhibiting vertical diplopia, this muscle is not likely to be damaged due to its lateral location within the orbit.

Choice C (Detached retina) is incorrect. A detached retina is often seen following trauma due to inflammation that pulls the sensory retina away from the retinal pigment epithelium. However, retinal detachment would lead to vision loss and blindness, not the vertical diplopia seen in this patient. **Choice D** (Paralysis of superior oblique muscle) is incorrect. The superior oblique muscle of the orbit is the only muscle innervated by the trochlear nerve (CN IV). This muscle would pull the eye inferolaterally, but it is clinically tested by asking the patient to look down after the eye is placed in an adducted position. Paralysis of the superior oblique muscle would lead to diplopia as well as clumsiness when descending stairs. However, due to the blowout fracture site in the floor of the orbital rim, this muscle is not likely to be damaged due to its superior location within the orbit. **Choice E** (Damage to infraorbital nerve) is incorrect. The infraorbital nerve, a branch of the second (maxillary) division of trigeminal nerve (CN V$_2$), courses through the superior aspect (roof) of the maxillary sinus, and due to its location, it would be the most likely damaged nerve during the blowout fracture of the inferior floor of the orbit. However, the infraorbital nerve supplies sensory innervation to the maxillary sinus as well as the skin of the inferior eyelid, lateral nose, and upper lip. Damage to the infraorbital nerve causes paresthesia and numbness in the areas of cutaneous (sensory) distribution for this nerve; however, damage to this nerve would not cause the vertical diplopia seen in this patient.

18 **The answer is D: Masseter.** Damage to the facial nerve would lead to loss of innervation to the muscles of facial expression, and the masseter muscle, a muscle of mastication, is the only listed muscle that will continue to function in a patient diagnosed with facial nerve (CN VII or Bell) palsy. The mandibular (third) division of the trigeminal nerve (CN V$_3$) supplies the four muscles of mastication (masseter, temporalis, lateral pterygoid, and medial pterygoid) and four additional muscles: **M**ylohoid, **A**nterior belly of the Digastric, **T**ensor Tympani, and **T**ensor Veli Palatini (mnemonic = "MATT"). The masseter muscle primarily works to close the jaw, though its superficial fibers may play a limited role in protrusion of the mandible. It is the only muscle on this list of options that would continue to function in facial nerve palsy. **Choice A** (Zygomaticus major) is incorrect. The zygomaticus major is a muscle of facial expression, so it would be paralyzed in facial nerve palsy. It functions as a dilator of the oral fissure by elevating the corners of mouth, as in smiling when the muscle contracts bilaterally or sneering to show disdain when the muscle contracts unilaterally. It originates on the lateral aspect of the zygomatic bone, which is how it receives its name. **Choice B** (Levator labii superioris) is incorrect. The levator labii superioris is a muscle of facial expression, so it would be paralyzed in facial nerve palsy. It functions as a dilator of the oral fissure by retracting (elevating) the upper lip to show the upper teeth and deepens the nasolabial sulcus. It originates on the infraorbital margin of maxilla, above, and therefore covers, the infraorbital foramen. **Choice C** (Buccinator) is incorrect. The buccinator is a muscle of facial expression, so it would be paralyzed in facial nerve palsy. It originates on the alveolar ridges of maxillary and mandibular molar teeth and contracts to give tension to the cheek to keep food between the occlusal surfaces of the teeth. The tone of the buccinator muscle provides resistance to keep teeth from tilting laterally and prevents patients from looking like a hamster, with food lodged in the oral vestibule, when they

chew food. **Choice E** (Platysma) is incorrect. The platysma is a muscle of facial expression, so it would be paralyzed in facial nerve palsy. It resides in the neck and lower face to depress the mandible and wrinkle the skin of neck, as seen when a person is placed in a stressful situation. The platysma originates in the subcutaneous tissue near the clavicle and inserts into the modiolus, lateral to the labial commissures.

19 **The answer is C: Sternocleidomastoid.** The sternocleidomastoid muscle (SCM) is abnormally shortened and/or excessively contracting in this baby girl with congenital torticollis (**L**: twisted neck). The etiology of congenital torticollis is unknown, but it is thought to be due to damage to the SCM during birth or intrauterine malposition. In this baby, the congenital torticollis presents with the head tilted (or laterally bent) toward the affected SCM (right side in this patient) and the chin is elevated and turned toward the contralateral (left) side. Bilateral contraction of the SCM causes flexion of the neck to move the chin toward the sternum. When the right SCM contracts alone, it functions to bring the mastoid process of the temporal bone closer to the sternum, which results in tilting the head toward the right side and elevation of the chin to the left. The excessive contraction (or tone) of the right SCM causes the inability of this baby to have her head turned to the right side. The accessory nerve (CN XI) provides motor innervation to the trapezius and SCMs, and the congenital torticollis, seen in this patient, is due to shortening or excessive contraction of the right SCM. **Choice A** (Platysma) is incorrect. The platysma is a muscle of facial expression that resides in the neck and lower face to depress the mandible and wrinkle the skin of neck, as seen when a person is placed in a stressful situation. The platysma originates in the subcutaneous tissue near the clavicle and inserts into the modiolus, lateral to the labial commissures. This muscle is innervated by the cervical branch of the main branch of the facial nerve (CN VII). Due to its superficial origin in the subcutaneous fascia, this muscle can only wrinkle the skin of the neck, not abnormally twist it. This baby has congenital torticollis due to the shortening or excessive contraction of the SCM. **Choice B** (Trapezius) is incorrect. Damage to the trapezius muscle would lead to asymmetry when shrugging the shoulders or "drooping" of the affected shoulder because the actions of this muscle include elevation and lateral rotation of the scapula during abduction of the upper limb to greater than 90 degrees. The accessory nerve (CN XI) provides motor innervation to the trapezius and SCMs; however, the congenital torticollis, seen in this patient, is due to the shortening or excessive contraction of the SCM. **Choice D** (Masseter) is incorrect. The masseter muscle primarily works to close the jaw, though its superficial fibers may play a limited role in protrusion of the mandible. The mandibular (third) division of the trigeminal nerve (CN V$_3$) supplies this muscle of mastication, which would have no role in the abnormal twisting of the neck and head posture seen in this newborn. **Choice E** (Digastric) is incorrect. The digastric muscle is a suprahyoid muscle that attaches to the body and greater horn of the hyoid bone and lies below the body of the mandible. This muscle consists of two muscle bellies, anterior and posterior, which are innervated by the mandibular (third) division of the trigeminal nerve (CN V$_3$) and facial nerve (CN VII), respectively. When it contracts, the digastric muscle acts to elevate the hyoid bone, which is important in swallowing (or deglutition); it is not involved with rotation and lateral bending of the neck.

20 **The answer is A: Zygomaticus major.** The zygomaticus major functions as a dilator of the oral fissure by elevating the labial commissures (corners of the mouth), in order to smile when the muscles contract bilaterally. The contraction of the zygomaticus major muscle bilaterally would be the proper facial expression after scoring a perfect score on the anatomy portion of her board examination. Interestingly, this muscle can also produce a sneer when this muscle contracts unilaterally to show disdain. Study hard for your examination, so you can make this muscle contract bilaterally. The zygomaticus major muscle originates on the lateral aspect of the zygomatic bone to insert into the labial commissures. It is a muscle of facial expression that is innervated by the facial nerve (CN VII), which innervates all of muscles of facial expression derived from the mesoderm of the second pharyngeal (branchial) arch. **Choice B** (Zygomaticus minor) is incorrect. The zygomaticus minor is also a muscle of facial expression innervated by the facial nerve (CN VII). It functions as a dilator of the oral fissure by retracting (elevating) the upper lip to show the upper teeth, which also deepens the nasolabial sulcus. It originates from the orbicular oris muscle and the zygomatic bone of the lateral face to insert into the upper lip. It has similar functions as the levator labii superioris muscle. It would not enable this professional student to smile after seeing her examination scores because it does not elevate the labial commissures specifically. **Choice C** (Levator labii superioris) is incorrect. The levator labii superioris is also a muscle of facial expression innervated by the facial nerve (CN VII). It functions as a dilator of the oral fissure by retracting (elevating) the upper lip to show the upper teeth, which also and deepens the nasolabial sulcus. It originates on the infraorbital margin of the maxilla, above, and therefore covers, the infraorbital foramen. It would not enable this professional student to smile after seeing her examination scores because it does not elevate the labial commissures specifically. **Choice D** (Buccinator) is incorrect. The buccinator is also a muscle of facial expression innervated by the facial nerve (CN VII). It originates on the alveolar ridges of the maxillary and mandibular molar teeth and contracts to gives tension to the cheek to keep food between the occlusal surfaces of the teeth. The tone of the buccinator muscle provides resistance to keep teeth from tilting laterally and prevents patients from looking like a hamster, with food lodged in the oral vestibule, when they chew food. It would not enable this professional student to smile after seeing her examination scores. **Choice E** (Orbicularis oris) is incorrect. The orbicularis oris is also a muscle of facial expression innervated by the facial nerve (CN VII). It encircles the mouth to act as the important sphincter of the oral fissure, and in performing this task, it functions to close the oral fissure as when protruding the lips to kiss, whistle, or suck. It also resists distension as when blowing into a brass instrument, like a trumpet. The orbicularis oris muscle originates on the incisive fossae of the mandible and maxilla and attaches to the modiolus, a convergence of several muscles of facial expression at the corners of mouth. It would not enable this professional student to smile after seeing her examination scores.

21 **The answer is D: Failure of fusion of retinal fissure.** Coloboma of the iris results from failure of fusion of the retinal (or choroidal) fissure, a ventral groove formed by the invagination of the optic cup and its stalk by vascular mesenchyme, during the sixth week of development. It is characterized by a defect of the inferior portion of the iris in the pupillary margin, which gives the pupil a keyhole appearance. This congenital defect can be an autosomal dominant malformation, which may or may not affect vision. **Choice A** (Traumatic damage to the sphincter muscle of the pupil) is incorrect. The keyhole defect in the right iris appears as an irregular pupil that can be caused by damage to the iris itself, loss of innervation to the sphincter or dilator muscle of the pupil, or insults to the central nervous system. In this patient, the iris coloboma was congenital, so traumatic damage to the sphincter muscle of the pupil can be ruled out. **Choice B** (Interruption of neural crest cell migration) is incorrect. The iris and its dilator and sphincter muscles of the pupil are derived from neuroectoderm, so the interruption of neural crest cell migration would not cause coloboma of the iris. **Choice C** (Persistent pupillary membrane) is incorrect. Remnants of the pupillary membrane, which covers the anterior surface of the lens in the embryo, may persist in the pupils of newborns, especially premature infants. A persistent pupillary membrane appears as web-like strands of connective tissue over the pupil, but this tissue tends to atrophy over time. In this patient, a defect in the iris was seen in a 21-year-old woman, so a persistent pupillary membrane is unlikely. **Choice E** (Lack of fusion of inner and outer layers of the optic cup) is incorrect. Failure of fusion of the inner and outer layers of the optic cup may lead to a congenital detachment of the retina due to the persistent intraretinal space, which impairs vision and would be surgically repaired (if possible) after birth. A detached retina would not lead to the defect of the iris seen in this 21-year-old patient.

22 **The answer is E: Hair cells in the base of the cochlea.** The hair cells in the base of the cochlea detect high frequency sound tones, so the factory worker's inability to detect these types of sounds implies damage to these specific sensory receptors. Being detected in the basal turn of the cochlea, high-frequency sounds travel the shortest distance in the cochlea while low-frequency sounds travel the farthest to reach the apex of the cochlea. People with high-frequency hearing loss would have trouble detecting consonant sounds, such as distinguishing between the words "thaw", "raw", and "law", because consonants are high-frequency sound components of human speech. Based upon his age and occupation, his sensorineural hearing loss is probably due to extended exposure to loud equipment, which has damaged the hair cells specifically at the base of the cochlea. **Choice A** (Tympanic membrane) is incorrect. A tear within the tympanic membrane that would separate the outer and middle ear would represent a conductive hearing loss where the patient would have trouble hearing sounds with low amplitudes irrespective of the frequency. Because this patient is unable to detect only sounds at high frequencies, a conductive hearing loss is not likely. **Choice B** (External acoustic meatus) is incorrect. A blockage of the external acoustic meatus, a part of the outer ear, would represent a conductive hearing loss where the patient would have trouble hearing sounds with low amplitudes irrespective of the frequency. Because this patient is unable to detect only sounds at high frequencies, a conductive hearing loss is not likely. **Choice C** (Hair cells in the apex of the cochlea) is incorrect. The hair cells in the apex of the cochlea detect low-frequency sound tones because these sounds travel farther. Whales communicate with low-frequency vocalizations that can be heard over great distances, and this fact enables a student to remember that low-frequency sounds travel farther within the cochlea. Though this patient is experiencing a sensorineural hearing loss, it is the hair cells in the base of the cochlea that are damaged because he is unable to detect high-frequency sounds. **Choice D** (Hair cells located in the middle of the cochlea) is incorrect. The hair cells in the middle of the cochlea would detect sounds in the middle of a human's hearing capacity for sound frequencies. However, based upon the patient's inability to hear high-frequency sounds, these particular hair cells would not be damaged in this case of sensorineural hearing loss.

23 **The answer is C: Noncommunicating hydrocephalus.** Noncommunicating hydrocephalus, or obstructive hydrocephalus, is caused by an obstruction of CSF flow between or within the ventricles of the brain, which prevents CSF from entering the subarachnoid space. In this 4-year-old girl, the medulloblastoma obstructs the 4th ventricle, preventing CSF arriving into the fourth ventricle via the cerebral aqueduct (of Sylvius) from entering the subarachnoid space via the 4th ventricular outlets (paired lateral foramina of Luschka and median foramen of Magendie). This acquired noncommunicating hydrocephalus (*G*: water in the head) is causing the associated abnormalities in the cerebral hemispheres (dilation of the third and lateral ventricles, shallow cortex, and effaced sulci). The girl's symptoms are mainly secondary due to the increased intracranial pressure (ICP), which is due to the blockage of the 4th ventricle and CSF flow. Papilledema is optic disc swelling caused by increased ICP, and it can be observed with an ophthalmoscope in a fundoscopic examination. Brain tumors are the second most common malignancy among children less than 20 years of age, and they are often located infratentorially (or beneath the cerebellum tentorium, a dural fold, which separates the occipital lobe of the brain from the cerebellum). **Choice A** (Dandy-Walker syndrome) is incorrect. Dandy-Walker syndrome is a congenital brain malformation characterized by the absence of the cerebellar vermis, leading to the enlargement of the 4th ventricle. In this patient, the presence of the medulloblastoma causes an acquired noncommunicating hydrocephalus, as noted on the MRI. **Choice B** (Chiari malformation) is incorrect. A Chiari malformation (or Arnold-Chiari malformation) is a downward displacement of the cerebellar tonsils and medulla through the magnum foramen, which may cause hydrocephalus. Chiari I malformations are more common in women, and the average age for diagnosis is approximately 27 years of age. Chiari II malformations generally present with open spinal dysraphism at birth. Because the downward displacement of the cerebellar tonsils, characteristic of the Chiari malformation, was not noted, a noncommunicating hydrocephalus is the better diagnosis. **Choice D** (Congenital communicating hydrocephalus) is incorrect. A communicating hydrocephalus, or nonobstructive hydrocephalus, is caused by an impairment of CSF resorption at the arachnoid granulations, located along the superior sagittal sinus. Conditions leading to a communicating hydrocephalus include subarachnoid hemorrhage, meningitis, Chiari malformation, or congenital absence of the arachnoid granulations. However, the medulloblastoma is blocking flow of CSF between the ventricles of the brain, which is the definition of a noncommunicating (obstructive) hydrocephalus. **Choice E** (Acquired communicating hydrocephalus) is incorrect. A communicating hydrocephalus, or nonobstructive hydrocephalus, is caused by an impairment of CSF resorption at the arachnoid granulations, located along the superior sagittal sinus. Conditions leading to a communicating hydrocephalus include subarachnoid hemorrhage, meningitis, Chiari malformation, or congenital absence of the arachnoid granulations. However, the medulloblastoma is blocking flow of CSF in the fourth ventricle, which is the definition of a noncommunicating (obstructive) hydrocephalus.

24 **The answer is B: Thyroid nodule.** A thyroid nodule refers to any abnormal growth that forms within the thyroid gland. Adult women (4% to 8%) are particularly prone to thyroid nodules, but, fortunately, only 10% of thyroid nodules are reported to be cancerous. The majority of thyroid nodules are asymptomatic; however, if the cells of the thyroid nodule are producing thyroid hormones, either thyroxine (T4) or triiodothyronine (T3), a thyroid nodule can lead to hyperthyroidism. Patient with hyperthyroidism may present with heart palpitations, weight loss, anxiety, insomnia, fatigue, heat intolerance, excessive sweating, exophthalmos (protruding eyes), and even amenorrhea (an absence of menstrual flow). Due to the symptoms of this patient and the mass being located at the location of the thyroid gland, a thyroid nodule is most likely diagnosis in this patient. **Choice A** (Enlarged deep cervical lymph node) is incorrect. The deep cervical lymph nodes lie within or in close proximity to the carotid sheath correlating in location with the internal jugular vein. While a few of the deep cervical lymph nodes could reside near the location of the mass, an enlarged deep cervical lymph node would not lead to the symptoms that brought this patient to the doctor, which were characteristic of hyperthyroidism. **Choice C** (Benign parathyroid adenoma) is incorrect. A parathyroid adenoma is a benign tumor of the parathyroid glands, which usually increases the circulation of parathyroid hormone (PTH). This condition of hyperparathyroidism leads to an increase in blood calcium levels due to elevated resorption of bone and may be asymptomatic in many patients. Symptomatic patients would present with lethargy, muscle pain, nausea, constipation, confusion, kidney stones, and even an increased risk of bone fractures due to the increased bone resorption. A physician can perform blood tests to test for calcium, chloride, potassium, and bicarbonate levels, and women over the age of 60 have the highest risk for developing hyperparathyroidism. The presence of a parathyroid adenoma has been reported in 80% to 85% of patients who present with hyperparathyroidism; however, the symptoms of this patient do not correlate with the presence of a parathyroid adenoma. **Choice D** (Thyroglossal duct cyst) is incorrect. The thyroid gland first appears as a single, ventromedian diverticulum (thyroid diverticulum) off the floor of the embryonic pharynx, between the tuberculum impar and copula of the incipient tongue. It descends along the midline, anterior to the gut tube, remaining connected to the tongue by a narrow canal (the thyroglossal duct). The thyroglossal duct usually solidifies and is obliterated after the final descent of the thyroid gland into its normal terminal position. A thyroglossal cyst is a cystic remnant of the thyroglossal duct. It is always located in or close to the midline of the neck. Most commonly (~50%), it is found near the body of the hyoid bone. Because the mass in this patient is located off the midline, a thyroglossal duct cyst is unlikely. Moreover, a thyroglossal cyst would not cause the symptoms seen in this patient. **Choice E** (Branchial cyst) is incorrect. Branchial cysts are located along the anterior border of the sternocleidomastoid muscle. Most often, these cysts are the remnants of the second pharyngeal cleft, located just below the angle of the mandible. Second branchial cleft cysts represent approximately 67% to 93% of all pharyngeal apparatus anomalies. However, branchial cysts may be found anywhere along the anterior margin of the sternocleidomastoid muscle. Very frequently, branchial cysts are inconspicuous at birth, becoming evident as they enlarge throughout childhood. Due to the location of the mass, symptoms of the patient, and age of the patient, a branchial cyst can be ruled out in this patient.

25   The answer is D: Infraorbital. The infraorbital nerve is a terminal branch of the maxillary (second) division of the trigeminal nerve (CN V$_2$). This nerve passes through the superior aspect (roof) of the maxillary sinus and emerges from the infraorbital foramen. It supplies the maxillary incisor, canine, and premolar teeth via its anterior and middle superior alveolar branches in the roof of the maxillary sinus. Ultimately, it supplies the inferior eyelid, cheek, lateral nose, and upper lip via its terminal branches in the face. In the described regional nerve block, the tip of the syringe needle is placed at the infraorbital foramen and the area is flooded with anesthetic, resulting in an infraorbital nerve block. The anesthetic agent also percolates through the thin maxillary bone to block the anterior and middle superior alveolar nerves. The infraorbital nerve is the only nerve listed, which could cause the extent of numbness and paresthesia described. **Choice A** (Anterior superior alveolar) is incorrect. The anterior superior alveolar nerve branches off the infraorbital nerve in the superior aspect (roof) of the maxillary sinus. It descends in a canal in the anterior wall of the maxillary sinus to supply the maxillary incisor and canine teeth. Blocking this nerve would numb most of the targeted dental area in this patient but would not account for the affected cutaneous region. In fact, the infraorbital nerve block is often administered following failure to block only the anterior superior alveolar nerve. **Choice B** (External nasal) is incorrect. The external nasal nerve is a terminal branch of the anterior ethmoidal nerve from the ophthalmic (first) division of the trigeminal nerve (CN V$_1$). It emerges between the bone and cartilage of the external nose to supply the tip of the nose. The external nasal nerve would not be responsible for the paresthesia and numbness described in this patient. **Choice C** (Infratrochlear) is incorrect. The infratrochlear nerve arises from the nasociliary nerve of the ophthalmic (first) division of the trigeminal nerve (CN V$_1$). It runs along the superior border of the medial rectus muscle, an extraocular muscle within the orbit, to supply cutaneous (sensory) innervation to the skin of the medial eyelids and bridge of the nose. It also supplies the conjunctiva, lacrimal sac, and caruncle of the eye. The infratrochlear nerve would not be responsible for the paresthesia and numbness described in this patient. **Choice E** (Nasopalatine) is incorrect. The nasopalatine nerve arises off the posterior superior nasal branches of the maxillary (second) division of the trigeminal nerve (CN V$_2$). It runs antero-inferior between the mucous membrane and periosteum of the nasal septum to enter the incisive canal in the roof of the mouth. It supplies the hard palate posterior to the maxillary incisor and canine teeth. The nasopalatine nerve would not be responsible for the paresthesia and numbness described in this patient.

26   The answer is A: Ethmoid. A fracture of the ethmoid bone, specifically its cribiform plate, which separates the nasal cavity from the anterior cranial fossa, would enable cerebrospinal fluid (CSF), the clear discharge that tests positive for glucose, to leak from the nose. The traumatic blow to the head has broken the cribiform plate of the ethmoid bone, which caused a communication between the patient's anterior cranial fossa and nasal cavity, which is noted by the black arrow in the given sagittal CT scan. This patient presents with CSF rhinorrhea, when can lead to meningitis and other intracranial complications, and this condition can be lethal if not properly treated. The given sagittal CT shows several fracture sites, including within the cribiform plate of the ethmoid bone as well as fractures of the anterior and posterior walls of the frontal sinus. The cribiform plate is fractured in several locations, and one of these fracture sites is indicated by the white arrow in the given CT. **Choice B** (Vomer) is incorrect. The unpaired vomer bone forms the bony posteroinferior component of the nasal septum. So, fracturing the vomer bone would not lead to the CSF rhinorrhea presentation of this patient. **Choice C** (Sphenoid) is incorrect. Portions of the sphenoid bone, specifically the crest and anterior part of the sphenoid body, do form a small component of the posterior roof of the nasal cavity. When a patient presents with CSF rhinorrhea, the cribiform plate of the ethmoid bone is the most likely fracture site, which will lead to a communication between the anterior cranial fossa and the nasal cavity. The given CT was added for visual evidence of this type of fracture. It should be noted that the sphenoid bone is fractured in this individual, which is typical of this type of trauma to the anterior skull base. Remember that the thinness of the cribiform plate of the ethmoid bone makes it more susceptible to injury, so the sphenoid bone is not the best answer for this question. **Choice D** (Maxilla) is incorrect. The maxilla contributes to the anterolateral walls of the nasal cavity and forms most of the boundary between the nasal and oral cavities. Though it is susceptible to injury, fracturing the maxilla would not provide a communication between the anterior cranial fossa and the nasal cavity or the CSF rhinorrhea seen in this patient. **Choice E** (Frontal) is incorrect. The nasal spine of the frontal bone does form a small part of the roof of the nasal cavity. However, this bone is not the BEST selection for this question as it does not contribute nearly as much to the roof as the ethmoid bone. The thinness of the cribiform plate of the ethmoid bone makes it a more likely candidate to cause CSF rhinorrhea after a fracture. The given CT was added for visual evidence of a fracture to the cribiform plate of the ethmoid bone. It should be noted that the frontal bone, specifically the anterior and posterior walls of the frontal sinus, is fractured in this individual.

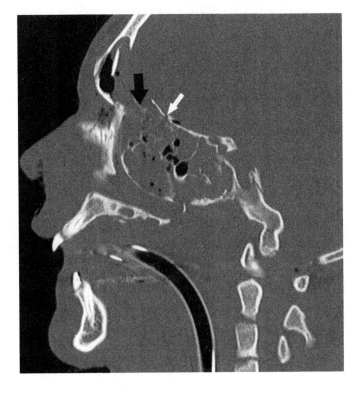

27 **The answer is B: Accessory.** The accessory nerve (CN XI) passes deep to the sternocleidomastoid muscle and to the investing layer of deep cervical fascia and courses postero-laterally into the lateral cervical region (posterior triangle of the neck). Due to its superficial course, it is at risk during a lymph node biopsy, cannulation of the internal jugular vein, carotid endartectomy, stab wounds, or removal of a mela-noma in the lateral cervical region. CN XI innervates only the sternocleidomastoid muscle and the trapezius muscle, which are primarily involved in head and shoulder movements. Specifically, the left sternocleidomastoid muscle contracts to bring the mastoid process of the temporal bone closer to the sternum, which results in tilting the head toward the left side and elevation of the chin to the right. The elevation of the chin to the right is the action being tested by this physi-cian, so the accessory nerve is the correct answer. **Choice A** (Hypoglossal nerve) is incorrect. The left hypoglossal nerve (CN XII) is located in the anterior cervical region, so it would not be damaged by a lymph node biopsy in the lateral cervi-cal region, or posterior triangle of the neck. Moreover, CN XII innervates all of the intrinsic muscles of the tongue and most of its extrinsic muscles with the lone exception being the palatoglossus muscle, innervated by the vagus nerve (CN X). Therefore, damage to the left CN XII would cause ipsi-lateral deviation of the tongue during protrusion and cause dysarthria, or difficulty speaking. In this patient, the doctor is testing the rotation of the head to the right, so the hypo-glossal nerve is not being assessed. **Choice C** (Mandibular division of trigeminal) is incorrect. The mandibular (third) division of the trigeminal nerve (CN V₃) is the only division of the trigeminal nerve (CN V) that supplies motor innerva-tion. It supplies the muscles derived from the mesoderm of the first pharyngeal arch, including the four muscles of mas-tication (temporalis, masseter, lateral pterygoid, and medial pterygoid) and four additional muscles: **M**ylohoid, **A**nterior belly of the Digastric, **T**ensor Tympani, and **T**ensor Veli Pala-tini (mnemonic = "MATT"). These muscles play no role in rotation of the head, and CN V₃ is not located in the lateral cervical triangle where the biopsy occurred. **Choice D** (Great auricular) is incorrect. The great auricular nerve does course through the lateral cervical region; however, it is a cutaneous (sensory) nerve supplying the skin over the mastoid process of the temporal bone, parotid gland, and auricle. It does not provide any motor innervation, so this nerve would not be involved with rotation of the head to the right side. **Choice E** (Upper trunk of the brachial plexus) is incorrect. The upper trunk of the brachial plexus is comprised of the anterior (ven-tral) rami of C5 and C6, and it emerges between the anterior and middle scalene muscles in the lateral cervical region (pos-terior triangle of neck). However, damage to the upper trunk of the brachial plexus would result in an abnormal postural presentation of the upper limb known as the "waiter's tip" deformity (or Erb-Duchenne palsy). The upper trunk of the brachial plexus is not involved with rotation of the head to the right side.

28 **The answer is E: Glossopharyngeal.** The glossopharyngeal nerve (CN IX) is responsible for visceral sensation to the posterior one third of the tongue, palatine tonsils, soft pal-ate, pharyngotympanic tube, tympanic (or middle ear) cav-ity, and pharynx. Therefore, CN IX would be responsible for the pain associated with the boy's earache and sore throat.

The palatine tonsillitis may be blocking the opening of the pharyngotympanic tube (auditory or eustachian), exacerbat-ing the symptoms of the patient. The glossopharyngeal nerve is also responsible for the afferent limb of the gag reflex. **Choice A** (Greater palatine) is incorrect. The greater pala-tine nerve, a branch off the maxillary (second) division of the trigeminal nerve (CN V₂), supplies sensory innervation to the mucosa and gingivae of the hard palate. It would not be responsible for the pain associated with the boy's earache and sore throat. **Choice B** (Lesser palatine) is incorrect. The lesser palatine nerve, a branch of the maxillary division of the trigeminal nerve (CN V₂), supplies sensory innervation to the soft palate and aspects of the palatine tonsil. However, it would not be responsible for the pain associated with the boy's earache and sore throat. **Choice C** (Vagus) is incorrect. The vagus nerve (CN X) serves as the efferent limb of the gag reflex because it gives motor innervation to a majority of muscles serving the soft palate, pharynx, and larynx. CN X does provide sensory (afferent) innervation in the larynx but not the areas affected in this patient. **Choice D** (Posterior superior alveolar) is incorrect. The posterior superior alveo-lar nerve, which branches off the maxillary division of the trigeminal nerve (CN V₂), supplies sensory innervation to the gingivae and posterior teeth of maxilla. This nerve would not be responsible for the pain associated with the boy's earache and sore throat.

29 **The answer is B: Branchial cyst.** The second pharyngeal (branchial) arch normally overgrows the more caudal pharyn-geal arches and merges with the epicardial ridge in the lower part of the developing neck region. This development causes the second, third, and fourth pharyngeal clefts (grooves) to lose contact with the surface of the neck and coalesce into a common cervical sinus. The cervical sinus is usually obliter-ated early in development. However, if the second arch does not properly grow caudally, remnants of the second, third, and/or fourth clefts may persist as a branchial cyst (lateral cer-vical cyst; cervical lymphoepithelial cyst) along the lateral side of the neck. This type of cyst may or may not be connected to the surface by a small drainage canal (branchial fistula). Thus, branchial cysts are the remnants of the cervical sinus and its duct. They are located along the anterior border of the SCM. Most often, these cysts are the remnants of the second pharyngeal cleft, located just below the angle of the mandible. Second branchial cleft cysts represent approximately 67% to 93% of all pharyngeal apparatus anomalies. However, bran-chial cysts may be found anywhere along the anterior margin of the SCM. Very frequently, branchial cysts are inconspicuous at birth, becoming evident as they enlarge throughout child-hood. **Choice A** (Thyroglossal cyst) is incorrect. The thyroid gland first appears as a single, ventromedian diverticulum (thyroid diverticulum) off the floor of the embryonic pharynx, between the tuberculum impar and copula of the incipient tongue. It descends along the midline, anterior to the gut tube, remaining connected to the tongue by a narrow canal (the thy-roglossal duct). The thyroglossal duct usually solidifies and is obliterated after the final descent of the thyroid gland into its normal terminal position. A thyroglossal cyst is a cystic rem-nant of the thyroglossal duct. It is always located in or close to the midline of the neck. Most commonly (~50%), it is found near the body of the hyoid bone. However, a thyroglossal cyst may lie anywhere along the normal migratory route of the thyroid gland. **Choice C** (Undescended thymus) is incorrect.

The thymus gland begins as epithelial primordia in the ventral wings of both the paired third pharyngeal (branchial) pouches. Losing their connections with the pharyngeal walls, these epithelial primordia descend caudally and medially and ultimately migrate into the upper anterior thorax where they fuse with each other. Sometimes, the tail portion of one or both of the descending primordia may persist in the neck. In such cases, thymic tissue may be embedded in the thyroid gland or may be found as isolated thymic pockets near the midline. Partial or complete absence of the thymus gland is a third pharyngeal pouch component of DiGeorge syndrome, a complex collection of craniofacial and cardiovascular anomalies. **Choice D** (Preauricular cyst) is incorrect. The auricle (pinna) of the external ear develops from multiple proliferations (auricular hillocks) in the dorsal ends of the first and second pharyngeal (branchial) arches, surrounding the opening of the first pharyngeal cleft. Its initial position is in the incipient neck region, with development of the neck and mandible causing the auricle to ascend to its final position at the side of the head. Development of the auricle is complicated, and congenital abnormalities of the auricle (preauricular cysts and pits, auricular sinuses, skin tags) are common. Importantly, auricular malformations are often associated with other congenital disorders. **Choice E** (Ectopic palatine tonsil) is incorrect. The fossa, epithelium, and crypts of the palatine tonsils are derived from the second pharyngeal (branchial) pouches and are related to the developing oropharyngeal region. The lymphoid tissue of the tonsil is a secondary infiltration of that bed. Ectopic lymphoid tissue may be found in small nodules near the tonsillar fossa.

30   **The answer is C: Maxillary bones.**   Neural crest cells arise in association with the neuroectoderm of the developing brain, and migrate into the pharyngeal arches, around the forebrain, and into the facial region. In these regions, neural crest cells account for numerous skeletal and other structures, including cartilage, tendon, dentin, dermis, sensory ganglia, and the arachnoid and pia mater. Therefore, development and migration of sufficient numbers of neural crest cells are critical for formation of much of the head and neck, especially the craniofacial region. Because neural crest cells also contribute significantly to heart formation, many infants with craniofacial defects also exhibit cardiac malformations. Unfortunately, neural crest cells are highly sensitive to environmental teratogens such as alcohol and retinoic acid. Overexposure to these substances (e.g., in fetal alcohol syndrome) may reduce production, kill, and/or limit the migration of the neural crest cells into their target regions. Neural crest cells form virtually all the facial skeleton, including the frontal, maxillary, zygomatic, squamous temporal, and mandibular bones, plus other smaller bones. Neural crest insufficiency is the major cause of palatofacial clefts that result from failure of fusion of facial primordia. **Choice A** (Laryngeal cartilages) is incorrect. Although neural crest cells form most of the skeletal structures (bone and cartilage) derived from the pharyngeal arches, the laryngeal cartilages are notable exceptions, derived from the lateral plate mesoderm of the fourth and sixth arches. **Choice B** (Parietal bones) is incorrect. Most of the cranial vault (including the parietal, occipital, and petrous portion of the temporal bones) and the cranial floor are formed from paraxial mesoderm (somites and somitomeres). **Choice D** (Common carotid arteries) is incorrect.

In general, the aortic arches that run within the pharyngeal arches are derived from the mesoderm of the pharyngeal arches, along with the muscles that originate there. Thus, the arteries derived from the aortic arches, including the common carotid arteries, have mesodermal origins. **Choice E** (Thyroid gland) is incorrect. The thyroid gland originates as an epithelial (endodermal) growth in the floor of the embryonic pharynx. It proliferates as a single, ventromedian diverticulum (thyroid diverticulum) off the pharynx, and descends into the neck.

31   **The answer is A: Maxillary and medial nasal processes.**   The face and palate are formed from the differentiation, growth, and merging of five facial primordia (facial prominences; facial swellings; facial processes): the single frontal (frontonasal) prominence and the paired maxillary and mandibular prominences (see figure on next page). The frontal prominence secondarily gives rise to paired nasal placodes and their bordering medial and lateral nasal prominences. Failure of the facial prominences to merge and fuse results in gaps (clefts) left remaining between primordial tissue zones. These gaps are the basis for palatofacial clefts of varying location and severity. The infant in this case suffers an anterior palatal cleft (cleft lip; harelip). Anterior clefts are located anterior to the incisive foramen. That location plus its position lateral to the midline indicates the defect was caused by incomplete fusion of the maxillary and medial nasal processes. Here, the defect is relatively small and unilateral. In more severe cases, the cleft may extend deeper and/or occur bilaterally. Cleft lip is a relatively common condition (1:1,000 births) that occurs more often in males and has an incidence that increases slightly with maternal age. Unilateral cleft lip is the most common craniofacial congenital defect. **Choice B** (Opposite maxillary processes) is incorrect. The opposite maxillary processes normally develop horizontal palatine shelves that fuse with each another in the midline to form the secondary palate (i.e., the bulk of the hard and soft palate). Defects in this fusion are termed posterior clefts (cleft palate) because they are located posterior to the incisive foramen. They vary in degree from relatively minor (cleft of only the uvula) to severe (cleft of the entire secondary palate). Posterior clefts occur less often than anterior clefts (1:2,500 births), occur more often in females, and are not related to maternal age. **Choice C** (Medial and lateral nasal processes) is incorrect. The medial and lateral nasal processes border each nasal placode. The tissue between each pair of nasal processes invaginates and canalizes to eventually form a nasal passage (i.e., the airway from naris to choana). Thus, the nasal processes fuse with each other only at their upper and lower margins to allow formation of the nasal passages. **Choice D** (Maxillary and lateral nasal processes) is incorrect. The maxillary prominence normally overgrows the nasolacrimal groove to fuse with its matching lateral nasal prominence. This development causes the nasolacrimal groove to sink into the face, where it canalizes and forms the nasolacrimal duct. Failure of this fusion is rare. When occurring, the result is an oblique facial cleft. In this craniofacial malformation, the defect runs from the medial canthus of the eye into the upper lip, with the nasolacrimal duct typically exposed to the surface. **Choice E** (Opposite medial nasal processes) is incorrect. The two medial nasal processes normally fuse in the midline to form the bridge of the nose, the nasal septum, and the intermaxillary segment of the face (philtrum of the upper lip; premaxilla; primary palate). Failure in this fusion is rare. The resultant malformation may be a midline grooved or cleft (bifid) nose and/or defects in the intermaxillary segment of

the face. Such conditions may indicate a more extensive loss of midline tissue (including neural tissue), characteristic of holoprosencephaly.

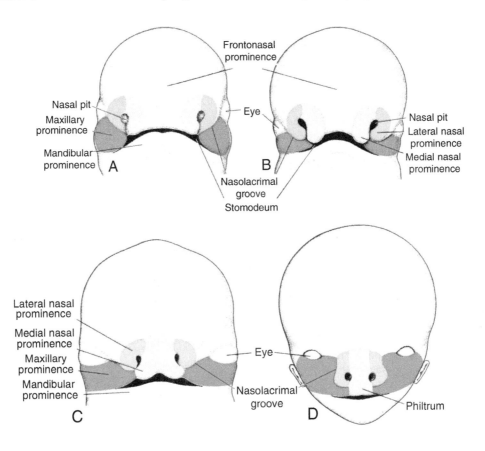

32 **The answer is B: Tensor tympani.** The masseter muscle is innervated by the masseteric branch of the mandibular division of the trigeminal nerve (CN V$_3$). The mandibular division of the trigeminal supplies all the skeletal muscles derived from the first pharyngeal arch. Thus, axonal degeneration in the masseter may indicate more widespread neural problems affecting any of the first arch muscles. These muscles, derived from the mesoderm of the first pharyngeal arch and innervated by the mandibular division of the trigeminal nerve (CN V$_3$), include the four muscles of mastication (temporalis, masseter, lateral pterygoid, and medial pterygoid) and four additional muscles: **M**ylohoid, **A**nterior belly of the Digastric, **T**ensor Veli Palatini, and **T**ensor Tympani (mnemonic = "MATT"). The tensor tympani muscle attaches to the malleus, a middle ear ossicle, and acts to adjust the tension of the tympanic membrane (eardrum). The malleus is also derived from the first pharyngeal arch, along with the incus. Further, the tympanic membrane forms partly from the epithelium of the first pharyngeal pouch. The other muscle in the middle ear, the stapedius, is derived from the second pharyngeal arch, attaches onto the stapes (also formed from the second arch), and is supplied by the facial nerve. One way to remember the innervation relations of the tensor tympani and tensor veli palatini is to recall the 3T's: the **T**rigeminal supplies the **T**ensors, which have distinct **T**endons. **Choice A** (Genioglossus) is incorrect. The genioglossus muscle is one of the extrinsic muscles of the tongue. All the extrinsic and intrinsic muscles of the tongue are supplied by the hypoglossal nerve (CN XII), with only one exception, the palatoglossus muscles, which are

supplied by the vagus nerve (CN X). These muscles of the tongue are derived from occipital somites. **Choice C** (Orbicularis oris) is incorrect. The orbicularis oris is one of the facial muscles (or muscles of facial expression). All of these muscles are derived from the mesoderm of the second (hyoid) pharyngeal arch and are supplied by the facial nerve (CN VII). **Choice D** (Levator veli palatini) is incorrect. The levator veli palatini is related to both the soft palate and the pharyngotympanic tube. It is derived from the fourth pharyngeal arch and is innervated by a pharyngeal branch of the vagus nerve (CN X). **Choice E** (Stylopharyngeus) is incorrect. The stylopharyngeus is a pharyngeal muscle. It is the sole skeletal muscle derived from the mesoderm of the third pharyngeal arch, and it is supplied by the glossopharyngeal nerve (CN IX).

33 **The answer is B: Second pharyngeal arch.** The asymmetry in the neck is due to an absence or underdevelopment of the platysma muscle on the patient's right side. The platysma is one of the facial muscles (or muscles of facial expression), even though it is located predominantly in the neck. The defining feature of the facial muscles is their origin or insertion into the subcutaneous tissue, which enables these muscles to convey facial expressions as well as alter the form of the facial orifices (orbits, nostrils, mouth, and external ears). All the facial muscles are derived from the mesoderm of the second pharyngeal (hyoid) arch and are innervated by the facial nerve (CN VII). Additional muscles derived from the second arch include the posterior belly of the digastric, stylohyoid, and stapedius. **Choice A** (First pharyngeal arch) is incorrect. The first pharyngeal (mandibular) arch folds on itself to form two parts: a dorsal maxillary process and a ventral mandibular process. This complex gives rise to the four muscles of mastication (temporalis, masseter, lateral pterygoid, and medial pterygoid) and four additional muscles: **M**ylohoid, **A**nterior belly of the Digastric, **T**ensor Veli Palatini, and **T**ensor Tympani (mnemonic = "MATT"). All are supplied by the mandibular division of the trigeminal nerve (CN V₃). **Choice C** (Third pharyngeal arch) is incorrect. The third pharyngeal arch gives rise to only a single skeletal muscle, the stylopharyngeus. This muscle is innervated by the glossopharyngeal nerve (CN IX). **Choice D** (Fourth pharyngeal arch) is incorrect. The fourth pharyngeal arch is the source of muscles of the soft palate (levator veli palatini, palatopharyngeus, muscle of uvula), pharynx (pharyngeal constrictors, salpingopharyngeus), tongue (palatoglossus), and larynx (cricothyroid). All are supplied by the superior laryngeal branch of the vagus nerve (CN X). **Choice E** (Fifth pharyngeal arch) is incorrect. The fifth pharyngeal arch is a rudimentary structure, along with the fifth pharyngeal pouch. These pharyngeal arch derivatives regress and disappear early in development. The absence of the fifth arch brings the sixth arch into such a close relationship with the fourth arch, and these pharyngeal arches are often considered a combined 4–6 arch complex. The sixth arch gives rise to most of the intrinsic laryngeal muscles and the esophageal skeletal musculature. The link between the fourth and sixth arches is reinforced by the innervation of the sixth arch by the recurrent laryngeal branch of the vagus nerve. Thus, the vagus nerve supplies both the fourth and sixth arch musculature.

34 **The answer is E: Inferior margin of the body of the mandible.** After originating from external carotid artery, the facial artery ascends in the upper neck deep to the posterior belly of the digastric and stylohyoid muscles and the submandibular gland. The facial artery then crosses the body of the mandible anterior to the masseter muscle to enter the face. Its pulse can be readily palpated at the point where it crosses the inferior margin of the body of the mandible, at the anterior border of the masseter muscle. The artery continues ascending across the face, taking a tortuous (or winding) path relatively close to the angle of the mouth. The folding of the vessel allows it to accommodate being stretched during wide opening of the mouth. It gives branches to the lips and side of the nose, finally terminating at the medial canthus (angle) of the eye. **Choice A** (Lateral side of the body of the hyoid bone) is incorrect. The facial artery arises from the external carotid artery in the upper neck. It courses superior to the hyoid bone. **Choice B** (Inferior edge of the zygomatic arch) is incorrect. The transverse facial artery arises within the parotid gland as a small branch of the superficial temporal artery. As it runs anterior, the transverse facial artery crosses the masseter muscle and is located just above the parotid duct and below the zygomatic arch. **Choice C** (Apex of the zygomatic bone) is incorrect. This bony feature is the point of the "cheek bone." No significant vessels reside at this location, so taking a pulse at the apex of the zygomatic bone is not possible. **Choice D** (Lateral surface of the nasal bone) is incorrect. As it ascends across the face, that facial artery gives branches to the ala and side of the nose (lateral nasal artery) and its terminal branch to the medial angle (canthus) of the eye (angular artery). However, these vessels are small and do not normally give pulse points.

35 **The answer is D: Philtrum.** The intermaxillary segment of the face is derived from the fused medial nasal processes of the facial primordia. It is the midline segment of the upper jaw and is composed of three parts: (1) the philtrum of the upper lip, (2) the premaxilla, and (3) the primary palate. The philtrum is the midline section of the upper lip that normally appears as a small fossa directly under the nasal aperture. The premaxilla is the bony segment that carries the four upper incisors. The primary palate is the small triangular shelf of bone directly posterior to the upper incisors. Its apex is the incisive foramen. Anterior palatal clefts typically lie along one or both lateral edges of the intermaxillary segment, where the medial nasal process would have fused with the maxillary process. Developmental failure of the medial nasal processes to merge causes a midline defect that may include absence of the entire intermaxillary segment (premaxillary agenesis). **Choice A** (Nasal bones) is incorrect. The nasal bones are derived from the frontonasal process primordial element, perhaps including the medial nasal processes. However, the nasal bones are not components of the intermaxillary segment of the face forming parts of the upper jaw. **Choice B** (Soft palate) is incorrect. The soft palate is formed from the posterior portion of the secondary palate. The secondary palate is derived from the palatine shelves of the maxillary processes. Posterior palatal clefts are located posterior to the intermaxillary segment and may include defects in the soft palate. **Choice C** (Inferior nasal conchae) is incorrect. These delicate bones are located on the inferolateral sides of the nasal cavities. Each is derived from the maxillary process, which also gives rise to the maxillary and zygomatic bones in the face and the lateral part of the upper lip, lateral to the philtrum. **Choice E** (Mandibular incisors) is incorrect. These teeth are located in the lower jaw. However, the upper incisors are held in the premaxillary part of the upper jaw and would be affected by premaxillary agenesis.

36 **The answer is B: Dense connective tissue.** The second layer of the scalp is composed of dense fibrous connective tissue, and this layer houses the main networks of nerves and vessels that enter the scalp from its periphery. The walls of the arteries within the scalp are tightly attached to the surrounding connective tissue bed. As a result, scalp lesions that penetrate the second layer tend to bleed profusely because the fibrous tissue holds apart the cut ends of the severed vessels. Conveniently, the scalp can be divided into five structural/functional layers, which create a mnemonic "SCALP" when moving from superficial to deep zones. Layer 1 (most superficial) is **S**kin. Layer 2 is the (dense) **C**onnective tissue highlighted in this question. Layer 3 is **A**poneurosis of the epicranius muscle (or the epicranial aponeurosis). Layer 4 is **L**oose (areolar) connective tissue that enables free movement of the first three layers of the scalp over the calvaria. Layer 5 is **P**ericranium (external periosteum), which is a dense layer of connective tissue fused to the outer surfaces of the neurocranium. The mnemonic "SCALP" can enable a student to recall the five layers of the scalp. **Choice A** (Skin) is incorrect. Skin is the first layer of the scalp, and it is the typically hair-bearing epidermis rich in sebaceous glands. **Choice C** (Epicranial aponeurosis) is incorrect. The epicranius (occipitofrontalis) muscle is formed by the frontalis and occipitalis muscles and the expansive aponeurosis that binds them together. This unit forms the third layer of the scalp. It is responsible for movement of the scalp by the actions of its muscular ends. Deep scalp wounds through the epicranius (especially the aponeurotic part in the frontal plane) tend to gape widely because the frontalis and occipitalis muscles pull in opposite directions and widen the lesion. **Choice D** (Loose connective tissue) is incorrect. Loose (areolar) connective tissue is the fourth layer of the scalp, and it forms the sub-aponeurotic space of the scalp, which becomes the plane of movement enabling the first three layers of the scalp to slide as a unit relative to the underlying pericranium. This loose connective tissue is also considered the danger layer of the scalp because infectious matter (blood, pus) can spread easily and widely through this fourth layer of the scalp. Also, infections can move from this layer through emissary (epiploic) veins into the intracranial dural venous sinuses. **Choice E** (Pericranium) is incorrect. The deepest (fifth) layer of the scalp is the pericranium (or external periosteum), which is a dense layer of connective tissue fused to the outer surfaces of the bones of the cranial vault.

37 **The answer is B: Auriculotemporal nerve.** The parotid is the largest salivary gland, occupying much of the retromandibular space. It is enclosed by two capsules: (1) the connective tissue capsule of the gland itself and (2) a dense fibrous capsule derived from the investing layer of deep cervical fascia. As a result, inflammation and swelling of the parotid, caused by mumps in this patient, can increase pressure significantly within the tightly bound glandular mass. Several structures are contained within the parotid as they pass across the face. Each of these structures is subject to undue pressure in disease conditions and must be carefully considered in surgery of this salivary gland. The auriculotemporal nerve, a branch of the mandibular division of the trigeminal nerve (CN V$_3$), traverses the substance of the parotid in its course from the infratemporal fossa to the lateral scalp. This nerve is the major sensory supply across the mandibular region, provides the parasympathetic secretomotor route to the parotid, and innervates the connective tissue within the gland itself. Irritation of the auriculotemporal nerve due to inflammation and swelling of the parotid produces severe pain. Pain would also be derived from the great auricular nerve, a branch of the cervical plexus composed of fibers from the C2 and C3 spinal nerves, which innervates the parotid sheath as well as the skin overlying the angle of the mandible and inferior lobe of the auricle. Other structures contained within the parotid include the facial nerve, the formation of the retromandibular vein (superficial temporal, maxillary, and retromandibular veins), and the termination of the external carotid artery (external carotid, superficial temporal, and maxillary arteries). **Choice A** (Buccal nerve of CN V$_3$) is incorrect. The buccal nerve is a sensory (afferent) branch of the mandibular division of the trigeminal nerve (CN V$_3$). It passes anterior through the infratemporal fossa, emerges from under the masseter muscle, and distributes across the cheek. Dentists often refer to this nerve as the long buccal nerve. In this case, it lies anterior to the parotid gland and its enveloping capsules. **Choice C** (Posterior belly of the digastric muscle) is incorrect. The posterior belly of the digastric originates from the deep aspect of the mastoid process and passes into the neck to attach to the hyoid bone. It would not be directly compressed by the inflammation of the parotid sheath due to its location inferior to the parotid gland. **Choice D** (External jugular vein) is incorrect. The external jugular vein is formed in the upper neck by the union of the

posterior branch of the retromandibular vein with the posterior auricular vein inferior to the parotid gland. It would not be directly compressed by the inflammation of the parotid sheath. **Choice E** (Facial artery) is incorrect. The facial artery originates in the upper neck, from the external carotid artery. It ascends to cross the mandible at the anterior edge of the masseter muscle, anterior to the parotid gland, to enter the face.

38 **The answer is D: Orbicularis oris.** The orbicularis oris is a muscle of facial expression (mimetic muscle), and these muscles insert or originate in the subcutaneous tissue of the skin, which enables them to convey mood via facial expressions as well as alter the form of the facial orifices. All the muscles of facial expression are derived from the mesoderm of the second pharyngeal (hyoid) arch and innervated by the facial nerve (CN VII). Most of these muscles are located within the face; however, a few extend into the scalp (e.g., epicranius) or the neck (platysma). The most important, and therefore most clinically relevant, role of the facial muscles is to control and operate the facial orifices, that is, the eyes, nose, mouth, and ears. Facial expression is a secondary byproduct of the ability to finely control the facial orifices. The mouth is controlled by an extensive, interweaving array of facial muscles that influence feeding, respiration, and articulate speech. The orbicularis oris is a broad, very complex muscle that encircles the mouth in a sphincter-like fashion. It interacts with the other orofacial muscles to modify the form and tension of the lips and their margins. By itself, it acts to close the mouth by bringing the lips together tightly. **Choice A** (Zygomaticus major) is incorrect. The zygomaticus major is an elongated muscle of facial expression that originates on the lateral aspect of the zygomatic bone and attaches into the angle of the mouth. It contracts to dilate oral fissure, but it also elevates the labial commissures bilaterally to smile (show happiness) or unilaterally to sneer (show disdain). **Choice B** (Buccinator) is incorrect. The buccinator (L: trumpeter) muscle is a wide, thin muscle of facial expression that lies relatively deep in the cheek, coursing from the pterygopalatine raphe and the alveolar ridges of maxillary and mandibular molar teeth to insert into the orbicularis oris at the angle of the mouth. The buccinator compresses the cheeks and lips against the teeth and gums, provides resistance to keep the teeth from tilting laterally, and prevents patients from looking like a hamster when they chew food. This muscle is important in all phases of feeding. During mastication, it assists in positioning food between the occlusal surfaces of the teeth. In suckling, it creates pressure within the oral cavity. This pressure also serves in blowing air, as when playing a wind instrument. **Choice C** (Levator labii superioris) is incorrect. The levator labii superioris is a relatively large muscle of facial expression that runs from the infraorbital margin of the maxilla into the upper lip. Acting in concert with its neighbors, it dilates the oral fissure by elevating and everting the upper lip to show the upper (maxillary) teeth. It also deepens nasolabial sulcus to show sadness. Please note that this muscle covers the infraorbital foramen, lying over the emerging infraorbital nerve and vessels. **Choice E** (Mentalis) is incorrect. The mentalis is a small, conical muscle of facial expression that originates on the incisive fossa of the mandible and inserts into the skin of the chin and the base of the lower lip. When pouting, this muscle raises, protrudes, and everts the lower lip. This muscle also elevates the skin of the chin to show doubt.

39 **The answer is C: Vertebral artery.** The stenosis of the right subclavian artery depicted in the MRA causes reduced blood flow to the right upper limb, leading to weakness. This stenosis causes the anatomical subclavian steal syndrome, in which the right vertebral artery, which is dilated in the provided MRA, delivers blood back into the occluded subclavian artery. With the stenosis of the proximal end of the right subclavian artery, the resulting arterial pressure differentials enable blood to enter the right vertebral artery after being "stolen" from the left (contralateral) internal carotid tract via the cerebral arterial circle (of Willis) and basilar circulation within the skull. In this patient, blood would travel retrograde within the right vertebral artery to circumvent the stenosis in the proximal right subclavian artery and re-establish blood flow to the right limb. This collateral pathway enables continued use of the right limb; however, the blood being diverted away from the brain can cause brainstem and/or cerebral ischemia, and possibly lead to a stroke. The symptoms seen in this patient, including dizziness, ataxia, vertigo, and aphasia, are indicators of the vertebrobasilar insufficiency, which tells the physician that the collateral circulation is emanating from the cranial circulation. A mnemonic for the four branches of the subclavian artery is "VITamin C," which stands for the Vertebral artery, Internal thoracic artery, Thyrocervical trunk, and Costocervical trunk. **Choice A** (Internal thoracic artery) is incorrect. The internal thoracic (internal mammary) artery arises from the subclavian artery as its second branch, typically distal to the origin of the vertebral artery. It descends into the thorax along the edge of the sternum to supply the thoracic and abdominal walls, and it receives extensive and important collateral connections along its course. Theoretically, the internal thoracic artery could contribute to bypassing the stenosis of the subclavian artery; however, this artery is not dilated in the provided MRA and its involvement in this case of anatomical subclavian steal syndrome would not account for the cranial ischemia and resulting symptoms. **Choice B** (Common carotid artery) is incorrect. The brachiocephalic trunk ends by dividing into its terminal branches, the right common carotid and right subclavian arteries. The stenosis depicted in the given MRA is distal to the origin of the common carotid artery, so it would not deter blood from entering into the common carotid artery and would not set up the arterial pressure differentials needed for reverse flow within it. The common carotid artery has no direct connections distal to the stenosis of the subclavian artery, so this artery is unable to bypass the occlusion. **Choice D** (Superior thyroid artery) is incorrect. The superior thyroid artery is the first branch of the external carotid artery, which supplies the thyroid gland and neighboring muscles. If blood traveled retrograde through the superior thyroid artery, it would travel back toward the common carotid artery, which is located proximal to the stenosis of the right subclavian artery. **Choice E** (Suprascapular artery) is incorrect. The thyrocervical trunk arises as the third branch of the first part of the subclavian artery, proximal to the anterior scalene muscle. The thyrocervical trunk typically divides into four branches: suprascapular, inferior thyroid, ascending cervical, and transverse cervical arteries. The suprascapular artery runs across the root of the neck to the superior border of the scapula where it supplies blood to the dorsal aspect of the scapula. It does not have any relations to the branching pattern needed to compensate for the stenosis of the subclavian artery in this anatomical subclavian steal syndrome.

40 **The answer is A: Maxillary process.** The muscles in question are located in the midface/lateral upper lip region. This area is formed around the maxillary process of the first pharyngeal arch. The atrophied muscles in this patient are derived from mesoderm of the second pharyngeal arch, which migrates into all the facial primordia. However, the underlying midfacial skeleton is derived from neural crest cells that migrate into the maxillary process portion of the first pharyngeal arch. Overall, the maxillary process gives rise to the lateral part of the upper lip, the midface, and the secondary palate. **Choice B** (Mandibular process) is incorrect. The mandibular process, the lower portion of the first pharyngeal arch, gives rise to the lower face region, including the entire lower lip and lower jaw. **Choice C** (Frontal process) is incorrect. The frontal (frontonasal) process is the only facial primordial component not derived from the first pharyngeal arch. Rather, this unpaired element forms from mesenchymal proliferation ventral to the forebrain vesicle (prosencephalon). The frontal process gives rise to the upper face (forehead) and part of the nose (bridge and tip of the nose and rostral nasal septum). **Choice D** (Lateral nasal process) is incorrect. The nasal processes are the elevated rims of the nasal placodes that form in the frontal process. The lateral nasal process gives rise to a small part of the face, the sides of the nose and the alae. **Choice E** (Medial nasal process) is incorrect. The medial nasal process gives rise to significant structures in the midline of the face, including contributions to the bridge and tip of the nose and nasal septum and the entire intermaxillary segment of the face.

41 **The answer is E: Arterial supply to the dura mater is reduced.** The indicated opening is the foramen spinosum. This small foramen conveys the middle meningeal artery (a branch of the maxillary artery) and the spinous nerve (a branch of the mandibular division of the trigeminal nerve, or CN V_3) from the infratemporal fossa into the cranium, in the floor of the middle cranial fossa. The middle meningeal artery provides the major blood supply to the dura mater and the cranial bones. It does not supply the brain. The middle meningeal artery is often involved with epidural hematomas. **Choice A** (Venous drainage from the base of the brain is obstructed) is incorrect. The main venous drainage of the brain is through the dural venous sinuses into the internal jugular veins, which exit the cranial cavity through the jugular foramina. This primary drainage route is supplemented by several emissary veins that pass through various other openings in the skull, including the foramen ovale and carotid canal in the floor of the middle cranial fossa. However, the foramen spinosum does not normally carry emissary veins. **Choice B** (Mucus secretion in the oral floor is reduced) is incorrect. Mucus secretion in the oral floor is controlled by parasympathetic neurons within the chorda tympani nerve. The chorda tympani branches from the facial nerve in the facial canal, passes through the tympanic (middle ear) cavity, and leaves that space through a small opening (petrotympanic fissure) to enter the infratemporal fossa. **Choice C** (Sensation from the mandibular teeth is lost) is incorrect. Afferent neurons from the mandibular teeth are carried in the inferior alveolar nerve, a branch of the mandibular division of the trigeminal nerve (CN V_3). CN V_3 passes through the foramen ovale in the base of the skull. The inferior alveolar nerve passes through the mandibular foramen as it leaves the mandible conveying sensation from the mandibular teeth. **Choice D** (Motor control of the pharyngeal constrictor muscles is lost) is incorrect. Motor control of the pharyngeal constrictor muscles is from branches of the vagus nerve (CN X). The vagus exits the cranial cavity through the jugular foramen, in company with the glossopharyngeal (CN IX) and accessory (CN XI) nerves.

42 **The answer is A: Internal acoustic meatus.** The loss of facial expression and drooping corner of the mouth indicate paralysis of the facial muscles and damage to the facial nerve (CN VII). The intact ability to clench the jaw and chew denotes proper functioning of the muscles of mastication and an intact mandibular division of the trigeminal nerve (CN V_3). The hearing loss and unsteady balance indicate failure in the inner ear complex implicating the right vestibulocochlear nerve (CN VIII; auditory nerve). The absence of the blink reflex is related to loss of the orbicularis oculi muscle, the facial muscle responsible for closing the eyelids, and this evidence reinforces a problem with the facial nerve. Normal cutaneous sensation across the face indicates the entire trigeminal pathway is intact. Therefore, the suspected tumor affects both CN VII and CN VIII, but not the trigeminal nerve (CN V). The only location where CN VII and CN VIII can be affected simultaneously is at the internal acoustic meatus (in the wall of the posterior cranial fossa), where the paired nerves leave the cranial cavity to enter the petrous part of the temporal bone. Very quickly thereafter, the nerves diverge and follow separate pathways to their target regions. The given contrast-enhanced T1-weighted MRI demonstrates a right-sided vestibular schwannoma (acoustic neuroma), located at the internal acoustic meatus and identified by the arrow, which confirms this diagnosis. This vestibular schwannoma, which is clearly seen in white due to the gadolinium-based intravenous contrast, resides at the cerebellopontine angle and affects the facial and vestibulocochlear nerves as they emerge from this location. This tumor would also increase intracranial pressure potentially causing pontomedullary brain stem compression. **Choice B** (Foramen ovale) is incorrect. The mandibular division of the trigeminal nerve (CN V_3) passes through the foramen ovale in the floor of the middle cranial fossa. At this location, a tumor would affect the muscles of mastication and cutaneous sensation over the mandibular region of the face, which is not evident in this patient. **Choice C** (Foramen rotundum) is incorrect. The maxillary division of the trigeminal nerve (CN V_2) passes through this opening in the anterior wall of the middle cranial fossa. Nerve damage here would affect cutaneous sensation across the midfacial region, which is not evident in this patient. **Choice D** (Geniculum of the facial canal) is incorrect. The facial nerve travels through the facial canal within the petrous part of the temporal bone, including the knee-like bend (geniculum) of the canal. Thus, tumor growth in this location would affect the facial nerve and produce the facial paralysis described in this case. However, the vestibulocochlear nerve would not be affected at this site, as it has already separated from the facial nerve. **Choice E** (Stylomastoid foramen) is incorrect. The main branch of the facial nerve exits the skull through the stylomastoid foramen at the base of the skull. Tumor growth here would affect the facial nerve, producing the described facial paralysis. However, the vestibulocochlear nerve would not be affected by problems at this location.

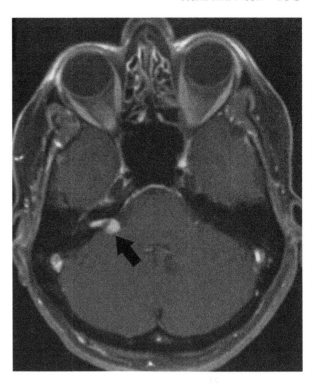

43 **The answer is E: Jugular foramen.** The jugular foramen is a large opening that connects the posterior cranial fossa with the exterior base of the skull. It is divided into an anterior and a posterior compartment for its major contents. The anterior compartment transmits a bundle of three cranial nerves out of the cranial cavity: the glossopharyngeal nerve (CN IX), the vagus nerve (CN X), and the (spinal) accessory nerve (CN XI). The superior ganglia of the glossopharyngeal and vagus nerves are located within the jugular foramen, whereas the inferior ganglia are situated just outside it. Upon exiting the jugular foramen, the nerves immediately diverge from one another to pass to their target regions. The posterior compartment transmits the internal jugular vein. This large vessel originates at the terminal end of the sigmoid dural sinus, at the internal opening of the jugular foramen. Thus, trauma to the jugular foramen can have significant and widespread vascular and neural consequences. **Choice A** (Foramen ovale) is incorrect. This large, oval-shaped opening connects the middle cranial fossa with the exterior base of the skull. It transmits the mandibular division of the trigeminal nerve (CN V_3) from the trigeminal ganglion into the infratemporal fossa. A small accessory meningeal artery (a branch of the maxillary artery) typically accompanies the nerve through the foramen ovale. **Choice B** (Foramen spinosum) is incorrect. This small foramen conveys the middle meningeal artery (a branch of the maxillary artery) and the spinous nerve (a branch of the mandibular division of the trigeminal nerve) from the infratemporal fossa into the cranium. **Choice C** (Foramen lacerum) is incorrect. The foramen lacerum is a large opening that connects the floor of the middle cranial fossa with the exterior base of the skull. Its irregular form gives the appearance of a roughly torn area (a laceration) in the skull, hence its name. However, in life, it is almost entirely filled with cartilage, and the true foramen is very small. The greater petrosal nerve (a parasympathetic branch of the facial nerve) traverses this foramen lacerum in passing from the floor of the middle cranial fossa to the mouth of the pterygoid canal at its anterior margin.

Also, small lymphatic vessels and perhaps small emissary veins pass through this cranial foramen. **Choice D** (Carotid canal) is incorrect. The carotid canal is a large, obliquely running passage through the base of the skull. It carries the internal carotid artery from the deep, upper neck into the middle cranial fossa. The carotid canal merges with the internal opening of the foramen lacerum within the skull to bring the internal carotid into position at the side of the sella turcica.

44   **The answer is C: Inability to close the eyelids.**   The stylomastoid foramen is located in a well-protected position between the styloid and mastoid processes, at the base of the skull. It is the terminal opening of the facial canal, transmitting the main branch of the facial nerve out of the petrous temporal bone to the exterior base of the skull. From there, the facial nerve sends sensory branches to the external ear, motor branches to small muscles in the upper neck (stylohyoid and posterior belly of the digastric), and terminal motor branches to the facial muscles (muscles of facial expression). However, the mastoid process is not developed at birth, leaving the stylomastoid foramen and the emerging facial nerve exposed. Undue pressure applied to the mastoid area (as from misapplied obstetric forceps) may entrap and damage the facial nerve. In this case, crush injury to the facial nerve would produce unilateral paralysis of the facial muscles, including the orbicularis oculi. This sphincter-like muscle surrounds the orbit, acting to close the eyelids. **Choice A** (Reduced blood flow to the inner ear) is incorrect. Vascular supply to the inner ear is provided by small labyrinthine vessels that accompany the facial and vestibulocochlear nerves through the internal acoustic meatus. Supply to the external ear is mainly from branches of the posterior auricular and superficial temporal arteries. The posterior auricular arterial branching is susceptible to damage in this scenario. Supply to the middle ear is mainly from branches of the maxillary artery. These vessels are unlikely to be affected by compression around the incipient mastoid process. **Choice B** (No sensation in the external acoustic meatus) is incorrect. The external ear receives afferent innervation from a plethora of cranial nerves, including trigeminal (CN V), facial (CN VII), vagus (CN X), and possibly even the glossopharyngeal (CN IX). The trigeminal and vagus are the major nerves, supplying most of the sensory fibers to this region, including the external acoustic meatus. The facial nerve provides relatively small contributions to the sensation of the external acoustic meatus because its sensory innervation is concentrated on the auricle. **Choice D** (Lack of taste on the body of the tongue) is incorrect. The facial nerve provides taste fibers to the body (anterior two thirds) of the tongue and parasympathetic fibers to the oral floor via its chorda tympani branch. However, the chorda tympani nerve leaves the facial nerve within the facial canal, traverses the tympanic (middle ear) cavity, and exits the base of the skull near the temporomandibular joint (TMJ). Therefore, this forceps injury would not affect the taste or parasympathetic functions governed by the facial nerve. **Choice E** (Inability to tense the eardrum) is incorrect. The tensor tympani muscle attaches to the handle of the malleus, acting to pull this ear ossicle medially and tense the tympanic membrane (eardrum). This muscle is innervated by the mandibular division of the trigeminal nerve (CN V_3). The stapedius muscle attaches to the stapes, acting to tighten the oval window. This muscle is controlled by the facial nerve, via a branch off the facial canal, proximal to the stylomastoid foramen.

45   **The answer is D: Petrous portion of temporal bone.**   The petrous portion of the temporal bone is a large wedge-shaped structure extending from the side of the skull toward the midline, forming much of the boundary between the middle and posterior cranial fossae. It is the densest bone in the body, being composed almost entirely of compact bone tissue. As a result, it forms a strong radiopaque image in plain films and CT scans. The image here is a PA (Posterior-Anterior) plain film (X-ray) of the head. The petrous part of the temporal bone appears as a distinct opaque structure with a sharp upper margin (petrous ridge) across the lower aspect of the orbit. Thus, it serves as a notable orientation structure in this view. **Choice A** (Superior orbital rim) is incorrect. The upper rim of the orbit is part of the frontal bone. It forms a distinct radiopaque curve well above the petrous ridge in the PA view. **Choice B** (Squamous part of temporal bone) is incorrect. The squamous portion of the temporal bone is a relatively thin, flat plate on the side of the skull. The curvature of the skull, plus the angle of this view, accounts for the opaque edge seen here. **Choice C** (Mastoid process) is incorrect. The mastoid process is a breast-like appendage of the temporal bone, housing the extensive mastoid air cells (mastoid sinuses). This pneumatic composition results in the mastoid process appearing as a ghost-like, nearly radiolucent image in the PA view. **Choice E** (Upper alveolar margin) is incorrect. The upper alveolar margin is the tooth-bearing part of the maxillary bone. It forms a horseshoe-shaped arch under the nasal cavity in this view. The appearance of the arcade may be intensified by the presence of dental fillings.

46   **The answer is E: Tympanic cavity.**   Evagination of the first pharyngeal pouch forms an elongate diverticulum off the pharynx (the tubotympanic recess). The distal part of this recess widens to form the tympanic (or middle ear) cavity. The proximal part remains more tubular and forms the pharyngotympanic (auditory; eustachian) tube. Development of the tubotympanic recess induces the formation of the overlying first pharyngeal cleft (groove), which forms the external acoustic meatus. The closing plate (pharyngeal membrane) between the tubotympanic recess and the first pharyngeal groove (i.e., the tissue interface between the two) forms the tympanic membrane (eardrum). **Choice A** (Thyroid gland) is incorrect. The thyroid gland first forms as a single, ventromedian diverticulum (thyroid diverticulum) off the floor of the embryonic pharynx, between the tuberculum impar and copula of the incipient tongue. It descends caudally along the midline, anterior to the gut tube, until achieving its final location in the neck. The thyroid gland is not derived from the pharyngeal pouches, so it can be easily eliminated as an answer. **Choice B** (Thymus gland) is incorrect. The thymus gland begins as bilateral epithelial primordia in the ventral portions of the third pharyngeal (branchial) pouches, which lose their connections with the pharyngeal walls, descend caudally and medially, and ultimately migrate into the upper anterior thorax where they fuse with each other. Descent of the thymic primordia is notably influenced by shifting of the embryonic heart into the differentiating thorax. **Choice C** (Parathyroid glands) is incorrect. The parathyroid glands develop from the epithelia of both the third and fourth pharyngeal pouches. The inferior parathyroid appears in the dorsal part of the third pouch, near the incipient thymus gland. The parathyroid is drawn caudally with the migration of the thymic tissue, eventually fixing into place near the caudal dorsal aspect of the thyroid gland. The superior parathyroid first forms in the dorsal part of the fourth pharyngeal pouch. This tissue attaches to the migrating thyroid gland and takes position in the more cranial dorsal aspect of the thyroid. **Choice D** (Facial muscles) is incorrect. The facial muscles (muscles of facial expression) are small skeletal muscles that form from the mesoderm of the second (hyoid) pharyngeal arch. Other muscles derived from the second arch include the stapedius (in the middle ear), and the stylohyoid and posterior belly of the digastric (in the upper neck). All the second arch muscles are supplied by the facial nerve (CN VII).

47 **The answer is C: Middle nasal meatus.** The lateral nasal wall is formed largely by three nasal conchae (turbinate bones). The superior and middle conchae are parts of the ethmoid bone. The inferior concha is an independent bone. The conchae divide the nasal passage into four air channels: the sphenoethmoidal recess (above the superior concha), the superior meatus (below the superior concha), the middle meatus (below the middle concha), and the inferior meatus (below the inferior concha). The paranasal sinuses open into the nasal passage on its lateral wall, in specific relations to the conchae and meati. The maxillary sinus is the largest paranasal sinus, occupying much of the maxillary bone. Infections there may affect the upper teeth, causing a toothache, because the sinus cavity is separated from the roots of the teeth by only a very thin layer of bone. The maxillary sinus opens into the most posterior part of the semilunar hiatus in the middle meatus. The frontal, anterior ethmoidal, and middle ethmoidal sinuses also open nearby into the middle meatus. **Choice A** (Sphenoethmoidal recess) is incorrect. The sphenoethmoidal recess receives the drainage of the sphenoidal sinus. **Choice B** (Superior nasal meatus) is incorrect. The superior nasal meatus contains the opening of the posterior ethmoidal sinuses (air cells). **Choice D** (Inferior nasal meatus) is incorrect. The inferior nasal meatus does not receive the opening of any paranasal sinus. Instead, it contains the opening of the nasolacrimal duct, thus receiving drainage of tears from the eye. **Choice E** (Pharyngotympanic tube) is incorrect. The pharyngotympanic (auditory; eustachian) tube opens into the nasopharynx, posterior to the nasal passage. It is not a component of any nasal meatus.

48 **The answer is C: Superficial temporal.** The superficial temporal artery is the smaller terminal branch of the external carotid artery. It ascends through the parotid gland, anterior to the auricle, and crosses the zygomatic arch to reach the temporal fossa and scalp. Its pulse (the temporal pulse) can be palpated anterior to the tragus of the external ear where the artery lies against the underlying zygomatic arch. **Choice A** (Maxillary) is incorrect. The maxillary artery is the larger terminal branch of the external carotid artery. From its origin within the substance of the parotid gland, it passes anterior, deep to the ramus of the mandible, to enter the infratemporal fossa. Its deep location makes this artery an unlikely candidate for taking a pulse. **Choice B** (Posterior auricular) is incorrect. The posterior auricular artery is a branch of the external carotid artery that runs posterior, near the styloid process to pass behind the ear. It supplies the auricle and the scalp, posterior to the auricle. It does not provide a palpable pulse location. **Choice D** (Facial) is incorrect. The facial artery is another branch of the external carotid artery.

It ascends anterior, deep to the posterior belly of the digastric and stylohyoid muscles and the submandibular gland, and crosses the mandible to enter the face. Its pulse can be readily palpated at the point where it crosses the inferior margin of the body of the mandible, at the anterior border of the masseter muscle. However, the pulse was taken anterior to the tragus of the auricle. **Choice E** (Internal carotid) is incorrect. This large vessel is one of the terminal branches of the common carotid artery. It arises deep in the upper neck and ascends into the base of the skull. Whereas the common carotid can be palpated lower in the neck, the internal carotid is too deep to detect a pulse.

49 **The answer is A: Lacrimal punctum.** The lacrimal apparatus is composed of the lacrimal gland, lacrimal canaliculi, lacrimal sac, and nasolacrimal duct. The lacrimal gland, located in the upper lateral corner of the orbit, secretes tears into the superolateral conjunctival fornix. Tears are spread across the eye by the blinking actions of the eyelids and accumulate in the medial corner (canthus) of the eye. They drain into the paired lacrimal canaliculi by passing through the lacrimal puncta (pores). This photo shows a silicone plug present in the inferior punctum of the patient's left eye. If permitted to enter the punctum, tears pass through the lacrimal canaliculus, the lacrimal sac, through the nasolacrimal duct, and enter the nasal cavity via inferior nasal meatus. Obstruction of a punctum with a silicone plug effectively closes the doorway into a canaliculus and prevents normal tear drainage. This plug placement would keep tears within the eye to lubricate and protect the cornea, which is altered in LASIK surgery to improve visual acuity. **Choice B** (Lacrimal canaliculus) is incorrect. The lacrimal canaliculi are paired canals into which the puncta drain in the margin of the eyelids, at their medial corners. The lacrimal punctum is obstructed with the silicone plug, so tears would not enter the lacrimal canaliculus. **Choice C** (Lacrimal sac) is incorrect. The lacrimal sac is the slightly dilated upper end of the nasolacrimal duct. It collects tears from the canaliculi. Because the lacrimal punctum is obstructed with the silicone plug, tears would not reach the lacrimal canaliculus or the lacrimal sac. **Choice D** (Nasolacrimal duct) is incorrect. The nasolacrimal duct extends from the lacrimal sac to its termination on the lateral nasal wall, which opens into the inferior meatus. Because the lacrimal punctum is obstructed with the silicone plug, tears would not reach the nasolacrimal duct of the lacrimal apparatus. **Choice E** (Inferior nasal meatus) is incorrect. The inferior nasal meatus receives the drainage of the lacrimal apparatus. However, due to placement of the silicone plug, tears would not drain into the nasal cavity. Remember that the inferior nasal meatus does not contain the drainage points of any of the four paranasal sinuses, unlike the other nasal meati.

50 **The answer is D: Paralysis of several infrahyoid (strap) muscles.** The ansa cervicalis is a motor nerve loop derived from the cervical plexus. It is formed by the union of its two parts: the superior root (descendens hypoglossi, from C1) and the inferior root (descendens cervicalis, from C2 and C3). This delicate structure normally lies on the superficial surface of the carotid sheath, with its inferior margin at about the level of the cricoid cartilage. The ansa cervicalis innervates most of the infrahyoid (strap) muscles (omohyoid, sternohyoid, sternothyroid). The exception is the thyrohyoid muscle being supplied by C1 via the hypoglossal nerve. **Choice A** (Decreased blood flow to the larynx) is incorrect. The ansa cervicalis is a motor nerve route to skeletal muscles in the neck. It does not carry autonomic fibers that influence vasomotor control. These fibers are derived from the cervical sympathetic chain. **Choice B** (Lymphedema in the carotid triangle of the neck) is incorrect. The ansa cervicalis is located mainly in the carotid triangle. However, it does not regulate lymphatic flow. Removal of lymph nodes in this region may produce some degree of lymphedema due to removal of the lymphatic channels, but that result is not related to lesion of the ansa cervicalis. **Choice C** (Reduced sensation in the skin over the posterior triangle of the neck) is incorrect. The ansa cervicalis does not convey cutaneous sensation. The cutaneous branches of the cervical plexus emerge together from under the posterior border of the sternocleidomastoid muscle, at a point termed the "punctum nervosum" (nerve point of the neck). From this location, the cutaneous nerves of the cervical plexus distribute across the skin of the anterior and posterior triangles of the neck, posterior scalp, lower face, and anterior shoulder. **Choice E** (Paralysis of the intrinsic laryngeal muscles) is incorrect. The intrinsic muscles controlling the larynx are all supplied by branches of the vagus nerve (CN X). Most are innervated by the recurrent laryngeal nerve of CN X. The cricothyroid muscle is supplied by the external laryngeal nerve off the superior laryngeal nerve of CN X.

51 **The answer is B: Pedicle.** The image is a lateral plane film (X-ray) of the cervical component of the vertebral column. This type of radiological imaging is used commonly for general evaluation of the neck, especially in severe neck injuries where fractures may be suspected. The pedicle is the constricted "foot" of the vertebral arch that links the neural arch with the body of a vertebra, and it is identified by the white leader line from the letter "B" in the labeled X-ray provided. In this view, the opposite pedicles are superimposed upon one another. Thus, these small structures produce a distinct radiodensity (radiopacity) in the film. **Choice A** (Vertebral body) is incorrect. The body is the large, block-like structure at the anterior aspect of the column, and it is identified by the white leader line from the letter "A" in the labeled X-ray provided. The margins of the cervical bodies typically present a smooth curvature on both the anterior and posterior aspects. Deviations of the normal curvature of the vertebral bodies may suggest a possible fracture and/or torn ligaments. **Choice C** (Intervertebral disc space) is incorrect. This radiolucent area, identified by the white leader line from the letter "C" in the labeled X-ray provided, is located between the vertebral bodies and is occupied by the intervertebral disc. The height of this space decreases with degeneration of the disc (from either pathology or aging), thus approximating the vertebral bodies. **Choice D** (Superior articular process) is incorrect. Because the articular processes in the cervical region are positioned at oblique inclinations, they appear as seemingly sharply pointed structures in the lateral view, which can be misinterpreted as displaced bone fragments. The superior articular process, identified by the white leader line from the letter "D" in the labeled X-ray provided, is an upwardly projecting element, and it articulates with the inferior articular process of the more superior vertebra to create a zygapophysial (or facet) joint between the vertebral arches. **Choice E** (Inferior articular process) is incorrect. The inferior articular process, identified by the white leader line from the letter "E" in the labeled

X-ray, can be seen projecting inferior in the lateral view. The inferior articular process articulates with the superior articular process of the more inferior vertebra to create a zygapophysial (or facet) joint between the vertebral arches. The articular processes are outgrowths of the vertebral arch at the junction of the pedicle and the lamina.

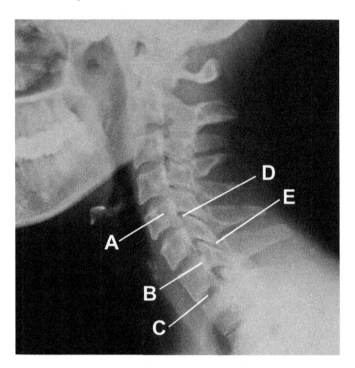

52 **The answer is D: Surgical removal of the thyroid gland.** The true vocal folds are controlled by the inferior laryngeal nerves, the terminal branches of the recurrent laryngeal nerves off the vagus nerve (CN X). The right recurrent laryngeal nerve branches from the right vagus nerve high in the superior mediastinum, loops under the right subclavian artery, and ascends through the neck along the tracheoesophageal groove. In its course, it runs on the deep aspect of the thyroid gland, where it is vulnerable to injury during thyroidectomy. Lesion of the recurrent laryngeal nerve paralyzes the ipsilateral intrinsic laryngeal muscles (except the cricothyroid) and eliminates sensation below the true vocal fold. **Choice A** (Repair of a patent ductus arteriosus) is incorrect. The ductus arteriosus is a fetal shunt connecting the root of the left pulmonary artery with the inferior side of the arch of the aorta. It normally closes soon after birth, becoming the ligamentum arteriosum. However, it may remain patent after birth, especially in premature infants, and may require surgical repair. The left recurrent laryngeal nerve branches from the left vagus nerve at the inferior edge of the arch of the aorta, loops under the arch immediately lateral to the ductus arteriosus, and ascends through the neck on a pathway mirroring the right recurrent laryngeal nerve. Because of its close relation to the ductus arteriosus, the left recurrent laryngeal nerve is vulnerable to injury during surgery related to the ductus arteriosus. **Choice B** (Repair of an aortic aneurysm) is incorrect. The aorta ascends from the heart, curves to the left to form the arch of the aorta, and descends into the thorax offset on the left side of the vertebral column. The left recurrent laryngeal nerve is closely related to the arch of the aorta from its origin to its initial ascent into the neck. It is vulnerable in an aneurysm of the aortic arch, where it may be stretched, and in surgical repair of the aneurysm. Remember that the right recurrent laryngeal nerve is not closely related to the aorta. **Choice C** (A gunshot wound below the second rib) is incorrect. A penetrating wound directly into the right side of the chest is normally too low to affect the right recurrent laryngeal nerve due to the nerve's high point of origin. However, a similar wound on the left side might affect the left recurrent laryngeal nerve. **Choice E** (Obstruction of the thoracic duct) is incorrect. The thoracic duct ascends through the thorax, diverges to the left side in the superior mediastinum, and joins the left venous angle (i.e., the junction of the left internal jugular and subclavian veins) in the root of the neck. It is not closely related to the right recurrent laryngeal nerve.

53   **The answer is A: Occipital triangle.**   The neck can be demarcated into anterior and lateral cervical regions by the obliquely running sternocleidomastoid (SCM) muscle. Both of these regions can be further subdivided into smaller triangular areas relative to the SCM and other neck muscles. This schematic plan allows a topographic organization of the structures within the neck. The lateral cervical region (or posterior cervical) triangle is demarcated by the posterior border of the SCM, anterior border of the trapezius, and the middle part of the clavicle. It is subdivided into an upper, larger occipital triangle and a lower, smaller omoclavicular (subclavian or supraclavicular) triangle by the course of the inferior belly of the omohyoid muscle. The roots of the brachial plexus emerge from the interscalene triangle (scalene hiatus) to form the three trunks of the brachial plexus in the occipital triangle. These trunks descend through the occipital triangle and form the divisions of the plexus as they approach the clavicle. Penetrating wounds into the occipital triangle are highly likely to contact some part of the trunks of the brachial plexus. **Choice B** (Omoclavicular triangle) is incorrect. The omoclavicular (subclavian or supraclavicular) triangle is the lower, smaller part of the lateral cervical region (or posterior cervical triangle). Its major contents include the third part of the subclavian artery, the suprascapular artery, and supraclavicular lymph nodes. A deep penetrating wound here may damage the divisions of the brachial plexus. **Choice C** (Submandibular triangle) is incorrect. The anterior cervical region (or triangle) is demarcated by the anterior border of the SCM, inferior border of the mandible, and the anterior midline of the neck. It is subdivided into four regions (or triangles) by the courses of the superior belly of the omohyoid and both bellies of the digastric muscles: the submandibular, submental, carotid, and muscular triangles. The submandibular (digastric) triangle is bounded by the mandible and the two bellies of the digastric muscle. Its major contents include the submandibular salivary gland, hypoglossal nerve (CN XII), and portions of the facial artery and vein. Trauma with this triangle would not affect the brachial plexus. **Choice D** (Carotid triangle) is incorrect. The carotid triangle represents a crowded region that is bounded by the SCM, superior belly of the omohyoid, and posterior belly of the digastric muscles. It houses several major neurovascular structures, including the common carotid artery and its branches, internal jugular vein, vagus and hypoglossal nerves, ansa cervicalis, and deep cervical lymph nodes. Trauma with this triangle would not affect the brachial plexus. **Choice E** (Muscular triangle) is incorrect. The muscular triangle is a large area demarcated by the SCM, superior belly of the omohyoid, and the anterior midline of the neck. It is occupied mainly by the infrahyoid (strap) muscles, and also includes the larynx and the thyroid and parathyroid glands. Trauma with this triangle would not affect the brachial plexus.

54   **The answer is B: Inferior oblique.**   Paralysis of one or more of the extraocular muscles causes a lack of coordinated eye movements, often resulting in diplopia (double vision). Clinical evaluation of the muscles includes step-wise positioning of the eye in such a way as to test each individual muscle at its position of greatest mechanical efficiency (relative to the visual axis) to determine if that muscle is functioning properly. Testing begins from the rest position, with the patient looking straight ahead. In this case, the first step (looking inward; adduction) tests the action of the medial rectus, the primary adductor of the eye. At the adducted position, the superior and inferior oblique muscles are aligned along their primary lines of action. The second step (looking upward; elevation) tests for function of the inferior oblique, which elevates the eye. Failure of either step indicates possible damage to the oculomotor nerve (CN III), which supplies both of these muscles. The inferior oblique and inferior rectus muscles can be impinged in head trauma cases when the floor of the orbit is fractured. These orbital (blowout) fractures lead to the downward herniation of orbital contents into the maxillary sinus, leading to the potential entrapment of these two extraocular muscles. The integrity of the inferior oblique muscle was tested in this question. **Choice A** (Superior oblique) is incorrect. Testing the superior oblique includes the same first step as for the inferior oblique, that is, adducting the eye to test the medial rectus and to position the oblique muscles along their primary lines of action. In this case, the second step is to look downward (depression) to test the superior oblique, which depresses the eye. Failure of this step indicates possible damage to the trochlear nerve (CN IV), which supplies only the superior oblique muscle. **Choice C** (Lateral rectus) is incorrect. The lateral rectus is the primary abductor of the eye from the rest position. Asking the patient to look outward (away from the nose) tests the ability of the lateral rectus to abduct at its position of greatest efficiency. Failure of this test indicates possible damage to the abducent nerve (CN VI), which supplies only the lateral rectus. Furthermore, at the adducted position, the superior and inferior rectus muscles are aligned along their primary lines of action and are set in best testing position. **Choice D** (Inferior rectus) is incorrect. At the abducted position, asking the patient to look downward tests the function of the inferior rectus, which depresses the eye. Failure to accomplish this task indicates possible damage to the oculomotor nerve, which supplies the inferior rectus muscle. **Choice E** (Superior rectus) is incorrect. From the abducted position, asking the patient to look upward tests the superior rectus, which elevates the eye. Failure to accomplish this task is another indicator of possible damage to the oculomotor nerve, which supplies the superior rectus muscle.

55   **The answer is B: Odontoid process.**   The image is an anteroposterior (AP) view of the upper cervical spine through the open mouth. This transoral radiological imaging view is valuable for evaluation of this region, especially for relations of the C1 and C2 vertebrae. The odontoid process (or dens) of C2 is a distinctive, tooth-like projection situated between the lateral masses of C1. It articulates with the anterior arch of C1, with the resultant middle atlantoaxial joint producing the major degrees of rotation within the cervical spine. Developmentally, the odontoid process begins as the body of the C1 vertebra. It separates from C1, migrates caudally, and joins the body of C2 to form the odontoid process. Thus, C1 is left with no body and possesses only the small anterior arch at that origin site. **Choice A** (Base of skull) is incorrect. The skull is divided into two main parts: (1) the neurocranium, forming the brain case; (2) the viscerocranium, forming the facial skeleton. The neurocranium is subdivided into two parts based on topographic and developmental features: (1) the chondrocranium (cartilaginous neurocranium), formed by endochondral ossification and composing the base of the skull; (2) the membranous neurocranium, formed by membranous ossification and composing the flat bones of the cranial vault. The base of the skull indicated in the X-ray is the occipital region, a part of the chondrocranium. It develops from occipital sclerotomes derived from the paraxial mesoderm. **Choice C** (Inferior articular facet of C1) is incorrect. The inferior articular facet (process) of C1 develops as an outgrowth from the vertebral (neural) arch of its incipient vertebral element. **Choice D** (Spinous process of C2) is incorrect. The spinous process of C2 develops as an outgrowth from the vertebral (neural) arch of its incipient vertebral element. **Choice E** (Transverse process of C1) is incorrect. In the cervical region, the transverse process of C1 is formed by contributions from both the vertebral arch and costal process elements.

56   **The answer is B: Paresthesia of the lower lip.** The inferior alveolar nerve, a branch of the mandibular division of the trigeminal nerve (CN V$_3$), leaves the ramus of the mandible after traveling through the extent of that bone, conveying afferent fibers from the mandibular teeth. Its mental nerve branch enters the mandible through the mental foramen after supplying sensory (cutaneous) innervation to the skin overlying the mandible, including the lower lip. Due to its location within the mandible and close relation to the dental arcade, the inferior alveolar nerve may be damaged during dental extractions, especially more complicated extractions of impacted third molars ("wisdom teeth"). Thus, paresthesia in the lower lip may result from such procedures. **Choice A** (Inability to compress the cheek) is incorrect. Compression of the cheek is an important action in all aspects of feeding and in other oral functions as well, and it is produced by the contraction of the buccinator muscle, one of the facial muscles. Being a muscle of facial expression, the buccinator is controlled by the facial nerve (CN VII), through its terminal facial branches. **Choice C** (Weakness in closing the jaw) is incorrect. Chewing is the result of the complex interactions of the muscles of mastication, which are controlled by the motor branches of the mandibular division of the trigeminal nerve (CN V$_3$). Of these four mastication muscles, the masseter, temporalis, and medial pterygoid muscles act in closing the jaw. The lateral pterygoid and anterior belly of the digastric muscles act in the opening of the oral fissure by depressing the mandible. The inferior alveolar nerve gives rise to the mylohyoid nerve before it enters the mandible via the mandibular foramen. The mylohyoid nerve supplies the anterior belly of the digastric and mylohyoid muscles. Therefore, while damage to the proximal part of the inferior alveolar nerve may influence jaw opening by affecting the anterior digastric muscle, damage to its distal (intramandibular) part does not affect any muscles of

mastication, sparing both opening and closing of the mandible. **Choice D** (Decreased salivary flow) is incorrect. Secretomotor control of the submandibular and sublingual salivary glands is governed by parasympathetic neurons that originate in the facial nerve through its chorda tympani branch and ultimately reach the oral floor via the lingual nerve, a branch of the mandibular division of the trigeminal nerve (CN V$_3$). Control of the parotid salivary gland is conveyed through parasympathetic fibers that originate in the glossopharyngeal nerve, travel through its tympanic and lesser petrosal branches, and ultimately reach the parotid through the auriculotemporal nerve (another branch of CN V$_3$). **Choice E** (Reduced taste in the body of the tongue) is incorrect. Taste fibers in the body (anterior two thirds) of the tongue are provided by the facial nerve via its chorda tympani branch. General sensory fibers to the same area are supplied by the lingual nerve, a branch of the mandibular division of the trigeminal nerve (CN V$_3$). The chorda tympani nerve unites with the lingual nerve within the infratemporal fossa. Thus, whereas the taste and general sensory components to the body of the tongue arise from separate cranial nerve pathways, they share a final common pathway to their target region. Remember that the parasympathetic supply to the oral floor (submandibular and sublingual salivary glands; oral floor mucus glands) also shares most of the chorda tympani/lingual nerve pathway. However, the autonomic fibers leave the lingual nerve in the oral floor to synapse in the submandibular ganglion.

57   **The answer is D: Superior cerebral veins.** Following traumatic impact to the front of the head, the superior cerebral veins may be torn as they drain into the superior sagittal sinus. Tearing of the superior cerebral veins leads to a subdural (or dural border) hemorrhage, which was pictured on the provided CT. Eight to ten superior cerebral veins drain the superior aspect of the cortical hemisphere, and these vessels can be damaged following impact to the front of the skull due to the resulting coup and countercoup movements of the brain within the skull following impact. This violent force on these bridging veins shears the superior cerebral veins entering the superior sagittal sinus, resulting in the pictured cerebral hematoma. The CT scan shows the characteristic crescent-shaped subdural hematoma, with its concave surface away from the cranium. **Choice A** (Middle meningeal artery) is incorrect. The middle meningeal artery is often torn following impact to the side of the head, fracturing the skull in the area of the pterion. The middle meningeal artery, specifically its anterior division, runs in close proximity to the pterion, so a fracture of this weakened area of the lateral skull may lacerate the middle meningeal artery, which leads to an epidural hemorrhage as the blood pools between the endosteal layer of the dura mater and the calvaria. In this patient, the cerebral hematoma resulted due to traumatic impact to the front of the skull, and the CT verified a hematoma in the area of the superior cerebral veins, within the subdural space (between the dura and arachnoid layers). **Choice B** (Superficial temporal artery) is incorrect. The superficial temporal artery, the terminal branch of the external carotid artery, lies outside of the skull. If this artery were lacerated, bleeding of the scalp would be profuse. Due to the extracranial location of the superficial temporal artery, damage to this artery would not cause intracranial hematoma noted on the CT. **Choice C** (Cerebral arterial circle) is incorrect. The cerebral arterial circle (of Willis) is an anastomoses of arteries located on the ventral surface of the brain in the area of the interpeduncular fossa, optic chiasm, and hypothalamus. These vessels are prone to saccular (berry) aneurysm, particularly where the arteries join together. Upon rupturing, blood spills into the subarachnoid space because all major vessels of the brain travel within the subarachnoid space. Subarachnoid hemorrhages are often seen in the absence of trauma, and the three cardinal signs and symptoms of a subarachnoid hemorrhage are (1) loss of consciousness (lethargy), (2) nuchal rigidity (stiff neck), and (3) a sudden onset of the "worst headache of your life," which were not present in this patient. This patient experienced a traumatic blow to the front of her head, and the hematoma, illustrated on the CT, confirmed a subdural hematoma, implicating the superior cerebral veins as the source of the bleed. **Choice E** (Occipital artery) is incorrect. The occipital artery, a branch of the external carotid artery, lies outside of the skull. If this artery were lacerated, bleeding of the scalp would be profuse; however, damage to this artery would not cause intracranial hematoma noted on the CT.

58 **The answer is A: Buccinator.** The buccinator muscle is pierced by the duct of the parotid gland as it passes toward the oral cavity to drain in the oral vestibule via a small opening opposite the second maxillary molar teeth. The muscular tone of the buccinator muscle can create a stenosis of the parotid duct, and it is the most likely site for a sialolith or calculus (*L.* pebble) of the parotid duct. The parotid duct arises from the anterior aspect of the parotid gland, and it courses across the superficial surface of the masseter muscle. Then, it dives medially to pierce the buccinator muscle and enters the oral cavity to drain at the second maxillary molar tooth. If sialolithiasis is confirmed, having a patient eat sour foods may dislodge the sialolith; however, surgical intervention may also be required to remove the calculus from the parotid duct. **Choice B** (Mentalis) is incorrect. The mentalis is a muscle of facial expression located on the chin that elevates and protrudes the lower lip or elevates the skin of the chin. It originates from the incisive fossa of the mandible and contracts to show doubt in a patient. This muscle is not pierced by the duct of the parotid gland, so it plays no role in the stenosis of the parotid duct or its obstruction by the sialolith. **Choice C** (Temporalis) is incorrect. The temporalis is a muscle of mastication that elevates the mandible in closing of the mouth, and its posterior, horizontally-oriented fibers serve as the primary means of retruding (retracting) the mandible when it is in a protruded (protracted) position. This muscle arises from the temporal fossa and inserts into the tip and medial border of the coronoid process of the mandible. This muscle is not pierced by the duct of the parotid gland, so it would play no role in the stenosis of the parotid duct or its obstruction by the sialolith. **Choice D** (Orbicularis oris) is incorrect. The orbicularis oris is a muscle of facial expression that encircles the mouth to act as the sphincter of the oral fissure. It originates from the incisive fossae of the mandible and maxilla and contracts in a patient to close the oral fissure, protrude the lips (as in kissing, whistling, or sucking), and resists distension when blowing (as seen when playing the trumpet). This muscle is not pierced by the duct of the parotid gland, so it would play no role in the stenosis of the parotid duct or its obstruction by the sialolith. **Choice E** (Masseter) is incorrect. The masseter is a muscle of mastication that primarily works to close the jaw, but its superficial fibers also play a limited role in protrusion

of the mandible. The duct of the parotid gland does course across the superficial surface of the masseter muscle, but this muscle would play no role in the stenosis of the parotid duct because the masseter is not pierced by it.

59 **The answer is C: Hypophyseal fossa.** This patient is exhibiting symptoms associated with Cushing disease, which results from the presence of a noncancerous tumor (adenoma) in the pituitary gland. The pituitary gland (or hypophysis) lies in the hypophyseal fossa of the sphenoid bone, which is identified by the "C" in this standard lateral plane film (X-ray) of the head. This fossa is part of the sella turcica, a complexly shaped part of the sphenoid located in the center of the floor of the cranial cavity. Cushing disease, also called pituitary adrenocorticotropic hormone (ACTH) hypersecretion, causes elevated cortisol levels, which lead to rapid weight gain, particularly in the face and trunk with sparing of the limbs (central obesity), excess sweating, thinning of the skin, muscle weakness, and hirsutism (facial hair growth). These symptoms are all part of Cushing syndrome, but Cushing disease refers specifically to the presence of a pituitary adenoma. The presence of a pituitary adenoma can be confirmed with an MRI of the pituitary gland. In this patient, the expanding pituitary adenoma expands upward out of the hypophyseal fossa to impinge about the optic chiasm, causing the bitemporal hemianopsia (tunnel vision). This visual deficit further implicates the pituitary gland as the location of the mass. The pituitary fossa (and its bounding parts of the sella turcica) is clearly defined and serves as a major orientation point in a lateral X-ray of the head. **Choice A** (Frontal sinus) is incorrect. The paranasal sinuses are radiolucent areas that may be mistaken for cranial fossae in some cases. The frontal sinus is located within the frontal bone. It may be more or less distinct, depending on its size and the thickness of its walls. Due to the signs and symptoms of this patient, the frontal sinuses would have no involvement in the diagnosis of Cushing disease. **Choice B** (Floor of the anterior cranial fossa) is incorrect. This obliquely lying plate of bone is formed mainly by the lesser wing of the sphenoid and the orbital plate of the frontal bone. It forms both the floor of the anterior cranial fossa and the roof of the orbit. In this view, it extends anterosuperior from the sella turcica. Due to the signs and symptoms of this patient, the floor of the anterior cranial fossa would have no involvement in the diagnosis of Cushing disease. **Choice D** (Sphenoidal sinus) is incorrect. This paranasal sinus lies within the body of the sphenoid bone, inferior to the hypophyseal fossa. Notice that the transnasal approach to the pituitary gland requires the surgeon to penetrate the sphenoid sinus but only as a means to reach the hypophyseal fossa. Due to the signs and symptoms of this patient, the sphenoidal sinus would have no involvement in the diagnosis of Cushing disease. **Choice E** (Mastoid sinuses) is incorrect. The mastoid sinuses are not paranasal sinuses. The mastoid sinuses are a complex of air cells within the mastoid part of the temporal bone, which connect with the tympanic (middle ear) cavity. Due to the signs and symptoms of this patient, the mastoid sinuses would have no involvement in the diagnosis of Cushing disease.

60 **The answer is E: Facial nerve.** The tympanic (middle ear) cavity is a small air-filled space within the petrous part of the temporal bone. Its position, shape, and relations make for challenging spatial concepts in anatomy because it is buried so deeply within the skull. It has six walls: the roof (tegmental wall), floor (jugular wall), anterior (carotid) wall, posterior (mastoid) wall, medial (labyrinthine) wall, and lateral (membranous) wall. Each wall has a close relationship to one or more significant neighboring structures. The upper part of the posterior wall contains an opening (aditus) that leads to the mastoid antrum and air cells. The distal limb of the facial canal (containing the main branch of the facial nerve) descends below the aditus, behind the posterior wall, on its way to its termination at the stylomastoid foramen. Thus, a tumor piercing the posterior wall may invade the facial canal and/or the mastoid air sinuses. **Choice A** (Internal jugular vein) is incorrect. The superior bulb of the internal jugular vein lies beneath the floor (jugular wall) of the tympanic cavity. Because this tumor is embedded in the posterior wall of the middle ear cavity, the internal jugular vein would not be affected. **Choice B** (Tympanic membrane) is incorrect. The tympanic membrane (eardrum) forms most of the lateral (membranous) wall. The epitympanic recess, situated above the tympanic membrane, completes the lateral wall. The handle of the malleus and the crossing chorda tympani nerve lie against the inside of the tympanic membrane. Because this tumor is embedded in the posterior wall of the tympanic cavity, the tympanic membrane would not be affected. **Choice C** (Internal carotid artery) is incorrect. The carotid canal (containing the internal carotid artery) lies outside the anterior (carotid) wall. Also, the pharyngotympanic (auditory) tube and the canal for the tensor tympani muscle open into the upper part of the anterior wall. Because this tumor is embedded in the posterior wall of the tympanic cavity, the internal carotid artery would not be affected. **Choice D** (Brain) is incorrect. The roof (tegmental wall) of the tympanic cavity is the tegmen tympani (roof of tympanum). This thin bony layer forms part of the floor of the middle cranial fossa, separating the dura mater and temporal lobe of the brain from the middle ear. Thus, fractures here may result in leakage of cerebrospinal fluid into the tympanic cavity and subsequently into the nasopharynx (via the pharyngotympanic tube) or external acoustic meatus (if the tympanic membrane is ruptured). The sixth wall (medial; labyrinthine) separates the middle ear from the internal ear. Its main features are the promontory, oval window, and round window.

61   **The answer is D: Thyroglossal duct cyst.**   A thyroglossal duct cyst is a fibrous cyst that forms within the thyroglossal duct, so it is located in, or close to, the midline of the neck. Most commonly (~50%), it is found near the body of the hyoid bone; however, the thyroglossal cyst in this patient is located inferior to this point. The thyroglossal cyst is usually painless and smooth, and this mass moves upward during swallowing or protrusion of the tongue, as reported in this patient. The thyroglossal duct is a remnant of the descent of the thyroid gland, which first appears as a single, ventromedian diverticulum (thyroid diverticulum) off the floor of the embryonic pharynx between the tuberculum impar and copula of the incipient tongue. As the thyroid gland descends along the midline, anterior to the gut tube, it remains connected to the tongue by a narrow canal called the thyroglossal duct. The thyroglossal duct usually solidifies and is obliterated after the final descent of the thyroid gland; however, if it persists, a thyroglossal cyst may develop, usually in individuals under the age of 20. **Choice A** (Enlarged deep cervical lymph node) is incorrect. The deep cervical lymph nodes lie within or in close proximity to the carotid sheath correlating in location with the internal jugular vein. While a few of the deep cervi-

cal lymph nodes could reside near the location of the mass, they do not tend to be found superficially on the midline of the neck and an enlarged deep cervical lymph node would not lead to the dysphagia (or difficulty swallowing) seen in this patient. **Choice B** (Thyroid nodule) is incorrect. A thyroid nodule refers to any abnormal growth that forms within the thyroid gland. Adult women (4% to 8%) are particularly prone to thyroid nodules, but fortunately, only 10% of thyroid nodules are reported to be cancerous. The majority of thyroid nodules are asymptomatic; however, if the cells of the thyroid nodule are producing thyroid hormones, either thyroxine (T4) or triiodothyronine (T3), a thyroid nodule can lead to hyperthyroidism. Patients with hyperthyroidism may present with heart palpitations, weight loss, anxiety, insomnia, fatigue, heat intolerance, excessive sweating, exophthalmos (protruding eyes), and even amenorrhea (an absence of menstrual flow). Due to the midline location of this mass, lack of hyperthyroidism symptoms, and age of this patient, a thyroglossal cyst is the most likely diagnosis. **Choice C** (Benign parathyroid adenoma) is incorrect. A parathyroid adenoma is a benign tumor of the parathyroid glands, which usually increases the circulation of parathyroid hormone (PTH). This condition of hyperparathyroidism leads to an increase in blood calcium levels due to elevated resorption of bone and may be asymptomatic in many patients. Symptomatic patients would present with lethargy, muscle pain, nausea, constipation, confusion, kidney stones, and even an increased risk of bone fractures due to the increased bone resorption. A physician can perform blood tests to test for calcium, chloride, potassium, and bicarbonate levels, and women over the age of 60 have the highest risk for developing hyperparathyroidism. The presence of a parathyroid adenoma has been reported in 80% to 85% of patients who present with hyperparathyroidism; however, the symptoms and age of this patient do not correlate with the presence of a parathyroid adenoma. **Choice E** (Branchial cyst) is incorrect. Branchial cysts are located along the anterior border of the sternocleidomastoid muscle. Most often, these cysts are the remnants of the second pharyngeal cleft, located just below the angle of the mandible. Second branchial cleft cysts represent approximately 67% to 93% of all pharyngeal apparatus anomalies. However, branchial cysts may be found anywhere along the anterior margin of the sternocleidomastoid muscle but not on the anterior midline of the neck. Very frequently, branchial cysts are inconspicuous at birth, becoming evident as they enlarge throughout childhood. Due to the midline location of this mass, a branchial cyst can be ruled out in this patient.

62   **The answer is B: Greater wing of the sphenoid bone.**   The pterion is a significant craniometric landmark point in the temporal fossa on the lateral aspect of the skull. It is the roughly H-shaped junction of four bones: greater wing of the sphenoid, frontal, parietal, and squamous parts of the temporal. The pterion is clinically significant in that the bones here are relatively thin and susceptible to fracture from impact. Furthermore, the anterior branch of the middle meningeal artery typically lies tightly grooved against the interior of the skull at this point. The middle meningeal artery is the major vessel supplying the dura mater and the bones of the cranial vault. It can be readily ruptured in trauma to the pterion, and the middle meningeal artery is the primary vessel implicated in epidural hemorrhage. **Choice A** (Zygomatic process of the temporal bone) is incorrect. The zygomatic process of the temporal bone is an anterior projection articulating with the zygomatic bone. Together, these two components form the zygomatic arch. **Choice C** (Mastoid process of the temporal bone) is incorrect. The mastoid process of the temporal bone is a breast-like projection extending inferior from the temporal bone behind the external acoustic meatus. It forms part of the posterior boundary of the infratemporal fossa. Additionally, it is the attachment site for certain neck muscles (e.g., sternocleidomastoid) and is largely hollowed by the mastoid air cells. **Choice D** (Lateral pterygoid plate of the sphenoid bone) is incorrect. The lateral pterygoid plate is a thin, wing-like, inferior extension of the sphenoid bone. It forms the medial (deep) boundary of the infratemporal fossa and provides attachment for portions of the medial and lateral pterygoid muscles. **Choice E** (Coronoid process of the mandible) is incorrect. The coronoid process of the mandible is a thin, blade-like, superior projection from the anterior aspect of the ramus of the mandible. It serves as the insertion area for the large temporalis muscle, a muscle of mastication.

63 **The answer is B: Sagittal.** Premature closure of the sagittal suture leads to scaphocephaly (G: boat-shaped head), or dolichocephaly, which presents with a disproportionately long and narrow skull. This marked increase in head length with narrowed width is particularly common in infants who are born prematurely. Surgical intervention is needed to treat scaphocephaly to remove bone from the sagittal suture. Craniosynostosis is the term that refers generally to the premature fusion of the cranial sutures. **Choice A** (Coronal) is incorrect. Premature closure of the coronal suture leads to brachycephaly (G: short head), which involves a disproportionately wide skull with a short occipitofrontal diameter. Babies with brachycephaly have a characteristic square-shaped skull due to the short occipitofrontal diameter seen following premature closure of the coronal suture. Brachycephaly is more common in females, and surgical intervention can be implemented to remove bone from the coronal suture. If only one side of the coronal suture closes prematurely, the infant presents with an asymmetric cranium, a condition known as plagiocephaly. In this baby boy, the long and narrow shape of the skull indicates premature closure of the sagittal suture. **Choice C** (Lambdoid) is incorrect. The lambdoid suture is a dense, fibrous connective tissue joint located on the back of the skull that connects the occipital bone with the posterior aspect of the parietal bone and petrous portion of the temporal bone. If only one side of the lambdoid suture closes prematurely, the infant presents with a twisted and asymmetric cranium, a condition known as plagiocephaly. In this baby boy, the long and narrow shape of the skull indicates premature closure of the sagittal suture. **Choice D** (Metopic) is incorrect. The metopic (or frontal) suture is a dense, fibrous connective tissue joint located between the two halves of the frontal bone. This suture usually begins fusion of the frontal bones at age 2 and disappears by age 6. If the metopic suture is not present at birth, trigonacephaly, a type of craniosynostosis, results in a keel-shaped deformity. In this baby boy, the long and narrow shape of the skull indicates premature closure of the sagittal suture. **Choice E** (Squamous) is incorrect. The squamous suture is a dense, fibrous connective tissue joint, which arches between the parietal bone and the squamous portion of the temporal bone, reaching anterior to the pterion. This suture is usually the last cranial suture to close around ages 35 to 39.

In this baby boy, the long and narrow shape of the skull indicates premature closure of the sagittal suture.

64 **The answer is B: Sphenopalatine.** The maxillary and superficial temporal arteries are the terminal branches of the external carotid artery. The maxillary artery is the larger and deeper running of the two. It provides a wide distribution to the lateral and deep aspects of the head as it courses anterior across the infratemporal fossa and through the pterygomaxillary fissure into the pterygopalatine fossa. Thus, the pterygomaxillary fissure is the narrow opening from the deep, anterior part of the infratemporal fossa into the lateral aspect of the pterygopalatine fossa. The maxillary artery is divided into three parts by its relation to the lateral pterygoid muscle: first (retromandibular or prepterygoid) part, second (pterygoid) part, third (pterygopalatine; postpterygoid) part. The first part of the maxillary artery supplies the external ear, temporomandibular joint (TMJ), dura mater, calvaria, and lower jaw. The second part of this artery supplies muscles of mastication and the cheek. The third part of the maxillary artery is the most difficult to envision because of its deep, distal location. It supplies the upper jaw, midface, palate, nasopharynx, and nasal passages. The sphenopalatine artery is one of the terminal branches off the third part of the maxillary artery (the other being the infraorbital artery). It arises within the pterygopalatine fossa; passes through the sphenopalatine foramen; and supplies the nasal septum, lateral nasal wall, and adjacent paranasal sinuses. **Choice A** (Superficial temporal) is incorrect. The superficial temporal artery is the smaller, more superficially running of the terminal branches of the external carotid artery. It ascends anterior to the tragus of the auricle to supply the lateral scalp. **Choice C** (Inferior alveolar) is incorrect. The inferior alveolar artery branches from the first part of the maxillary artery, in the infratemporal fossa. It travels with the inferior alveolar nerve to enter the mandible. It supplies the mandible, mandibular teeth and associated gingivae, and overlying skin. **Choice D** (Middle meningeal) is incorrect. This middle meningeal artery is a notable artery arising from the first part of the maxillary artery, just in front of the TMJ. It ascends through the foramen spinosum, enters the floor of the middle cranial fossa, and supplies the dura mater and calvaria. **Choice E** (Ophthalmic) is incorrect. The ophthalmic artery branches from the internal carotid artery within the cranium. It passes through the optic canal with the optic nerve supply the orbit and forehead.

65 **The answer is E: Temporalis.** The posterior fibers of the temporalis muscle run in a horizontal plane, and during contraction, enable retrusion (or retraction) of the mandible allowing it to return to its normal position in the TMJ. By pulling the mandible down, the dentist frees the mandibular condyle from its stuck position on the articular eminence of the temporal bone. The temporalis muscle is also involved with closing of the mouth (elevation of the mandible); however, its posterior, horizontally oriented fibers are the primary retractors of the mandible. **Choice A** (Lateral pterygoid) is incorrect. The lateral pterygoid muscle acts on the TMJ to allow protrusion (or protraction) of the mandible. During contraction of the lateral pterygoid muscle, the mandibular condyle slides anterior (translation) to be located inferior to the articular eminence of the temporal bone, which enables the mouth to open due to the effects of gravity. It has no role in the retraction of the mandible.

In this patient, the tone of the temporalis muscle returned the mandibular condyle to the TMJ. **Choice B** (Masseter) is incorrect. The masseter muscle primarily works to close the jaw, but its superficial fibers also play a limited role in protrusion of the mandible. The vertical (deep) fibers of this muscle may also play a limited role in the retrusion of the mandible; however, the temporalis muscle is the prime mover in retrusion at the TMJ. **Choice C** (Medial pterygoid) is incorrect. The medial pterygoid muscle elevates the mandible and contributes to protrusion. Therefore, it does not function in the retraction of the mandible, which is the action that returned the mandibular condyle to the TMJ in this patient. **Choice D** (Stylohyoid) is incorrect. The stylohyoid is a suprahyoid muscle that depresses the mandible against resistance when the infrahyoid muscles have the hyoid bone fixed in position. It would not be involved in correcting the anterior dislocation of the TMJ seen in this patient.

66 **The answer is D: Middle pharyngeal constrictor.** Fracture of the hyoid bone can be accomplished by blunt trauma to the anterior neck region. Because it is the attachment site for 10 muscles in the neck, pharynx, and oral floor, loss of movement of the hyoid may impair swallowing and normal separation of the GI and respiratory passages. The three pharyngeal constrictor muscles form a circular series that collectively attach in an overlapping fashion along the posteromedian raphe of the pharynx. However, each has a distinctly separate origin. The middle constrictor arises from the greater and lesser horns of the hyoid bone. Thus, fracture of the hyoid disrupts the compressive action of the middle pharyngeal constrictor muscle in swallowing (or deglutition). **Choice A** (Palatopharyngeus) is incorrect. The palatopharyngeus muscle descends from the palate to attach into the pharyngeal wall and thyroid cartilage. It constricts the nasopharynx and elevates the pharynx and larynx during swallowing. It does not have a direct connection to the hyoid bone and would be only peripherally affected in this patient. **Choice B** (Stylopharyngeus) is incorrect. The stylopharyngeus muscle is the only skeletal muscle derived from the mesoderm of the third pharyngeal arch and innervated by the glossopharyngeal nerve (CN IX). It arises from the styloid process, descends through the pharyngeal wall between the superior and middle pharyngeal constrictors, and inserts into the thyroid cartilage to assist in elevating the pharynx and larynx during swallowing. It does not have a direct connection to the hyoid bone and would be only peripherally affected in this patient. **Choice C** (Superior pharyngeal constrictor) is incorrect. The superior pharyngeal constrictor muscle arises from the pterygoid region on the base of the skull, the pterygomandibular raphe, and the mandible. It acts to compress the upper pharynx during swallowing. However, this muscle does not have a direct connection to the hyoid bone and would be only peripherally affected in this patient. **Choice E** (Inferior pharyngeal constrictor) is incorrect. The inferior pharyngeal constrictor muscle originates from the thyroid and cricoid cartilages of the larynx to compress the lower pharynx during swallowing. This muscle does not have a direct connection to the hyoid bone and would be only peripherally affected in this patient.

67 **The answer is B: Taste in the anterior two thirds of tongue.** The chorda tympani nerve, a terminal branch of the facial nerve (CN VII), conveys taste sensation to the anterior two thirds of the tongue and carries presynaptic (preganglionic)

parasympathetic fibers to the submandibular and sublingual glands to enable salivation. CN VII enters the skull through the internal acoustic meatus, and in this coronal CT, the margins of this foramen remain intact and are not involved in this presentation. Therefore, the tumor in the posterior cranial fossa is not currently affecting CN VII and its chorda tympani branch, which exits the skull via the petrotympanic fissure. This image shows a massive lesion within the right petrous temporal bone at the right jugular foramen with gross bone destruction. Involvement of the hypoglossal canal was also noted, though not shown on this particular CT. Therefore, the functions of the glossopharyngeal (CN IX), vagus (CN X), accessory nerve (CN XI), and hypoglossal (CN XII) nerves would be lost. Taste supplied to the anterior two thirds of the tongue by the chorda tympani nerve of CN VII would be the only function remaining intact. **Choice A** (Control of the true vocal fold) is incorrect. All of the intrinsic laryngeal muscles are controlled by branches of the vagus nerve (CN X). Specifically, all of these muscles are supplied by the recurrent laryngeal nerve of CN X, except for the cricothyroid muscle, which is innervated by the external laryngeal nerve off the superior laryngeal nerve of CN X. The pictured lesion has caused gross bone destruction within the right petrous temporal bone at the right jugular foramen. Therefore, the main stem of the vagus nerve is compromised at the right jugular foramen, causing loss of control and sensation in the entire right side of the larynx. Remember that the glossopharyngeal (CN IX), vagus (CN X), and (spinal) accessory (CN XI) nerves emerge from the cranium through the jugular foremen, and the given CT showed erosion of this bony canal by the invading tumor. **Choice C** (Symmetric protrusion of the tongue) is incorrect. The hypoglossal nerve (CN XII) innervates all of the intrinsic muscles of the tongue and most of its extrinsic muscles with the lone exception being the palatoglossus muscle, innervated by the vagus nerve (CN X). Therefore, damage to the right CN XII would produce ipsilateral deviation of the tongue during protrusion due to the unopposed muscular contractions of the contralateral genioglossus muscle. The mnemonic "The tongue licks the wound" will help you remember that the tongue deviates to the ipsilateral side in a lower motor neuron lesion of CN XII. A patient with a CN XII deficit would also display dysarthria and fasciculations within the tongue musculature, and the right CN XII would have been damaged in this patient due to the invading tumor destroying the hypoglossal canal, as noted in the clinical case. **Choice D** (Sensation in the tympanic cavity) is incorrect. Sensation from the walls of the tympanic (middle ear) cavity is carried by the branches of the tympanic nerve, a branch of the glossopharyngeal nerve (CN IX). This lesion has caused gross bone destruction at the right jugular foramen, resulting in damage to CN IX. The invading nature of this tumor would cause a sensory deficit in the right tympanic cavity. Remember that the glossopharyngeal (CN IX), vagus (CN X), and accessory (CN XI) nerves emerge from the cranium through the jugular foramen, and this tumor would lead to functional loss of these three cranial nerves. **Choice E** (Elevation of the shoulder) is incorrect. The (spinal) accessory nerve (CN XI) innervates the trapezius and sternocleidomastoid muscles. The trapezius elevates, retracts, depresses, and rotates the scapula. Thus, damage to CN XI at the jugular foramen results in notable deficits in shoulder action, including elevation. Remember that the glossopharyngeal (CN IX), vagus (CN X), and accessory (CN XI) nerves emerge from the cranium through the jugular foramen, and the given CT showed erosion of this canal by the invading tumor.

68 **The answer is D: Tension of the vocal cord.** The superior thyroid artery accompanies the external laryngeal nerve (or external branch of the superior laryngeal nerve) as they descend from their origins high in the neck. The artery supplies the superior pole of the thyroid gland while the external laryngeal nerve innervates the cricothyroid muscle in the larynx and the lower part of the inferior pharyngeal constrictor. The cricothyroid muscle tilts the thyroid cartilage forward (anterior), causing elongation, tension, and adduction of the vocal cords. Thus, compression of the external laryngeal nerve may reduce the tension of the ipsilateral vocal cord, causing a weakened voice, slight hoarseness, and difficulty raising the pitch of the voice. **Choice A** (Sensation above the true vocal fold) is incorrect. The true vocal folds (or simply vocal folds) mark the line of separation between the two sensory fields within the larynx. Sensation from the mucosa above the vocal fold (i.e., lining the inlet, vestibule, vestibular folds, and ventricle) is carried by the internal laryngeal nerve, a terminal branch of the superior laryngeal nerve. The external laryngeal nerve is the other terminal branch of the superior laryngeal nerve, and it innervates the cricothyroid and lower part of the inferior pharyngeal constrictor muscles. **Choice B** (Sensation below the true vocal fold) is incorrect. The (true) vocal folds mark the line of separation between the two sensory fields within the larynx. Sensation from the mucosa below the vocal fold (i.e., lining the infraglottic cavity) is carried by the inferior laryngeal nerve, the terminal branch of the recurrent laryngeal nerve. **Choice C** (Abduction of the vocal cord) is incorrect. Abduction of the vocal cord (i.e., opening of the rima glottidis) is caused by the contraction of the posterior cricoarytenoid muscle, which laterally rotates the arytenoid cartilage. This muscle is controlled by the inferior laryngeal nerve. Remember that the inferior laryngeal (recurrent laryngeal) nerve supplies all the intrinsic laryngeal muscles except one, the cricothyroid. **Choice E** (Depression of the hyoid bone) is incorrect. Depression of the hyoid is caused by the actions of the four infrahyoid (strap) muscles (**T**hyrohyoid, **O**mohyoid, **S**ternohyoid, and **S**ternothyroid). The mnemonic to remember the infrahyoid muscles is "TOSS". Three of the muscles (the "OSS" of the "TOSS") are innervated by the ansa cervicalis, a branch of the cervical plexus. The lone remaining muscle, the thyrohyoid muscle, is innervated by a C1 branch off the hypoglossal nerve (CN XII).

69 **The answer is A: Superior sagittal sinus.** The dural venous sinuses (dural sinuses) are valveless venous channels formed between the layers of the dura mater. All the blood from the brain drains into the dural sinuses and then out of the cranium via true veins. Most of the blood from the brain drains through the dural sinuses to the internal jugular veins. The cerebral hemispheres drain through various dural sinuses to the confluence of dural venous sinuses or confluens sinuum, a common collection pool at the junction of these three dural septa: falx cerebri, falx cerebelli, and tentorium cerebelli. Blood within the confluence of sinuses, located in close proximity to the internal occipital protuberance, flows into the transverse sinuses to the sigmoid sinuses to the internal jugular veins. The superior sagittal sinus is a large venous channel located along the attached border of the falx cerebri. It drains the more superficial cerebral veins directly to the confluence of sinuses. Obstruction of the confluence of sinuses prevents proper drainage through the superior sagittal sinus, resulting in backpressure buildup in that channel. **Choice B** (Transverse sinus) is incorrect. The transverse sinuses are large venous channels within the attached border of the tentorium cerebelli. They drain blood from the confluence of sinuses into the sigmoid sinuses. Because the transverse sinus is distal to the confluence of sinuses, compression at this location would not hinder drainage through the transverse sinus; however, it will reduce the amount of blood draining through the transverse sinuses. **Choice C** (Cavernous sinus) is incorrect. The basal veins from the brainstem drain primarily to the cavernous sinuses, located on either side of the sella turcica. The cavernous sinuses drain to the internal jugular veins via the superior and inferior petrosal sinuses. It should be mentioned that multiple important alternative connections between the cavernous sinuses and other pericranial veins can exist. Compression of the confluence of sinuses would not directly affect blood draining from the cavernous sinuses because their connections to the internal jugular veins are well distal to the confluence of the sinuses. **Choice D** (Superior petrosal sinus) is incorrect. The superior petrosal sinus lies along the crest of the petrous part of the temporal bone and carries blood from the cavernous sinus into the distal part of the transverse sinus. Normal flow through this channel would not be compromised because it is located distal to the compressed confluence of the sinuses. **Choice E** (Inferior petrosal sinus) is incorrect. The inferior petrosal sinus runs in close proximity to the junction of the clivus of the sphenoid bone and the petrous temporal bone. It carries blood from the cavernous sinus to the distal end of the sigmoid sinus or directly into the origin of the internal jugular vein. This drainage path is located well distal to the confluence of the sinuses and would not be obstructed by this tumor.

70 **The answer is C: Mastoiditis.** Mastoiditis, an infection of the air cells within the mastoid process, is the most likely diagnosis due to the symptoms (pain, tenderness, and inflammation) being localized posterior to the right auricle, where the mastoid process of the temporal bone resides. Before the invention of antibiotics, mastoiditis was the leading cause of child mortality; today, however, it is rarely seen in developed countries. In this patient, mastoiditis could be confirmed with imaging studies. In the coronal CT located on the next page, the indicated fluid accumulation can be seen within the right mastoid air cells and mastoid antrum and the extracranial inflammation located behind the auricle, characteristic of mastoiditis, can be visualized lateral to the encircled mastoid process. **Choice A** (Otitis externa) is incorrect. Otitis externa (or swimmer's ear) is a bacterial infection affecting skin lining the external acoustic meatus, which results from polluted water being trapped within this meatus. It presents with pain, inflammation, itchiness, and ear discharge; these symptoms may lead to temporary conductive hearing loss if inflammation and discharge block the external acoustic meatus. When otitis externa is suspected, a physician can push on the tragus of the external ear to see if the intensity of pain increases, which is how swimmer's ear is diagnosed. This patient presented with pain, inflammation, and tenderness; however, these symptoms were localized posterior to her right auricle, not within the external acoustic meatus. **Choice B** (Blockage of pharyngotympanic tube) is incorrect. The pharyngotympanic (auditory; eustachian) tube connects the nasopharynx to the tympanic (middle ear) cavity, which can provide a route for infection into the tympanic cavity. When it is occluded, the tympanic cavity is prone to middle ear infections (otitis media). This patient had a history of otitis media, which presents with pain and inflammation due to a collection of fluid located deep to the tympanic membrane. Because her symptoms (pain, inflammation, and tenderness) were localized posterior to her right auricle, mastoiditis is a more accurate diagnosis. **Choice D** (Perforated tympanic membrane) is incorrect. A perforated tympanic membrane is often seen secondary to severe otitis media (middle ear infection). A ruptured tympanic membrane would cause a conductive hearing loss, which was not evident in this patient. **Choice E** (Ménière syndrome) is incorrect. Ménière syndrome affects the inner ear, and it presents with periodic episodes of vertigo and dizziness, tinnitus, and fluctuating, progressive sensori neural hearing loss. It is caused by blockage of the cochlear aqueduct, which affects the drainage of endolymph within the inner ear. These symptoms were not seen in this patient.

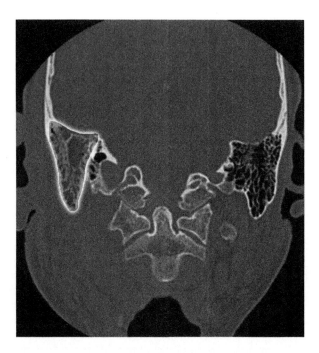

71 **The answer is D: Masseter.** The masseter muscle, one of four muscles of mastication, is a powerful elevator (adductor) of the mandible, acting to close the mouth and approximate the occlusal surfaces of the teeth. The provided CT shows the left mandible is fractured slightly superior to the mandibular angle, causing the associated edema evident on the image. The masseter muscle, lying laterally to the fracture, originates from the inferior border and medial surface of the zygomatic arch and inserts into the angle, lower lateral surface of the ramus, and posterior aspect of the body of the mandible. This mandibular fracture is located in the midpoint of the insertion of the masseter, which is more clearly seen on the right (unaffected) side of the CT scan. Because a large part of the insertion of the masseter inserts distal to the fracture site, it is capable of closing the mouth making it difficult to remove the mouthpiece. Of note, the medial pterygoid muscle is a deep mirror of the masseter in its insertion and action, so both the masseter and medial pterygoid muscles would be acting to close the mouth in this boxer. **Choice A** (Temporalis) is incorrect. The temporalis muscle, another muscle of mastication, runs from the temporal

fossa to the coronoid process and anterior edge of the ramus of the mandible. It also acts as an elevator (adductor) of the mandible, to close the mouth. In this CT, the fracture is distal to the attachment of the temporalis, so this muscle could only elevate the fractured ramus of the mandible, which would not effectively close the mouth and approximate the occlusal surfaces of the teeth. Due to the fracture site, the spasticity of the masseter muscle would result in the closing of the mouth making it difficult to remove the mouthpiece. **Choice B** (Lateral pterygoid) is incorrect. The lateral pterygoid is a muscle of mastication which acts to protract (or protrude) the mandible. It plays a significant role in opening of the mouth and medial-lateral excursion. In this case, the lateral pterygoid can move the proximal detached segment of the jaw because of its attachment above the fracture, to the neck of the mandible and the jaw joint capsule and disc. **Choice C** (Zygomaticus major) is incorrect. The zygomaticus major is a muscle of facial expression. It originates on the lateral aspect of the zygomatic bone (explaining its name) and inserts into the skin and other facial muscles at the corner of the mouth. It functions as a dilator of the oral fissure by elevating the corners of mouth, as in smiling when the muscle contracts bilaterally or sneering to show disdain when the muscle contracts unilaterally. This muscle would be paralyzed in facial nerve palsy, but it would not be affected by this mandibular fracture. **Choice E** (Posterior digastric) is incorrect. The posterior digastric (or posterior belly of the digastric) is a suprahyoid muscle, not a muscle of mastication. It runs from the mastoid part of the skull to the hyoid bone, and acts to stabilize and elevate the hyoid during swallowing. Its counterpart, the anterior digastric, may play a role in opening the mouth, especially against resistance.

72 **The answer is B: Opening of the parotid duct.** The vestibule of the mouth is the narrow space between the cheeks and lips and the hard wall of teeth and related gingivae (gums). The duct of the parotid gland drains into the vestibule, opposite the upper (maxillary) second molar tooth. The opening of the parotid duct can be visualized in an oral examination and readily located by the tongue. The integrity of the wall of the oral vestibule is critical in food handling and articulate speech. Also, the vestibule is important in oral hygiene as food and other materials may collect and fester there if the area is not cleaned properly. **Choice A** (Lingual frenulum) is incorrect. The lingual frenulum is a thin, midline fold of tissue that anchors the underside of the tongue to the floor of the oral cavity proper. Abnormal shortening of the frenulum results in ankyloglossia (tongue-tie). In this condition, the tongue has limited mobility, which may impact food handling and speech, potentially producing a speech impediment. **Choice C** (Opening of the submandibular duct) is incorrect. The submandibular duct runs forward across the oral floor and drains at the sublingual papilla (caruncle) on the side of the lingual frenulum. **Choice D** (Uvula) is incorrect. The uvula is the soft midline extension of the soft palate that is most often identified as "that thing that hangs down in the back of the mouth." It serves to assist in sealing off the nasopharynx during swallowing so that food does not regurgitate into the nasal passages. Deviation of the uvula during phonation (saying "Ah") indicates lesion of the vagus nerve (CN X), which innervates the muscle of the uvula (musculus uvulae). **Choice E** (Palatine tonsil) is incorrect. The palatine tonsil lies on the side of the oropharynx, between the palatoglossal and palatopharyngeal arches. It is highly vascular and may bleed profusely during tonsillectomy.

73 **The answer is C: Third.** The thymus and inferior parathyroid glands are derived from the third pharyngeal pouch. Therefore, migration of neural crest cells into the third pharyngeal pouch has been diminished in this patient with DiGeorge (22q11.2 deletion) syndrome. The patient would present with immunodeficiency due to an absence of the thymus, and hypocalcemia (low blood calcium levels) due to the absence of inferior parathyroid glands. DiGeorge syndrome is also characterized by conotruncal hearts defects, such as tetralogy of Fallot or interrupted aortic arch. Moreover, facial anomalies usually resemble first arch syndrome with the patient presenting with a hypoplastic mandible, low-set ears, hypertelorism (increased distance between the eyes), and microstomia (abnormally small mouth). **Choice A** (First) is incorrect. Evagination of the first pharyngeal pouch forms an elongated diverticulum off the pharynx (the tubotympanic recess). The distal part of this recess widens to form the tympanic (middle ear) cavity. The proximal part remains more tubular and forms the pharyngotympanic (auditory; eustachian) tube. Therefore, agenesis of the thymus and inferior parathyroid glands is not due to maldevelopment of the first pharyngeal pouch. **Choice B** (Second) is incorrect. The second pharyngeal pouch helps to form the tonsillar fossa and surface epithelium of the palatine tonsil. Secondarily, lymphatic tissue, which becomes the palatine tonsils, is incorporated into the second pharyngeal pouch. Maldevelopment of the second pharyngeal pouch does not cause agenesis of the thymus and inferior parathyroid glands. **Choice D** (Fourth) is incorrect. The fourth pharyngeal pouch forms the superior parathyroid gland and the ultimobranchial body, which gives rise to the parafollicular (C) cells of the thyroid gland. Maldevelopment of the fourth pharyngeal pouch does not cause agenesis of the thymus and inferior parathyroid glands. **Choice E** (Fifth) is incorrect. The fifth pharyngeal pouch only exists transiently in human embryologic growth and development. No adult structures are derived from the fifth pharyngeal pouch, so this option can be easily eliminated.

74 **The answer is E: Ophthalmic division of trigeminal.** The ophthalmic (first) division of trigeminal nerve (CN V$_1$) supplies sensory (cutaneous) innervation to the skin of the upper eyelid, anterior aspect of the nose, forehead, and anterior scalp. CN V$_1$ enters the middle cranial fossa through the superior orbital fissure, and its three terminal branches (lacrimal, nasociliary, and frontal nerves) are distributed throughout the orbit, anterior cranial fossa, anterior scalp, and nasal cavity. Other cranial nerves traverse the superior orbital fissure, including the oculomotor (CN III), trochlear (CN IV), and abducent (CN VI) nerves, to supply extraocular eye muscles. The superior orbital fissure also contains the superior and inferior ophthalmic veins and sympathetic fibers from the carotid plexus. With the broken pool cue residing in close proximity to the superior orbital fissure, the ophthalmic division of the trigeminal nerve is most likely damaged in this question. **Choice A** (Optic nerve) is incorrect. The optic nerve (CN II) leaves the orbit via the optic canal to relay vision from the retina to the brain. Because only the superior orbital fissure is involved in this patient, the optic nerve is not likely damaged. **Choice B** (Facial nerve) is incorrect. The facial nerve enters the petrous temporal bone through the internal acoustic meatus, traveling through this foramen with the vestibulocochlear nerve (CN VII). It has three terminal branches (chorda tympani, greater petrosal, and the main branch of the facial nerve), and none of

these branches traverse the superior orbital fissure, which was involved in this patient. **Choice C** (Mandibular division of trigeminal nerve) is incorrect. The mandibular (third) division of the trigeminal nerve (CN V$_3$) supplies general sensation to the skin of the lower lip, chin, cheek, and even the anterior auricular and lateral scalp. This sensory innervation is supplied via three cutaneous nerves: mental, buccal, and auriculotemporal. The mandibular division of the trigeminal nerve also supplies innervation to the mandibular teeth and gingivae via the inferior alveolar nerve, and it is the only division of CN V that supplies motor innervation. CN V$_3$ enters the middle cranial fossa through the foramen ovale, so it would not be affected by damage in the superior orbital fissure. **Choice D** (Maxillary division of trigeminal nerve) is incorrect. The maxillary (second) division of the trigeminal nerve (CN V$_2$) supplies sensory (cutaneous) innervation to the skin to the lower eyelid, cheek, upper lip, upper dentition and gingivae, and lateral aspects of the nose. CN V$_2$ enters the middle cranial fossa through the foramen rotundum, so it would not be affected by damage in the superior orbital fissure.

75 **The answer is D: Fourth.** This patient is exhibiting atrophy of the muscles on the left side of the soft palate, which are derived from the mesoderm of the fourth pharyngeal arch. In this patient, the palatal arch droops on the affected (left) side, and the uvula deviates to the unaffected (right) side as a result of the unopposed action of the intact (contralateral) muscles acting on the soft palate. This patient presentation would be indicative of a left vagus nerve (CN X) injury. Remember that the pharyngeal branches of CN X innervate all of the musculature of the soft palate, except the tensor veli palatini (tensor of the soft palate), which is innervated by the mandibular division of the trigeminal nerve (CN V$_3$). Besides forming most of the muscles of the soft palate, the mesoderm of the fourth pharyngeal arch would give rise to the muscles of the pharynx (with the exception of the stylopharyngeus muscle) and the cricothyroid, a muscle of the larynx. **Choice A** (First) is incorrect. The muscles derived from the mesoderm of the first pharyngeal arch include four muscles of mastication (temporalis, masseter, lateral pterygoid, and medial pterygoid) and four additional muscles: **M**ylohoid, **A**nterior belly of the Digastric, **T**ensor Tympani, and **T**ensor Veli Palatini (mnemonic = "MATT"). The tensor veli palatini muscle is the only muscle of the soft palate derived from the first pharyngeal arch. However, damage to the first pharyangeal arch musculature would not affect elevation of the soft palate or deviation of the uvula. **Choice B** (Second) is incorrect. The muscles derived from the mesoderm of the second pharyngeal arch include the muscles of facial expression and three additional muscles: posterior belly of digastric, stylohyoid, and stapedius. None of these listed muscles are associated with the soft palate, so they play no role in this patient's presentation. **Choice C** (Third) is incorrect. The only muscle derived from the mesoderm of the third pharyngeal arch is the stylopharyngeus, a muscle of the pharynx. The stylopharyngeus is the only muscle innervated by the glossopharyngeal nerve (CN IX). Because this muscle is not associated with the soft palate, it plays no role in this patient's presentation. **Choice E** (Sixth) is incorrect. The muscles derived from the mesoderm of the sixth pharyngeal arch include the intrinsic muscles of the larynx and the skeletal muscle of the upper esophagus. Because these muscles are not involved with the soft palate, they play no role in this patient's presentation.

Chapter 10

Cranial Nerves

QUESTIONS

Select the single best answer.

1　After asking a 47-year-old woman to open her mouth wide and say "Ah," the physician notes deviation of the uvula to the left side and asymmetry in the elevation of the soft palate, with the right side of the palate sagging, as noted in the figure. What specific nerve is most likely damaged?

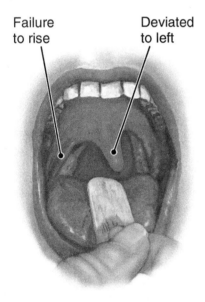

Failure to rise   Deviated to left

(A)　Left glossopharyngeal nerve
(B)　Left vagus nerve
(C)　Right vagus nerve
(D)　Left hypoglossal nerve
(E)　Right hypoglossal nerve

2　A 59-year-old man went to his doctor unable to close his right eye. The physical examination also revealed asymmetry in his smile and an inability to wrinkle the right side of his forehead, as seen in the figure. What cranial nerve is affected in this patient?

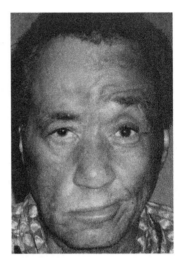

(A)　Trigeminal nerve
(B)　Facial nerve
(C)　Glossopharyngeal nerve
(D)　Vagus nerve
(E)　Hypoglossal nerve

3　A 23-year-old man reports to physician due to shoulder weakness and instability. After removing his shirt, his left shoulder appears to reside lower than his right shoulder, asymmetry noted in the figure. During an examination, the patient is unable to abduct his left arm over his head and shows an inability to shrug (or elevate) his left shoulder against resistance. What nerve was most likely damaged in this patient?

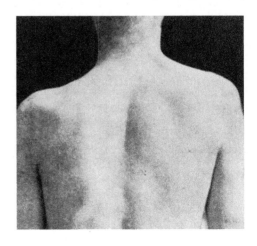

(A) Facial nerve
(B) Glossopharyngeal nerve
(C) Vagus nerve
(D) Accessory nerve
(E) Hypoglossal nerve

4 A 10-year-old boy underwent surgery, a bilateral palatine ton-sillectomy. During a postoperative examination, the doctor noted the boy did not possess a gag reflex on the right side on the posterior tongue. He also complained of abnormal taste sensations in the back of his oral cavity. The soft palate elevated symmetrically when the gag reflex was tested. No other signs or symptoms were noted. What cranial nerve was damaged during the tonsillectomy?
(A) Trigeminal nerve
(B) Facial nerve
(C) Glossopharyngeal nerve
(D) Vagus nerve
(E) Hypoglossal nerve

5 A 23-year-old man has an impacted left third mandibular molar (or wisdom) tooth extracted. Following the surgery, the patient reports numbness in the anterior aspect of his tongue. Which of the following nerves is damaged?
(A) Chorda tympani nerve
(B) Mylohyoid nerve
(C) Inferior alveolar nerve
(D) Lingual nerve
(E) Glossopharyngeal nerve

6 A 47-year-old woman with a history of multiple sclerosis comes to her doctor complaining of sudden bursts (paroxysms) of pain in her mandible, especially in the lower lip, mandibular teeth and gingivae, and cheek on her right side. This debilitating pain is often triggered by eating, talking, or brushing her teeth and often gets worse as the day progresses. Which nerve is the source of her pain?
(A) First division of trigeminal nerve
(B) Second division of trigeminal nerve
(C) Third division of trigeminal nerve
(D) Buccal branch of facial nerve
(E) Marginal mandibular branch of facial nerve

7 A 45-year-old man goes to his physician complaining of having trouble with his speech (dysarthria) and involuntary contractions (fasciculations) within his tongue muscles. The doctor notes that his tongue deviates to the right when the patient attempts to protrude his tongue, as seen in the figure. What nerve is most likely damaged in this patient?

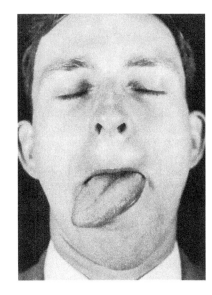

(A) Left hypoglossal nerve
(B) Right hypoglossal nerve
(C) Left glossopharyngeal nerve
(D) Left vagus nerve
(E) Right vagus nerve

8 An 18-year-old male skier is brought to the emergency room after a high-speed collision with a tree. His forehead absorbed much of the impact, resulting in multiple fractures and lacerations. His ER physician noted a clear nasal discharge, which tested positive for glucose. Given the patient's presentation, what cranial nerve was most likely damaged?
(A) Olfactory nerve
(B) Optic nerve
(C) Abducent nerve
(D) Facial nerve
(E) Hypoglossal nerve

9 A 54-year-old man comes to his doctor complaining of an inability to open his left eye. When he physically pries open his affected eye with his fingers (see photo), the gaze of his left eye is directed inferiorly and laterally, causing diplopia. His left pupil is also dilated in comparison to the right one. What nerve is most likely affected in this patient?

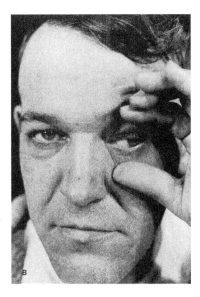

(A) Left oculomotor nerve
(B) Right oculomotor nerve
(C) Left abducent nerve
(D) Right abducent nerve
(E) Left trochlear nerve

10 A 24-year-old man came to his physician with a history of chronic maxillary sinusitis. A computed tomography (CT) scan reveals a soft-tissue mass in the superior aspect (or roof) of the right maxillary sinus. Functional endoscopic sinus surgery (FESS) was performed to biopsy the mass. Postoperatively, the patient experiences paresthesia and numbness of the skin of the right inferior eyelid and upper lip. Which nerve was most likely damaged during the surgery?
(A) First division of trigeminal nerve
(B) Second division of trigeminal nerve
(C) Third division of trigeminal nerve
(D) Zygomatic branch of facial nerve
(E) Buccal branch of facial nerve

11 A 38-year-old woman comes to her family physician complaining of repeatedly tripping and double vision when descending stairs. While testing the eye movements in a cranial nerve examination, she was unable to move her left eye inferiorly when she followed the physician's finger to her right side, as seen in the given figure. What specific nerve is most likely damaged?

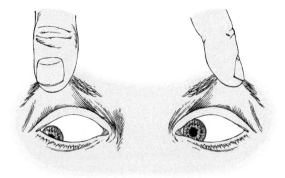

(A) Left oculomotor nerve
(B) Right oculomotor nerve
(C) Left abducent nerve
(D) Right abducent nerve
(E) Left trochlear nerve

12 A 68-year-old woman with thyroid cancer undergoes a total thyroidectomy. Postoperatively, the surgeon notes hoarseness and dysphonia, or altered voice production, while conversing with the patient. What nerve was damaged during the thyroidectomy?
(A) Lingual branch of glossopharyngeal nerve
(B) Accessory nerve
(C) Superior laryngeal nerve
(D) Recurrent laryngeal nerve
(E) Hypoglossal nerve

13 A 67-year-old man presents with shingles on his left forehead, upper eyelid, and bridge of the nose as shown in the figure. Shingles (or herpes zoster) is caused by the varicella zoster virus, which causes chickenpox in children and young adults.

After the initial chickenpox outbreak, this virus usually resides latent in sensory ganglia in the body for many years. When a patient is immunocompromised, this virus can cause shingles unilaterally along the infected nerve's dermatome distribution. What sensory ganglion is most likely affected in this patient?

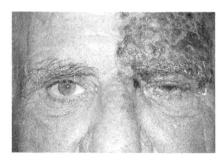

(A) Otic ganglion
(B) Trigeminal ganglion
(C) Superior cervical ganglion
(D) Ciliary ganglion
(E) Submandibular ganglion

14 A 13-year-old girl visits her pediatrician complaining of loss of sensitivity in her lower eyelid, the skin below her right eye, and in her upper lip and teeth. Which of the following sites is the most likely location for the nerve lesion responsible for these signs and symptoms?
(A) Foramen rotundum
(B) Foramen spinosum
(C) Superior orbital fissure
(D) Foramen ovale
(E) Optic canal

15 A 12-year-old boy suffers a fracture of the floor of the right side of the middle cranial fossa during an automobile accident. Subsequent physical examination reveals he is devoid of emotional tearing on the ipsilateral side. Which of the following nerves is most likely damaged?
(A) Greater petrosal nerve
(B) Lesser petrosal nerve
(C) Deep petrosal nerve
(D) Lacrimal nerve
(E) Chorda tympani nerve

16 A 42-year-old woman noticed that her right upper eyelid was drooping and her right pupil was constricted (see the given photo). She goes to her physician where a thorough examination revealed ptosis, miosis, anhydrosis, flushing of her face, and narrowing of the palpebral fissure (the slit between the upper and lower eyelids) on the right side of the patient. Which of the following structure is most likely damaged in this patient?

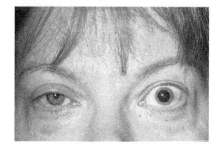

(A) Superior division of the oculomotor nerve
(B) Superior cervical ganglion
(C) Nerve of the pterygoid canal
(D) Ciliary ganglion
(E) Ophthalmic division of trigeminal nerve

17 A 32-year-old man presents with unilateral paralysis of the muscles of mastication on the right side. This condition has resulted in facial asymmetry as noted in the figure. Though he is uncomfortable with his appearance and has difficulty when chewing his food, his chief complaint is his difficulty swallowing (dysphagia). What muscle is most likely involved in his dysphagia?

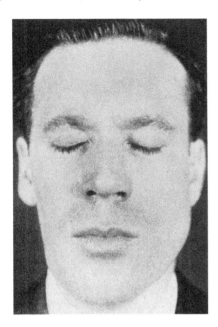

(A) Sternohyoid
(B) Stylohyoid
(C) Cricothyroid
(D) Stylopharyngeus
(E) Mylohyoid

18 A 27-year-old woman with green eyes comes to her physician with noted asymmetry in her pupils (as seen in the figure). Her right pupil is abnormally dilated, and on examination, the right eye is slow to respond to light stimuli. Her visual acuity is not impaired, and no other signs and symptoms are noted. What structure is most likely affected in this patient?

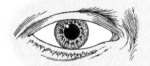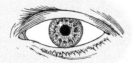

(A) Superior cervical ganglion
(B) Optic nerve
(C) Oculomotor nerve
(D) Trochlear nerve
(E) Abducent nerve

19 To differentiate between idiopathic unilateral paralysis of the muscles of facial expression (Bell palsy) and a herpes zoster infection of CN VII, the physician must look for small herpetic lesions (vesicles or blisters). Where are these skin lesions located in a herpes zoster infection involving the facial nerve?
(A) Mental region of the mandible
(B) Temporal and parietal region of the scalp
(C) Upper lip and cheek of the face
(D) Auricle of the external ear
(E) Bridge and tip of the external nose

20 A 37-year-old man presented with decreased emotional tearing on the right side and intermittent headaches. Magnetic resonance images (MRIs) revealed a facial nerve schwannoma located within the right pterygoid (vidian) canal. What nerve fibers are most likely injured by this tumor?
(A) Taste fibers to the anterior two thirds of the tongue
(B) Parasympathetic innervation to the submandibular and sublingual glands
(C) Presynaptic sympathetic fibers
(D) Presynaptic parasympathetic fibers
(E) Postsynaptic parasympathetic fibers

21 A 57-year-old woman presents with right unilateral facial paralysis and dizziness. During an examination, the physician also notes a loss of hearing on the right side. An MRI of the patient's head reveals a brain tumor, as noted by the asterisk in the figure. Based upon the patient's presentation and MRI, where is the tumor located?

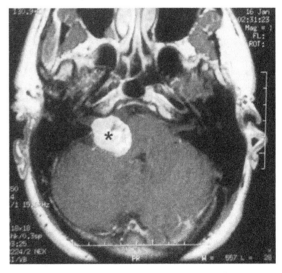

(A) Foramen rotundum
(B) Foramen ovale
(C) Internal acoustic meatus
(D) Facial canal
(E) Stylomastoid foramen

22 A 3-year-old girl presents with headache, vomiting, and papilledema. A sagittal MRI of the patient's head reveals a large craniopharyngioma, or a tumor arising from the remnants of Rathke pouch, as noted in the figure. This suprasellar tumor, located above the diaphragm sellae, is compressing the pituitary gland. Given the location and size of this tumor, what visual disturbances are likely to be seen in this patient?

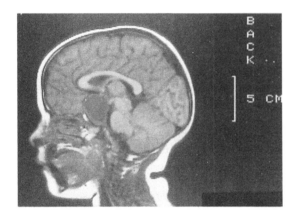

(A) Monocular blindness
(B) Binasal hemianopsia
(C) Bitemporal hemianopsia
(D) Right homonymous hemianopsia
(E) Left homonymous hemianopsia

23   A patient damages the cranial nerve indicated by the arrow in the figure. What signs or symptoms would be evident in a patient with this nerve lesion?

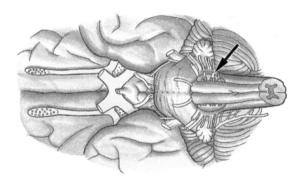

(A) Inability to elevate the ipsilateral shoulder
(B) Deviation of the uvula to the contralateral side
(C) Loss of gag reflex on the ipsilateral side
(D) Ipsilateral loss of parotid gland secretion
(E) Deviation of the tongue to the ipsilateral side

24   In the provided X-ray, an opening in the skull is identified at the tip of the red arrow. If the nerve that traverses this cranial opening were damaged, what signs or symptoms would most likely be seen in the patient?

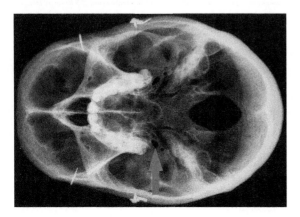

(A) Unilateral muscles of facial expression paralysis
(B) Unilateral muscles of mastication paralysis
(C) Paresthesia of the upper lip, cheek, and lower eyelid
(D) Decreased salivation of the submandibular gland
(E) Decreased salivation of the parotid gland

25   A 27-year-old man comes to his family physician complaining of double vision. While sitting face-to-face, the doctor notes the patient exhibits strabismus, especially esotropia of the left eye, which gives the patient a "cross-eyed" appearance. When asked to follow the doctor's index finger with only his eyes, the patient is unable to look laterally, as illustrated in the figure. No other visual deficits are noted. What specific nerve is most likely damaged?

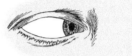

(A) Left oculomotor nerve
(B) Right oculomotor nerve
(C) Left abducent nerve
(D) Right abducent nerve
(E) Left trochlear nerve

26   A 25-year-old professional boxer loses a fight when he is rendered unconscious by his opponent. After he regains consciousness, the ringside physician notes the boxer has a severe headache, nausea, and even vomiting. Being concerned about intracranial trauma, what cranial nerve can be observed by the physician, without the aid of radiographic imaging, to gain more information on whether the boxer has increased intracranial pressure?
(A) Optic nerve
(B) Oculomotor nerve
(C) Olfactory nerve
(D) Trigeminal nerve
(E) Trochlear nerve

27   A 14-year-old girl presents with Horner syndrome, after surgical removal of a mass growing in her posterior mediastinum. What nerve would be affected by the loss of sympathetic innervation to the head?
(A) Lesser petrosal
(B) Deep petrosal
(C) Greater petrosal
(D) Chorda tympani
(E) Optic

28   While planning a delicious dinner for his former anatomy professors, a doctor finds himself salivating at the thought of the feast. What description accurately describes the secretomotor pathway for innervation of the submandibular gland?
(A) Parasympathetic fibers via the inferior alveolar nerve
(B) Sympathetic fibers via the lingual nerve
(C) Parasympathetic fibers via the mandibular branch of the facial nerve
(D) Sympathetic fibers via the hypoglossal nerve
(E) Parasympathetic fibers via the chorda tympani nerve

29 A 70-year-old woman goes to her physician complaining of headache, nausea, and vomiting. A head MRI reveals a tumor disrupting the visceral afferent fibers running into the solitary nucleus located within the medulla. What signs or symptoms would be manifested following the degeneration of these nerve fibers entering the solitary nucleus?

(A) Blindness
(B) Loss of sensation from the cornea
(C) Loss of equilibrium
(D) Altered taste
(E) Deafness

30 In the provided CT scan of the head, an opening in the skull is identified at the tip of the black arrow. What cranial nerve exits the cranium via this opening?

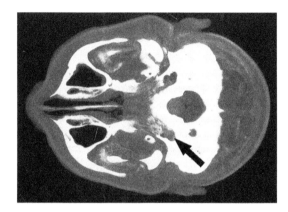

(A) Trochlear nerve
(B) Trigeminal nerve
(C) Facial nerve
(D) Glossopharyngeal nerve
(E) Hypoglossal nerve

31 A 46-year-old woman was cut on the right side of her face by a window that shattered. Her laceration was located at the anterior border of the inferior part of the masseter muscle. When she returns to her doctor to have the stitches removed, her physician notes asymmetry in her lower lip when she grimaces as seen in the figure. Damage to what nerve would cause the facial asymmetry seen in this patient?

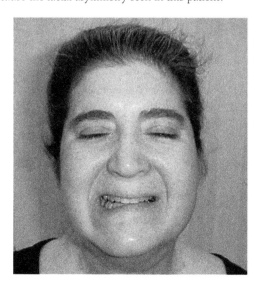

(A) Zygomatic branch of facial nerve
(B) Temporal branch of facial nerve
(C) Cervical branch of facial nerve
(D) Buccal branch of facial nerve
(E) Marginal mandibular branch of facial nerve

32 A male 1st-year medical student mistakenly enters the women's locker room and finds a group of his female colleagues changing their clothes. He is shocked and embarrassed by his mistake and immediately runs away with his heart pounding. Given his agitated state, what ganglion, housing neuron cell bodies, is experiencing an extremely high rate of activity?

(A) Ciliary ganglion
(B) Trigeminal ganglion
(C) Inferior (nodose) vagal ganglion
(D) Superior cervical ganglion
(E) Pterygopalatine ganglion

33 A physician directs a small light into only the left eye of a patient to test pupillary constriction. The left pupil does not respond to the light; however, the right pupil constricts. What nerve is most likely damaged in this patient?

(A) Right optic nerve
(B) Left optic nerve
(C) Right ophthalmic nerve
(D) Right oculomotor nerve
(E) Left oculomotor nerve

34 An MRI of the right internal carotid artery reveals atherosclerotic plaques causing stenosis of the vessel's lumen within the cavernous sinus. The stenosis is causing increased pressure within the internal carotid artery as it courses through the cavernous sinus, resulting in an aneurysm. Given its location, what cranial nerve would most likely be damaged?

(A) Trochlear nerve
(B) Abducent nerve
(C) Maxillary nerve
(D) Ophthalmic nerve
(E) Oculomotor nerve

35 Most senior citizens dislike the bass audio frequencies augmented by a large subwoofer in a teenager's car. But, one 68-year-old man came to his doctor complaining of hyperacusis, or heightened sensitivity to these loud, low-frequency sounds. The results from an audiometer hearing test reveal normal hearing for a man of his age. Given the presentation, what cranial nerve is most likely involved with his hyperacusis?

(A) Facial nerve
(B) Vestibulocochlear nerve
(C) Glossopharyngeal nerve
(D) Vagus nerve
(E) Hypoglossal nerve

ANSWERS AND DISCUSSION

1 **The answer is C: Right vagus nerve.** Damage to the right vagus nerve is causing asymmetry in soft palate elevation and contralateral deviation of the uvula of the soft palate to the left side. The pharyngeal branches of the vagus nerve innervate all the musculature of the soft palate, except the tensor veli palatini (tensor of the soft palate), which is innervated by the mandibular division of the trigeminal nerve (CN V_3). On examination, the arch of the soft palate droops on the affected side (right side) and the uvula deviates to the unaffected side (left side) as a result of the unopposed action of the intact muscles acting on the soft palate. This patient may report dysphagia, difficulty in swallowing, and nasal regurgitation, due to reduced muscular tone within the soft palate. **Choice A** (Left glossopharyngeal nerve) is incorrect. The glossopharyngeal nerve only innervates one muscle, the stylopharyngeus, which is a pharyngeal muscle. Because it does not innervate any muscles of the soft palate, the glossopharyngeal nerve is unable to affect the elevation of the soft palate or deviation of the uvula. **Choice B** (Left vagus nerve) is incorrect. The left vagus nerve is not injured because the patient's uvula deviates to the left, a sign that the contralateral (right) vagus nerve is damaged. **Choice D** (Left hypoglossal nerve) is incorrect. The left hypoglossal nerve does not innervate any muscles of the soft palate, so it would not be involved in the deviation of the uvula. Damage to the left hypoglossal nerve causes the tongue to deviate ipsilaterally (to the left side) when the patient protrudes the tongue. **Choice E** (Right hypoglossal nerve) is incorrect. The right hypoglossal nerve does not innervate any muscles of the soft palate and would not cause the deviation of the uvula. A lesion of the right hypoglossal nerve causes the tongue to deviate ipsilaterally (to the right side) when the patient protrudes the tongue.

2 **The answer is B: Facial nerve.** The main trunk of the facial nerve (CN VII) exits the stylomastoid foramen and runs anteriorly in close relationship to (or within) the parotid gland. This nerve branches into five terminal branches: **T**emporal, **Z**ygomatic, **B**uccal, **M**arginal mandibular, and **C**ervical. These branches innervate the muscles of facial expression derived from the mesoderm of the second pharyngeal arch and can be remembered by the mnemonics "Two Zebras Bit My Cheek" or "To Zanzibar By Motor Car". Damage to the main trunk of the facial nerve causes unilateral facial paralysis due to loss of innervation to these muscles. The patient would present ipsilaterally with an inability to close the eye (due to the loss of the sphincter of the eye, the orbicularis oculi muscle), inability to wrinkle the forehead (due to loss of the frontalis muscle), and asymmetry in the smile (due to the loss of many muscles acting on the labial commissure and upper lip). Unilateral facial paralysis is seen following damage to the facial nerve following a nerve lesion, brain tumor, stroke, or even Lyme disease. When no specific cause (idiopathic) can be found, it is called facial (Bell or CN VII) palsy. **Choice A** (Trigeminal nerve) is incorrect. The trigeminal nerve (CN V) is the main sensory nerve for the face and scalp, and it has three divisions, namely, the ophthalmic (CN V_1), maxillary (CN V_2), and mandibular (CN V_3). CN V_3 is the only division of the trigeminal nerve (CN V) that supplies motor innervation. It supplies the eight muscles derived from the mesoderm of the first pharyngeal arch, including the muscles of mastication. Losing innervation to the muscles supplied by CN V_3 would not cause ipsilateral facial paralysis. **Choice C** (Glossopharyngeal nerve) is incorrect. The glossopharyngeal nerve (CN IX) supplies only one muscle, the stylopharyngeus, derived from the mesoderm of the third pharyngeal arch. Losing innervation to the stylopharyngeus, a muscle of the pharynx, would not cause ipsilateral facial paralysis. **Choice D** (Vagus nerve) is incorrect. The vagus nerve (CN X) supplies the muscles derived from the mesoderm of the fourth and sixth pharyngeal arches, including all the muscles of the larynx as well as most of the muscles of soft palate (exception = tensor veli palatini of CN V_3) and pharynx (exception = stylopharyngeus of CN IX). Despite its extensive motor innervation, damage to the vagus nerve would not cause ipsilateral facial paralysis. However, it would result in dysphagia, or difficulty swallowing. **Choice E** (Hypoglossal nerve) is incorrect. The hypoglossal nerve (CN XII) innervates the intrinsic and (most of the) extrinsic muscles of tongue (exception = palatoglossus muscle of CN X). Losing innervation to the muscles of the tongue would not cause ipsilateral facial paralysis.

3 **The answer is D: Accessory nerve.** The accessory nerve (CN XI) provides motor innervation to the sternocleidomastoid muscle and the trapezius muscle. The asymmetry of the shoulders (shown in the figure) suggests paralysis of the left trapezius muscle. Actions of the trapezius include elevation of the scapula and lateral rotation of the scapula during abduction greater than 90 degrees. Both of these actions were affected in this patient. Damage to the accessory nerve also leads to "drooping" of the affected shoulder due to loss of innervation and subsequent loss of muscle tone (atrophy) of the trapezius muscle. **Choice A** (Facial nerve) is incorrect. Damage to the facial nerve (CN VII) could result in the loss of taste sensation to the anterior two thirds of the tongue, decreased salivation due its innervation of the submandibular and sublingual salivary glands, unilateral facial paralysis, hyperacusis due to loss of stapedius muscle function, and even dysphagia due to its innervation of the posterior belly of the digastric and stylohyoid muscles, which have attachments to the hyoid bone. These signs or symptoms were not noted in this patient. **Choice B** (Glossopharyngeal nerve) is incorrect. Damage to the glossopharyngeal nerve (CN IX) could result in decreased salivation due to its innervation of the parotid gland and loss of taste and visceral sensation to the posterior one third of the tongue. Therefore, a lesion compromising this nerve would result in a dry mouth, abnormal taste sensations, and dysphagia due to loss of a gag reflex and loss of innervation to the stylopharyngeus muscle. These signs or symptoms were not noted in this patient. However, glossopharyngeal nerve dysfunction may be encountered along with accessory nerve dysfunction because they exit the skull through the same opening, the jugular foramen. **Choice C** (Vagus nerve) is incorrect. Damage to the vagus nerve could result in problems with speech (dysphonia) and swallowing (deglutition) due to loss of the efferent limb of the gag reflex and loss of motor innervation to the majority of palatal, pharyngeal, and laryngeal musculature. These symptoms were not noted in this patient. However, vagus nerve dysfunction may be encountered along with accessory nerve dysfunction because they exit the skull through the same opening, the jugular foramen. **Choice E** (Hypoglossal nerve) is incorrect. The hypoglossal nerve is responsible for innervation of all of the intrinsic and extrinsic muscles of the tongue, except the palatoglossus (innervated by the vagus nerve). Damage to CN XII would not alter the actions of the left trapezius muscle, but it would affect the musculature of the tongue.

4 **The answer is C: Glossopharyngeal nerve.** The lingual and tonsillar branches of the glossopharyngeal nerve (CN IX) reside in the palatine tonsillar bed between the palatoglossal and palatopharyngeal folds. At this location, these branches of CN IX are susceptible to damage during a tonsillectomy, which would compromise taste and visceral sensation to the posterior one third of the tongue. Therefore, damage to CN IX at this location results in abnormal taste sensations and a loss of the afferent limb (CN IX) of the gag reflex on the ipsilateral side, respectively. These signs and symptoms were noted in this patient. **Choice A** (Trigeminal nerve) is incorrect. The trigeminal nerve (CN V) provides general sensation to the anterior two thirds of the tongue via the lingual nerve; however, in this patient, the right posterior part of the tongue is affected. **Choice B** (Facial nerve) is incorrect. Compromising the chorda tympani branch of the facial nerve leads to loss of taste sensation to the anterior two thirds of the tongue and decreased salivation due its parasympathetic innervation of the submandibular and sublingual salivary glands. The chorda tympani branch of the facial nerve performs these actions by joining the lingual nerve of the mandibular division of the trigeminal nerve (CN V$_3$) to reach the oral cavity. However, the facial nerve is not involved in the gag reflex and does not supply taste to the posterior aspect of the tongue. **Choice D** (Vagus nerve) is incorrect. The vagus nerve does provide taste sensations in the area of the epiglottis and serves as the efferent limb of the gag reflex; however, CN X is not involved in this patient's signs and symptoms due to the symmetry in elevation of the soft palate noted during the postoperative examination. **Choice E** (Hypoglossal nerve) is incorrect. The hypoglossal nerve is responsible for innervation of all of the intrinsic and extrinsic muscles of the tongue, except the palatoglossus (innervated by the vagus nerve). Damage to CN XII would not affect the gag reflex or lead to abnormal taste sensations, but it would affect the musculature of the tongue.

5 **The answer is D: Lingual nerve.** The lingual nerve is a branch of the mandibular division of the trigeminal nerve (CN V$_3$), which traverses the foramen ovale and resides in the infratemporal fossa. This nerve supplies general sensation to the anterior two thirds of the tongue, and this nerve is at risk during extraction of an impacted third mandibular molar tooth. **Choice A** (Chorda tympani nerve) is incorrect. The chorda tympani, a branch of the facial nerve (CN VII), joins the lingual branch of the mandibular nerve in the infratemporal fossa. The chorda tympani nerve conveys taste sensation to the anterior two thirds of the tongue and carries presynaptic parasympathetic fibers to the submandibular ganglion for innervation of the submandibular and sublingual salivary glands. While the chorda tympani nerve merges with the lingual nerve to reach its effector region, cutting the chorda tympani nerve would not result in numbness on the tip of the tongue. **Choice B** (Mylohyoid nerve) is incorrect. The mylohyoid nerve, a branch of the mandibular division of the trigeminal nerve (CN V$_3$), supplies motor innervation to the anterior belly of the digastric muscle and the mylohyoid muscles. The mylohyoid nerve branches off the inferior alveolar nerve prior to the latter nerve

entering the mandibular foramen to supply sensory innervation to the inferior dentition. Cutting the mylohyoid nerve would not result in numbness on the tip of the tongue, but it would result in paralysis of the mylohyoid and anterior belly of the digastric muscles. **Choice C** (Inferior alveolar nerve) is incorrect. The inferior alveolar nerve, a branch off the mandibular division of the trigeminal nerve (CN V$_3$), enters the mandibular foramen to supply the lower teeth, periosteum, and gingivae of the mandible. The mental nerve, a terminal branch of the inferior alveolar nerve, supplies the skin and mucosa of the lower lip and chin. Though the inferior alveolar nerve may be damaged during this procedure, it is not responsible for giving general sensation to the anterior aspect of the tongue. **Choice E** (Glossopharyngeal nerve) is incorrect. The lingual branch of the glossopharyngeal nerve (CN IX) enters the tongue to provide sensory and taste information to the posterior one third of the tongue. It also gives off a tonsillar branch, which gives sensation to the mucosa of the oropharynx, including the palatine tonsil. This nerve would not be responsible for the numbness on the tip of the tongue described in this patient.

6 **The answer is C: Third division of trigeminal nerve.** The third (mandibular) division of the trigeminal nerve (CN V$_3$) supplies general sensation to the skin of the lower lip, chin, cheek, and even the anterior auricle and the lateral scalp. This sensory innervation is supplied via three cutaneous nerves: mental, buccal, and auriculotemporal. The mandibular division of the trigeminal nerve also supplies innervation to the mandibular teeth and gingivae via the inferior alveolar nerve. This patient is suffering from trigeminal neuralgia (or tic douloureux), often seen in patients suffering from demyelinating diseases such as multiple sclerosis, affecting CN V$_3$. Trigeminal neuralgia is characterized by episodes of pain that occur suddenly, and debilitating pain can often be triggered by stimuli within the distribution area of the nerve affected, which was seen following eating, talking, or brushing her teeth in this patient. **Choice A** (First division of the trigeminal nerve) is incorrect. The first (ophthalmic) division of the trigeminal nerve (CN V$_1$) supplies sensory (cutaneous) innervation to the skin of the upper eyelid, anterior aspect of the nose, forehead, and anterior scalp. The sensory distribution of the ophthalmic division of the trigeminal nerve does not correlate to the areas of the face affected in this patient, so this option can be eliminated. **Choice B** (Second division of trigeminal nerve) is incorrect. The second (maxillary) division of the trigeminal nerve (CN V$_2$) supplies sensory (cutaneous) innervation to the skin to the lower eyelid, cheek, and upper lip, upper dentition and gingivae, maxillary sinus, and lateral aspect of the nose. The sensory distribution of the maxillary division of the trigeminal nerve does not correlate to the areas of the face affected in this patient, so this option can be eliminated. **Choice D** (Buccal branch of facial nerve) is incorrect. The buccal branch of the facial nerve (CN VII) is one of five terminal branches of the main trunk of CN VII, which supplies the muscles of facial expression and other muscles derived from mesoderm in the embryonic second pharyngeal arch. This buccal branch is entirely efferent (motor) in its innervation supplying the buccinator muscle and muscles of the upper lip. It does not have a sensory component, so this nerve would not be the source of this patient's pain. **Choice E** (Marginal mandibular branch of the facial nerve) is incorrect. The marginal mandibular branch of the facial nerve (CN VII) is another one of five terminal branches of the main trunk of CN VII. This nerve only has an efferent (motor) component supplying the muscles of lower lip and chin. It does not have a sensory component, so this nerve would not be the source of this patient's pain.

7   **The answer is B: Right hypoglossal nerve.**   The hypoglossal nerve (CN XII) innervates all of the intrinsic muscles of the tongue and most of its extrinsic muscles with the lone exception being the palatoglossus muscle, innervated by the vagus nerve (CN X). Damage to the right CN XII produces the dysarthria and fasciculations within the tongue musculature, noted in the patient. The ipsilateral deviation of the tongue is due to the unopposed muscular contractions of the left (contralateral) genioglossus muscle. The mnemonic "The tongue licks the wound" will help you remember that the tongue deviates to the ipsilateral side in a lower motor lesion of CN XII. **Choice A** (Left hypoglossal nerve) is incorrect. The hypoglossal nerve (CN XII) innervates all of the intrinsic muscles of the tongue and most of its extrinsic muscles with the lone exception being the palatoglossus muscle, innervated by the vagus nerve (CN X). Therefore, the cutting of the left CN XII produces dysarthria and fasciculations, noted in this patient; however, the tongue would deviate to the left side during protrusion due to the unopposed muscular contractions of the right genioglossus muscle. **Choice C** (Left glossopharyngeal nerve) is incorrect. The glossopharyngeal nerve only innervates one muscle, the stylopharyngeus, which is a muscle of the pharynx. Without innervating a muscle of the tongue, the glossopharyngeal nerve is unable to affect the deviation of the tongue. **Choice D** (Left vagus nerve) is incorrect. Damage to the left vagus nerve causes asymmetry in soft palate elevation and contralateral deviation of the uvula to the right. These deficits result because pharyngeal branches of the vagus nerve innervate all of the musculature of the soft palate, except the tensor veli palatini (tensor of the soft palate), which is innervated by the mandibular division of the trigeminal nerve (CN V_3). Within the tongue, the vagus nerve supplies only the palatoglossus muscle, which elevates the posterior aspect of the tongue during swallowing. Therefore, a lesion of the left vagus nerve would not affect tongue protrusion or result in ipsilateral tongue deviation. **Choice E** (Right vagus nerve) is incorrect. Damage to the right vagus nerve causes asymmetry in soft palate elevation and contralateral deviation of the uvula to the left. The pharyngeal branches of the vagus nerve innervate all of the musculature of the soft palate, except the tensor veli palatini (tensor of the soft palate), which is innervated by the mandibular division of the trigeminal nerve (CN V_3). Within the tongue, the vagus nerve supplies only the palatoglossus muscle, which elevates the posterior aspect of the tongue during swallowing. Therefore, a lesion on the right vagus nerve would not affect tongue protrusion or result in ipsilateral tongue deviation.

8   **The answer is A: Olfactory nerve.**   The traumatic impact to the forehead caused a defect (or communication) in the floor of the patient's anterior cranial fossa. The cribiform plate of the ethmoid bone, which physically separates the nasal cavity from the anterior cranial fossa, was fractured due to the patient's presentation with cerebrospinal fluid (CSF) rhinorrhea, as the clear nasal discharge that tested positive for glucose would imply. Olfactory nerve (CN I) fibers descend into the nasal cavity via the foramina within the cribiform plate of

the ethmoid bone, so when this bone is fractured the olfactory nerve is most likely damaged. During a cranial nerve examination, the patient exhibited anosmia (loss of smell) and may even experience alteration of taste perceptions due to the complex interactions between the olfaction and gustatory sensory pathways. Severe head trauma often results in anosmia due to the delicate olfactory nerves traversing the foramina within the cribiform plate of the ethmoid bone. **Choice B** (Optic nerve) is incorrect. Damage to the optic nerve (CN II) causes ipsilateral blindness or other visual deficits of the affected eye. This finding was not reported in this patient. **Choice C** (Abducent nerve) is incorrect. Damage to the abducent nerve (CN VI) causes ipsilateral paralysis to the lateral rectus muscle, which is the only extraocular muscle innervated by CN VI. When the abducent nerve is damaged, the patient displays diplopia, and the ipsilateral eye rests in the adducted position due to the unopposed action of the other extraocular muscles. The abducent nerve is the cranial nerve with the longest intradural course, and it can often be damaged (impinged) as it arches over the crest of the petrous part of the temporal bone or by an aneurysm of the internal carotid artery in the cavernous sinus. This nerve lesion can occur following increased intracranial pressure from a supratentorial (above the cerebellum tentorium) space-occupying lesion in the brain, which could result from a tumor, hemorrhage, or blockage of CSF. Because this patient presented with CSF rhinorrhea, the olfactory nerve is the cranial nerve most likely damaged. **Choice D** (Facial nerve) is incorrect. Damage to the facial nerve (CN VII) causes the following sequelae of signs and symptoms: ipsilateral paralysis of the muscles of facial expression, hyperacusis (sensitivity to noise), loss of taste to the anterior two thirds of the tongue, loss of secretion from the submandibular and sublingual salivary glands, and loss of emotional tearing. However, none of these findings were reported in this patient. **Choice E** (Hypoglossal nerve) is incorrect. Damage to the hypoglossal nerve (CN XII) causes ipsilateral deviation of the tongue during protrusion, dysarthria (difficulty speaking), and fasciculations (involuntary twitching of muscle fibers). However, none of these findings were reported in this patient.

9   **The answer is A: Left oculomotor nerve.**   The left oculomotor nerve, CN III, innervates four (of six) extraocular eye muscles and the levator palpebrae superioris in the ipsilateral (left) eye. Damage to the left CN III leads to ptosis (or drooping) of the left upper eyelid due to loss of innervation to the levator palpebrae superioris muscle, which is why the patient is having trouble opening his left eye without assistance from his fingers. His left eye is also located in an abducted and lateral position due to loss of innervation to the four extraocular muscles. Due to the unopposed muscular contractions of the lateral rectus muscle, innervated by the abducent nerve (CN VI), and the superior oblique muscle, innervated by the trochlear nerve (CN IV), the eye resides in this abnormal "down and out" position causing diplopia (or double vision). Finally, the oculomotor nerve also has a parasympathetic component that enables accommodation of the eye, which involves pupillary constriction. Damage to the parasympathetic component of CN III causes pupillary dilation due to the unopposed sympathetic innervation to the dilator pupillae muscle of the iris. All of these signs and symptoms are evident in the left eye of this patient, which implies damage to the left CN III. **Choice B** (Right oculomotor nerve) is incorrect. Damage to the right

CN III leads to diplopia (due to the right pupil resting in an abducted and lateral position), ptosis of the upper eyelid, and pupillary dilation, which is noted in this patient. However, the left eye is affected in this patient, which implies involvement of the left CN III. **Choice C** (Left abducent nerve) is incorrect. The only extraocular muscle innervated by the left abducent nerve, CN VI, is the left lateral rectus muscle, which turns the left globe laterally. If this nerve were damaged, the patient would display diplopia, and the left pupil would be resting in the adducted position due to the unopposed action of the other extraocular muscles. **Choice D** (Right abducent nerve) is incorrect. The only extraocular muscle innervated by the right abducent nerve, CN VI, is the right lateral rectus muscle, which turns the right globe laterally. If this nerve were damaged, the patient would display diplopia, and the right pupil would be resting in the adducted position due to the unopposed action of the other extraocular muscles. Because extraocular eye movements were affected in the left eye of this patient, this option can be easily eliminated. **Choice E** (Left trochlear nerve) is incorrect. The left trochlear nerve innervates only one muscle, the superior oblique muscle, in the orbit. This muscle pulls the eye inferolaterally; however, this nerve is tested clinically by asking the patient to look inferiorly after the left eye is placed in an adducted position. While a patient with left trochlear nerve damage would experience diplopia, especially when looking inferiorly, this answer does not explain the ptosis and pupillary dilation seen in this patient.

10 **The answer is B: Second division of trigeminal nerve.** The second (maxillary) division of the trigeminal nerve (CN V$_2$) supplies the skin of the inferior eyelid and upper lip through the infraorbital nerve that courses through the superior aspect (roof) of the maxillary sinus, and due to its location, this nerve is most likely damaged during the biopsy. Damage to the infraorbital nerve causes paresthesia and numbness in the areas of cutaneous (sensory) distribution for this nerve. **Choice A** (First division of trigeminal nerve) is incorrect. The first (ophthalmic) division of the trigeminal nerve (CN V$_1$) supplies the skin of the upper eyelid, forehead, and scalp. CN V$_1$ enters the middle cranial fossa via the superior orbital fissure, and its branches are distributed within the orbit, anterior cranial fossa, and nasal cavity. CN V$_1$ does not supply sensory innervation to the maxillary sinus, so it would be spared during this FESS. However, the ophthalmic division of the trigeminal nerve does innervate three other paranasal sinuses (ethmoidal, frontal, and sphenoidal). **Choice C** (Third division of trigeminal nerve) is incorrect. The third (mandibular) division of the trigeminal nerve (CN V$_3$) supplies the skin of the lower lip, chin, cheek, anterior auricle, and aspects of the lateral scalp. CN V$_3$ leaves the middle cranial fossa via the foramen ovale, and it does NOT have a significant branch, which courses through the superior aspect (roof) of the maxillary sinus. Therefore, it could not be damaged in this patient. **Choice D** (Zygomatic branch of facial nerve) is incorrect. The zygomatic branch of the facial nerve (CN VII) is a terminal branch of the main trunk of CN VII. This nerve has only motor innervation, supplying the inferior part of the orbicularis oculi and other muscles of facial expression located below the orbit. Because it does not pass through the maxillary sinus or supply cutaneous innervation to any region, the zygomatic nerve of CN VII could not cause the numbness and paresthesia seen in this patient. **Choice E** (Buccal branch of facial nerve) is incorrect. The buccal branch of the facial nerve (CN VII) is a terminal branch of the main trunk of CN VII. This nerve has only motor innervation, supplying the risorius and muscles of the upper lip. Because it does not pass through the maxillary sinus or supply cutaneous innervation to any region, the buccal nerve of CN VII could not cause the numbness and paresthesia seen in this patient.

11 **The answer is E: Left trochlear nerve.** The left trochlear nerve innervates only one muscle, the superior oblique, located in the orbit. Acting individually, this muscle pulls the eye inferolaterally, but it would be hard to distinguish this movement from the combined movements of the inferior rectus muscle (innervated by the oculomotor nerve) and the lateral rectus muscle (innervated by the abducent nerve), which also move the globe inferior and lateral, respectively. Therefore, the left trochlear nerve is clinically tested by asking the patient to look inferiorly after the left eye is placed in an adducted position. Due to its course and involvement with the trochlea of the superior oblique muscle, this extraocular muscle is the only muscle that can strongly direct the gaze of the adducted eye inferiorly. Damage to this nerve also explains her diplopia, or double vision, and clumsiness when descending stairs. **Choice A** (Left oculomotor nerve) is incorrect. The left oculomotor nerve, CN III, innervates most of the extraocular eye muscles (with the exception of superior oblique and lateral rectus muscles) and the levator palpebrae superioris (which elevates the eyelid) in the ipsilateral (left) eye. Damage to the left CN III leads to diplopia (due to the left pupil resting in an abducted and lateral position) and ptosis (drooping of the eyelid) associated with the left eye. **Choice B** (Right oculomotor nerve) is incorrect. The right oculomotor nerve, CN III, innervates most of the extraocular eye muscles (with the exception of superior oblique and lateral rectus muscles) and the levator palpebrae superioris (which elevates the eyelid) in the ipsilateral (right) eye. Damage to the right CN III leads to diplopia (due to the right pupil resting in an abducted and lateral position) and ptosis (drooping of the eyelid) associated with the right eye. However, abnormal positioning of the resting pupil and ptosis were not seen in this patient. **Choice C** (Left abducent nerve) is incorrect. The only extraocular muscle innervated by the left abducent nerve, CN VI, is the left lateral rectus muscle, which directs the left globe laterally. If the left abducent nerve were damaged, the patient would display diplopia, and the left pupil would be resting in the adducted position due to the unopposed action of the other extraocular muscles. **Choice D** (Right abducent nerve) is incorrect. The only extraocular muscle innervated by the right abducent nerve, CN VI, is the right lateral rectus muscle, which directs the right globe laterally. If this nerve were damaged, the patient would display diplopia, and the right pupil would be resting in the adducted position due to the unopposed action of the other extraocular muscles. Because extraocular eye movements were affected in the left eye of this patient, this option can be easily eliminated.

12 **The answer is D: Recurrent laryngeal nerve.** The recurrent laryngeal nerve, a branch of the vagus nerve (CN X), passes posterior to the thyroid gland as it ascends in the neck to innervate most of the muscles of the larynx. Iatrogenic damage to the recurrent laryngeal nerve occurs in approximately 1% to 2% of thyroid surgeries and leads to the patient's hoarseness and dysphonia due to ipsilateral paralysis of all the muscles of the larynx, except the cricothyroid muscle. **Choice A** (Lingual branch of glossopharyngeal nerve) is incorrect. The lingual branch of the glossopharyngeal nerve (CN IX) provides sensation and taste to the posterior one third of the tongue. Damage to the lingual branch of the glossopharyngeal nerve (CN IX) would not cause the speech difficulties displayed in this patient. **Choice B** (Accessory nerve) is incorrect. The accessory nerve (CN XI) innervates the sternocleidomastoid and trapezius muscles, so damage to CN XI would cause an inability to shrug the shoulders and weakness turning the head to the contralateral side. These signs and symptoms were not seen in this patient. **Choice C** (Superior laryngeal nerve) is incorrect. Cutting the superior laryngeal nerve of the vagus nerve (CN X) produces numbness of the superior part of the larynx above the vestibular (false) vocal folds. It also innervates the cricothyroid muscle, a muscle of the larynx, involved in increasing the length of the true vocal folds. Though this muscle is important in increasing the pitch of the voice, it would not produce the hoarseness and dysphonia seen in this patient. **Choice E** (Hypoglossal nerve) is incorrect. The hypoglossal nerve (CN XII) is located in the anterior cervical region, and it innervates all of the intrinsic and most of the extrinsic muscles of the tongue, with the lone exception being the palatoglossus muscle, innervated by the vagus nerve (CN X). Cutting CN XII produces a speech impediment and deviation of the tongue to the ipsilateral side during protrusion due to atrophy of the tongue musculature. However, these deficits were not seen in this patient.

13   **The answer is B: Trigeminal ganglion.**   As seen in the photo, shingles is evident in the dermatome distribution pattern of the ophthalmic division of the left trigeminal nerve (CN V$_1$). Therefore, the trigeminal (or semilunar) ganglion is the most probable ganglion infected by the varicella zoster virus. There are two types of cranial ganglia: sensory (afferent) and autonomic. The sensory ganglia, which are most often affected by shingles, are equivalent to the spinal (dorsal root) ganglia of spinal nerves in that they house typical pseudounipolar cell bodies of afferent neurons and do not contain synapses. Other cranial sensory ganglia include the geniculate (CN VII), vestibular and spiral (CN VIII), superior and inferior glossopharyngeal (CN IX), and superior and inferior vagal (CN X) ganglia; however, shingles would be present in their dermatome distribution patterns if these ganglia were infected by the varicella zoster virus. **Choice A** (Otic ganglion) is incorrect. The otic ganglion is an autonomic ganglion, which houses the postsynaptic (postganglionic) parasympathetic cell bodies that provide secretomotor fibers to the parotid gland. This ganglion is located deep within the infratemporal fossa, adjacent to the mandibular division of the trigeminal nerve (CN V$_3$). The otic ganglion receives presynaptic (preganglionic) parasympathetic fibers from the lesser petrosal nerve of the glossopharyngeal nerve (CN IX). Because it is an autonomic ganglion, it is unlikely to be infected by the varicella zoster virus, which causes shingles unilaterally. **Choice C** (Superior cervical ganglion) is incorrect. The superior cervical ganglion is also an autonomic ganglion; specifically, it is a component of the sympathetic system. This autonomic ganglion is located at the cranial end of the sympathetic chain, near the base of the skull. There are two superior cervical ganglia, located bilaterally, which contain the cell bodies for all the postsynaptic sympathetic fibers that supply the head. Because it is an autonomic ganglion, it is unlikely to be infected by the varicella zoster

virus, which causes shingles unilaterally. **Choice D** (Ciliary ganglion) is incorrect. The ciliary ganglion is another parasympathetic autonomic ganglion. It is located in the orbit and carries fibers related to the oculomotor nerve (CN III). Because it is an autonomic ganglion, it is unlikely to be infected by the varicella zoster virus, which causes shingles unilaterally. **Choice E** (Submandibular ganglion) is incorrect. The submandibular ganglion is a parasympathetic autonomic ganglion. It is located in the posterolateral oral floor and carries fibers related to the facial nerve (CN VII) to supply secretomotor fibers to the submandibular and sublingual glands. Because it is an autonomic ganglion, it is unlikely to be infected by the varicella zoster virus, which causes shingles unilaterally.

14   **The answer is A: Foramen rotundum.**   The foramen rotundum is an opening in the greater wing of the sphenoid bone that enables the maxillary (second) division of the trigeminal nerve (CN V$_2$) to pass into the middle cranial fossa. CN V$_2$ supplies sensory (cutaneous) innervation to the skin to the lower eyelid, cheek, upper lip, upper dentition and gingivae, and lateral aspects of the nose. Due to the sensory deficits within this patient, this nerve is damaged along its route, and the foramen rotundum is the most likely location. **Choice B** (Foramen spinosum) is incorrect. The foramen spinosum conveys the middle meningeal artery and the meningeal branch (nervus spinosum) of the mandibular division of the trigeminal nerve (CN V$_3$). This artery and nerve supply the dura mater in the cranial cavity. Thus, this site has no relation to the deficits in this patient. **Choice C** (Superior orbital fissure) is incorrect. The superior orbital fissure is a large opening that conveys the oculomotor (CN III), trochlear (CN IV), ophthalmic division of the trigeminal (CN V$_1$), and abducent (CN VI) nerves as well as the superior ophthalmic veins into the orbit. None of these structures have a functional role in the deficits in question. **Choice D** (Foramen ovale) is incorrect. The foramen ovale (or oval foramen) is an opening in the greater wing of the sphenoid bone that enables the mandibular (third) division of the trigeminal nerve (CN V$_3$) and a small meningeal artery to pass into the middle cranial fossa. CN V$_3$ supplies cutaneous (general) sensation to the lower lip, chin, cheek, and anterior auricular and posterior temporal regions. This sensory innervation is supplied via three cutaneous nerves: mental, buccal, and auriculotemporal. The mandibular division of the trigeminal nerve also supplies innervation to the mandibular teeth and gingivae via the inferior alveolar nerve. Due to the listed sensory deficits in this patient, this nerve would not have been damaged along its route. **Choice E** (Optic canal) is incorrect. The optic canal carries the optic nerve (CN II) and ophthalmic artery into the orbit. Again, these structures have no bearing on the deficits in this patient.

15   **The answer is A: Greater petrosal nerve.**   Secretomotor control of the lacrimal gland is provided by parasympathetic neurons derived from the facial nerve. These fibers branch from the facial nerve as the greater petrosal nerve at the geniculum of the facial canal, within the petrous part of the temporal bone. This parasympathetic nerve leaves the temporal bone and courses along the floor of the middle cranial fossa on its way to the foramen lacerum, pterygoid canal, and pterygopalatine fossa. It is readily damaged in trauma to the floor of the middle cranial fossa. Lesion of the nerve will result in loss of emotional tearing plus reduced mucus secretion in the nasal cavity (dry nasal passages). **Choice B** (Lesser petrosal nerve) is incorrect. The lesser petrosal nerve is a parasympathetic bundle derived from the tympanic branch of the glossopharyngeal nerve in the middle ear. It is the presynaptic (preganglionic) element in the secretomotor pathway to the parotid gland via the otic ganglion. **Choice C** (Deep petrosal nerve) is incorrect. The deep petrosal nerve is a sympathetic bundle that branches off the carotid plexus at the exterior base of the skull. It joins with the greater petrosal nerve to form the nerve of the pterygoid canal that travels through the pterygoid canal into the pterygopalatine fossa. The deep petrosal nerve may be damaged in a fracture of the floor of the middle cranial fossa. However, it does not control lacrimation, and thus is not the element related to the deficit here. Obviously, you must take care to differentiate the three petrosal nerves in accounting for autonomic relations in the head. **Choice D** (Lacrimal nerve) is incorrect. The lacrimal nerve is a branch of the ophthalmic division of the trigeminal nerve within the orbit. It conveys general sensory fibers from the upper eyelid, conjunctiva, and lacrimal sac. Further, its distal portion carries the postsynaptic parasympathetic secretomotor fibers to the lacrimal gland. However, the lacrimal nerve itself would not be damaged by a fracture within the middle cranial fossa. **Choice E** (Chorda tympani nerve) is incorrect. The chorda tympani nerve is a branch of the facial nerve that runs through the middle ear cavity and continues into the infratemporal fossa. It carries parasympathetic secretomotor fibers to two salivary glands, the submandibular and sublingual glands, via the submandibular ganglion. It also conveys taste sensation from the anterior part of the tongue.

16 **The answer is B: Superior cervical ganglion.** The family of deficits described in this patient comprises a classic generalized sympathetic innervation deficit known as Horner syndrome. Normal sympathetic functions in the head include elevation of the upper eyelid (by the superior tarsal muscle), vasoconstriction of cutaneous arteries, sweat gland secretion, pupillary dilatation (via the dilator pupillae muscle), and forward positioning of the eyeball in the orbit (via the orbital muscle sling). Loss of sympathetic input results in ptosis (drooping of the eyelid), miosis (constricted or "pin-point" pupil), anhydrosis (warm, flushed, dry skin), and enophthalmosis (sunken eye). Such widespread deficits indicate damage at the source point of sympathetic input to the head, and the superior cervical ganglion is the only choice involved in sympathetic innervation. **Choice A** (Superior division of the oculomotor nerve) is incorrect. This nerve conveys motor fibers to the superior rectus muscle of the eyeball and the levator palpebrae superioris in the upper eyelid. Both are skeletal muscles and are not affected by loss of autonomic supply. The levator palpebrae superioris is the major elevator of the upper eyelid. Loss of its motor control does produce ptosis of the upper eyelid, but not the other deficits described in this patient. **Choice C** (Nerve of the pterygoid canal) is incorrect. The nerve of the pterygoid canal is a combination of sympathetic fibers (from the deep petrosal nerve) and parasympathetic fibers (from the greater petrosal nerve). It runs into the pterygopalatine ganglion, with eventual distribution to the lacrimal gland, nasal cavity, and oral roof. Damage to the nerve of the pterygoid canal would result in loss of lacrimation, dry nasal walls, and dilation of vessels along the course of the maxillary nerve. **Choice D** (Ciliary ganglion) is incorrect. The ciliary ganglion is the synapse point for parasympathetic input to the eyeball. These fibers, derived from the oculomotor nerve, control the sphincter pupillae and ciliary muscles. Sympathetic fibers also pass through the ciliary ganglion on their way to the dilator pupillae muscle. Damage to this ganglion would disrupt autonomic functions in the eye, but would not produce the extraocular deficits seen in this case. **Choice E** (Ophthalmic division of trigeminal nerve) is incorrect. The ophthalmic division of the trigeminal nerve (CN V_1) conveys general sensory axons from the forehead, upper eyelid, orbit, and eye. Lesion of this nerve would result in a cutaneous deficit in the upper face, and sensory loss in the orbit and cornea.

17 **The answer is E: Mylohyoid.** The mylohyoid muscle is innervated by the mandibular division of the trigeminal nerve (CN V_3), and this nerve is damaged in this patient due to the right-sided paralysis of the muscles of mastication, facial asymmetry (noted in the figure), and dysphagia. The mandibular division of the trigeminal nerve (CN V_3) is the only division of the trigeminal nerve (CN V) that supplies motor innervation. It supplies the muscles derived from the mesoderm of the first pharyngeal arch, including the four muscles of mastication (temporalis, masseter, lateral pterygoid, and medial pterygoid) and four additional muscles: **M**ylohoid, **A**nterior belly of the Digastric, **T**ensor Tympani, and **T**ensor Veli Palatini (mnemonic = "MATT"). The mylohyoid muscle is a suprahyoid muscle that depresses the mandible against resistance when the infrahyoid muscles fix or depress the hyoid bone. Movement of the hyoid bone is crucial during swallowing (or deglutition), so paralysis of the mylohyoid and anterior belly of the digastric muscles causes dysphagia in a patient with damage to CN V_3. **Choice A** (Sternohyoid) is incorrect. The sternohyoid is innervated by the ansa cervicalis from the cervical plexus (C1-3). This muscle would not be affected by paralysis of the muscles of mastication, which is caused by damage to the mandibular division of the trigeminal nerve (CN V_3). The sternohyoid muscle is an infrahyoid (strap) muscle that anchors and depresses the hyoid bone, so paralysis of this muscle may cause dysphagia. However, this muscle is not the best selection, as it is not innervated by the mandibular division of the trigeminal nerve (CN V_3). **Choice B** (Stylohyoid) is incorrect. The stylohyoid is a suprahyoid muscle that fixes and depresses the hyoid bone during swallowing, so losing this muscle may cause dysphagia noted in this patient. However, the patient presents with unilateral paralysis of the muscles of mastication on the right side, which implies damage to the mandibular division of the trigeminal nerve (CN V_3). Damage to CN V_3 would not involve the stylohyoid muscle because this muscle is derived from the mesoderm of the second pharyngeal (hyoid) arch and is therefore innervated by the facial nerve (CN VII). **Choice C** (Cricothyroid) is incorrect. The cricothyroid muscle is innervated by the external branch of the superior laryngeal nerve (from CN X), and it acts in lengthening and tensing the vocal ligament by pulling the thyroid cartilage anteroinferiorly. Paralysis of this muscle would change the pitch of the patient's voice but would not cause the dysphagia seen in this patient. **Choice D** (Stylopharyngeus) is incorrect. The stylopharyngeus muscle is innervated by the glossopharyngeal nerve (CN IX). Loss of this muscle's function would affect deglutition (swallowing) as it elevates the pharynx, but it is not the best choice due to its innervation by the glossopharyngeal nerve (CN IX). Moreover, it would not be affected by damage to the mandibular division of the trigeminal nerve (CN V_3).

18   **The answer is C: Oculomotor nerve.**   The slowness of the right pupil to respond to light stimuli is the first sign of compression of the oculomotor nerve (CN III). In this patient, it is the parasympathetic component of the right oculomotor nerve that is affected due to the loss of the sphincter pupillae muscle, which results in dilation of her right pupil. When a patient has an ipsilateral dilation of the pupil and lethargy (the latter symptom was not noted in this patient), a physician must rule out a supratentorial (above the tentorium cerebelli) brain lesion causing increased intracranial pressure (ICP). This type of lesion could result from a blockage of cerebrospinal fluid (CSF) flow, an intracranial bleed (hemorrhage), or a supratentorial tumor, and these lesions often affect the parasympathetic component of CN III by impinging this nerve component at the tentorial notch, often seen in an uncal herniation. **Choice A** (Superior cervical ganglion) is incorrect. Damage to the superior cervical ganglion results in loss of sympathetic innervation to the head. If this structure were damaged, a patient would exhibit miosis (constriction of the pupil), ptosis (drooping of the eyelid), and anhydrosis (inability to sweat) on the affected side, which is characterized as Horner syndrome, or loss of sympathetic innervation to the head. In this patient, the right pupil is dilated, so the sympathetic innervation is intact but unopposed by the loss of the parasympathetic component of the oculomotor nerve. **Choice B** (Optic nerve) is incorrect. If the right optic nerve were compromised, the patient would be blind in his right eye. The optic nerve is not affected because the visual acuity of the patient is not impaired. **Choice D** (Trochlear nerve) is incorrect. The right trochlear nerve provides innervation to the superior oblique muscle in the orbit solely. This muscle pulls the eye inferolaterally, but it is tested clinically by putting the eye in an adducted position because the superior oblique muscle is the only extraocular muscle that can direct the gaze of the adducted eye inferiorly. Damage to the trochlear nerve leads to diplopia, or double vision. However, it would not account for the asymmetric pupils seen in this patient. **Choice E** (Abducent nerve) is incorrect. The lateral rectus muscle is the only extraocular muscle innervated by the abducent nerve. If this nerve were cut, the patient would display diplopia. However, involvement of the abducent nerve would not account for the asymmetric pupils seen in this patient.

19   **The answer is D: Auricle of the external ear.**   Unilateral facial paralysis can result from brain tumor, stroke, or a virus, such as herpes zoster. When no specific cause can be found (idiopathic), the condition is called facial (Bell or CN VII) palsy. When differentiating between unilateral facial paralysis and herpes zoster infection of CN VII, the physician must immediately look for herpetic lesions in the skin supplied by the cutaneous innervation of the facial nerve. CN VII supplies cutaneous innervation to only a small portion of the auricle of the external ear, via the posterior division of the main trunk of the facial nerve. The geniculate ganglion of the facial nerve would be affected by the viral infection known as herpes zoster, or varicella zoster virus. This virus causes chickenpox, and after exposure to chickenpox, this virus can reside latent in ganglia of an individual for years. If this individual becomes immunocompromised, the skin (or dermatomes supplied by the infected ganglia) can develop shingles, a painful skin rash, which blisters, breaks open, crusts over, and then disappears. For CN VII, these herpetic lesions are found in the auricle

of the external ear, which is the only cutaneous distribution site for the facial nerve. In Ramsay Hunt syndrome, a patient presents with Zoster eruptions in the auricle or external acoustic meatus of the ear and unilateral facial paralysis. This syndrome is often associated with other CN VII and CN VIII symptoms, including loss of taste to the anterior two thirds of the tongue (CN VII), tinnitus (CN VIII), vertigo (CN VIII), or hearing loss (CN VIII). **Choice A** (Mental region of the mandible) is incorrect. The mental region of the mandible is supplied by the mental nerve, a cutaneous nerve off the mandibular division of the trigeminal nerve (CN V_3). If the herpes zoster virus infected the trigeminal (or semilunar) ganglion, herpetic lesions could be found along the sensory distribution pattern of CN V_3; however, in this patient, the facial nerve (CN VII) was affected due to unilateral paralysis of the facial muscles. **Choice B** (Temporal and parietal region of the scalp) is incorrect. The temporal and parietal regions of the scalp are supplied by the auriculotemporal nerve, a cutaneous nerve off the mandibular division of the trigeminal nerve (CN V_3). If the herpes zoster virus infected the trigeminal (or semilunar) ganglion, herpetic lesions could be found along the sensory distribution pattern of CN V_3; however, in this patient, the facial nerve (CN VII) was affected due to unilateral paralysis of the facial muscles. **Choice C** (Upper lip and cheek of the face) is incorrect. The upper lip and cheek of the face are supplied by the infraorbital nerve, a cutaneous nerve off the maxillary division of the trigeminal nerve (CN V_2). If the herpes zoster virus infected the trigeminal (or semilunar) ganglion, herpetic lesions could be found along the sensory distribution pattern of CN V_2; however, in this patient, the facial nerve (CN VII) was affected due to unilateral paralysis of the facial muscles. **Choice E** (Bridge and tip of the external nose) is incorrect. The bridge and tip of the external nose are supplied by the infratrochlear and external nasal nerves, respectively. These two nerves are cutaneous branches off the ophthalmic division of the trigeminal nerve (CN V_1). If the herpes zoster virus infected the trigeminal (or semilunar) ganglion, herpetic lesions could be found along the sensory distribution pattern of CN V_1; however, in this patient, the facial nerve (CN VII) was affected due to unilateral paralysis of the facial muscles.

20   **The answer is D: Presynaptic parasympathetic fibers.**   The nerve of the pterygoid (vidian) canal consists of presynaptic parasympathetic fibers from the greater petrosal nerve of the facial nerve (CN VII) and postsynaptic sympathetic fibers from the deep petrosal nerve, derived from the periarterial arterial plexus enveloping the internal carotid artery. The presynaptic parasympathetic fibers follow the greater petrosal nerve (of CN VII), traverse the pterygoid canal, enter the pterygopalatine fossa to synapse in the pterygopalatine ganglion, and carry the postsynaptic parasympathetic fibers to the lacrimal gland via branches of the first two divisions of the trigeminal nerve (CN V_1 and CN V_2). The parasympathetic fibers of CN VII produce emotional tears from the lacrimal glands. **Choice A** (Taste fibers to the anterior two thirds of the tongue) is incorrect. The chorda tympani, a branch of the facial nerve (CN VII), joins the lingual branch of the mandibular nerve (CN V_3) in the infratemporal fossa. The chorda tympani nerve conveys taste sensation from the anterior two thirds of the tongue and carries presynaptic parasympathetic fibers to the submandibular ganglion for innervation of the submandibular and sublingual salivary glands. However, the chorda tympani nerve is not associated with the pterygoid canal, so it would not be damaged by a facial nerve schwannoma at this location. **Choice B** (Parasympathetic innervation to the submandibular and sublingual glands) is incorrect. The chorda tympani, a branch of the facial nerve (CN VII), joins the lingual branch of the mandibular nerve (CN V$_3$) in the infratemporal fossa. The chorda tympani nerve conveys taste sensation to the anterior two thirds of the tongue and carries presynaptic parasympathetic fibers to the submandibular ganglion for innervation of the submandibular and sublingual salivary glands. However, the chorda tympani nerve is not associated with the pterygoid canal, so it would not be damaged by a facial nerve schwannoma at this location. **Choice C** (Presynaptic sympathetic fibers) is incorrect. All sympathetic fibers in the head are postsynaptic because they synapse in the superior cervical ganglion before reaching their targets in the head. Therefore, the sympathetic fibers traveling in the pterygoid canal are postsynaptic. These postsynaptic sympathetic fibers control the smooth muscle tone (vasodilation and vasoconstriction) of the blood vessels lying underneath the nasal mucosa. **Choice E** (Postsynaptic parasympathetic fibers) is incorrect. The parasympathetic fibers derived from the greater petrosal nerve (of CN VII) do not synapse until after they have left the pterygoid (vidian) canal. After leaving this canal, these presynaptic parasympathetic fibers synapse in the pterygopalatine ganglion distal to the pterygoid canal. Therefore, the parasympathetic fibers in the pterygoid (vidian) canal are presynaptic. These fibers serve to increase emotional tearing of the lacrimal glands.

21 **The answer is C: Internal acoustic meatus.** This patient is displaying deficits associated with the facial nerve (CN VII), explaining the unilateral facial paralysis, and the vestibulocochlear nerve (CN VIII), evident from the dizziness and hearing loss on her right side. The internal acoustic meatus is the only location where both CN VII and CN VIII travel together. The MRI demonstrates a right-sided vestibular schwannoma (acoustic neuroma) located at the internal acoustic meatus, which confirms this diagnosis. This vestibular schwannoma resides at the cerebellopontine angle and affects the facial and vestibulocochlear nerves as they emerge from this location. This tumor would also increase intracranial pressure, potentially causing pontomedullary brain stem compression. **Choice A** (Foramen rotundum) is incorrect. The maxillary (second) division of the trigeminal nerve (CN V$_2$) passes through the foramen rotundum carrying sensation from the cheek, lower eyelid, and upper lip. The facial and vestibulocochlear nerves, which show deficits in this patient, do not reside in this location. **Choice B** (Foramen ovale) is incorrect. The mandibular (third) division of the trigeminal nerve (CN V$_3$) passes through the foramen ovale carrying cutaneous (sensory) information from the lower lip, chin, parotid region, anterior auricle, and lateral aspects of the scalp. CN V$_3$ is the only division of the trigeminal nerve to carry motor (efferent) information, supplying the muscles of mastication derived from the mesoderm of first pharyngeal (branchial) arch. The facial and vestibulocochlear nerves, deficient in this patient, do not reside in this location. **Choice D** (Facial canal) is incorrect. A tumor at this site would not impinge on the vestibulocochlear nerve, so hearing would not be impaired. A tumor in the facial canal would present with facial muscle paralysis and loss of the efferent limb of the corneal reflex, but would not explain

the unilateral hearing impairment. **Choice E** (Stylomastoid foramen) is incorrect. A tumor located at this site would show facial muscle paralysis due to the involvement of the facial nerve; however, this lesion would not explain the involvement of the vestibulocochlear nerve (unilateral hearing loss).

22 **The answer is C: Bitemporal hemianopsia.** Bitemporal hemianopsia is commonly called "tunnel vision" due to the loss of vision in the temporal visual fields of both eyes. This visual impairment occurs when the medial retinal fibers are impinged while crossing within the optic chiasm. Tumors, such as pituitary adenomas, meningiomas, or craniopharyngiomas (as seen in this patient), are the most common cause of a lesion to the optic chiasm due to its midline location sitting superior to the sella turcica, which houses the pituitary gland. The craniopharyngioma seen on the MRI is compressing the pituitary gland, and it is most likely impinging the medial retinal fibers crossing within the optic chiasm, leading to bitemporal hemianopsia. **Choice A** (Monocular blindness) is incorrect. Monocular blindness results from a lesion of the left or right optic nerve (CN II), which contains the retinal ganglion cell axons passing from the retina of the eye to the brain traversing the optic canal. The craniopharyngioma shown in this sagittal MRI is not extending anteriorly toward the termination of the optic nerves, so it is unlikely that this tumor would cause monocular blindness. **Choice B** (Binasal hemianopsia) is incorrect. Binasal hemianopsia, or loss of half the vision specifically in the nasal visual fields of both eyes, occurs when the uncrossed, lateral retinal fibers are impinged. Binasal hemianopsia is rarely seen, but can result due to congenital hydrocephalus or calcification of both internal carotid arteries. The suprasellar craniopharyngioma in this patient would most likely impinge the medial retinal fibers, leading to bitemporal hemianopsia. **Choice D** (Right homonymous hemianopsia) is incorrect. Right homonymous hemianopsia results from a lesion of the left optic tract, left geniculocalcarine tract, or the left visual cortex. These structures are located too far posteriorly to be affected by the suprasellar craniopharyngioma seen in this patient. The word "homonymous" means same sided, so a right homonymous hemianopsia would refer to visual defects in both right halves of the visual field of each eye. **Choice E** (Left homonymous hemianopsia) is incorrect. Left homonymous hemianopsia, a visual deficit in the left halves of the visual fields in each eye, results from a lesion of the right optic tract, right geniculocalcarine tract, or the right visual cortex. These structures are located too far posteriorly to be affected by the suprasellar craniopharyngioma seen in this patient.

23 **The answer is E: Deviation of the tongue to the ipsilateral side.** One of the rootlets of the hypoglossal nerve (CN XII) is identified in this photo. CN XII emerges from the brainstem in the medulla between the pyramid medially and the olive (inferior olivary nucleus) laterally. The hypoglossal nerve innervates all of the intrinsic muscles of the tongue and most of its extrinsic muscles with the lone exception being the palatoglossus muscle are innervated by the vagus nerve (CN X). Damage to CN XII produces ipsilateral deviation of the tongue due to the unopposed muscular contractions of the genioglossus muscle contralaterally. The mnemonic "The tongue licks the wound" will help you remember that the tongue deviates to the ipsilateral side in a lower motor lesion of CN XII. **Choice A** (Inability to elevate the ipsilateral shoulder) is incorrect. The accessory nerve (CN XI) emerges from the cervical aspect of the spinal cord, ascends through the magnum foramen, and leaves the cranial cavity through the jugular foramen, accompanying the glossopharyngeal (CN IX) and vagus (CN X) nerves. It provides motor innervation to the ipsilateral sternocleidomastoid and trapezius muscles. Damage to CN XI causes an inability to elevate the shoulder leading to "drooping" of the ipsilateral shoulder due to paralysis of the trapezius muscle. A CN XI lesion also affects lateral rotation of the scapula causing an inability to abduct the upper limb greater than 90 degrees. Loss of innervation to the sternocleidomastoid muscle causes paresis (weakness) in turning the head to the contralateral side. However, the hypoglossal nerve (CN XII) was identified in the photo. **Choice B** (Deviation of the uvula to the contralateral side) is incorrect. The vagus nerve (CN X) emerges from the brainstem in the medulla posterior to the olive. Damage to CN X causes asymmetry in soft palate elevation and contralateral deviation of the uvula. The pharyngeal branches of the vagus nerve innervate all of the musculature of the soft palate, except the tensor veli palatini (tensor of the soft palate), which is innervated by the mandibular division of the trigeminal nerve (CN V$_3$). On examination, the arch of the soft palate droops on the affected side and the uvula deviates to the unaffected side as a result of the unopposed actions of the intact muscles acting on the soft palate on the unaffected (contralateral) side. However, the hypoglossal nerve (CN XII) was identified in the photo. **Choice C** (Loss of gag reflex on the ipsilateral side) is incorrect. The gag (or pharyngeal) reflex prevents foreign objects from entering the pharynx, except during normal swallowing (deglutition). The afferent limb of the gag reflex is supplied by the glossopharyngeal nerve (CN IX), and the efferent limb is supplied by the vagus nerve (CN X). Both the glossopharyngeal and vagus nerves emerge from the brainstem in the medulla posterior to the olive. Due to the hypoglossal being identified in this figure, the gag reflex would not be affected on the ipsilateral side. **Choice D** (Ipsilateral loss of parotid gland secretion) is incorrect. The parotid gland is supplied by the parasympathetic fibers from the glossopharyngeal nerve (CN IX) that enable secretions of this salivary gland. The glossopharyngeal nerve (CN IX) emerges from the brainstem in the medulla posterior to the olive, so this cranial nerve is not identified in this photo and ipsilateral loss of parotid gland secretions would not be seen in this patient.

24   **The answer is B: Unilateral muscles of mastication paralysis.** The foramen identified in the figure is the foramen ovale (oval foramen), which transmits the mandibular (third) division of the trigeminal nerve (CN V$_3$). This nerve provides cutaneous (general) sensation to the skin of the lower lip, chin, cheek, anterior auricle, and lateral scalp. It also supplies motor innervation to the muscles derived from the mesoderm of the first pharyngeal arch, including the four muscles of mastication (temporalis, masseter, lateral pterygoid, and medial pterygoid) and four additional muscles: **M**ylohoid, **A**nterior belly of the Digastric, **T**ensor Tympani, and **T**ensor Veli Palatini (mnemonic = "MATT"). Therefore, a lesion at the foramen ovale produces unilateral paralysis of the muscles of mastication. **Choice A** (Unilateral muscles of facial expression paralysis) is incorrect. The muscles of facial expression are supplied by the main trunk of the facial nerve, which leaves the cranium via the stylomastoid foramen. This foramen is not identified in the X-ray, so unilateral

paralysis of the muscles of facial expression is not likely. **Choice C** (Paresthesia of the upper lip, cheek, and lower eyelid) is incorrect. The cutaneous (general) sensation to the skin of the upper lip, cheek, and lower eyelid is supplied by the maxillary (second) division of the trigeminal nerve (CN V$_2$). CN V$_2$ enters the infratemporal fossa via the foramen rotundum to reach the middle cranial fossa. The foramen rotundum was not identified in the X-ray, so paresthesia in these areas is unlikely. **Choice D** (Decreased salivation of the submandibular gland) is incorrect. The chorda tympani nerve, a terminal branch of the facial nerve (CN VII), conveys taste sensation to the anterior two thirds of the tongue and carries presynaptic (preganglionic) parasympathetic that will cause salivation of the submandibular (and sublingual) gland(s). The chorda tympani nerve exits the skull via the petrotympanic fissure, which is located in the infratemporal fossa. The petrotympanic fissure was not identified in the X-ray, so loss of salivation from the submandibular gland is unlikely. **Choice E** (Decreased salivation of the parotid gland) is incorrect. The lesser petrosal nerve, a branch of the glossopharyngeal nerve (CN IX), carries presynaptic parasympathetic fibers that will cause salivation of the parotid gland. The lesser petrosal nerve may sometimes traverse the foramen ovale, which is identified in the figure; however, it more often goes through other openings (petrosal foramen or sphenopetrosal fissure). Therefore, unilateral paralysis of the muscles of mastication is more likely.

25   **The answer is C: Left abducent nerve.** The only extraocular muscle innervated by the left abducent nerve, CN VI, is the left lateral rectus muscle, which enables the left globe to move laterally following the doctor's index finger. When the left abducent nerve is damaged, the patient would display strabismus, causing diplopia, because the left pupil would rest in the adducted position, termed esotropia, due to the unopposed action of the medial rectus muscle. Because this patient displays these symptoms, particularly the inability to abduct the left eye, the left abducent nerve is damaged. **Choice A** (Left oculomotor nerve) is incorrect. The left oculomotor nerve, CN III, innervates most of the extraocular eye muscles (with the exception of superior oblique and lateral rectus muscles) and the levator palpebrae superioris (which elevates the eyelid) in the ipsilateral (left) eye. Damage to the left CN III leads to diplopia (due to the left pupil resting in an abducted and lateral position) and ptosis (drooping of the eyelid) associated with the left eye. Because of the esotropia evident in this patient without ptosis, this option can be eliminated. **Choice B** (Right oculomotor nerve) is incorrect. The right oculomotor nerve, CN III, innervates most of the extraocular eye muscles (with the exception of superior oblique and lateral rectus muscles) and the levator palpebrae superioris (which elevates the eyelid) in the ipsilateral (right) eye. Damage to the right CN III leads to diplopia (due to the right pupil resting in an abducted and lateral position) and ptosis (drooping of the eyelid) associated with the right eye. Because of the esotropia evident in this patient without ptosis, this option can be eliminated. Moreover, the left eye was affected in this patient. **Choice D** (Right abducent nerve) is incorrect. The only extraocular muscle innervated by the right abducent nerve, CN VI, is the right lateral rectus muscle, which directs the right globe laterally. If this nerve were damaged, the patient would display diplopia, and the right pupil would be resting in the adducted position due to the unopposed action of the other extraocular muscles.

However, the left eye was affected in this patient. **Choice E** (Left trochlear nerve) is incorrect. The left trochlear nerve innervates only one muscle, the superior oblique muscle, in the orbit. This muscle pulls the eye inferolaterally, but it is hard to distinguish this movement from the combined movements of the inferior rectus muscle (innervated by the oculomotor nerve) and the lateral rectus muscle (innervated by the abducent nerve), which move the globe inferior and lateral, respectively. Therefore, the left trochlear nerve is clinically tested by asking the patient to look inferiorly after the left eye is placed in an adducted position. Damage to this nerve also causes diplopia, or double vision, especially when the gaze is directed inferiorly and medially, but the esotropia is not evident in the left eye of this patient.

26 **The answer is A: Optic nerve.** Unlike other cranial nerves, the optic nerve (CN II) develops as an anterior extension of the diencephalon, part of the forebrain. Due to this unique embryological origin, the optic nerve is enveloped with extension of the cranial meninges (dura, arachnoid, and pia mater) and contains cerebrospinal (CSF) fluid in its subarachnoid space. The optic nerve is formed when the axons of the retinal ganglion cells coalescence at the optic disc. A physician can view the optic disc by performing a fundoscopic examination of the back of the eye (or fundus) with an ophthalmoscope. This boxer exhibits signs of increased intracranial pressure (ICP), such as headache, nausea, and vomiting, so the physician can look at the optic disc to look for papilledema, or swelling of the optic disc, which is another sign of increased ICP. If the optic disc is elevated, swollen, darker than normal, or its edges are blurred, then the fundoscopic examination can reveal evidence of increased ICP. These changes in the optic disc are due to the pressure transmitted via the CSF within the optic nerve. **Choice B** (Oculomotor nerve) is incorrect. The oculomotor nerve, CN III, innervates most of the extraocular eye muscles (with the exception of superior oblique and lateral rectus muscles) and the levator palpebrae superioris, which elevates the upper eyelid. Damage to the left CN III leads to diplopia (due to the left pupil resting in an abducted and lateral position) and ptosis (drooping of the eyelid) associated with the left eye. However, the physician would be unable to correlate damage to the oculomotor nerve with increased ICP. **Choice C** (Olfactory nerve) is incorrect. The olfactory nerve, CN I, provides olfaction (or a sense of smell) to the patient. Damage to this nerve causes anosmia, or loss of olfaction, which is frequently seen in patients with severe head trauma due to the delicate olfactory nerves traversing the cribiform plate of the ethmoid bone to enter the olfactory bulb. However, damage to CN I would imply head trauma due to the punches the boxer received, not increased ICP. **Choice D** (Trigeminal nerve) is incorrect. The trigeminal nerve (CN V) is the main sensory nerve for the face and scalp, and it has three divisions: the ophthalmic (CN V₁), maxillary (CN V₂), and mandibular (CN V₃). CN V₃ is the only division of the trigeminal nerve (CN V) that supplies motor innervation. It supplies the eight muscles derived from the mesoderm of the first pharyngeal arch, including the muscles of mastication. Damage to the trigeminal nerve causes numbness (paresthesia) and paralysis of the muscles of mastication; however, it would not give additional information concerning increased ICP. **Choice E** (Trochlear nerve) is incorrect. The trochlear nerve, CN IV, innervates only one muscle, the superior oblique muscle, in the orbit. This muscle pulls the eye inferolaterally, but it

is clinically tested by asking the patient to look inferiorly after the left eye is placed in an adducted position. Damage to this nerve would lead to diplopia, but it would not give additional information concerning increased ICP.

27 **The answer is B: Deep petrosal.** The deep petrosal nerve is a sympathetic bundle that branches off the internal carotid plexus at the exterior of the base of the skull. It joins with the greater petrosal nerve to form the nerve of the pterygoid (vidian) canal. This nerve enters the pterygopalatine fossa where it joins the pterygopalatine ganglion. The postsynaptic sympathetic fibers, derived from the deep petrosal nerve, pass through the pterygopalatine ganglion without synapsing and supply the mucosal glands of the nasal cavity as well as the smooth muscle controlling vasomotion (vasoconstriction and vasodilation) of the arteries supplying the nasal cavity. Disruption of sympathetic fibers in the sympathetic chain causing Horner syndrome would greatly affect the deep petrosal nerve. **Choice A** (Lesser petrosal) is incorrect. The lesser petrosal nerve carries presynaptic parasympathetic nerve fibers derived from the glossopharyngeal nerve. It runs from the tympanic plexus in the middle ear to the otic ganglion in the infratemporal fossa, where it synapses. Then, the postsynaptic parasympathetic fibers follow the auriculotemporal nerve (a branch of the mandibular division of the trigeminal nerve) into the parotid gland, where they provide the secretomotor control for this salivary gland. Loss of sympathetic innervation to the head (Horner syndrome) would not affect this nerve. **Choice C** (Greater petrosal) is incorrect. The greater petrosal nerve branches off the facial nerve at the geniculum of the facial canal and carries presynaptic parasympathetic innervation. It coalesces with the deep petrosal nerve to form the nerve of the pterygoid (vidian) canal and synapses within the pterygopalatine ganglion. The postsynaptic parasympathetic fibers follow branches of the maxillary nerve to supply the emotional tearing to the lacrimal gland as well as other glands in the nasal cavity and palate. Loss of sympathetic innervation to the head (Horner syndrome) would not affect this nerve. **Choice D** (Chorda tympani) is incorrect. The chorda tympani nerve, a branch of the facial nerve, carries taste and presynaptic parasympathetic fibers to the tongue and oral floor. It originates from the distal part of the facial nerve, runs across the middle ear cavity, enters the infratemporal fossa, and joins the lingual nerve (a branch of the mandibular division of the trigeminal nerve). Ultimately, the taste fibers distribute into the anterior two thirds of the tongue. The parasympathetic fibers synapse in the submandibular ganglion, with the postsynaptic fibers passing to the submandibular and sublingual salivary glands and to mucus glands in the oral floor. Loss of sympathetic innervation to the head (Horner syndrome) would not affect this nerve. **Choice E** (Optic) is incorrect. The optic nerve is one of the few cranial nerves (along with the olfactory, vestibulocochlear, and spinal accessory nerves), which do not transport autonomic fibers at some point in its distribution. This nerve (really the optic tract) extends from the retina traversing the optic canal to reach the diencephalon of the brain.

28 **The answer is E: Parasympathetic fibers via the chorda tympani nerve.** All the salivary glands receive their secretomotor innervation from the parasympathetic nervous system. Both the submandibular and sublingual salivary glands are supplied by the facial nerve by way of its chorda tympani branch.

The chorda tympani nerve originates from the distal part of the main trunk of the facial nerve and runs across the middle ear cavity. It earns its name at this location by its thread-like form lying across the deep surface of the tympanic membrane and the handle of the malleus. The nerve then enters the infratemporal fossa and merges with the lingual nerve (a branch of the mandibular division of the trigeminal nerve, or CN V_3). The parasympathetic fibers synapse in the submandibular ganglion, with the postsynaptic fibers passing to the submandibular and sublingual salivary glands and to mucus glands in the oral floor. Remember, the chorda tympani nerve also carries taste fibers from the anterior two thirds of the tongue. The remaining salivary gland, the parotid, is supplied by the glossopharyngeal nerve, by way of the following pathway: tympanic nerve/lesser petrosal nerve/otic ganglion/auriculotemporal nerve. **Choice A** (Parasympathetic fibers via the inferior alveolar nerve) is incorrect. The inferior alveolar nerve is a branch of the mandibular division of the trigeminal nerve (CN V_3) within the infratemporal fossa. It gives off the mylohyoid nerve, which innervates the mylohyoid and anterior digastric muscles, and then enters the mandible traversing the mandibular foramen. Most of its distribution is concerned with general sensation in the lower jaw (including the teeth and gums) and the skin overlying the mandible, including the lower lip. It has no direct role in secretion of any salivary gland. **Choice B** (Sympathetic fibers via the lingual nerve) is incorrect. Sympathetic neurons do not supply the salivary glands. The lingual nerve does carry autonomic fibers to the submandibular and sublingual salivary glands. However, this autonomic innervation is derived from parasympathetic fibers of the facial nerve/chorda tympani nerve pathway. **Choice C** (Parasympathetic fibers via the mandibular branch of the facial nerve) is incorrect. The (marginal) mandibular branch of the facial nerve is one of the five terminal branches of the main trunk of the facial nerve innervating the muscles of facial expression. The (marginal) mandibular branch of the facial nerve does not carry autonomic fibers to any salivary glands despite the fact that this nerve transverses the parotid gland. **Choice D** (Sympathetic fibers via the hypoglossal nerve) is incorrect. Again, the sympathetic division does not supply the salivary glands. The hypoglossal nerve may carry a small hitchhiking sympathetic bundle for part of its course. However, its dominant content is motor fibers to the intrinsic and most of the extrinsic skeletal muscles of the tongue.

29 **The answer is D: Altered taste.** The tumor impinges on the afferent fibers entering the solitary nucleus, which include visceral sensation and taste from the facial (CN VII), glossopharyngeal (CN IX), and vagus (CN X) nerves. Altered taste perceptions would most likely be present in this patient. These taste fibers are sometimes referred to as special visceral afferent (SVA) neurons, which relay the special senses of taste and olfaction. Damage to the taste information going to the solitary nucleus and carried by CN VII, CN IX, and CN X would result in altered taste. Moreover, the solitary nucleus receives visceral sensory inputs, which include chemoreceptors and baroreceptors located at the termination of the common carotid artery, and these nerve fibers would be involved with many reflexes within the head region, including the carotid sinus and aortic reflexes. **Choice A** (Blindness) is incorrect. Vision is a special sense that is relayed by the optic nerve (CN II). CN II input provides whole body (somatic) position and orientation in space (the external environment). This afferent

information carried by CN II is referred to as special sensory (special somatic afferent or SSA) neurons, and it is not related to the solitary nucleus. **Choice B** (Loss of sensation from the cornea) is incorrect. Developmentally, the cornea is derived from surface ectoderm (i.e., the body soma). Sensory information from the cornea would be classified as general sensory (general somatic afferent or GSA) fibers, and this information is carried by the ophthalmic division of the trigeminal nerve (CN V_1). This sensory information is not related to the solitary nucleus. **Choice C** (Loss of equilibrium) is incorrect. As with vision, equilibrium and balance are related to whole body orientation in space. Thus, these senses receive the special sensory (SSA) designation. This sensory information carried by the vestibular portion of the vestibulocochlear nerve (CN VIII) is not related to the solitary nucleus. **Choice E** (Deafness) is incorrect. As with vision, auditory sensations are related to whole body orientation in space. Thus, hearing receives the special sensory (SSA) designation. This sensory information carried by the cochlear portion of the vestibulocochlear nerve (CN VIII) is not related to the solitary nucleus.

30 **The answer is D: Glossopharyngeal nerve.** The jugular foramen is identified in this CT, and this cranial opening transmits the glossopharyngeal (CN IX), vagus (CN X), and accessory (CN XI) nerves. The glossopharyngeal nerve (CN IX) is the only nerve listed in this question that exits the posterior cranial fossa via the jugular foramen. **Choice A** (Trochlear nerve) is incorrect. The trochlear nerve (CN IV) is the only cranial nerve that emerges from the posterior surface of the midbrain, and it has the longest intracranial course of any cranial nerve. CN IV courses anteriorly to reach the orbit after traversing the superior orbital fissure. However, the jugular foramen was identified in the CT scan. **Choice B** (Trigeminal nerve) is incorrect. The trigeminal nerve (CN V) is the main sensory nerve for the face and scalp, and it has three divisions, namely, the ophthalmic (CN V_1), maxillary (CN V_2), and mandibular (CN V_3). CN V_1 travels from the orbit entering the middle cranial fossa via the superior orbital fissure. CN V_2 travels through the foramen rotundum. Finally, CN V_3 traverses the foramen ovale to reach the infratemporal region. However, the jugular foramen was identified in the CT scan. **Choice C** (Facial nerve) is incorrect. The facial nerve (CN VII) exits the posterior cranial fossa through the internal acoustic meatus, along with the vestibulocochlear nerve (CN VIII). However, the jugular foramen was identified in the CT scan. **Choice E** (Hypoglossal nerve) is incorrect. The hypoglossal nerve (CN XII) exits the posterior cranial fossa through the hypoglossal canal. However, the jugular foramen was identified in the CT scan.

31 **The answer is E: Marginal mandibular branch of facial nerve.** The marginal mandibular branch of the facial nerve (CN VII) is one of five terminal branches of the main trunk of CN VII that supply the muscles of facial expression. This nerve supplies muscles of the lower lip and chin, including the depressor anguli oris, depressor labii inferioris, and mentalis muscles. The loss of muscular tone in the lower lip of this patient is causing asymmetry in her facial expression. Therefore, the marginal mandibular branch of the facial nerve was damaged by the broken glass. Remember, the main trunk of the facial nerve (CN VII) branches into five terminal branches, named in order: (1) **T**emporal, (2) **Z**ygomatic, **B**uccal, **M**arginal mandibular, and **C**ervical; they can be remembered by the mnemonics

"Two Zebras Bit My Cheek" or "To Zanzibar By Motor Car". **Choice A** (Zygomatic branch of facial nerve) is incorrect. The zygomatic branch of the facial nerve (CN VII) innervates primarily the inferior part of the orbicularis oculi muscle to close the lower eyelid ipsilaterally. In this patient, asymmetry in the lower lip was noted, so the zygomatic branch of the facial nerve was not injured. **Choice B** (Temporal branch of facial nerve) is incorrect. The temporal branch of the facial nerve (CN VII) innervates muscles that move the auricle as well as the frontalis muscle and the superior part of the orbicularis oculi. The frontalis muscle raises the eyebrows and wrinkles the skin of the forehead. The orbicularis oculi acts as the sphincter of the orbit by closing the eyelids to cover the eye. In this patient, asymmetry in the lower lip was noted, so the temporal branch of the facial nerve was not injured. **Choice C** (Cervical branch of facial nerve) is incorrect. The cervical branch of the facial nerve (CN VII) innervates the platysma muscle, which wrinkles the skin of the inferior face and neck, which is often seen when a person is under stress. In this patient, asymmetry in the lower lip was noted, so the cervical branch of the facial nerve was not injured. **Choice D** (Buccal branch of facial nerve) is incorrect. The buccal branch of facial nerve (CN VII) supplies the buccinator, orbicularis oris, and muscles of upper lip. Damage to this nerve results in the loss of muscular tone within the cheek and an inability to elevate the labial commissure, purse the upper lip, or show the upper teeth ipsilaterally. In this patient, asymmetry in the lower lip was noted, so the buccal branch of the facial nerve was not injured.

32 **The answer is D: Superior cervical ganglion.** The student's reaction is a classic sympathetic "fight, fright, flight" response. All sympathetic fibers destined for the head synapse in the superior cervical ganglion. This ganglion marks the cranial end of the sympathetic chain, and is located near the base of the skull, at about vertebral level C2. Presynaptic neurons ascend through the sympathetic chain to the superior cervical ganglion. There, they synapse with postsynaptic neuron cell bodies that distribute their axonal processes throughout the head. These sympathetic fibers head control vasomotion, pilomotion, and sudomotion. **Choice A** (Ciliary ganglion) is incorrect. The ciliary ganglion is a parasympathetic ganglion, located in the orbit. The fibers that synapse in this ganglion supply the ciliary and sphincter pupillae muscles in the eye. It has no input into this sympathetic response. **Choice B** (Trigeminal ganglion) is incorrect. The trigeminal (semilunar) ganglion is a sensory ganglion. It houses the cell bodies of the pseudounipolar neurons carrying general sensory information from the trigeminal nerve (CN V). It has no input into this sympathetic response. **Choice C** (Inferior [nodose] vagal ganglion) is incorrect. The vagus nerve possesses two ganglia, superior and inferior, which are sensory ganglia. The superior vagal ganglion houses cell bodies of general sensory neurons. The inferior vagal ganglion houses the cell bodies of visceral afferent neurons. It has no input into this sympathetic response. **Choice E** (Pterygopalatine ganglion) is incorrect. The pterygopalatine ganglion is a parasympathetic ganglion, located within the pterygopalatine fossa. It sends fibers to the lacrimal gland and glands within the nasal cavity. It has no input into this sympathetic response.

33 **The answer is E: Left oculomotor nerve.** The left oculomotor nerve (CN III) is damaged in this patient. The physician is performing the pupillary light reflex, which tests the integrity of the sensory and motor functions of the eye. The afferent limb of the reflex is the optic nerve, and the efferent limb is the oculomotor nerve. In this patient, the constriction of the right pupil (a consensual response to the light) implies the afferent limb (left optic nerve) of the light reflex is intact because one of the pupils responded to the light. However, the efferent limb of the left eye is likely damaged due to the lack of a direct response (pupillary constriction) to the light. Under normal circumstances, both pupils constrict in response to increased light intensity due to a bilateral projection from the pretectal nucleus within the upper medulla to the Edinger-Westphal nucleus, which then projects its parasympathetic fibers along the oculomotor nerve causing pupillary constriction. **Choice A** (Right optic nerve) is incorrect. Because the physician did not direct the light into the right eye, the integrity of the right optic nerve was not tested. To test this afferent limb of the pupillary light reflex, the physician must shine the light directly into the right eye. Because there was no direct response (pupillary constriction) of the left eye, the physician did confirm damage to the left oculomotor nerve. **Choice B** (Left optic nerve) is incorrect. The left optic nerve is intact in this patient because the right pupil constricted (a consensual response), which implies the patient's left optic nerve recognized the increase in light intensity. **Choice C** (Right ophthalmic nerve) is incorrect. The ophthalmic nerve (or first division of the trigeminal nerve) supplies sensory (cutaneous) innervation to the skin of the upper eyelid, cornea, anterior aspect of the nose, forehead, and anterior scalp. This nerve did not participate in the pupillary light reflex, so this option can be eliminated. **Choice D** (Right oculomotor nerve) is incorrect. The right oculomotor nerve is intact because the right pupil constricted in response to the increased luminescence. The bilateral projections within the pupillary light response pathway enable this consensual response.

34 **The answer is B: Abducent nerve.** All of the listed nerves travel within the cavernous sinus; however, the abducent nerve (CN VI) parallels the course of the internal carotid artery within the cavernous sinus, which makes it the most likely nerve to be damaged. The internal carotid artery and abducent nerve are located medially as they traverse the cavernous sinus. In the given figure, the other nerves that travel through the cavernous sinus (CNs III, IV, V_1, and V_2) lie laterally. Therefore, the increased pressure, seen within the internal carotid artery due to the atherosclerotic plaque causing the stenosis and resulting aneurysm, would most likely affect the abducent nerve. **Choice A** (Trochlear nerve) is incorrect. The trochlear nerve (CN IV) traverses the cavernous sinus; however, it lies along the lateral wall of the sinus. The abducent nerve, which parallels the internal carotid artery, would most likely be affected by increased pressure within this vessel due to the stenosis and subsequent aneurysm. **Choice C** (Maxillary nerve) is incorrect. The maxillary nerve (or second division of the trigeminal nerve) traverses the cavernous sinus; however, it lies along the lateral wall of the sinus. The abducent nerve, which parallels the internal carotid artery, would most likely be affected by increased pressure within this vessel due to the stenosis and subsequent aneurysm. **Choice D** (Ophthalmic nerve) is incorrect. The ophthalmic nerve (or first division of the trigeminal nerve) traverses the cavernous sinus; however, it lies along the lateral wall of the sinus. The abducent nerve, which parallels the internal carotid artery, would most likely be affected by increased pressure within this vessel due to the stenosis and subsequent aneurysm. **Choice E** (Oculomotor nerve) is incorrect. The oculomotor nerve (CN III) traverses the cavernous sinus; however, it lies along the lateral wall of the sinus. The abducent nerve, which parallels the internal carotid artery, would most likely be affected by increased pressure within this vessel due to the stenosis and subsequent aneurysm.

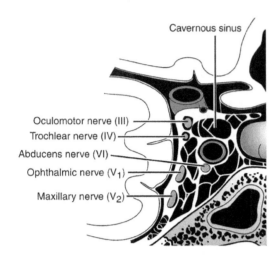

Cavernous sinus

Oculomotor nerve (III)
Trochlear nerve (IV)
Abducens nerve (VI)
Ophthalmic nerve (V$_1$)
Maxillary nerve (V$_2$)

35 **The answer is A: Facial nerve.** Along with the muscles of facial expression, posterior belly of the digastric, and stylohyoid muscles, the facial nerve also innervates the stapedius muscle, which contracts to pull the stapes away from the oval window of the cochlea. This action lowers the amplitude of sounds waves and decreases the transmission of vibrations to the cochlea. Paralysis of the stapedius results in hyperacusis due to heightened reaction of the stapes to sound vibration. Therefore, a person would be more sensitive to loud sounds, particular low-frequency sounds, like the bass emitted from a subwoofer. The stapedius muscle contracts involuntarily, along the tensor tympani muscle innervated by CN V$_3$, in response to high intensity sound waves, forming the acoustic reflex. **Choice B** (Vestibulocochlear nerve) is incorrect. Because of the normal results from the audiometer hearing examination, the vestibulocochlear nerve (CN VIII) has not been damaged. However, the stapedius muscle, which decreases the impact of the footplate of the stapes on the oval window of the cochlea, has been injured. Given this patient's loss of the acoustic reflex, extended exposure to loud sounds could damage the cochlea in the future. **Choice C** (Glossopharyngeal nerve) is incorrect. The glossopharyngeal nerve (CN IX) supplies only one muscle, the stylopharyngeus, and it is not involved with the acoustic reflex or sound transduction. So, the hyperacusis seen in this patient is not due to CN IX. **Choice D** (Vagus nerve) is incorrect. The vagus nerve (CN X) supplies all the muscles of the larynx as well as most of the muscles of soft palate (exception = tensor veli palatini of CN V$_3$) and pharynx (exception = stylopharyngeus of CN IX). Despite its extensive motor innervation, the vagus nerve does not play a role in the acoustic reflex or sound conduction. **Choice E** (Hypoglossal nerve) is incorrect. The hypoglossal nerve (CN XII) innervates the intrinsic and (most of the) extrinsic muscles of tongue (exception = palatoglossus muscle of CN X). Losing innervation to the muscles of the tongue would cause ipsilateral tongue deviation, but would not cause hyperacusis.

Figure Credits

Chapter 1

Q1-21: Image from Moore KL, Agur AMR. *Essential Clinical Anatomy.* 2nd ed. Philadelphia: Lippincott Williams & Wilkins, 2002. Modified as per sketch courtesy of Lawrence E. Wineski, PhD, Dept. of Pathology and Anatomy, Morehouse School of Medicine.

Q1-27: LifeART image copyright (c) Lippincott Williams & Wilkins.

A1-1: Image from Moore KL, Dalley AF, Agur AMR. *Clinical Oriented Anatomy.* 6th ed. Baltimore: Lippincott Williams & Wilkins, 2010, Figures I-1 and I-11.

A1-2: Image from Moore KL, Dalley AF, Agur AMR. *Clinical Oriented Anatomy.* 6th ed. Baltimore: Lippincott Williams & Wilkins, 2010, Figure I-2.

A1-3: Image from Moore KL, Dalley AF, Agur AMR. *Clinical Oriented Anatomy.* 6th ed. Baltimore: Lippincott Williams & Wilkins, 2010, Figure I-2(A).

A1-4: Image from Moore KL, Dalley AF, Agur AMR. *Clinical Oriented Anatomy.* 6th ed. Baltimore: Lippincott Williams & Wilkins, 2010, Figure I-2(C).

A1-7: Image from Moore KL, Dalley AF, Agur AMR. *Clinical Oriented Anatomy.* 6th ed. Baltimore: Lippincott Williams & Wilkins, 2010, Figure I-14(A).

A1-9: Image from Moore KL, Dalley AF, Agur AMR. *Clinical Oriented Anatomy.* 6th ed. Baltimore: Lippincott Williams & Wilkins, 2010, Figure I-16(B).

A1-12: Image from Moore KL, Dalley AF, Agur AMR. *Clinical Oriented Anatomy.* 6th ed. Baltimore: Lippincott Williams & Wilkins, 2010, Figure I-6.

A1-14: Image from Oatis CA. *Kinesiology—The Mechanics and Pathomechanics of Human Movement.* Baltimore: Lippincott Williams & Wilkins, 2004, Figure 17-7.

A1-18: Image from Smeltzer SC, Bare BG, Hinkle JL, et al. *Brunner & Suddarth's Textbook of Medical-Surgical Nursing.* 11th ed. Philadelphia: Lippincott Williams & Wilkins, 2006, Figure 60-11.

A1-29: Image provided by Lawrence E. Wineski, PhD, Dept. of Pathology and Anatomy, Morehouse School of Medicine.

A1-30: Image from Moore KL, Dalley AF, Agur AMR. *Clinical Oriented Anatomy.* 6th ed. Baltimore: Lippincott Williams & Wilkins, 2010, Figure I-51(A).

Chapter 2

Q2-2: Sketch courtesy of Lawrence E. Wineski, PhD, Dept. of Pathology and Anatomy, Morehouse School of Medicine. Adapted from Sadler TW. *Langman's Medical Embryology.* 9th ed. Baltimore: Lippincott Williams & Wilkins, 2003, Figure 2-11.

Q2-6: Image from Anatomical Chart Company. Philadelphia: Lippincott Williams & Wilkins.

Q2-9: Image from Sadler TW. *Langman's Medical Embryology.* 11th ed. Baltimore: Lippincott Williams & Wilkins, 2010, Figure 6-4A.

Q2-12: Image from Fleisher GR, Ludwig S, Baskin MN. *Atlas of Pediatric Emergency Medicine.* Philadelphia: Lippincott Williams & Wilkins, 2004, Figure 15-25.

Q2-15: Image from MacDonald MG, Mullett MD, Seshia MM. *Avery's Neonatology: Pathophysiology & Management of the Newborn.* 6th ed. Philadelphia: Lippincott Williams & Wilkins, 2005, Figure 44-21.

Q2-18: Image from Premkumar K. *The Massage Connection Anatomy and Physiology.* Baltimore: Lippincott Williams & Wilkins, 2004, Figure 7-8A.

A2-3: Image from McConnell TH. *The Nature of Disease: Pathology for the Health Professions.* Philadelphia: Lippincott Williams & Wilkins, 2007, Figure 7-12.

A2-8: Image from Sadler TW. *Langman's Medical Embryology.* 9th ed. Baltimore: Lippincott Williams & Wilkins, 2003, Figure 4-3B.

Chapter 3

Q3-1: Image from Campbell W. *DeJong's The Neurologic Examination.* 6th ed. Philadelphia: Lippincott Williams & Wilkins, 2005, Figure 14-20.

Q3-3: Image from Baim DS. *Grossman's Cardiac Catheterization, Angiography, and Intervention.* 7th ed. Philadelphia: Lippincott Williams & Wilkins, 2006, Figure 29-8(A).

Q3-5: Image from Eisenberg RL. *Clinical Imaging: An Atlas of Differential Diagnosis.* 4th ed. Philadelphia: Lippincott Williams & Wilkins, 2003, Figure C 3-1(A).

Q3-7: Image provided by Lawrence E. Wineski, PhD, Dept. of Pathology and Anatomy, Morehouse School of Medicine.

Q3-9: Image from Berg D, Worzala K. *Atlas of Adult Physical Diagnosis.* Philadelphia: Lippincott Williams & Wilkins, 2006, Figure 4-1.

Q3-11: Image provided by Jeffery P. Hogg, MD, Depts. of Radiology, Neurosurgery, and Neurology, West Virginia University School of Medicine.

Q3-13: Image from MacDonald MG, Mullett MD, Seshia MM. *Avery's Neonatology: Pathophysiology & Management of the Newborn.* 6th ed. Philadelphia: Lippincott Williams & Wilkins, 2005, Figure 33-35.

Q3-15: Image provided by Jeffery P. Hogg, MD, Depts. of Radiology, Neurosurgery, and Neurology, West Virginia University School of Medicine.

Q3-17: Image provided by Lawrence E. Wineski, PhD, Dept. of Pathology and Anatomy, Morehouse School of Medicine.

Q3-19: Image from MacDonald MG, Mullett MD, Seshia MM. *Avery's Neonatology: Pathophysiology & Management of the Newborn.* 6th ed. Philadelphia: Lippincott Williams & Wilkins, 2005, Figure 33-38.

Q3-21: Image from Eisenberg RL. *Clinical Imaging: An Atlas of Differential Diagnosis.* 4th ed. Philadelphia: Lippincott Williams & Wilkins, 2003, Figure C 25-1(B).

Q3-23: Image provided by Lawrence E. Wineski, PhD, Dept. of Pathology and Anatomy, Morehouse School of Medicine.

Q3-25: Image from McConnell TH. *The Nature of Disease Pathology for the Health Professionals.* 1st ed. Philadelphia: Lippincott Williams & Wilkins, 2007, Figure 13-21.

Q3-27: Image from MacDonald MG, Mullett MD, Seshia MM. *Avery's Neonatology: Pathophysiology & Management of the Newborn.* 6th ed. Philadelphia: Lippincott Williams & Wilkins, 2005, Figure 33-43.

Q3-30: LifeART image copyright (c) Lippincott Williams & Wilkins.

Q3-33: Image adapted from Bickley LS, Szilagyi PG. *Bates' Guide to Physical Examination and History Taking.* 8th ed. Philadelphia: Lippincott Williams & Wilkins, 2004, Figure 2-19.

Q3-36: Image from Daffner RH. *Clinical Radiology: The Essentials.* 3rd ed. Philadelphia: Lippincott Williams & Wilkins, 2007, Figure 5-53.

Q3-39: Image from Gorbach SL, Barlett JG, Backlow NR. *Infectious Diseases.* 3rd ed. Philadelphia: Lippincott Williams & Wilkins, 2004, Figure 89-1.

Q3-42: Image provided by Jeffery P. Hogg, MD, Depts. of Radiology, Neurosurgery, and Neurology, West Virginia University School of Medicine.

A3-4: Image from Blackbourne LH. *Advanced Surgical Recall.* 2nd ed. Baltimore: Lippincott Williams & Wilkins, 2004, Figure 68-20.

A3-9: Image from Bickley LS, Szilagyi PG. *Bates' Guide to Physical Examination and History Taking.* 8th ed. Philadelphia: Lippincott Williams & Wilkins, 2003, Figure 2-19.

A3-18: Image from Mills SE. *Histology for Pathologists.* 3rd ed. Philadelphia: Lippincott Williams & Wilkins, 2007, Figure 22-5.

A3-23: Image provided by Lawrence E. Wineski, PhD, Dept. of Pathology and Anatomy, Morehouse School of Medicine.

A3-35: Image from Eisenberg RL. *Clinical Imaging: An Atlas of Differential Diagnosis.* 4th ed. Philadelphia: Lippincott Williams & Wilkins, 2003, Figure C 28-3(B).

A3-45: Image from Crapo JD, Glassroth JL, Karlinsky JB, King TE. *Baum's Textbook of Pulmonary Diseases.* 7th ed. Philadelphia: Lippincott Williams & Wilkins, 2004, Figure 19-6.

Chapter 4

Q4-1: Image from Leyendecker JR, Brown JJ. *Practical Guide to Abdominal and Pelvic MRI.* Philadelphia: Lippincott Williams & Wilkins, 2004, Plate 3-164.

Q4-4: Image from Daffner RH. *Clinical Radiology: The Essentials.* 3rd ed. Philadelphia: Lippincott Williams & Wilkins, 2007, Figure 8-4.

Q4-8: Image provided by Jeffery P. Hogg, MD, Depts. of Radiology, Neurosurgery, and Neurology, West Virginia University School of Medicine.

Q4-12: Image provided by Jeffery P. Hogg, MD, Depts. of Radiology, Neurosurgery, and Neurology, West Virginia University School of Medicine.

Q4-15: Image from Dean D, Herbener TE. *Cross-Sectional Human Anatomy.* Baltimore: Lippincott Williams & Wilkins, 2000, Plate 3-7.

Q4-18: Image from Eisenberg RL. *Clinical Imaging: An Atlas of Differential Diagnosis.* 4th ed. Philadelphia: Lippincott Williams & Wilkins, 2003, Figure GI 47-4.

Q4-21: Image from MacDonald MG, Mullett MD, Seshia MM. *Avery's Neonatology: Pathophysiology & Management of the Newborn.* 6th ed. Philadelphia: Lippincott Williams & Wilkins, 2005, Figure 12-19.

Q4-25: Image from Rubin E, Farber JL. *Pathology.* 3rd ed. Philadelphia: Lippincott Williams & Wilkins, 1999, Figure 40-8.

Q4-29: Image provided by Lawrence E. Wineski, PhD, Dept. of Pathology and Anatomy, Morehouse School of Medicine.

Q4-33: Image from *Stedman's Medical Dictionary*. Baltimore: Lippincott Williams & Wilkins, 2006.

Q4-36: Image provided by Jeffery P. Hogg, MD, Depts. of Radiology, Neurosurgery, and Neurology, West Virginia University School of Medicine.

Q4-38: Image provided by Lawrence E. Wineski, PhD, Dept. of Pathology and Anatomy, Morehouse School of Medicine.

Q4-40: Image from Rubin E, Farber JL. *Pathology*. 3rd ed. Philadelphia: Lippincott Williams & Wilkins, 1999, Figure 13-28.

Q4-42: Image from Fleisher GR, Ludwig S, Baskin MN. *Atlas of Pediatric Emergency Medicine*. Philadelphia: Lippincott Williams & Wilkins, 2004, Figure 9-4.

A4-6: Image from Fleisher GR, Ludwig S, Henretig FM. *Textbook of Pediatric Emergency Medicine*. 5th ed. Philadelphia: Lippincott Williams & Wilkins, 2006, Figure 108-4.

A4-7: Images from Sadler TW. *Langman's Medical Embryology*. 11th ed. Baltimore: Lippincott Williams & Wilkins, 2010, Figures 14-4 and 14-25(A).

A4-9: Image from Mulholland MW, Lillemoe KD, Doherty GM, et al. *Greenfield's Surgery: Scientific Principles and Practice*. 4th ed. Philadelphia: Lippincott Williams & Wilkins, 2006, Figure 110-38.

A4-12: Image provided by Jeffery P. Hogg, MD, Depts. of Radiology, Neurosurgery, and Neurology, West Virginia University School of Medicine.

A4-17: Image from Fleisher GR, Ludwig S, Baskin MN. *Atlas of Pediatric Emergency Medicine*. Philadelphia: Lippincott Williams & Wilkins, 2004, Figure 19-6.

A4-21: Image from O'Doherty N. *Atlas of the Newborn*. Philadelphia: JB Lippincott, 1979, Figure 13-40.

A4-27: Image from Hendrickson, T. *Massage for Orthopedic Conditions*. Philadelphia: Lippincott Williams & Wilkins, 2003, Figure 3-6.

A4-33: Image from Cohen BJ, Wood DL. *Memmler's The Human Body in Health and Disease*. 9th ed. Baltimore: Lippincott Williams and Wilkins, 2000, Figure 8-23.

A4-38: Image provided by Lawrence E. Wineski, PhD, Dept. of Pathology and Anatomy, Morehouse School of Medicine.

A4-42: Image from Chung KW, Chung, HM. *BRS Gross Anatomy*. 6th ed. Baltimore: Lippincott Williams & Wilkins, 2008, Figure 5-3A.

Chapter 5

Q5-2: Image from Cohen BJ. *Medical Terminology: An Illustrated Guide*. 4th ed. Philadelphia: Lippincott Williams & Wilkins, 2003, Figure 13-13.

Q5-4: Image from Berg D, Worzala K. *Atlas of Adult Physical Diagnosis*. Philadelphia: Lippincott Williams & Wilkins, 2006, Figure 3-12.

Q5-6: Image from Fleisher GR, Ludwig S, Baskin MN. *Atlas of Pediatric Emergency Medicine*. Philadelphia: Lippincott Williams & Wilkins, 2004, Figure 9-5.

Q5-8: Image from Wilkinson EJ, Stone IK. *Atlas of Vulvar Disease*. 1st ed. Philadelphia: Lippincott Williams & Wilkins, 1995, Figure 33-17.

Q5-10: Image from Daffner RH. *Clinical Radiology: The Essentials*. 3rd ed. Philadelphia: Lippincott Williams & Wilkins, 2007, Figure 11-106.

Q5-12: Image from Daffner RH. *Clinical Radiology: The Essentials*. 3rd ed. Philadelphia: Lippincott Williams & Wilkins, 2007, Figure 8-52.

Q5-14: Image from Smeltzer SC, Bare BG. *Brunner & Suddarth's Textbook of Medical-Surgical Nursing*. 9th ed. Philadelphia: Lippincott Williams & Wilkins, 2000, Figure 63-12a.

Q5-16: Image from Klossner NJ, Hatfield, NT. *Introductory Maternity and Pediatric Nursing*. 2nd ed. Philadelphia: Lippincott Williams & Wilkins, 2010, Figure 11-2(A).

Q5-18: Image from Pillitteri A. *Maternal and Child Nursing*. 4th ed. Philadelphia: Lippincott Williams & Wilkins, 2003, Figure 19-5.

Q5-20: Image from Sadler TW. *Langman's Medical Embryology*. 11th ed. Baltimore: Lippincott Williams & Wilkins, 2010, Figure 6-8D.

Q5-22: Image from Peitzman AB, Rhodes M, Schwab CW, Yealy DM, Fabian TC. *The Trauma Manual: Trauma and Acute Care Surgery*. 3rd ed. Philadelphia: Lippincott Williams & Wilkins, 2007, Figure 32-2C.

Q5-24: Image from Sadler TW. *Langman's Medical Embryology*. 11th ed. Baltimore: Lippincott Williams & Wilkins, 2010, Figure 15-35C.

Q5-26: Image provided by Patricia B. Stoltzfus, MD, Dept. of Radiology, West Virginia University School of Medicine.

Q5-28: Image provided by Patricia B. Stoltzfus, MD, Dept. of Radiology, West Virginia University School of Medicine.

Q5-30: Image from Leyendecker JR, Brown JJ. *Practical Guide to Abdominal and Pelvic MRI*. Philadelphia: Lippincott Williams & Wilkins, 2004, Figure 3-111.

Q5-32: Image from Bucholz RW, Heckman JD. *Rockwood & Green's Fractures in Adults*. 5th ed. Lippincott Williams & Wilkins, 2001, Figure 34-208.

Q5-34: Image from Fletcher MA. *Physical Diagnosis in Neonatology*. Philadelphia: Lippincott-Raven Publishers, 1998, Figure 17-81.

Q5-37: Image provided by Patricia B. Stoltzfus, MD, Dept. of Radiology, West Virginia University School of Medicine.

Q5-40: Image from Leyendecker JR, Brown JJ. *Practical Guide to Abdominal and Pelvic MRI*. Philadelphia: Lippincott Williams & Wilkins, 2004, Figure 3-205.

Q5-43: Image from Daffner RH. *Clinical Radiology: The Essentials*. 3rd ed. Philadelphia: Lippincott Williams & Wilkins, 2007, Figure 8-66B.

A5-5: Image from Weber J, Kelley J. *Health Assessment in Nursing*. 2nd ed. Philadelphia: Lippincott Williams & Wilkins, 2003, Figure 25-20.

A5-11: Image from Eisenberg RL. *Clinical Imaging: An Atlas of Differential Diagnosis*. 4th ed. Philadelphia: Lippincott Williams & Wilkins, 2003, Figure 1-29.

A5-16: Image from Moore KL, Dalley AF, Agur AMR. *Clinical Oriented Anatomy*. 6th ed. Baltimore: Lippincott Williams & Wilkins, 2010, Figure 3B-29.

A5-17: Image from Moore KL, Dalley AF, Agur AMR. *Clinical Oriented Anatomy*. 6th ed. Baltimore: Lippincott Williams & Wilkins, 2010, Figure 3-60.

A5-23: Image from Moore KL, Agur AMR. *Essential Clinical Anatomy*. 3rd ed. Baltimore: Lippincott Williams & Wilkins, 2007, Figure B3-1.

A5-29: Image from Moore KL, Agur AMR. *Essential Clinical Anatomy*. 3rd ed. Baltimore: Lippincott Williams & Wilkins, 2007, Figure 3-21B.

Chapter 6

Q6-2: Image from Daffner, RH. *Clinical Radiology: The Essentials*. 3rd ed. Philadelphia: Lippincott Williams & Wilkins, 2007, Figure 13-18a.

Q6-4: Image provided by Lawrence E. Wineski, PhD, Dept. of Pathology and Anatomy, Morehouse School of Medicine.

Q6-6: Image provided by Jeffery P. Hogg, MD, Depts. of Radiology, Neurosurgery, and Neurology, West Virginia University School of Medicine.

Q6-8: Image provided by Jeffery P. Hogg, MD, Depts. of Radiology, Neurosurgery, and Neurology, West Virginia University School of Medicine.

Q6-10: Image provided by Jeffery P. Hogg, MD, Professor, Depts. of Radiology, Neurosurgery, and Neurology, West Virginia University School of Medicine.

Q6-12: Image from Bickley LS, Szilagyi PG. *Bates' Guide to Physical Examination and History Taking*. 8th ed. Philadelphia: Lippincott Williams & Wilkins, 2003, Figure 7-58.

Q6-14: Image provided by Jeffery P. Hogg, MD, Depts. of Radiology, Neurosurgery, and Neurology, West Virginia University School of Medicine.

Q6-16: Image provided by Jeffery P. Hogg, MD, Depts. of Radiology, Neurosurgery, and Neurology, West Virginia University School of Medicine.

Q6-18: Image provided by Jeffery P. Hogg, MD, Depts. of Radiology, Neurosurgery, and Neurology, West Virginia University School of Medicine.

Q6-20: Image provided by Jeffery P. Hogg, MD, Depts. of Radiology, Neurosurgery, and Neurology, West Virginia University School of Medicine.

Q6-22: Image from Berg D, Worzala K. *Atlas of Adult Physical Diagnosis*. Philadelphia: Lippincott Williams & Wilkins, 2006, Figure 14-74.

Q6-24: Image provided by Jeffery P. Hogg, MD, Depts. of Radiology, Neurosurgery, and Neurology, West Virginia University School of Medicine.

Q6-26: Image from Daffner RH. *Clinical Radiology: The Essentials*. 3rd ed. Philadelphia: Lippincott Williams & Wilkins, 2007, Figure 10-12.

Q6-28: Image provided by Jeffery P. Hogg, MD, Depts. of Radiology, Neurosurgery, and Neurology, West Virginia University School of Medicine.

Q6-30: Image provided by Jeffery P. Hogg, MD, Depts. of Radiology, Neurosurgery, and Neurology, West Virginia University School of Medicine.

A6-7: Sketch courtesy of Lawrence E. Wineski, PhD, Dept. of Pathology and Anatomy, Morehouse School of Medicine.

A6-25: Image from Oatis CS. *Kinesiology—The Mechanics and Pathomechanics of Human Movement*. Baltimore: Lippincott Williams & Wilkins, 2004, Figure 7-5B.

A6-29-1: Image provided by Jeffery P. Hogg, MD, Depts. of Radiology, Neurosurgery, and Neurology, West Virginia University School of Medicine.

A6-29-2: Image provided by Jeffery P. Hogg, MD, Depts. of Radiology, Neurosurgery, and Neurology, West Virginia University School of Medicine.

Chapter 7

Q7-1: Photograph courtesy of Bruce Palmer, Dept. of Neurobiology and Anatomy, West Virginia University School of Medicine.

Q7-2: Image from Bucholz RW, Heckman JD. *Rockwood and Green's Fractures in Adults*. 5th ed. Philadelphia: Lippincott Williams & Wilkins, 2001, Figure 50-10.

Q7-3: Image from Yochum TR, Rowe LJ. *Yochum and Rowe's Essentials of Skeletal Radiology*. 3rd ed. Philadelphia: Lippincott Williams & Wilkins, 2004, Figure 9-139.

Q7-5: Photograph courtesy of Bruce Palmer, Dept. of Neurobiology and Anatomy, West Virginia University School of Medicine.

Q7-7: Photograph courtesy of Bruce Palmer, Dept. of Neurobiology and Anatomy, West Virginia University School of Medicine.

Q7-12: Image from Yochum TR, Rowe LJ. *Yochum and Rowe's Essentials of Skeletal Radiology.* 3rd ed. Philadelphia: Lippincott Williams & Wilkins, 2004, Figure 12-59.

Q7-15: Image from Yochum TR, Rowe LJ. *Yochum and Rowe's Essentials of Skeletal Radiology.* 3rd ed. Philadelphia: Lippincott Williams & Wilkins, 2004, Figure 9-115.

Q7-18: Photograph courtesy of Bruce Palmer, Dept. of Neurobiology and Anatomy, West Virginia University School of Medicine.

Q7-20: Photograph courtesy of Bruce Palmer, Dept. of Neurobiology and Anatomy, West Virginia University School of Medicine.

Q7-21: Image from Moore KL, Dalley AF. *Clinically Oriented Anatomy.* 4th ed. Baltimore: Lippincott Williams & Wilkins, 2001, Figure 5-25.

Q7-23: Image from Eisenberg RL. *Clinical Imaging: An Atlas of Differential Diagnosis.* 4th ed. Philadelphia: Lippincott Williams & Wilkins, 2003, Figure B 34-5.

Q7-24: Photograph courtesy of Bruce Palmer, Dept. of Neurobiology and Anatomy, West Virginia University School of Medicine.

Q7-28: Photograph courtesy of Bruce Palmer, Dept. of Neurobiology and Anatomy, West Virginia University School of Medicine.

Q7-32: Image from Koval KJ, Zuckerman, JD. *Atlas of Orthopaedic Surgery: A Multimedia Reference.* Philadelphia: Lippincott, Williams & Wilkins, 2004, Figure 21-8.

Q7-36: Image from Bucholz RW, Heckman JD. *Rockwood and Green's Fractures in Adults.* 5th ed. Philadelphia: Lippincott Williams & Wilkins, 2001, Figure 50-43.

Q7-38: Photograph courtesy of Bruce Palmer, Dept. of Neurobiology and Anatomy, West Virginia University School of Medicine.

Q7-44: Photograph courtesy of Bruce Palmer, Dept. of Neurobiology and Anatomy, West Virginia University School of Medicine.

Q7-46: Photograph courtesy of Bruce Palmer, Dept. of Neurobiology and Anatomy, West Virginia University School of Medicine.

Q7-47: Photograph courtesy of Bruce Palmer, Dept. of Neurobiology and Anatomy, West Virginia University School of Medicine.

Q7-50: Photograph courtesy of Bruce Palmer, Dept. of Neurobiology and Anatomy, West Virginia University School of Medicine.

A7-17: Image from Bucholz RW, Heckman JD. *Rockwood and Green's Fractures in Adults.* 5th ed. Philadelphia: Lippincott Williams & Wilkins, 2001, Figure 49-6A.

A7-31: Photograph courtesy of Bruce Palmer, Dept. of Neurobiology and Anatomy, West Virginia University School of Medicine.

A7-39: Image from Moore KL, Dalley AF, Agur AMR. *Clinically Oriented Anatomy.* 6th ed. Philadelphia: Lippincott Williams & Wilkins, 2010, Figure B5-19(B).

A7-43: Photograph courtesy of Bruce Palmer, Dept. of Neurobiology and Anatomy, West Virginia University School of Medicine.

Chapter 8

Q8-2: From Moore KL, Dalley AF. *Clinically Oriented Anatomy.* 5th ed. Baltimore: Lippincott Williams & Wilkins, 2006, Figure B6-12(A).

Q8-3: Photograph courtesy of Bruce Palmer, Dept. of Neurobiology and Anatomy, West Virginia University School of Medicine.

Q8-6: Photograph courtesy of Bruce Palmer, Dept. of Neurobiology and Anatomy, West Virginia University School of Medicine.

Q8-8: Image from Moore KL, Dalley AF. *Clinically Oriented Anatomy.* 5th ed. Baltimore: Lippincott Williams & Wilkins, 2006, Figure B6-5.

Q8-9: Image from Bucholz RW, Heckman JD. *Rockwood and Green's Fractures in Adults.* 5th ed. Philadelphia: Lippincott Williams & Wilkins, 2001, Figure 19-24(d).

Q8-10: Image from Koval KJ, Zuckerman JD. *Atlas of Orthopaedic Surgery: A Multimedia Reference.* Philadelphia: Lippincott Williams & Wilkins, 2001, Fig. 7-4A.

Q8-11: Photograph courtesy of Bruce Palmer, Dept. of Neurobiology and Anatomy, West Virginia University School of Medicine.

Q8-15: Photograph courtesy of Bruce Palmer, Dept. of Neurobiology and Anatomy, West Virginia University School of Medicine.

Q8-18: Photograph courtesy of Bruce Palmer, Dept. of Neurobiology and Anatomy, West Virginia University School of Medicine.

Q8-19: Photograph courtesy of Bruce Palmer, Dept. of Neurobiology and Anatomy, West Virginia University School of Medicine.

Q8-21: Image from Sadler TW. *Langman's Medical Embryology.* 10th ed. Baltimore: Lippincott Williams & Wilkins, 2006, Figure 9-19B.

Q8-22: Image from Berquist, TH. *Musculoskeletal Imaging Companion.* 2nd ed. Philadelphia: Lippincott Williams & Wilkins, 2007, Figure 8-19.

Q8-32: Image from Bucholz RW, Heckman JD. *Rockwood and Green's Fractures in Adults.* 5th ed. Philadelphia: Lippincott Williams & Wilkins, 2001, Figure 5-6.

Q8-37: Photograph courtesy of Bruce Palmer, Dept. of Neurobiology and Anatomy, West Virginia University School of Medicine.

Q8-43: Photograph courtesy of Bruce Palmer, Dept. of Neurobiology and Anatomy, West Virginia University School of Medicine.

Q8-46: Image from Koval KJ, Zuckerman JD. *Atlas of Orthopaedic Surgery: A Multimedia Reference.* Philadelphia: Lippincott Williams & Wilkins, 2001, Figure 7-4B.

Q8-49: Photograph courtesy of Bruce Palmer, Dept. of Neurobiology and Anatomy, West Virginia University School of Medicine.

Q8-50: Photograph courtesy of Bruce Palmer, Dept. of Neurobiology and Anatomy, West Virginia University School of Medicine.

A8-29: Photograph courtesy of Bruce Palmer, Dept. of Neurobiology and Anatomy, West Virginia University School of Medicine.

A8-51: Image from Moore KL, Dalley AF. *Clinically Oriented Anatomy.* 5th ed. Baltimore: Lippincott Williams & Wilkins, 2006, Figure B6-36(A).

Chapter 9

Q9-1: Image from Campbell W. *DeJong's The Neurologic Examination.* 6th ed. Philadelphia: Lippincott Williams & Wilkins, 2005, Figure 15-10.

Q9-3: Image from McConnell TH. *The Nature of Disease: Pathology for the Health Professions.* Philadelphia: Lippincott Williams & Wilkins, 2007, Figure 23-20.

Q9-5: Image from Fleisher GR, Ludwig S, Baskin MN. *Atlas of Pediatric Emergency Medicine.* Philadelphia: Lippincott Williams & Wilkins, 2004, Figure 15-23B.

Q9-7: Image from Tasman W, Jaeger EA. *The Wills Eye Hospital Atlas of Clinical Ophthalmology,* 2nd ed. Lippincott Williams & Wilkins, 2001, Figure 10-31A.

Q9-9: Image from Gold DH, Weingeist TA. *Color Atlas of the Eye in Systemic Disease.* Baltimore: Lippincott Williams & Wilkins, 2001.

Q9-11: Image provided by Jeffery P. Hogg, MD, Depts. of Radiology, Neurosurgery, and Neurology, West Virginia University School of Medicine.

Q9-13: Image provided by Jeffery P. Hogg, MD, Depts. of Radiology, Neurosurgery, and Neurology, West Virginia University School of Medicine.

Q9-15: Image from Anatomical Chart Company. Philadelphia: Lippincott Williams & Wilkins.

Q9-17: Image provided by Jeffery P. Hogg, MD, Depts. of Radiology, Neurosurgery, and Neurology, West Virginia University School of Medicine.

Q9-19: Image from Avery GB, Fletcher MA, MacDonald MG. *Neonatology: Pathophysiology and Management of the Newborn.* 5th ed. Philadelphia: Lippincott Williams & Wilkins, 1999, Figure 13-23.

Q9-21: Image from Tasman W, Jaeger EA. *The Wills Eye Hospital Atlas of Clinical Ophthalmology.* 2nd ed. Lippincott Williams & Wilkins, 2001, Figure 11-48A.

Q9-23: Image provided by Jeffery P. Hogg, MD, Depts. of Radiology, Neurosurgery, and Neurology, West Virginia University School of Medicine.

Q9-25: Image from Scheid RC. *Woelfel's Dental Anatomy: Its Relevance to Dentistry.* 7th ed. Philadelphia: Lippincott Williams & Wilkins, 2007, Figure 2-14.

Q9-27: Image from Berg D, Worzala K. *Atlas of Adult Physical Diagnosis.* Philadelphia: Lippincott Williams & Wilkins, 2006, Figure 7-26(B).

Q9-29: Image from Sadler TW. *Langman's Medical Embryology.* 9th ed. Baltimore: Lippincott Williams & Wilkins, 2003, Figure 15-15.

Q9-31: Image from Moore KL, Dalley AF, Agur AMR. *Clinical Oriented Anatomy.* 6th ed. Baltimore: Lippincott Williams & Wilkins, 2010, Figure B7-32.

Q9-33: Photograph courtesy of Bruce Palmer, Dept. of Neurobiology and Anatomy, West Virginia University School of Medicine.

Q9-35: Image from Sadler TW. *Langman's Medical Embryology.* 11th ed. Baltimore: Lippincott Williams & Wilkins, 2010, Figure 17-34.

Q9-37: Image from Fleisher GR, Ludwig S, Baskin MN. *Atlas of Pediatric Emergency Medicine.* Philadelphia: Lippincott Williams & Wilkins, 2004, Figure 15-24.

Q9-39: Image from Daffner RH. *Clinical Radiology: The Essentials.* 3rd ed. Philadelphia: Lippincott Williams & Wilkins, 2007, Figure 5-18A.

Q9-41: X-ray provided by Frank D. Reilly, PhD, Dept. of Neurobiology and Anatomy, West Virginia University School of Medicine.

Q9-43: Image adapted from Moore KL, Dalley AF, Agur AMR. *Clinical Oriented Anatomy.* 6th ed. Baltimore: Lippincott Williams & Wilkins, 2010, Figure 7-5B.

Q9-45: X-ray provided by Lawrence E. Wineski, PhD, Dept. of Pathology and Anatomy, Morehouse School of Medicine.

Q9-47: Image adapted from Moore KL, Agur AMR. *Essential Clinical Anatomy.* 3rd ed. Baltimore: Lippincott Williams & Wilkins, 2007, Figure 7-40(A).

Q9-49: Image from Tasman W, Jaeger EA. *The Wills Eye Hospital Atlas of Clinical Ophthalmology.* 2nd ed. Baltimore: Lippincott Williams & Wilkins, 2001, Figure 1-66.

Q9-51: X-ray provided by Lawrence E. Wineski, PhD, Dept. of Pathology and Anatomy, Morehouse School of Medicine.

Q9-53: Sketch courtesy of Lawrence E. Wineski, PhD, Dept. of Pathology and Anatomy, Morehouse School of Medicine.

Q9-55: X-ray provided by Lawrence E. Wineski, PhD, Dept. of Pathology and Anatomy, Morehouse School of Medicine.

Q9-57: Image provided by Jeffery P. Hogg, MD, Depts. of Radiology, Neurosurgery, and Neurology, West Virginia University School of Medicine.

Q9-59: X-ray provided by Lawrence E. Wineski, PhD, Dept. of Pathology and Anatomy, Morehouse School of Medicine.

Q9-61: Image from Moore KL, Dalley AF, Agur AMR. *Clinical Oriented Anatomy.* 6th ed. Baltimore: Lippincott Williams & Wilkins, 2010, Figure B8-6(B).

Q9-63: Image from Fletcher MA. *Physical Diagnosis in Neonatology.* Philadelphia: Lippincott–Raven, 1998, Figure 4-8.

Q9-65: Image from Anatomical Chart Company. Philadelphia: Lippincott Williams & Wilkins.

Q9-67: Image provided by Jeffery P. Hogg, MD, Depts. of Radiology, Neurosurgery, and Neurology, West Virginia University School of Medicine.

Q9-69: Image provided by Jeffery P. Hogg, MD, Depts. of Radiology, Neurosurgery, and Neurology, West Virginia University School of Medicine.

Q9-71: Image provided by Jeffery P. Hogg, MD, Depts. of Radiology, Neurosurgery, and Neurology, West Virginia University School of Medicine.

A9-6: Image from Moore KL, Dalley AF, Agur AMR. *Clinical Oriented Anatomy.* 6th ed. Baltimore: Lippincott Williams & Wilkins, 2010, Figure 7-105.

A9-26: Image provided by Jeffery P. Hogg, MD, Depts. of Radiology, Neurosurgery, and Neurology, West Virginia University School of Medicine.

A9-31: Image from Sadler TW. *Langman's Medical Embryology.* 6th ed. Baltimore: Lippincott Williams & Wilkins, 1990, Figures 16-19 and 16-20.

A9-42: Image provided by Jeffery P. Hogg, MD, Depts. of Radiology, Neurosurgery, and Neurology, West Virginia University School of Medicine.

A9-51: X-ray provided by Lawrence E. Wineski, PhD, Dept. of Pathology and Anatomy, Morehouse School of Medicine.

A9-70: Image provided by Jeffery P. Hogg, MD, Depts. of Radiology, Neurosurgery, and Neurology, West Virginia University School of Medicine.

Chapter 10

Q10-1: Image from Bickley LS, Szilagyi PG. *Bates' Guide to Physical Examination and History Taking.* 8th ed. Philadelphia: Lippincott Williams & Wilkins, 2003, Figure 7-47.

Q10-2: Image from Berg D, Worzala K. *Atlas of Adult Physical Diagnosis.* Philadelphia: Lippincott Williams & Wilkins, 2006, Figure 7-20.

Q10-3: Image from Campbell W. *DeJong's The Neurologic Examination.* 6th ed. Philadelphia: Lippincott Williams & Wilkins, 2005, Figure 19-3.

Q10-7: Image from Campbell W. *DeJong's The Neurologic Examination.* 6th ed. Philadelphia: Lippincott Williams & Wilkins, 2005, Figure 20-3.

Q10-9: Image from Campbell W. *DeJong's The Neurologic Examination.* 6th ed. Philadelphia: Lippincott Williams & Wilkins, 2005, Figure 14-12B.

Q10-11: Image from Weber J, Kelley J. *Health Assessment in Nursing.* 2nd ed. Philadelphia: Lippincott Williams & Wilkins, 2003, Figure 11-4.

Q10-13: Image from Tasman W, Jaeger EA. *The Wills Eye Hospital Atlas of Clinical Ophthalmology.* 2nd ed. Lippincott Williams & Wilkins, 2001, Figure 1-30.

Q10-16: Image from Tasman W, Jaeger EA. *The Wills Eye Hospital Atlas of Clinical Ophthalmology.* 2nd ed. Lippincott Williams & Wilkins, 2001, Figure 9-58.

Q10-17: Image from Campbell W. *DeJong's The Neurologic Examination.* 6th ed. Philadelphia: Lippincott Williams & Wilkins, 2005, Figure 15-8.

Q10-18: Image from Weber J, Kelley J. *Health Assessment in Nursing.* 2nd ed. Philadelphia: Lippincott Williams & Wilkins, 2003, Figure 11-8.

Q10-21: Image from Barker LR, Fiebach NH, Kern DE et al. *Principles of Ambulatory Medicine.* 7th ed. Philadelphia: Lippincott Williams & Wilkins, 2006, Figure 110-6.

Q10-22: Image from Becker KL, Bilezikian JP, Brenner WJ, et al. *Principles and Practice of Endocrinology and Metabolism.* 3rd ed. Philadelphia: Lippincott Williams & Wilkins, 2001, Figure 7-8A.

Q10-23: Image from Sadler TW. *Langman's Medical Embryology.* 9th ed. Baltimore: Lippincott Williams & Wilkins, 2004, Figure 10-2A.

Q10-24: X-ray provided by Frank D. Reilly, PhD, Dept. of Neurobiology and Anatomy, West Virginia University School of Medicine.

Q10-25: Image from Weber J, Kelley J. *Health Assessment in Nursing.* 2nd ed. Philadelphia: Lippincott Williams & Wilkins, 2003, Figure 11-40.

Q10-30: X-ray provided by Frank D. Reilly, PhD, Dept. of Neurobiology and Anatomy, West Virginia University School of Medicine.

Q10-31: Image from Oatis CA. *Kinesiology—The Mechanics and Pathomechanics of Human Movement.* Baltimore: Lippincott Williams & Wilkins, 2004, Figure 20-16.

A10-34: Image from Chung KW, Chung, HM. *BRS Gross Anatomy.* 6th ed. Baltimore: Lippincott Williams & Wilkins, 2008, Figure 8-26.

Index

Page numbers in *italics* denote figures